**Autoantibodies
and Autoimmunity**

Edited by
K. Michael Pollard

Related Titles

H. Kropshofer, A. B. Vogt (Eds.)

Antigen Presenting Cells

From Mechanisms to Drug Development

2005
ISBN 3-527-31108-4

J. R. Kalden, M. Herrmann (Eds.)

Apoptosis and Autoimmunity

From Mechanisms to Treatments

2003
ISBN 3-527-30442-8

A. Hamann, B. Engelhardt (Eds.)

Leukocyte Trafficking

Molecular Mechanisms, Therapeutic Targets, and Methods

2005
ISBN 3-527-31228-5

M. Lutz, N. Romani, A. Steinkasserer (Eds.)

Handbook of Dendritic Cells

Biology, Diseases and Therapies

2006
ISBN 3-527-31109-2

S. H. E. Kaufmann (Ed.)

Novel Vaccination Strategies

2004
ISBN 3-527-30523-8

R. Coico, G. Sunshine, E. Benjamini

Immunology

A Short Course

2004
ISBN 0-471-22689-0

L.-J. Eales

Immunology for Life Scientists

2003
ISBN 0-470-84523-6

R. A. Meyers (Ed.)

Encyclopedia of Molecular Cell Biology and Molecular Medicine

Second Edition

2005
ISBN 3-527-30542-4

Autoantibodies and Autoimmunity

Molecular Mechanisms in Health and Disease

Edited by
K. Michael Pollard

WILEY-VCH

WILEY-VCH Verlag GmbH & Co. KGaA

Editor

Prof. Dr. K. Michael Pollard
Department of Molecular
and Experimental Medicine
The Scripps Research Institute, MEM 131
10550 North Torrey Pines Road
La Jolla, CA 92037
USA

Cover
Front cover design in cooperation
with Janet Hightower, Digital Artist,
BioMedical Graphics Department,
The Scripps Research Institute.

Library of Congress Card No.: applied for

British Library Cataloguing-in-Publication Data
A catalogue record for this book is available
from the British Library

**Bibliographic information published by
Die Deutsche Bibliothek** Die Deutsche Bibliothek
lists this publication in the Deutsche National-
bibliografie; detailed bibliographic data is available
in the Internet at http://dnb.ddb.de

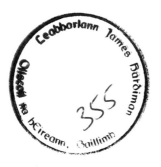

Typesetting K+V Fotosatz GmbH, Beerfelden
Printing betz-druck GmbH, Darmstadt
Binding J. Schäffer GmbH, Grünstadt

Printed in the Federal Republic of Germany
Printed on acid-free paper

ISBN-13: 978-3-527-31141-5
ISBN-10: 3-527-31141-6

Contents

Autoantibodies and Autoimmunity: Molecular Mechanisms
in Health and Disease. Edited by K. Michael Pollard
Copyright © 2006 WILEY-VCH Verlag GmbH & Co. KGaA, Weinheim
ISBN: 3-527-31141-6

Preface

The basis for this book was a chapter written for the 2nd edition of R. A. Meyers'
Encyclopedia of Molecular Cell Biology and Molecular Medicine. Entitled *Autoanti-bodies and Autoimmunity,* that chapter sought to take a different approach in re-viewing the broad field that encompasses autoimmunity. This was in part due
to my own research experiences, but also due to the realization that autoimmunity,
and autoantibodies in particular, have contributed to more than just the medical
sciences.

Historically autoantibodies have served as indicators of an autoimmune re-sponse and early studies focused on their clinical and diagnostic significance.
Today many autoantibody specificities contribute as diagnostic and prognostic
indicators in clinical medicine. The burgeoning numbers of known autoantibod-ies has revolutionized methods of detection leading to development of multiplex
assays capable of identifying numerous diagnostically important autoantibodies
in a single assay.

It remains unknown why distinct profiles of autoantibodies occur in autoim-mune diseases, particularly systemic autoimmune diseases. Experimental stud-ies suggest that both MHC and non-MHC genes contribute to disease specific
autoantibody profiles, and that the presence or absence of particular cytokines
may also play a role in determining autoantibody profiles. Nonetheless while it
is clear that disease specific autoantibodies are acting as "molecular reporters",
the message they are relaying is still garbled. Genetic research using animal
models will play an increasingly important role in deciphering the messages in-grained in autoantibody responses.

Ironically the movement toward high-throughput assays to detect autoantibod-ies threatens the clinical usefulness of the immunofluorescence test (IFT) which
was instrumental in the original description of many autoantibody specificities.
The dramatic visual images of antibodies binding to sub-cellular organelles and
substructures that are so readily revealed by this technique can be both stun-ningly beautiful and biologically significant. Once the purview of the clinical
Immunologist/Rheumatologist seeking to diagnose autoimmune diseases, the
IFT is increasingly found in the laboratories of cellular and molecular biologists
questing for answers at the very frontiers of biology.

Autoantibodies and Autoimmunity: Molecular Mechanisms in Health and Disease. Edited by K. Michael Pollard
Copyright © 2006 WILEY-VCH Verlag GmbH & Co. KGaA, Weinheim
ISBN: 3-527-31141-6

This book would not have been possible without the outstanding contributions of a group of highly talented and internationally respected authors. I am very grateful to each author for giving their valuable time and effort toward compilation of this book, and to Janet Hightower, Digital Artist in the BioMedical Graphics Department of The Scripps Research Institute, for the front cover art. I am indebted to Andreas Sendtko at Wiley-VCH for the initial suggestion that the *Encyclopedia* chapter might be the basis for a book. I am also grateful to Andreas Sendtko and his colleagues at Wiley-VCH for bringing the book to life.

La Jolla, October 2005   *Mike Pollard*

List of Contributors

Michael P. Bachmann
Institute of Immunology
Medical Faculty of the Technical
University Dresden
Fetscherstrasse 74
01307 Dresden
Germany

H. Bantel
Department of Gastroenterology,
Hepatology and Endocrinology
Hannover Medical School
Carl-Neuberg-Strasse 1
30623 Hannover
Germany

Susan J. Baserga
Department of Molecular Biophysics
and Biochemistry, Department
of Genetics, and Department
of Therapeutic Radiology
Yale University
333 Cedar Street
P.O. Box 208024
New Haven, CT 06520-8024
USA

Alan G. Baxter
Comparative Genomics Centre
Molecular Sciences Building 21
James Cook University
Townsville, QLD 4811
Australia

Marina Botto
Rheumatology Section
Faculty of Medicine
Imperial College
Hammersmith Campus
Du Cane Road
London W12 0NN
United Kingdom

Jean-Paul Briand
Unité Propre de Recherche 9021
Centre National de la Recherche
Scientifique
Institut de Biologie Moléculaire
et Cellulaire
15 rue René Descartes
67000 Strasbourg
France

Rufus W. Burlingame
INOVA Diagnostics, Inc.
9900 Old Grove Road
San Diego, CA 92131
USA

Livia Casciola-Rosen
Department of Medicine
and Department of Dermatology
Johns Hopkins University School
of Medicine
5200 Eastern Avenue
Baltimore, MD 21224
USA

Autoantibodies and Autoimmunity: Molecular Mechanisms in Health and Disease. Edited by K. Michael Pollard
Copyright © 2006 WILEY-VCH Verlag GmbH & Co. KGaA, Weinheim
ISBN: 3-527-31141-6

Carlos A. Casiano
Department of Biochemistry
and Microbiology, Center for
Molecular Biology and Gene Therapy,
and Department of Medicine
Section of Rheumatology
Loma Linda University School of
Medicine
Mortensen Hall 132
11085 Campus Street
Loma Linda, CA 92350
USA

Erica A. Champion
Department of Genetics
Yale University
333 Cedar Street
New Haven, CT 06520-8024
USA

Edward K. L. Chan
Department of Oral Biology
University of Florida
P.O. Box 100424
Gainesville, FL 32610-0424
USA

Michael R. Christie
Beta Cell Development and Function
Group
Division of Reproductive Health
Endocrinology and Development
2nd Floor Hodgkin Building
King's College London
Guy's Campus
London SE1 1UL
United Kingdom

Karsten Conrad
Institute of Immunology
Medical Faculty of the Technical
University Dresden
Fetscherstrasse 74
01307 Dresden
Germany

M. Eric Gershwin
Division of Rheumatology, Allergy,
and Clinical Immunology
University of California at Davis
Davis, CA 95616
USA

Tom P. Gordon
Department of Immunology,
Arthritis, and Allergy
Flinders University of South Australia
Bedford Park, South Australia 5042
Australia

Falk Hiepe
Charité – Medical School
Department of Internal Medicine
(Rheumatology and Clinical
Immunology)
Schumannstrasse 20/21
10117 Berlin
Germany

Per Hultman
Department of Molecular
and Immunological Pathology
Division of Molecular and
Clinical Medicine
Linköping University
58185 Linköping
Sweden

Pietro Invernizzi
Division of Internal Medicine
San Paolo School of Medicine
University of Milan
Via di Rudini 8
20142 Milan
Italy

Catherine L. Keech
Department of Microbiology
and Immunology
University of Melbourne
Melbourne, Victoria 3010
Australia

J. Kneser
Department of Gastroenterology,
Hepatology and Endocrinology
Hannover Medical School
Carl-Neuberg-Strasse 1
30623 Hannover
Germany

Dwight H. Kono
The Scripps Research Institute
Department of Immunology
10550 N. Torrey Pines Road
La Jolla, CA 92037
USA

Stuart M. Levine
Department of Medicine
Johns Hopkins University
School of Medicine
5200 Eastern Avenue
Baltimore, MD 21224
USA

Michael P. Manns
Department of Gastroenterology,
Hepatology and Endocrinology
Hannover Medical School
Carl-Neuberg-Strasse 1
30623 Hannover
Germany

Osvaldo Martinez
Department of Microbiology
Mount Sinai School of Medicine
1 Gustave L. Levy Place
New York, NY 10029
USA

James McCluskey
Department of Microbiology
and Immunology
University of Melbourne
Melbourne, Victoria 3010
Australia

Tsuneyo Mimori
Department of Rheumatology
and Clinical Immunology
Graduate School of Medicine
Kyoto University
54 Shogoin-Kawahara-cho
Sakyo-ku, Kyoto 606-8507
Japan

Sylviane Muller
Institut de Biologie Moléculaire
et Cellulaire (IBMC)
Immunologie et Chimie
Thérapeutiques
Unité Propre de Recherche 9021
15 rue René Descartes
67000 Strasbourg
France

Sabine Oertelt
Division of Rheumatology, Allergy,
and Clinical Immunology
University of California at Davis
Davis, CA 95616
USA

Fabio J. Pacheco
Department of Morphology
Federal University of São Paulo
Rua Botucatu, 740
04023-900 São Paulo
Brazil

Carol L. Peebles
INOVA Diagnostics, Inc.
9900 Old Grove Road
San Diego, CA 92131
USA

Stanford L. Peng
Department of Internal Medicine/
Rheumatology and Department
of Pathology and Immunology
Washington University School
of Medicine
660 S. Euclid Avenue
St. Louis, MO 63110
USA

Matthew C. Pickering
Rheumatology Section
Faculty of Medicine
Imperial College
Hammersmith Campus
Du Cane Road
London W12 0NN
United Kingdom

Mauro Podda
Division of Internal Medicine
San Paolo School of Medicine
University of Milan
Via di Rudini 8
20142 Milan
Italy

K. Michael Pollard
Department of Molecular
and Experimental Medicine
The Scripps Research Institute
MEM131
10550 North Torrey Pines Road
La Jolla, CA 92037
USA

Bellur S. Prabhakar
Department of Microbiology
and Immunology
University of Illinois at Chicago
835 South Wolcott Avenue
Chicago, IL 60612
USA

Ivan Raška
Institute of Cellular Biology
and Pathology
1st Medical Faculty
Charles University of Prague
Albertov 4
12800 Prague 2
Czech Republic

Antony Rosen
Department of Medicine, Department
of Dermatology, Department of
Cell Biology and Anatomy, and
Department of Pathology
Johns Hopkins University School
of Medicine
5200 Eastern Avenue
Baltimore, MD 21224
USA

Robert L. Rubin
Department of Molecular Genetics
and Microbiology
University of New Mexico School
of Medicine
915 Camino de Salud NE
Albuquerque, NM 87131
USA

Šárka Růžičková
Institute of Rheumatology
Department of Molecular Biology
and Immunogenetics
1st Medical Faculty
Charles University of Prague
Na Slupi 4
12850 Prague 2
Czech Republic

Barbara Schraml
Department of Internal Medicine/
Rheumatology and Department
of Pathology and Immunology
Washington University School
of Medicine
660 S. Euclid Avenue
St. Louis, MO 63110
USA

Carlo Selmi
Division of Rheumatology, Allergy,
and Clinical Immunology
University of California at Davis
Davis, CA 95616
USA

Yulius Y. Setiady
Department of Pathology
University of Virginia
P.O. Box 800168
Charlottesville, VA 22908
USA

Eng M. Tan
Department of Molecular
and Experimental Medicine
The Scripps Research Institute
10550 North Torrey Pines Road
La Jolla, CA 92037
USA

Argyrios N. Theofilopoulos
The Scripps Research Institute
Department of Immunology
10550 N. Torrey Pines Road
La Jolla, CA 92037
USA

Kenneth S. K. Tung
Department of Pathology
University of Virginia
P.O. Box 800168
Charlottesville, VA 22908
USA

Sarah M. Weenink
Beta Cell Development and
Function Group
Division of Reproductive Health
Endocrinology and Development
2nd Floor Hodgkin Building
King's College London
Guy's Campus
London SE1 1UL
United Kingdom

Part 1
Introductory Chapters

Autoantibodies and Autoimmunity: Molecular Mechanisms
in Health and Disease. Edited by K. Michael Pollard
Copyright © 2006 WILEY-VCH Verlag GmbH & Co. KGaA, Weinheim
ISBN: 3-527-31141-6

1
Introduction

K. Michael Pollard

1.1
Background

The stimulus for this book came from a chapter written for the second edition of R. A. Meyer's *Encyclopedia of Molecular Cell Biology and Molecular Medicine*. Appreciating that autoimmunity, and autoantibodies in particular, has contributed to more than just the medical sciences, that chapter approached its discussion of autoantibodies from four different directions. The conventional topics of autoimmunity and mechanisms of elicitation of autoantibodies were addressed. The contribution of autoantibodies to diagnostic markers was also discussed. In addition significant consideration was given to the important but often neglected role that autoantibodies have played as probes in molecular and cellular biology. The last area covered focused on the different types of animal models of autoimmune disease, the autoantibody specificities associated with those models, and the relevance of animal models to human idiopathic autoimmune disease.

The topics addressed in this book are based closely on the chapter in the *Encyclopedia of Molecular Cell Biology and Molecular Medicine*. However, individual contributors, selected for their expertise in well-defined areas of investigation, were given free range to articulate their views of a particular theme. The present chapter, which is an updated version of the chapter described above, has been included so that the reader can appreciate the background on which this book is based. The relevant literature has been updated and augmented from the original chapter. In addition I have noted in the text those areas that have been expanded upon by individual chapters from contributors.

In Chapter 2, Eng Tan summarizes a series of landmark observations that have defined the properties of epitopes recognized by autoantibodies, particularly those from patients with systemic autoimmune diseases. These properties, which include recognition of conserved protein structure and the involvement of regions close to, or including, functional domains of the antigen, are reoccurring themes throughout this book and serve to highlight some of the distinctive aspects of many autoantibody responses.

Autoantibodies and Autoimmunity: Molecular Mechanisms in Health and Disease. Edited by K. Michael Pollard
Copyright © 2006 WILEY-VCH Verlag GmbH & Co. KGaA, Weinheim
ISBN: 3-527-31141-6

1.2
Autoimmunity

An autoimmune response is an attack by the immune system on the host itself. In healthy individuals the immune system is "tolerant" of its host ("self") but attacks foreign ("non-self") constituents such as bacteria and viruses. The ability to distinguish self from non-self is considered to be the determining factor in whether the immune system responds to a suspected challenge. Although it may appear obvious, there is actually considerable debate over what constitutes "self" and "non-self" and what cellular/molecular mechanisms are involved. A fascinating historical perspective on self/non-self recognition has been written by Alan Baxter (see Chapter 3) and includes the often-forgotten point that Macfarlane Burnet used the phrase "self and not-self" when he first introduced the concept. Possible discriminators between "self" and "non(not)-self" include recognition of infection [1] or identification of danger signals [2]. The outcome of the debate on self/non-self discrimination not withstanding, autoimmunity represents an obvious disruption to the mechanism by which the immune system regulates its activities. Importantly, the responsible effector mechanisms appear to be no different from those used to combat exogenous infective reagents and include soluble products such as antibodies (humoral immunity) as well as direct cell-to-cell contact resulting in specific cell lysis (cell-mediated immunity). No single mechanism has been described that can account for the diversity of autoimmune responses, or the production of autoantibodies. Figure 1.1 outlines

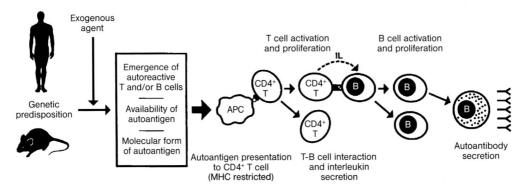

Fig. 1.1 Hypothetical pathway of autoantibody elicitation in human disease and experimental animal models. This model combines features from the most commonly accepted postulated mechanisms for autoantibody production. Genetically predisposed individuals may be triggered to begin the response by an exogenous agent such as exposure to a drug, chemical toxin, or other environmental influence. The events that follow (listed in large box) are poorly understood but must involve the emergence of autoreactive lymphoid cells and the presence of autoantigen in a molecular form reactive with autoreactive cells. Once the presentation of autoantigen has activated autoreactive lymphoid cells, the production of autoantibody proceeds essentially as it would for a nonautoimmune antibody response.

the common features of hypothetical models of autoantibody elicitation. Most models, particularly those relating to autoimmune disease in animals, include a genetic predisposition. Breeding experiments between inbred strains of mice have shown that the genetic control of autoantibody production is complex, involving multiple genes [3]. Although most of the required genetic elements remain to be characterized, it appears that both acceleration and suppression of autoimmune responses are under genetic control [4–6]. The most frequently observed genetic requirement involves the major histocompatibility complex (MHC) class II genes, which encode proteins responsible for the presentation of processed antigen to CD4$^+$ T cells via the T-cell receptor.

The most perplexing and challenging aspect of autoimmunity and autoantibody elicitation is the identification of the events involved in the initiation of the response. Although these early events are poorly understood for most autoimmune diseases, it is thought that an exogenous trigger can provide the first step in the initiation of some autoimmune responses. The best evidence for this comes from drug- and chemical-induced autoimmunity, which has been described in both human disease and animal models of autoimmunity [7]. However, even in exogenously induced autoimmunity, many of the events between the administration of a chemical or drug and the appearance of autoantibodies remain to be unveiled. Induction of autoantibodies by exogenous agents can take several weeks to many months. Drug-induced systemic autoimmunity in humans can take prolonged periods of time to develop and can be provoked by a large number of chemically unrelated drugs [7]. The autoantibody response, however, appears quite restricted, targeting histones and histone-DNA complexes, the components of chromatin [8, 9]. Complexes of drug and autoantigen are not the immunogens responsible for the autoantibody response, since the drug is not required for autoantibody interaction with autoantigen. Withdrawal of the drug often leads to cessation of clinical symptoms, clearly implicating the participation of the drug in some mechanism inciting the autoimmune response, although autoantibody may persist for months in the absence of the drug. In several animal models, exposure to chemicals–particularly inorganic forms of heavy metals such as mercury, silver, or gold–can lead to autoantibody expression within weeks [10]. In these murine models the autoantibody response is again restricted, but here the predominant targets are non-chromatin components of the nucleolus [11, 12]. The development of restricted autoantibody specificities in humans given many different drugs or in mice given heavy metals suggests that it is not the parent molecule that is important but rather the metabolic products of these compounds that lead on the one hand to anti-chromatin autoantibodies and on the other to anti-nucleolar antibodies. In human drug-induced autoimmunity, a common pathway of oxidative metabolism via the ubiquitous neutrophil has been suggested as a means of producing reactive drug metabolites that may perturb immune regulation sufficiently to produce autoimmune disease [13]. Another mechanism that has been proposed is disruption by drug metabolites of positive selection of T cells during their development in the thymus [14–16]. This mechanism has been shown to result in mature CD4$^+$ T cells that are able to respond to self-antigen, leading to T-cell proliferation as well as autoantibody production by B cells [16].

In Figure 1.1 the large boxed area highlights several concepts that form pivotal points in many hypothetical postulates of autoantibody elicitation but about which little is known. How do B and T cells, with receptors for autoantigen, emerge from and escape the regulatory mechanisms that normally keep them in check and then make their way to the secondary lymphoid tissues? Studies involving transgenic mice possessing neo-autoantigens suggest that possible mechanisms include avoidance of apoptotic elimination, escape from tolerance induction, and reversal of an anergic state [17]. Mechanisms of immune tolerance and how their disruption may lead to autoimmunity are discussed by Robert Rubin in Chapter 4.

Molecular identification of autoantigens, their presence in macromolecular complexes, the occurrence of autoantibodies to different components of the same complex, and the appearance of somatic mutations in the variable regions of autoantibodies have suggested that it is the autoantigen that drives the autoimmune response [18]. It remains unclear how autoantigens, particularly intracellular autoantigens, are made available to autoreactive lymphoid cells, and what molecular forms of these complex macromolecular structures interact with autoreactive lymphoid cells. One mechanism that has been proposed as a means by which autoantigens might be made available to the immune system is apoptotic cell death. The impetus for this hypothesis is the finding that many autoantigens undergo proteolytic cleavage during apoptotic cell death and that apoptotic bodies (debris from dying cells) contain multiple autoantigens [19]. Processing and presentation of such material by antigen-presenting cells (APCs) has been suggested as a means of providing antigen to autoreactive T cells [20]. However, uptake of apoptotic cellular material does not lead to the activation of APCs [21–24], which is necessary if APCs are to activate T cells. Inability of apoptotic material to activate APCs may stem from the observation that apoptosis is a descriptor for programmed cell death (PCD), which is a physiological process. This contrasts sharply with necrotic cell death, which is a non-physiological process that produces cellular material that activates APCs [25]. Also of note is that necrotic cell death induced by mercury leads to proteolytic cleavage of the autoantigen fibrillarin [26]. Immunization with the N-terminal fragment of such cleavage leads to autoantibodies against fibrillarin that possess some of the characteristics of the anti-fibrillarin response elicited by mercury alone [26]. In contrast the antibody response elicited by immunization with full-length fibrillarin does not mimic the mercury-induced response, suggesting that processing and presentation of fragmented autoantigens may allow loss of self/nonself discrimination. Examination of the molecular forms of autoantigens during and after cell death and their roles in activating both APCs and T cells will be fruitful areas of future research. An overview of the two major forms of cell death and the evidence supporting their role in autoimmunity are discussed by Carlos Casiano and Fabio Pacheco in Chapter 6. How autoantigen might become modified to generate novel, non-tolerized structures and the role that pro-

teolytic cleavage during cell death might have on such a process are analyzed by
Antony Rosen and colleagues in Chapter 7.

Roles in autoantibody production have been argued for pathways that either
are or are not dependent on the presence of T cells. A T cell–dependent response
is shown in Figure 1.1, with an APC supplying processed antigen to CD4$^+$ T cells.
An essential element in any model of autoantibody elicitation is the emergence of
antibody-secreting B cells, which recognize material derived from the host [27]. As
indicated in Figure 1.1 the interaction between T and B cells involves both soluble
(e.g., interleukin) and membrane-bound receptor–co-receptor interactions [28].
The effect of the presence, or absence, of these molecular interactions on autoimmunity is discussed by Barbara Schraml and Stanford Peng in Chapter 5. The
antibody secreted by a B cell is directed against a single region (or epitope) on
an antigen. An autoantibody response can target a number of epitopes on any
one antigen, clearly showing that multiple autoreactive B-cell clones are activated
during an autoimmune response. In the systemic autoimmune diseases, many
autoantigens are complexes of nucleic acid and/or protein, and an autoimmune
response may target several of the components of a complex [29]. It is unknown
whether the autoantibody responses to the components of a complex arise simultaneously, sequentially, independently, or through interrelated mechanisms. For a
detailed analysis of the T- and B-cell response against a self-antigen, see Chapter
19 by James McCluskey and colleagues.

In only a few diseases have autoantibodies been shown to be the causative
agents of pathogenesis (e.g., anti-acetylcholine receptor autoantibodies in
myasthenia gravis, anti-thyroid-stimulating hormone receptor autoantibodies in
Graves' disease) [30, 31]. It is noteworthy not only that these diseases are organ
specific but also that their autoantigens are extracellular or on the surface of cell
membranes and therefore easily targeted by the immune system. In some individuals the largest organ, the skin, can suffer insult from several blistering conditions now known to be autoimmune diseases characterized by autoantibodies
against products of keratinocytes [32]. The autoantigens involved are cell adhesion molecules that are important in maintaining the integrity of the skin by
cell-cell contact between the various cell layers in the epidermis and at the dermal-epidermal junction. In the non-organ-specific autoimmune disease systemic
lupus erythematosus (SLE), anti-double-stranded DNA (dsDNA) autoantibodies
have been shown to participate in pathogenic events by way of complexing with
their cognate antigen to cause immune complex–mediated inflammation [33,
34]. These examples show that in both the organ-specific and systemic autoimmune diseases, *in vivo* disposition of autoantibody in tissues and organs has
clinical significance inasmuch as it indicates sites of inflammation, which may
contribute to the pathological process. Moreover, detection of autoantibody
deposits in the organ-specific autoimmune diseases has particular significance
because some organ-specific autoantibodies have been found to be the direct
mediators of pathological lesions. In most autoimmune diseases, however, it
has not been determined whether autoantibodies cause or contribute to disease
or are merely a secondary consequence of the underlying clinical condition.

1.3
Autoantibodies as Diagnostic Markers

The diseases associated with autoantibodies can be divided into two broad groups: the organ-specific autoimmune diseases, in which autoantibodies have the ability to react with autoantigens from a particular organ or tissue, and the multi-system autoimmune diseases, in which autoantibodies react with common cellular components that appear to bear little relevance to the underlying clinical picture. In both cases particular autoantibody specificities can serve as diagnostic markers (Table 1.1). A synopsis of the methodology used to determine the presence of autoantibodies, including high-throughput multiplex assays, is covered by Rufus Burlingame and Carol Peebles in Chapter 8. Discussion of more specialized assay systems using synthetic peptides to detect autoantibodies is covered by Jean-Paul Briand and Sylviane Muller in Chapter 9.

In the multi-system autoimmune diseases, there are several features of the relationship between autoantibody specificity and diagnostic significance that bear consideration. Autoantigens in these diseases are components of macromolecular structures such as the nucleosome of chromatin and the small nuclear ribonucleoprotein (snRNP) particles of the spliceosome, among others. Autoantibodies to different components of the same macromolecular complex can be diagnostic for different clinical disorders [35, 36]. Thus, the core proteins B, B', D, and E, which are components of the U1, U2, and U4–U6 snRNPs and are antigenic targets in the anti-Smith antigen (Sm) response in SLE, are different from the U1 snRNP–specific proteins of 70 kDa, A and C, which are targets of the anti-nRNP response in mixed connective tissue disease (MCTD; see Table 1.1). It has also been observed that certain autoantibody responses are consistently associated with one another. The anti-Sm response, which is diagnostic of SLE, is commonly associated with the anti-nRNP response; but the anti-nRNP response can occur without the anti-Sm response, in which case it can be diagnostic of MCTD. These two observations suggest that the snRNP complexes responsible for the autoantibody response against the spliceosome in MCTD may differ from the snRNP complexes that produce the anti-spliceosome response in SLE. Other autoantibody responses demonstrate similar associations and restrictions. The anti-SS-A/Ro response (see Table 1.1) frequently occurs alone in SLE, but the anti-SS-B/La response in Sjögren's syndrome is almost always associated with the anti-SS-A/Ro response. Similarly, the anti-chromatin response occurs alone in drug-induced lupus [37] but is usually associated with the anti-dsDNA response in idiopathic SLE [38].

Autoantibody specificities may occur at different frequencies in a variety of diseases, and the resultant profile consisting of distinct groups of autoantibodies in different diseases can have diagnostic use [35]. In some cases the grouping of autoantibody specificities, such as the preponderance of anti-nucleolar autoantibodies in scleroderma (Table 1.1) [39], provides provocative but poorly understood relationships with clinical diagnosis. Unlike SLE, where a single patient may have multiple autoantibody specificities to a number of unrelated nuclear

Table 1.1 Examples of clinical diagnostic specificity of autoantibodies.

Autoantibody specificity [a]	Molecular specificity	Clinical association
Organ-specific autoimmune diseases		
Anti-acetylcholine receptor*	Acetylcholine receptor	Myasthenia gravis
Anti-TSH receptor*	TSH receptor	Graves' disease
Anti-thyroglobulin*	Thyroglobulin	Chronic thyroiditis
Anti-thyroid peroxidase*	Thyroid peroxidase	Chronic thyroiditis
Anti-mitochondria*	Pyruvate dehydrogenase complex	Primary biliary cirrhosis
Anti-keratinocyte*	Desmoplakin I homologue	Bullous pemphigoid
Anti-keratinocyte*	Desmoglein	Pemphigus foliaceus
Anti-GAD65	Glutamic acid decarboxylase, 65 kDa	Type 1 diabetes
Multi-system autoimmune diseases		
Anti-double-stranded DNA*	B form of DNA	SLE
Anti-Sm*	B, B', D, and E proteins of U1, U2, and U4–U6 snRNP	SLE
Anti-nRNP	70-kDa A and C proteins of U1-snRNP	MCTD, SLE
Anti-SS-A/Ro	60- and 52-kDa proteins associated with hY1-Y5 RNP complex	SS, neonatal lupus, SLE
Anti-SS-B/La	47-kDa phosphoprotein complexed with RNA polymerase III transcripts	SS, neonatal lupus, SLE
Anti-Jo-1*	Histidyl tRNA synthetase	Polymyositis
Anti-fibrillarin*	34-kDa protein of C/D box–containing snoRNP (U3, U8, etc.)	Scleroderma
Anti-RNA polymerase 1*	Subunits of RNA polymerase 1 complex	Scleroderma
Anti-DNA topoisomerase 1 (anti-Scl-70)*	100-kDa DNA topoisomerase I	Scleroderma
Anti-centromere*	Centromeric proteins CENP-A, -B, and -C	CREST (limited scleroderma)
cANCA	Serine proteinase (proteinase 3)	Wegener's vasculitis
Anti-CCP*	Cyclic citrullinated peptide	Rheumatoid arthritis

a) Disease-specific diagnostic marker antibodies indicated by asterisk.

Abbreviations: SLE = systemic lupus erythematosus; MCTD = mixed connective tissue disease; SS = Sjögren's syndrome; cANCA = cytoplasmic anti-neutrophil cytoplasmic antibody; TSH = thyroid-stimulating hormone; CREST = calcinosis, Raynaud's phenomenon, esophageal dysmotility, sclerodactyly, telangiectasia.

autoantigens (e.g., DNA, Sm, SS-A/Ro), scleroderma patients infrequently have multiple autoantibody specificities to nucleolar autoantigens that are unrelated at the macromolecular level (i.e., not part of the same macromolecular complex).

In planning the content of this book, it was decided that it was not possible to devote multiple chapters to discussion of disease-specific autoantibodies. Instead, a single chapter has been assigned to the two major forms of autoimmune disease (i.e., organ-specific and systemic), and two additional chapters have been allocated to cover the major diseases within each group. Karsten Conrad and Michael Bachmann have outlined autoantibodies and systemic autoimmune diseases (Chapter 10), while Falk Heipe has expanded upon autoantibodies in systemic lupus erythematosus (Chapter 11) and Tsuneyo Mimori has focused on autoantibodies in rheumatoid arthritis (Chapter 12). In the organ-specific disease section, Michael Manns and colleagues expand the discussion on autoantibodies and organ-specific autoimmunity (Chapter 13) by including comments on autoimmune liver diseases. Osvaldo Martines and Bellur Prabhakar provide an excellent analysis of autoantibodies in autoimmune thyroid disease (Chapter 14) including comments on functionally relevant epitopes. See Chapters 2 and 20 for more on this topic. Another excellent chapter on organ specific autoimmunity is that by Sarah Weenink and Michael Christie on autoantibodies in diabetes (Chapter 15). The material on T-cell responses in this chapter can be expanded upon by reading Chapters 19 and 21.

1.4
Autoantibodies as Molecular and Cellular Probes

Autoantibodies can be used for the detection of their cognate antigens using immunoprecipitation, immunoblotting, enzyme-linked immunosorbent assay (ELISA), and a variety of microscopy techniques including immunoelectron microscopy. The most visually impressive demonstration of the usefulness of autoantibodies as biological probes is the indirect immunofluorescence (IIF) test. In this technique (Fig. 1.2), a cell or tissue source containing the autoantigen of interest is permeabilized, to allow entry of the antibody into the cell, and fixed, to ensure that the target antigen is not leached away during the procedure. Although some procedures are inappropriate for particular antigens, workable means of cell permeabilization and fixation have been developed [40]. The cell substrate is incubated with the autoantibody to allow interaction with the antigen, and any excess is washed away. The location of the antigen-autoantibody complex within the cell is revealed by addition of an anti-antibody tagged with a fluorochrome. Fluorescence microscopy is then used to view the cells to determine the location of the antigen/autoantibody/fluorochrome-tagged anti-antibody complex. Using this technique, investigators are identifying an increasing number of autoantibody specificities that recognize cellular substructures and domains (Table 1.2, Figs. 1.3 and 1.4). Ivan Raska and Sarka Ruzickova discuss

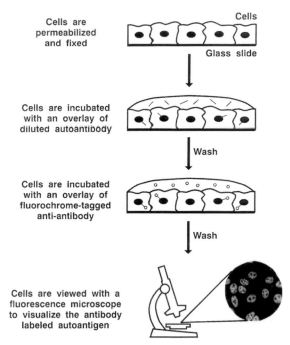

Cells are permeabilized and fixed

Cells

Glass slide

Cells are incubated with an overlay of diluted autoantibody

Wash

Cells are incubated with an overlay of fluorochrome-tagged anti-antibody

Wash

Cells are viewed with a fluorescence microscope to visualize the antibody labeled autoantigen

Fig. 1.2 Diagrammatic representation of the steps involved in the indirect immunofluorescence (IIF) test (see text for explanation).

how autoantibodies have helped to reveal novel substructures within the cell in Chapter 16.

The nucleus can be identified by a variety of autoantibodies such as those against chromatin and DNA or, as shown in Figure 1.3a, autoantibodies to the nuclear lamina, which underlies the nuclear envelope and produces a ringlike fluorescence around the nucleus. The nucleolus and its subdomains can also be identified by a variety of autoantibody specificities (Table 1.2). Autoantibodies against the 34-kDa protein fibrillarin, a component of the C/D box–containing small nucleolar ribonucleoprotein (snoRNP) particles, label the nucleolus in a distinctive "clumpy" pattern [41] (Fig. 1.3e). The list of autoantibodies that are able to distinguish subnuclear domains and compartments, some considerably smaller than the nucleolus, continues to grow. One example is the Cajal body, a small subnuclear structure described using light microscopy by the Spanish cytologist Santiago Ramon y Cajal in 1903 [42]. This nuclear domain can now be easily identified using human autoimmune sera that react with p80 coilin (Fig. 1.3d), a protein highly enriched in the Cajal body [43]. Using other autoantibodies, it has been found that Cajal bodies contain snRNP particles and fibrillarin (previously thought to be restricted to the nucleolus and prenucleolar bodies). Knowledge of the functional associations of these coiled-body constituents suggests that the Cajal body may play a role in RNA processing and/or the accumulation of components involved in RNA processing [43].

Table 1.2 Examples of subcellular structures and domains recognized by autoantibodies.

Autoantibody	Molecular specificity	Subcellular structure
Nuclear components		
Anti-chromatin	Nucleosomal and subnucleosomal complexes of histones and DNA	Chromatin
Antinuclear pore	210-kDa glycoprotein (gp210)	Nuclear pore
Anti-lamin	Nuclear lamins A, B, and C	Nuclear lamina
Anti-centromere	Centromere proteins (CENP) A, B, C, and F	Centromere
Anti-p80 coilin	p80-coilin (80-kDa protein)	Coiled body
Anti-PIKA	p23–25 kDa proteins	Polymorphic interphase karyosomal association (PIKA)
Anti-NuMA	238-kDa protein	Mitotic spindle apparatus
Nucleolar components		
Anti-fibrillarin	34-kDa fibrillarin	Dense fibrillar component of nucleolus
Anti-RNA polymerase 1	RNA polymerase 1	Fibrillari center of nucleolus
Anti-Pm-Scl	75- and 100-kDa proteins of Pm-Scl complex	Granular component of nucleolus
Anti-NOR 90	90-kDa doublet of (human) upstream binding factor (hUBF)	Nucleolar organizer region (NOR)
Cytosolic components		
Anti-mitochondria	Pyruvate dehydrogenase complex	Mitochondria
Anti-ribosome	Ribosomal P proteins (P_0, P_1, P_2)	Ribosomes
Anti-Golgi	95- and 160-kDa golgins	Golgi apparatus
Anti-endosome	180-kDa protein	Early endosomes
Anti-microsomal	Cytochrome P450 superfamily	Microsomes
cANCA	Serine proteinase (proteinase 3)	Lysosomes
Anti-midbody	38-kDa protein	Midbody
Anti-centrosome/centriole	Pericentrin (48 kDa)	Centrosome/centriole

Abbreviations: NuMA = nuclear mitotic apparatus; Pm-Scl = polymyositis-scleroderma; cANCA = cytoplasmic anti-neutrophil cytoplasmic antibody.

Many features of subcellular structures such as size, shape, and distribution can be studied by IIF during the cell cycle, viral infection, mitogenesis, or any cellular response that may result in changes in the distribution of an antigen or subcellular structure. As shown in Figure 1.3a (arrowheads) antinuclear lamin autoantibodies can be used to reveal re-formation of the lamina during telophase. Autoantibodies have identified unexpected protein distributions such as

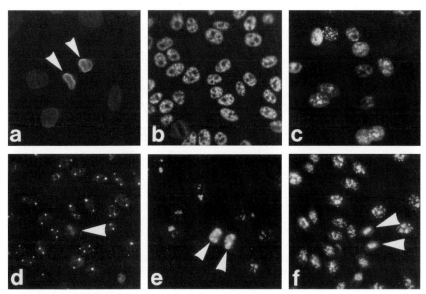

Fig. 1.3 Immunofluorescence patterns produced by autoantibodies recognizing structural and functional domains within the cell nucleus (magnification, 350×). (a) Antinuclear lamin B1 antibodies identify the periphery of the nucleus; arrowheads show the reformation of the nuclear envelope during late telophase. (b) Anti-Sm antibodies localize the U1, U2, and U4–U6 snRNP particles as a speckled nuclear pattern. (c) Anti-PCNA antibodies recognize the auxiliary protein of DNA polymerase delta during active DNA synthesis, producing different fluorescence patterns as cells progress through mitosis.

(d) Anti-p80 coilin antibodies highlight subnuclear domains known as Cajal bodies, which disappear during metaphase (arrowhead). (e) Anti-fibrillarin antibodies target the nucleolus and produce a characteristic clumpy pattern in interphase cells, decorating the chromosomes from late metaphase until cell division (arrowhead). (f) Antibodies to centromeric proteins A, B, and C produce a discrete speckling of the interphase nucleus and identify the centromeric region of the dividing chromosomes during cell division (arrowheads).

the localization of the nucleolar protein fibrillarin to the outer surface of the chromosomes during cell division (Fig. 1.3 e, arrowheads). The localization of some autoantigens during the cell cycle has aided in their identification. Detection of proliferating cell nuclear antigen (PCNA) in S-phase cells (Fig. 1.3 c) suggested its involvement in DNA synthesis [44], while the distribution of speckles along the metaphase plate produced by other autoantibodies (Fig. 1.3 f, arrowheads) was an important clue to their identification as autoantibodies to centromeric proteins A, B, and C [45].

The IIF test has also proved useful in the identification of autoantibodies that react with subcellular structures other than the nucleus. Figure 1.4 shows the IIF patterns produced by some of these autoantibodies. Prior knowledge of subcellular organelles and their relative cellular distribution was instrumental in identifying the structures recognized by these and other autoantibodies. In turn,

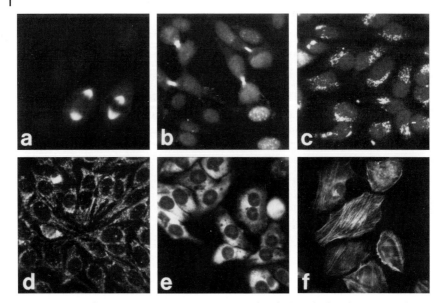

Fig. 1.4 Immunofluorescence patterns produced by autoantibodies recognizing intracellular structures other than the nucleus.
(a) Anti-mitotic spindle apparatus antibodies identify spindle poles and spindle fibers during cell division. (b) Anti-midbody antibodies react with the bridgelike midbody that connects daughter cells following chromosome segregation but before cell separation.
(c) Anti–Golgi complex antibodies decorate the Golgi apparatus, which in most cells is shown as an accumulation of fluorescence in a discrete cytoplasmic region. (d) Anti-mitochondrial antibodies demonstrate the presence of mitochondria throughout the cytoplasm; the discrete nuclear dots represent an additional autoantibody specificity in this serum unrelated to mitochondria. (e) Anti-ribosome antibodies produce a diffuse cytoplasmic staining pattern that spares the nucleus but may show some weak nucleolar fluorescence. (f) Anti-cytoskeletal antibodies react with a variety of cytoskeletal components; in this case the antibody reacts with non-muscle myosin. Magnification:
(a) 700 ×; (b–f) 350 ×.

autoantibodies, by virtue of their reactivity with individual autoantigens, have allowed cell and molecular biologists insight into the molecular constituents of the nucleus and other subcellular organelles. An excellent review of this field, including the birthing of the field of small RNP biology, is given by Erica Champion and Susan Baserga in Chapter 17.

Comparative studies using human autoantibodies, and nonhuman autoantibodies against specific cellular proteins, can be useful in determining the cellular distribution of a specific protein. This is achieved by using anti-human antibodies labeled with one chromophore and antibodies specific for the nonhuman antibody labeled with a different chromophore and comparing the fluorescence patterns. Immunolocalization of the snoRNP components recognized by monoclonal antibodies obtained from mice exposed to mercury was confirmed in this way by comparison of the IIF pattern of human autoimmune anti-fibrillarin sera, which recognizes a protein component of the box C/D snoRNPs [12].

One feature of autoantibodies that distinguishes them from antibodies raised by specific immunization, and underscores their uniqueness, is their ability to recognize their target antigen not only from the host but also from a variety of species. The extent of this species cross-reactivity is dependent on the evolutionary conservation of the autoantigen and is related to the conservation of protein sequence. One example is the snoRNP protein fibrillarin [11]. Using autoantibodies in a variety of immunological techniques, including IIF, this protein can be recognized from species as diverse as humans and the unicellular yeast *Saccharomyces cerevisiae*. cDNA cloning of fibrillarin has confirmed the expected high degree of conservation of the protein sequence [46].

The reactivity of autoantibodies with conserved sequence and conformational protein elements has made them useful reagents in the cloning of cDNAs of expressed proteins from cDNA libraries from a variety of species. However, because of their reactivity with the human protein, they have found most use in the cloning and characterization of the primary structure of numerous human cellular proteins [47, 48]. The diversity of targets that can be exploited by this approach is clearly illustrated in Tables 1.1 and 1.2. Using recent work from his own laboratory, Edward Chan points out the practical aspects to cDNA cloning using autoantibodies in Chapter 18.

Elucidation of the structure of the autoantigens that are the targets of autoantibodies from systemic autoimmune diseases has revealed that many are functional macromolecular complexes involved in nucleic acid and protein synthesis and processing (Table 1.3). A distinguishing feature of many of these complexes of nucleic acid and/or proteins is that autoantibodies do not recognize all the components of the complex. An extreme, but useful, example is the ribosome, which in eukaryotes may contain more than 70 proteins. However, only a small number of these proteins – predominantly the P proteins (P_0, P_1, and P_2), S10, and L12 – are recognized by autoantibodies [49]. Nonetheless, the use of autoantibodies that identify specific components of such complexes has aided in identifying other subunits of these complexes, with profound consequences. Thus, the initial identification of anti-Sm autoantibodies in SLE [50] led to the observation that they recognize some of the protein components of the snRNP particles [51], fueling subsequent studies that showed the snRNPs as components of the spliceosome complex that functions in pre-mRNA splicing [52].

As the functional associations of autoantigens have become known, attempts to uncover the role of the autoantigen itself have revealed that autoantibodies can directly inhibit the function of their target autoantigen (Table 1.3) [53]. Eric Gershwin and colleagues describe their experience with anti-mitochondrial antibodies to document the characteristics of autoantibodies directed against functional sites in Chapter 20. Although it remains to be determined, it seems likely that such inhibition reflects the involvement of conserved protein sequence or structure in functional activity. An increasing number of autoantibodies, many of unknown molecular specificity, recognize their autoantigen only in a particular functional state or phase of the cell cycle. Of the several examples known, the best characterized is PCNA, which is the auxiliary protein of DNA polymerase delta and is rec-

Table 1.3 Examples of the function of nuclear autoantigens and the effects of autoantibody on antigen function.

Autoantigen	Function	Autoantibody effect [a]
	Known function	
Sm/nRNP (U1, U2, U4–6 snRNP)	Pre-mRNA splicing	Inhibition of pre-mRNA splicing
PCNA (DNA polymerase delta auxiliary protein)	DNA replication	Inhibition of DNA replication and repair
RNA polymerase I	Transcription of rRNA	Inhibition of rRNA transcription
tRNA polymerase	Aminoacylation of tRNA	Inhibition of charging of tRNA
Ribosomal RNP	mRNA translation	Inhibition of protein synthesis
Centromere/kinetochore	Microtubule-based chromosome movement during mitosis	Inhibition of centromere formation and function
	Probable function	
Fibrillarin (box C/D snoRNP)	Processing and methylation of pre-rRNA	Blocks translocation of fibrillarin during the cell cycle, thereby influencing the ultrastructure of the nucleolus
NOR-90	Nucleolar transcription factor	Not tested

a) Inhibition of function has been demonstrated *in vitro* or following injection of autoantibody into living cells.

ognized by autoantibodies only during mitosis, even though PCNA is present throughout the cell cycle. When a population of cells at different stages of the cell cycle is used as substrate in the IIF test, anti-PCNA autoantibodies produce varying degrees of fluorescence intensity, being negative in G_0 cells and highly positive in S-phase cells (Fig. 1.3 c). These intriguing features of some autoantibodies have added new dimensions to the biological usefulness of these proteins and have suggested that functionally active macromolecular complexes may play a role in the elicitation of the autoantibody response [53].

The presence of multiple autoantibody specificities in the blood of individual human patients with autoimmune diseases poses a limitation on their use in studies involving a single autoantigen. Only infrequently are patients found whose autoantibody response is so restricted that they express autoreactivity to a single autoantigen or autoantigenic complex; such autoantibodies are termed monospecific. For some autoantibody specificities this condition has been overcome by the production of hybridomas secreting a monoclonal autoantibody. Some hybridomas have been produced by fusion of B cells from human patients, but most have come from fusion of lymphoid cells from animal models of autoimmunity, particularly inbred murine strains [54, 55]. Monoclonal antibody specificities include reactivity against the nucleic acids DNA and RNA, subunits of chromatin, protein components of snRNP particles, fibrillarin, and immunoglobulin.

1.5
Autoantibodies in Experimental Models of Autoimmunity

Research into mechanisms of autoimmunity and the antigenic specificity, and possible pathogenic role, of autoantibodies has been significantly advanced by the availability of animal models. Four different types of models have been used (Table 1.4). Specific antigen immunization models are produced by direct injection of purified antigen into animals to elicit autoantibody. Direct immunization has proven most useful when the autoantigen is extracellular or on the cell membrane. In such examples the elicited autoantibody response can produce pathological consequences such as the myasthenia gravis–like disease produced in rodents following immunization with purified acetylcholine receptor [56]. The animals used in this type of model are most often healthy, normal individuals with fully functional immune systems and are able to downregulate the autoimmune response produced by the immunization of autoantigen. As a result, direct immunization models often produce transient autoimmune responses and the animals return to a healthy state. Some of the most elegant studies in this area have been done with the autoimmune ovarian disease (AOD) model as described by Yulius Setiady and Kenneth Tung in Chapter 21.

Comparison of the autoantigenic reactivities of antibodies raised by immunization, especially to intracellular autoantigens, has revealed distinct differences in comparison to autoantibodies found in human autoimmune disease. Direct immunization requires a purified antigen, which means subjecting the antigen to rigorous biophysical, biochemical, and, sometimes, immunological separation techniques. The resulting preparation may therefore be partially or totally denatured and no longer in association with other cellular components that constitute its *in vivo* molecular form. Even if the native *in vivo* macromolecular complex can be purified, direct immunization experiments are "best guess" attempts to mimic the natural autoimmunization process, because the molecular structure of the putative autoimmunogen that contains the autoantigen of interest is unknown. A further complication is the use of adjuvants to boost the immune response [57]. As a result, direct immunization produces antibodies that, although reacting with the autoantigen, usually recognize a denatured form rather than the autoantigen in its native state; only rarely do they react with the autoantigen when it is in association with other cellular subunits that make up its *in vivo* molecular form [26]. Although direct immunization antibodies can recognize conformational epitopes, they do not appear to recognize conserved epitopes and therefore cannot exhibit the same lack of species specificity that allows, for example, anti-fibrillarin autoantibodies to recognize fibrillarin in all

Table 1.4 Examples of animal models of autoantibody production.

Model	Animal	Human disease	Autoantibody specificity
Spontaneous			
NZB	Mouse	Hemolytic anemia	Erythrocyte
(NZB×NZW) F_1	Mouse	SLE	Chromatin, DNA
MRL/Fas^{lpr}	Mouse	SLE	Chromatin, DNA, Sm, ribosome
MRL/Fas$^{+/+}$	Mouse	SLE	Chromatin, DNA, Sm
BXSB	Mouse	SLE	Chromatin, DNA
Obese strain (white leghorn chicken)	Bird	Thyroiditis	Thyroglobulin
Induced by exogenous agents			
Chronic GVHD	Mouse	SLE	DNA, chromatin, snRNP, ribosome
Mercuric chloride	Mouse (H–2^s)	Scleroderma[a] (immune-complex nephritis)	Fibrillarin (box C/D snoRNP)
Mercuric chloride	Mouse (non-H–2 restricted)	SLE	Chromatin
Mercuric chloride	Rat (RT1^n)	Immune-complex nephritis	GBM
Pristane	Mouse	SLE	DNA, Sm, RNP, Su
Direct immunization (antigen)			
EAT (thyroglobulin)	Rabbit, mouse (H–2$^{k, s, or q}$)	Thyroiditis	Thyroglobulin
GMB nephritis (GBM)	Sheep, mouse	Immune-complex nephritis	GBM
EMG (acetylcholine receptor)	Lewis rat	Myasthenia gravis	Acetylcholine receptor
Gene mutation			
C1q knockout	Mouse (MRL/Fas$^{+/+}$)	SLE	DNA, Rheumatoid factor
Dnase1 knockout	Mouse	SLE	Chromatin, DNA
SAP knockout	Mouse	SLE	Chromatin, DNA
c-mer knockout	Mouse	SLE	Chromatin
IFN-γ transgenic	Mouse	SLE	DNA, histones

a) Autoantibody specificity is specific for scleroderma, but a scleroderma-like disease has not been described in mice treated with mercuric chloride.

Abbreviations: GVHD = graft-versus-host disease; GMB = glomerular basement membrane; EAT = experimental autoimmune thyroiditis; EMG = experimental myasthenia gravis; C1q = component of serum complement; Dnase1 = deoxyribonuclease 1; SAP = serum amyloid P component; c-mer = tyrosine kinase.

species that contain this protein [11]. Lack of reaction against conserved epitopes means that direct immunization antibodies are less efficient at inhibiting the functional activity of their target autoantigen than are autoantibodies from patients with autoimmune diseases [53]. Animal models of other types, described next, can produce autoantibodies with reactivities that are extremely difficult to differentiate from those of human patients. As a result, such models more closely approximate their human counterparts.

The second type of model also involves the manipulation of normal, non autoimmune animals to produce an autoimmune response. In these cases the triggering event is the introduction into the animal of exogenous material that, unlike the case of direct immunization, may appear to bear little relationship to the ensuing autoimmune response. These mediators – which may include drugs, biologicals, and environmental agents such as hormones and microbes – and their role in inducing autoimmunity are discussed by Per Hultman in Chapter 22. An excellent example of this type of model is the autoimmunity induced by heavy metals [10]. Administration of mercury by several different routes and in several different forms (most notably, subcutaneous injection of mercuric chloride) produces in mice an autoantibody response that targets the nucleolus [12]. The principal autoantigen involved is the 34-kDa protein fibrillarin [58, 59], a protein component of the box C/D snoRNP particles. Mercury induces this autoantibody response in a restricted number of histocompatibility genotypes, most commonly H-2^s [60]. Although offspring of crosses between the autoimmune-sensitive H-2^s strains and the autoimmune-resistant strains such as C57BL/6 (H-2^b) or DBA/2 (H-2^d) are sensitive to anti-fibrillarin induction following HgCl$_2$ treatment, the response does not appear to be due solely to the product of a dominant *H-2* gene but involves multiple loci. This is supported by backcrossing of hybrids onto the autoimmune-sensitive H-2^s background, where the HgCl$_2$-induced anti-fibrillarin response is even less frequent, even though 50% of the mice would be expected to be homozygous for H-2^s. Although anti-fibrillarin autoantibodies are a marker for human scleroderma, mercury does not appear to produce a scleroderma-like disease in mice; the importance of the model lies instead in the similarity of this toxin-induced murine autoantibody response to the spontaneous anti-fibrillarin autoantibody in human scleroderma [11].

Another example of the exogenous factor type of model is murine graft-versus-host disease (GVHD). In this model the offspring of the mating of two inbred non-autoimmune mouse strains are injected (grafted) with lymphocytes from one of the parental strains. The injected lymphocytes recognize genetic differences in the host strain that are inherited from the other parental strain and are stimulated to mount a variety of immune responses against the host animal, hence the name "graft versus host." Unlike the case of direct immunization models, the autoimmunity produced in this type of model can lead to severe pathological consequences, including lethal immune complex disease. The immunological sequelae that occur during a GVHD response depend on the murine inbred strains used. Injection of DBA/2 lymphocytes into a cross between the DBA/2 and C57B16 mice produces a chronic GVHD, which results in an autoimmune response similar to human SLE, including the presence of autoantibodies against chromatin and DNA [61]. Injection of lymphocytes from the A/J strain into Balb/c×A/J hybrids also produces a chronic GVHD in which autoantibodies to snRNP particles including the U3 snoRNP are found [62]. The relationship of different autoantibody specificities to the use of different strains of inbred mice in the GVHD model again highlights the influence of genotype on autoimmunity and autoantibodies.

The third type of model does not require any manipulation of the animal at all, as the disease develops spontaneously. The best described of these are the murine strains BXSB, (NZB×NZW) F_1, NZM, MRL/Fas$^{+/+}$, and MRL/Fas^{lpr}, which develop forms of SLE that serve as excellent models of the autoantibody specificities and pathology of the human disease [63]. Dwight Kono provides an overview of the genetics leading to autoimmunity in these models in Chapter 23. While the variety of autoantibodies developed by these different strains continues to be investigated, the common autoantibody response, like human SLE, is against chromatin and its subcomponents including DNA [38, 64]. In the (NZB×NZW) F_1 strain, autoimmune disease and autoantibodies occur earlier and more frequently in female mice, a finding that has been revealed to be associated with the presence of female sex hormones. Because of this and other features, the (NZB×NZW) F_1 strain is considered the best animal model of human SLE. As noted above it is the genetic makeup of these inbred strains that has significant potential to address the genesis of the autoimmune response. A much-studied aspect of several of the spontaneous models of systemic autoimmune disease is the presence of single gene defects that accelerate or exacerbate autoimmunity in these already susceptible mouse strains. In the MRL substrains, the *Lpr* phenotype is responsible for massive lymphoproliferation of CD4$^-$, CD8$^-$, and B200$^+$ T cells and an accelerated occurrence of autoimmune phenomena compared to the MRL/Fas$^{+/+}$. Recent studies have indicated that the *Lpr* defect is due to a mutation in the *Fas* gene that leads to defective expression of *Fas* on T and B cells, which allows them to escape apoptotic elimination and reach the peripheral circulation [65]. Breeding experiments to impart the *Lpr* gene onto non-autoimmune genetic backgrounds have shown that the *Fas* defect does influence the development of autoimmunity and the expression of autoantibodies. A dominant role for *Fas* in the initiation of autoimmunity and autoantibodies is questionable, however, because the MRL/Fas$^{+/+}$, which does not have the *Fas* defect, does develop an autoantibody profile and immunopathological disease that is similar to the MRL/Fas^{lpr}, albeit at a much later age. Other genes that appear to play a role in acceleration of autoimmunity include *Gld*, the ligand for *Fas*, and *Yaa*, a sex-linked gene that produces a defect in B cells and is the accelerator gene of autoimmunity in the male BXSB mouse [66]. Exposure of lupus-prone strains to exogenous agents known to elicit autoimmunity in normal mice can result in accelerated appearance of disease features, including autoantibodies. In some cases the exogenous agent accelerates appearance of idiopathic disease, while in others the elicited disease has features of xenobiotic-induced disease. Thus, mercury exposure accelerates idio-pathic disease in BXSB mice, including anti-chromatin autoantibodies of the IgG2a subclass [67], while pristane injection into (NZB×NZW) F_1 mice elicits anti-Sm/RNP and Su autoantibodies, which are not part of the idiopathic dis-ease of the (NZB×NZW) F_1 but are found in pristane-induced autoimmunity [68]. These observations suggest not only that idiopathic and induced autoim-munity may arise by different mechanisms but also that exogenous triggers can influence disease expression.

The fourth type of model involves genetic manipulation in which a gene is de-leted ("knockout") or added ("transgenic") in order to influence the expression of autoimmunity. Both types of genetic modification can be used to study the influ-ence of single genes on the animal models described above. Perhaps not unexpect-edly, many gene deletions have little or no effect on the expression of autoimmu-nity and autoantibodies. Such negative effects need to be interpreted carefully, as they may indicate a genetically redundant process rather than an unimportant gene. Other gene deletions have been reported to influence differing aspects of autoimmunity in a gene-specific manner, although the extent of the effect may vary between experimental models. Some gene deletions exhibit highly consistent responses. Thus, deletion of the gene for the pleiotropic cytokine interferon-γ (IFN-γ) abrogates autoantibody production and immunopathology in mercury-in-duced autoimmunity of B10.S mice [69] and spontaneous autoimmunity in MRL/Fas^{lpr} mice [70]. The significance of IFN-γ in systemic autoimmunity has been demonstrated in non-autoimmune-prone mice made transgenic for IFN-γ expres-sion in the epidermis [71]. The increased expression of IFN-γ leads to a lupus-like disease characterized by production of autoantibodies and immune complex–mediated tissue damage [71]. Further evidence for the importance of IFN-γ has come from an examination of gene expression in the Nba2 locus of chromosome 1 of the mouse. Nba2 is a genetic interval identified as a locus of genetic suscep-tibility for lupus in the NZB strain. The offspring of Nba2 interval–specific con-genic C57BL/6 mice mated with NZW mice develop autoimmunity similar to the SLE-prone (NZB×NZW) F_1 mouse. Examination of gene expression by DNA array revealed a relationship between increased expression of interferon-in-ducible gene 202 (Ifi202) and features of systemic autoimmunity [72]. Importantly, the gene for Ifi202 lies within the Nba2 interval. Confirmation that increased ex-pression of Ifi202 occurs in other models of systemic lupus would significantly en-hance its stature as a lupus susceptibility gene. However, as susceptibility for SLE maps to multiple genetic loci, it is highly likely that additional genes contribute to full disease expression in the (NZB×NZW) F_1 mouse [4].

A number of other gene deletions are associated with expression of autoim-munity and autoantibodies. Some of these, such as deficiency of C1q, a compo-nent of the complement system, have particular relevance, as complement defi-ciencies in humans can lead to development of systemic lupus. Significantly, lack of C1q is not sufficient for development of murine lupus; this gene dele-tion must occur on genetic backgrounds carrying additional susceptibility genes for autoimmunity to occur [73]. It must also be noted that although many knockout and transgenic models exhibit features of autoimmunity, they may also exhibit other features that are not consistent with the known spectrum of clinical and immunological facets of autoimmune diseases [74]. More telling is the finding that many of the genetic mutations that lead to autoimmunity in mice are not necessary for the development of human systemic autoimmune disease. As described above, mutation in the *Fas* gene contributes significantly to the severity of murine SLE. However, mutations in the *Fas* gene are not associated with human SLE, but rather with autoimmune lymphoproliferative syndrome (ALPS). ALPS is characterized by lymphoproliferation of double-negative T cells and autoantibodies against DNA and cardiolipin [75], features found in mice with a *Fas* mutation but without other lupus susceptibility genes. Similarly, Dnase1-deficient mice develop a lupus-like disease with anti-chromatin autoantibodies [76], but deficiency of Dnase1 is not common in human systemic lupus. A nonsense mutation in exon 2 of the DNASE1 gene has been reported in two apparently unrelated young Japanese patients [77] but not in Caucasian SLE patients [78]. Matthew Pickering and Marina Botto present an overview of the most significant gene-targeted models of SLE, with special emphasis on complement deficiency, and how they have contributed to our knowledge of the pathogenesis of lupus in Chapter 24.

Although care must be taken in their interpretation, identification and characterization of genes that are associated with autoimmunity and autoantibody production constitute fertile ground for the molecular biologist [79]. Elucidation of the roles of the many genes that appear to contribute to the development of autoimmunity will help to define the critical molecular events in the disease process. The murine strains described above have proven to be valuable model systems for the study of many facets of autoimmunity and will play significant roles in future genetic studies. It will be important to focus attention not only on the genetic loci that impart susceptibility to autoimmunity but also on those that may allow an individual to resist development of autoimmune phenomena [5, 80].

1.6
Conclusions

Initially used as aids to clinical diagnosis, autoantibodies have become increasingly useful "reporter" molecules in the identification of structure-function relationships. New autoantigens continue to be discovered, while many described autoantigens remain to be characterized both structurally and functionally. Autoantibodies will figure prominently in these characterization studies. As the molecular structures of the interaction between autoantigen and autoantibody become known, it should be possible to design peptide configurations capable of perturbing the functional activity of numerous cellular processes.

Understanding the influence of genes and their products not only on susceptibility but also on resistance to autoimmunity and autoantibody expression is in its infancy. But the tools to mature this field (inbred animal models of spontaneous and induced autoimmunity, molecular techniques of transgenics and gene knockout) are already available. They await the complex but potentially fruitful identification and functional analysis of candidate genes.

References

1 Medzhitov, R., and C. A. Janeway, Jr. 2002. Decoding the patterns of self and nonself by the innate immune system. *Science* 296:298–300.

2 Matzinger, P. 2002. The danger model: a renewed sense of self. *Science* 296:301–305.

3 Theofilopoulos, A. N., and D. H. Kono. 2002. A genetic analysis of lupus. *Allergy* 57 Suppl 72:67–74.

4 Croker, B. P., G. Gilkeson, and L. Morel. 2003. Genetic interactions between susceptibility loci reveal epistatic pathogenic networks in murine lupus. *Genes Immun* 4:575–585.

5 Morel, L., X. H. Tian, B. P. Croker, and E. K. Wakeland. 1999. Epistatic modifiers of autoimmunity in a murine model of lupus nephritis. *Immunity* 11:131–139.

6 Marrack, P., J. Kappler, and B. L. Kotzin. 2001. Autoimmune disease: why and where it occurs. *Nat Med* 7:899–905.

7 Rubin, R. L. 1999. Etiology and mechanisms of drug-induced lupus. *Curr Opin Rheumatol* 11:357–363.

8 Rubin, R. L., S. A. Bell, and R. W. Burlingame. 1992. Autoantibodies associated with lupus induced by diverse drugs target a similar epitope in the (H2A-H2B)-DNA complex. *J Clin Invest* 90:165–173.

9 Burlingame, R. W., and R. L. Rubin. 1991. Drug-induced anti-histone autoantibodies display two patterns of reactivity with substructures of chromatin. *J Clin Invest* 88:680–690.

10 Pollard, K. M., and P. Hultman. 1997. Effects of mercury on the immune system. *Met Ions Biol Syst* 34:421–440.

11 Takeuchi, K., S. J. Turley, E. M. Tan, and K. M. Pollard. 1995. Analysis of the autoantibody response to fibrillarin in human disease and murine models of autoimmunity. *J Immunol* 154:961–971.

12 Yang, J. M., S. J. Baserga, S. J. Turley, and K. M. Pollard. 2001. Fibrillarin and other

snoRNP proteins are targets of autoantibodies in xenobiotic-induced autoimmunity. *Clin Immunol* 101:38–50.

13 Jiang, X., G. Khursigara, and R. L. Rubin. 1994. Transformation of lupus-inducing drugs to cytotoxic products by activated neutrophils. *Science* 266:810–813.

14 Kretz-Rommel, A., and R. L. Rubin. 1997. A metabolite of the lupus-inducing drug procainamide prevents anergy induction in T cell clones. *J Immunol* 158:4465–4470.

15 Kretz-Rommel, A., S. R. Duncan, and R. L. Rubin. 1997. Autoimmunity caused by disruption of central T cell tolerance. A murine model of drug-induced lupus. *J Clin Invest* 99:1888–1896.

16 Kretz-Rommel, A., and R. L. Rubin. 2000. Disruption of positive selection of thymocytes causes autoimmunity. *Nat Med* 6:298–305.

17 Goodnow, C. C. 1992. Transgenic mice and analysis of B-cell tolerance. *Annu Rev Immunol* 10:489–518.

18 Radic, M. Z., and M. Weigert. 1994. Genetic and structural evidence for antigen selection of anti-DNA antibodies. *Annu Rev Immunol* 12:487–520.

19 Rosen, A., L. Casciola-Rosen, and J. Ahearn. 1995. Novel packages of viral and self-antigens are generated during apoptosis. *J Exp Med* 181:1557–1561.

20 Navratil, J. S., J. M. Sabatine, and J. M. Ahearn. 2004. Apoptosis and immune responses to self. *Rheum Dis Clin North Am* 30:193–212.

21 Liu, K., T. Iyoda, M. Saternus, Y. Kimura, K. Inaba, and R. M. Steinman. 2002. Immune tolerance after delivery of dying cells to dendritic cells in situ. *J Exp Med* 196:1091–1097.

22 Steinman, R. M., S. Turley, I. Mellman, and K. Inaba. 2000. The induction of tolerance by dendritic cells that have cap-

tured apoptotic cells. *J Exp Med* 191:411–416.

23 Gallucci, S., M. Lolkema, and P. Matzinger. 1999. Natural adjuvants: endogenous activators of dendritic cells. *Nat Med* 5:1249–1255.

24 Huynh, M. L., V. A. Fadok, and P. M. Henson. 2002. Phosphatidylserine-dependent ingestion of apoptotic cells promotes TGF-beta1 secretion and the resolution of inflammation. *J Clin Invest* 109:41–50.

25 Reiter, I., B. Krammer, and G. Schwamberger. 1999. Cutting edge: differential effect of apoptotic versus necrotic tumor cells on macrophage antitumor activities. *J Immunol* 163:1730–1732.

26 Pollard, K. M., D. L. Pearson, M. Bluthner, and E. M. Tan. 2000. Proteolytic cleavage of a self-antigen following xenobiotic-induced cell death produces a fragment with novel immunogenic properties. *J Immunol* 165:2263–2270.

27 Shlomchik, M. J., J. E. Craft, and M. J. Mamula. 2001. From T to B and back again: positive feedback in systemic autoimmune disease. *Nat Rev Immunol* 1:147–153.

28 Baxter, A. G., and P. D. Hodgkin. 2002. Activation rules: the two-signal theories of immune activation. *Nat Rev Immunol* 2:439–446.

29 Yang, J. M., B. Hildebrandt, C. Luderschmidt, and K. M. Pollard. 2003. Human scleroderma sera contain autoantibodies to protein components specific to the U3 small nucleolar RNP complex. *Arthritis Rheum* 48:210–217.

30 Lang, B., and A. Vincent. 2003. Autoantibodies to ion channels at the neuromuscular junction. *Autoimmun Rev* 2:94–100.

31 Kohn, L. D., and N. Harii. 2003. Thyrotropin receptor autoantibodies (TSHRAbs): epitopes, origins and clinical significance. *Autoimmunity* 36:331–337.

32 Liu, Z., and L. A. Diaz. 2001. Bullous pemphigoid: end of the century overview. *J Dermatol* 28:647–650.

33 Giorgio Natali, P., and E. M. Tan. 1972. Experimental renal disease induced by DNA-anti-DNA immune complexes. *J Clin Invest* 51:345–355.

34 Tan, E. M., P. H. Schur, R. I. Carr, and H. G. Kunkel. 1966. Deoxybonucleic acid (DNA) and antibodies to DNA in the serum of patients with systemic lupus erythematosus. *J Clin Invest* 45:1732–1740.

35 Tan, E. M. 1989. Antinuclear antibodies: diagnostic markers for autoimmune diseases and probes for cell biology. *Adv Immunol* 44:93–151.

36 Tan, E. M., E. K. Chan, K. F. Sullivan, and R. L. Rubin. 1988. Antinuclear antibodies (ANAs): diagnostically specific immune markers and clues toward the understanding of systemic autoimmunity. *Clin Immunol Immunopathol* 47:121–141.

37 Burlingame, R. W. 1997. The clinical utility of antihistone antibodies. Autoantibodies reactive with chromatin in systemic lupus erythematosus and drug-induced lupus. *Clin Lab Med* 17:367–378.

38 Burlingame, R. W., M. L. Boey, G. Starkebaum, and R. L. Rubin. 1994. The central role of chromatin in autoimmune responses to histones and DNA in systemic lupus erythematosus. *J Clin Invest* 94:184–192.

39 Pollard, K. M., G. Reimer, and E. M. Tan. 1989. Autoantibodies in scleroderma. *Clin Exp Rheumatol* 7 Suppl 3:S57–62.

40 von Muhlen, C. A., and E. M. Tan. 1995. Autoantibodies in the diagnosis of systemic rheumatic diseases. *Semin Arthritis Rheum* 24:323–358.

41 Reimer, G., V. D. Steen, C. A. Penning, T. A. Medsger, Jr., and E. M. Tan. 1988. Correlates between autoantibodies to nucleolar antigens and clinical features in patients with systemic sclerosis (scleroderma). *Arthritis Rheum* 31:525–532.

42 Gall, J. G. 2000. Cajal bodies: the first 100 years. *Annu Rev Cell Dev Biol* 16:273–300.

43 Raska, I., R. L. Ochs, L. E. Andrade, E. K. Chan, R. Burlingame, C. Peebles, D. Gruol, and E. M. Tan. 1990. Association between the nucleolus and the coiled body. *J Struct Biol* 104:120–127.

44 Takasaki, Y., J. S. Deng, and E. M. Tan. 1981. A nuclear antigen associated with cell proliferation and blast transformation. *J Exp Med* 154:1899–1909.

45 Moroi, Y., C. Peebles, M. J. Fritzler, J. Steigerwald, and E. M. Tan. 1980.

Autoantibody to centromere (kineto-chore) in scleroderma sera. *Proc Natl Acad Sci USA* 77:1627–1631.

46 Turley, S.J., E.M. Tan, and K.M. Pollard. 1993. Molecular cloning and sequence analysis of U3 snoRNA-associated mouse fibrillarin. *Biochim Biophys Acta* 1216:119–122.

47 Pollard, K.M., E.K. Chan, B.J. Grant, K.F. Sullivan, E.M. Tan, and C.A. Glass. 1990. In vitro posttranslational modification of lamin B cloned from a human T-cell line. *Mol Cell Biol* 10:2164–2175.

48 Chan, E.K., K.F. Sullivan, R.I. Fox, and E.M. Tan. 1989. Sjogren's syndrome nuclear antigen B (La): cDNA cloning, structural domains, and autoepitopes. *J Autoimmun* 2:321–327.

49 Desbos, A., P. Gonzalo, J.C. Monier, J. Tebib, J.P. Reboud, H. Perrier, J. Bienvenu, and N. Fabien. 2002. Autoantibodies directed against ribosomal proteins in systemic lupus erythematosus and rheumatoid arthritis: a comparative study. *Autoimmunity* 35:427–434.

50 Tan, E.M., and H.G. Kunkel. 1966. Characteristics of a soluble nuclear antigen precipitating with sera of patients with systemic lupus erythematosus. *J Immunol* 96:464–471.

51 Lerner, M.R., J.A. Boyle, J.A. Hardin, and J.A. Steitz. 1981. Two novel classes of small ribonucleoproteins detected by antibodies associated with lupus erythematosus. *Science* 211:400–402.

52 Padgett, R.A., S.M. Mount, J.A. Steitz, and P.A. Sharp. 1983. Splicing of messenger RNA precursors is inhibited by antisera to small nuclear ribonucleoprotein. *Cell* 35:101–107.

53 Tan, E.M., Y. Muro, and K.M. Pollard. 1994. Autoantibody-defined epitopes on nuclear antigens are conserved, conformation-dependent and active site regions. *Clin Exp Rheumatol* 12 Suppl 11:S27–31.

54 Pollard, K.M., J.E. Jones, E.M. Tan, A.N. Theofilopoulos, F.J. Dixon, and R.L. Rubin. 1986. Polynucleotide specificities of murine monoclonal anti-DNA antibodies. *Clin Immunol Immunopathol* 40:197–208.

55 Reimer, G., K.M. Pollard, C.A. Penning, R.L. Ochs, M.A. Lischwe, H. Busch, and E.M. Tan. 1987. Monoclonal autoantibody from a (New Zealand black x New Zealand white) F1 mouse and some human scleroderma sera target an Mr 34,000 nucleolar protein of the U3 RNP particle. *Arthritis Rheum* 30:793–800.

56 Vincent, A., N. Willcox, M. Hill, J. Curnow, C. MacLennan, and D. Beeson. 1998. Determinant spreading and immune responses to acetylcholine receptors in myasthenia gravis. *Immunol Rev* 164:157–168.

57 Janeway, C.A., Jr. 1989. Approaching the asymptote? Evolution and revolution in immunology. *Cold Spring Harb Symp Quant Biol* 54 Pt 1:1–13.

58 Hultman, P., S. Enestrom, K.M. Pollard, and E.M. Tan. 1989. Anti-fibrillarin autoantibodies in mercury-treated mice. *Clin Exp Immunol* 78:470–477.

59 Reuter, R., G. Tessars, H.W. Vohr, E. Gleichmann, and R. Luhrmann. 1989. Mercuric chloride induces autoantibodies against U3 small nuclear ribonucleoprotein in susceptible mice. *Proc Natl Acad Sci USA* 86:237–241.

60 Hultman, P., L.J. Bell, S. Enestrom, and K.M. Pollard. 1992. Murine susceptibility to mercury. I. Autoantibody profiles and systemic immune deposits in inbred, congenic, and intra-H-2 recombinant strains. *Clin Immunol Immunopathol* 65:98–109.

61 Pollard, K.M., E.K. Chan, R.L. Rubin, and E.M. Tan. 1987. Monoclonal autoantibodies to nuclear antigens from murine graft-versus-host disease. *Clin Immunol Immunopathol* 44:31–44.

62 Gelpi, C., J.L. Rodriguez-Sanchez, M.A. Martinez, J. Craft, and J.A. Hardin. 1988. Murine graft vs host disease. A model for study of mechanisms that generate autoantibodies to ribonucleoproteins. *J Immunol* 140:4160–4166.

63 Kofler, R., F.J. Dixon, and A.N. Theofilopoulos. 1989. Genetic basis for autoantibody-production in murine models of systemic autoimmunity. *Contrib Microbiol Immunol* 11:206–230.

64 Burlingame, R.W., R.L. Rubin, R.S. Balderas, and A.N. Theofilopoulos. 1993.

Genesis and evolution of antichromatin autoantibodies in murine lupus implicates T-dependent immunization with self antigen. *J Clin Invest* 91:1687–1696.

65 Watanabe-Fukunaga, R., C.I. Brannan, N.G. Copeland, N.A. Jenkins, and S. Nagata. 1992. Lymphoproliferation disorder in mice explained by defects in Fas antigen that mediates apoptosis. *Nature* 356:314–317.

66 Kono, D.H., and A.N. Theofilopoulos. 2000. Genetics of systemic autoimmunity in mouse models of lupus. *Int Rev Immunol* 19:367–387.

67 Pollard, K.M., D.L. Pearson, P. Hultman, T.N. Deane, U. Lindh, and D.H. Kono. 2001. Xenobiotic acceleration of idiopathic systemic autoimmunity in lupus-prone bxsb mice. *Environ Health Perspect* 109:27–33.

68 Yoshida, H., M. Satoh, K.M. Behney, C.G. Lee, H.B. Richards, V.M. Shaheen, J.Q. Yang, R.R. Singh, and W.H. Reeves. 2002. Effect of an exogenous trigger on the pathogenesis of lupus in (NZB×NZW) F$_1$ mice. *Arthritis Rheum* 46:2235–2244.

69 Kono, D.H., D. Balomenos, D.L. Pearson, M.S. Park, B. Hildebrandt, P. Hultman, and K.M. Pollard. 1998. The prototypic Th2 autoimmunity induced by mercury is dependent on IFN-gamma and not Th1/Th2 imbalance. *J Immunol* 161:234–240.

70 Balomenos, D., R. Rumold, and A.N. Theofilopoulos. 1998. Interferon-gamma is required for lupus-like disease and lymphoaccumulation in MRL-lpr mice. *J Clin Invest* 101:364–371.

71 Seery, J.P., J.M. Carroll, V. Cattell, and F.M. Watt. 1997. Antinuclear autoantibodies and lupus nephritis in transgenic mice expressing interferon gamma in the epidermis. *J Exp Med* 186:1451–1459.

72 Rozzo, S.J., J.D. Allard, D. Choubey, T.J. Vyse, S. Izui, G. Peltz, and B.L. Kotzin. 2001. Evidence for an interferon-inducible gene, Ifi202, in the susceptibility to systemic lupus. *Immunity* 15:435–443.

73 Mitchell, D.A., M.C. Pickering, J. Warren, L. Fossati-Jimack, J. Cortes-Hernandez, H.T. Cook, M. Botto, and M.J. Walport. 2002. C1q deficiency and autoimmunity: the effects of genetic background on disease expression. *J Immunol* 168:2538–2543.

74 Scott, R.S., E.J. McMahon, S.M. Pop, E.A. Reap, R. Caricchio, P.L. Cohen, H.S. Earp, and G.K. Matsushima. 2001. Phagocytosis and clearance of apoptotic cells is mediated by MER. *Nature* 411:207–211.

75 Carter, L.B., J.L. Procter, J.K. Dale, S.E. Straus, and C.C. Cantilena. 2000. Description of serologic features in autoimmune lymphoproliferative syndrome. *Transfusion* 40:943–948.

76 Napirei, M., H. Karsunky, B. Zevnik, H. Stephan, H.G. Mannherz, and T. Moroy. 2000. Features of systemic lupus erythematosus in Dnase1-deficient mice. *Nat Genet* 25:177–181.

77 Yasutomo, K., T. Horiuchi, S. Kagami, H. Tsukamoto, C. Hashimura, M. Urushihara, and Y. Kuroda. 2001. Mutation of DNASE1 in people with systemic lupus erythematosus. *Nat Genet* 28:313–314.

78 Simmonds, M.J., J.M. Heward, M.A. Kelly, A. Allahabadia, H. Foxall, C. Gordon, J.A. Franklyn, and S.C. Gough. 2002. A nonsense mutation in exon 2 of the DNase I gene is not present in UK subjects with systemic lupus erythematosus and Graves' disease: Comment on the article by Rood et al. *Arthritis Rheum* 46:3109–3110.

79 Goodnow, C.C., R. Glynne, S. Akkaraju, J. Rayner, D. Mack, J.I. Healy, S. Chaudhry, L. Miosge, L. Wilson, P. Papathanasiou, and A. Loy. 2001. Autoimmunity, self-tolerance and immune homeostasis: from whole animal phenotypes to molecular pathways. *Adv Exp Med Biol* 490:33–40.

80 Kono, D.H., M.S. Park, A. Szydlik, K.M. Haraldsson, J.D. Kuan, D.L. Pearson, P. Hultman, and K.M. Pollard. 2001. Resistance to xenobiotic-induced autoimmunity maps to chromosome 1. *J Immunol* 167:2396–2403.

2
Prefatory Chapter:
The Importance of the Autoantibody-defined Epitope

Eng M. Tan

2.1
Introduction

Autoimmunity should be defined in the strict sense as an immune response by the host to a self-antigen, at either the humoral or cellular level or both. This definition distinguishes the autoimmune response per se from autoimmune disease where the humoral and/or cellular consequences of the immune response have resulted in pathophysiological abnormalities. In this sense, autoimmunity as a phenomenon is not uncommon, but the follow-through to autoimmune disease has been less common. This observation begs the question of whether there are autoimmune responses that are physiological and others that are pathological. In this chapter, I will describe the unique features of the autoantibody-defined epitope, or the antigenic determinant on the self-antigen, and how perhaps this knowledge might be useful in the context of designing reagents for immunotherapy.

Immunotherapy has been described as any approach aimed at mobilizing or manipulating a patient's immune system to treat or cure disease [1]. This has included therapeutic vaccines consisting of modified or unmodified self-antigens or peptides of such antigens in order to activate the patient's own immune response. Other approaches include the use of monoclonal antibodies targeting autoantigens, cytokines, or cell receptors shown to be involved in tissue pathology. Immunotherapy in the form of monoclonal antibodies to TNFα or as secretory subunits of TNFα have been strikingly successful in the treatment of rheumatoid arthritis [2], but other forms of immunotherapy have not been as successful. The problems encountered have included unacceptable side effects of autoimmune hyperthyroidism in multiple sclerosis patients treated with monoclonal antibody to CD52 [3, 4] and minimal responsiveness using cancer immunotherapy based on peptide antigens [5, 6]. These and other difficulties have led some investigators to say that human immunotherapy is currently "bewildered" about how to stimulate the immune system and what new directions to pursue [1].

Autoantibodies and Autoimmunity: Molecular Mechanisms in Health and Disease. Edited by K. Michael Pollard
Copyright © 2006 WILEY-VCH Verlag GmbH & Co. KGaA, Weinheim
ISBN: 3-527-31141-6

It is not a point of contention to say that there is very little proven knowledge concerning the mechanisms leading to an autoimmune response to a molecule that is part of self. Our understanding of mechanisms leading to the immune processing of a foreign antigen such as a purified foreign protein is fairly comprehensive, but the knowledge concerning immune processing of a self-protein is at present rudimentary and speculative. There are multiple and complex reasons for this state of our ignorance, not the least of which are uncertainties as to how self-proteins or other self-molecules are recognized as foreign by the immune system. Some of these questions addressed in this book include apoptosis and cell necrosis in the intracellular degradation of potential autoantigens (see Chapters 6 and 7), but these may be but the tip of a hidden iceberg of many mechanisms.

One of the hallmarks of many autoimmune diseases is the production of autoantibodies to specific cassettes of cellular autoantigens. This is abundantly demonstrated not only in systemic autoimmune diseases such as lupus but also in organ-specific autoimmune diseases such as type 1 diabetes, autoimmune thyroid disease, and others as described by several authors in this book. Autoantibodies to these disease-specific autoantigens have become clinically useful as diagnostic markers in medicine. What has been not as fully appreciated is the fact that there is valuable information to be gained from analyzing the reactive epitopes of autoantigens. In essence, the immune system of the patient is saying that in the case of a particular self-molecule, its own immune system is able to mount an immune response to one particular region but is unable to make a response to another. In the design of antigen-specific immunotherapy, it would be important to capitalize on this information and not design antigens to which the immune system has been non-responsive.

2.2
The Uniqueness of the Autoantibody-defined Antigenic Determinant or the Autoepitope

In the 1960s there was great interest and activity in identification of autoantibodies in the systemic rheumatic diseases (reviewed in [7]). One of the standard methods for the identification of such autoantibodies was with the use of immunofluorescence microscopy for detection of autoantibodies reacting with nucleus and cytoplasm of tissue cryosections or tissue culture cells. This immunohistochemical technique revealed that different autoantibodies would display different patterns of fluorescence in nucleus, nucleolus, and cytoplasm. One of the key observations was that autoantibodies from patients with many systemic rheumatic diseases not only reacted with nuclear, nucleolar, or cytoplasmic constituents of human origin but also were reactive with tissues or tissue culture cells across a wide range of species. These observations gave rise to the concept that autoantibodies were reacting with antigens that were highly conserved in evolution. It was not immediately apparent at that time that there was a more profound significance to these findings. The antigenic determinant that was re-acting with autoantibodies was a unique region of the antigen. The special characteristics of the antigenic determinant or the autoepitope are described below.

2.2.1
The Highly Conserved Nature of the Autoepitope

Patients with Sjögren's syndrome produce autoantibodies to a nuclear protein that is transiently associated with a number of small RNA species in the form of a complex of ribonucleoprotein particles. This nuclear protein called SS-B/La was isolated from bovine thymus extracts and purified as an antigen-antibody complex using autoantibodies from Sjögren's syndrome patients [8]. The SS-B/La immune complex was used to immunize mice and the immune response was analyzed using immunoprecipitation, Western blotting, and immunohisto-chemistry. The sera from these mice as well as monoclonal antibodies generated from spleen cells were compared in their immunoreactivity with a standard human autoantibody to SS-B/La obtained from the Centers for Disease Control and Prevention (CDC) in Atlanta. Five monoclonal antibodies to SS-B/La were examined for immunological reactivities to full-length native SS-B/La and SS-B/La fragments obtained from *S. aureus* V8 digestion. It was observed that all five monoclonal antibodies showed different patterns of reactivity from the human autoantibody, indicating that although experimentally induced antibodies and the human autoantibody were all reactive with the full-length protein, they were recognizing different antigenic determinants. The crucial finding was in immu-nohistochemistry, using tissue culture cell lines from different species including human, monkey, rabbit, bovine, hamster, rat, mouse, and rat kangaroo (Table 2.1). The experimentally induced murine monoclonal antibodies were reactive in immunohistochemistry with the nuclei of cells from human, monkey, rabbit, and bovine cells but were non-reactive with nuclei of hamster, rat, mouse, and rat kangaroo. In contrast, the human autoantibody was equally reactive with nu-clear SS-B/La in all of the species tested. This experiment clearly demonstrated that the epitope on SS-B/La reactive with human autoantibody was a region that was more highly conserved than other regions of the molecules. This special property was exhibited by sera from all Sjögren's syndrome patients tested.

2.2.2
The Autoepitope Resides at or in Close Proximity to the Functional Region
or Binding Site of the Antigen

Studies were continued comparing the properties of human autoantibodies to antibodies experimentally produced by immunization. Proliferating cell nuclear antigen (PCNA) was first observed in an immunoprecipitation reaction between lupus serum and an antigen in thymus extracts [9]. It was noted that activated lymphocytes undergoing proliferation contained high amounts of the antigen and hence the designation of PCNA given to this antigen. PCNA was shown to

Table 2.1 Species-specific reactivities of monoclonal antibodies to
SS-B/La antigen as detected by immunofluorescence (taken from [8]).

Species	Cell line origin	Immunofluorescence [a]					
		Murine monoclonal antibodies					Human sera Ze [b]
		A1	A2	A3	A4	A5	
Human	Hep-2, larynx	+	+	+	–	–	+
Human	HeLa, cervix	+	+	+	–	–	+
Human	Raji, Burkitt lymphoma	+	+	+	–	–	+
Monkey	Vero, kidney	+	+	+	–	–	+
Rabbit	R9ab, lung	+	+	+	–	–	+
Bovine	MDBK, kidney	+	+	+	–	–	+
Hamster	BHK-21, kidney	–	–	–	–	–	+
Rat	6m2, kidney	–	–	–	–	–	+
Mouse	3T3, fibroblast	–	–	–	–	–	+
Rat kangaroo	PtK2, kidney	–	–	–	–	–	+

a)   Cells were grown in Lab-Tek tissue culture chambers and fixed
     in a mixture of acetone and methanol (3:1) at –20 °C for 2 min.
b)   Ze serum is the CDC reference serum for anti-SS-B/La specificity.

be identical to the auxiliary protein of DNA polymerase δ and was an essential component of DNA synthesis in replicating cells [10]. The properties of two murine monoclonal antibodies to PCNA and a rabbit polyclonal antibody raised against an N-terminal peptide were examined in a comparative study with human autoantibody. The ability of DNA polymerase δ to utilize template/primers containing long stretches of single-stranded nucleotides was inhibited by the human autoantibody, whereas the two murine monoclonal antibodies and the rabbit anti-peptide antibody were ineffective [11]. This observation was consistent with immunostaining, which showed that human autoantibodies to PCNA reacted with the nuclei of tissue culture cells in the late G1 and the S phases of the cell cycle. The areas of antibody immunolocalization coincided with uptake of radiolabeled thymidine, indicating that these areas were the sites of DNA replication.

The ability of human autoantibodies to inhibit function was demonstrated in a study using serum from a patient with polymyositis that contained autoantibody to threonyl-tRNA synthetase [12]. Antibodies to a few classes of tRNA synthetases are a feature of patients with polymyositis. The human autoantibody to threonyl-tRNA synthetase was examined together with an experimentally induced antibody against highly purified rabbit reticulocyte threonyl-tRNA synthetase. The human autoantibody specifically inhibited threonyl-tRNA synthetase activity, whereas the experimentally induced antibody had no effect on aminoacylation. It was inferred that the epitopes recognized by the human auto-antibody were formed by the tertiary structure of the enzyme and were associated with the catalytic site of the synthetase, whereas the experimentally induced antibody recognized epitopes not related to the catalytic function of the synthetase.

Many studies have shown that autoantibodies with specific reactivities for a number of nuclear antigens with known functions have the same capability of inhibiting such functions. These include antibodies to small nuclear ribonucleo protein particles such as antibodies to Sm and to U1-snRNP, which are able to inhibit pre-mRNA splicing. Human autoantibodies to specific antigens are able to inhibit functions of DNA topoisomerase 1, DNA topoisomerase 2, and RNA polymerase 1.

2.2.3
The Autoepitope is Composed of Conformation-dependent
Discontinuous Sequences of the Antigen

The molecular structure of the autoepitope of PCNA was further analyzed with human autoantibody and experimentally induced antibodies. Epitope mapping of full-length human PCNA as well as *in vitro*–translated protein products with carboxy-terminal or amino-terminal deletions were performed [13–15]. From analysis of the patterns of reactivity of 14 different human anti-PCNA autoanti-bodies, it was deduced that the apparent heterogeneity of human autoantibodies to PCNA could be explained by immune responses to conformational epitopes. It was postulated that these conformational epitopes may be related to protein folding or to association of PCNA with other intranuclear proteins or nucleic acids as might occur when PCNA is complexed with other molecules in the functional state. This hypothesis was further examined by the use of compound peptides of PCNA, which consisted of joining of discontinuous regions of the primary amino acid sequence. Several such compound peptides were synthe-sized and used to immunize rabbits to produce antibodies. These antibodies were then examined in various parameters including immunoprecipitation, im-munoblotting, and immunohistochemistry. One compound peptide, composed of amino acid sequences 159–165 joined to sequence 255–261, induced an anti-body response remarkably similar to that demonstrated by human anti-PCNA autoantibody. Figure 2.1 compares the immunohistochemistry of antibody to this compound peptide with that of human anti-PCNA. Double immunofluores-cent labeling with fluorescein isothiocyanate and rhodamine demonstrated that anti-compound peptide (Fig. 2.1 A) and human antibody (Fig. 2.1 B) decorated nuclei of the same cells. Fig. 2.1 C, D shows labeling of a different field with anti-compound peptide (Fig. 2.1 C) and BrdU (Fig. 2.1 D). This study supports the observations from epitope mapping by showing that a peptide composed of discontinuous sequences of PCNA was able to induce antibody with reactivities similar to those of human autoantibody.

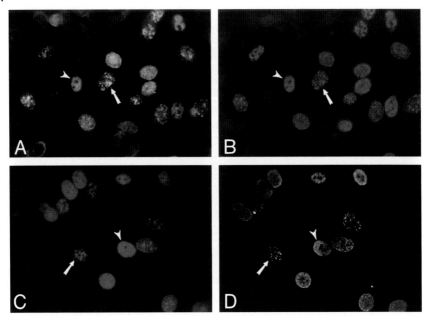

Fig. 2.1 Characterization by immunohisto-chemistry of nuclear staining by antiserum to compound peptide. Frames A and B are double immunofluorescent labeling of the same field (yellow-green: fluorescein isothio-cyanate; red: rhodamine) with antiserum to compound peptide (A) and with human anti-PCNA autoantibody (B). This is a non-syn-chronized tissue culture cell preparation showing that cells undergoing DNA synthe-sis (arrow for early S phase and arrowhead for late S phase) are recognized in a similar fashion by both sera. Frames C and D com-pare another field showing staining with anti-compound peptide (C) and BrdU stain-ing (D), the latter showing that nuclei in DNA synthesis are also those recognized by anti-compound peptide antibody (from [15]).

Extensive studies by others have also demonstrated that the majority of B-cell epitopes are discontinuous and conformational [16]. Antibodies against discon-tinuous regions of a picornavirus protein have been demonstrated in foot and mouth disease of cattle [17]. In human choriogonadotropin, a region of the α subunit (residues 41–60) was joined to a region of the β subunit (residues 101–121), and antibodies to the compound peptide inhibited the binding of human choriogonadotropin to its receptor [18]. Autoreactive epitopes defined by type 1 diabetes–associated human monoclonal antibodies have been mapped to the middle and C-terminal domains of GAD65 [19, 20].

2.3
Conclusions

Autoimmunity and autoimmune disease continue to be puzzles that are receiv-ing intensive scrutiny by many research laboratories worldwide. In this chapter, I have focused on the humoral arm of the autoimmune response and reviewed observations made in human autoimmune diseases including systemic lupus erythematosus, Sjögren's syndrome, polymyositis, and related autoimmune rheumatic diseases. These studies have shown that the autoantibody response to a self-antigen may be unlike an immune response to a foreign antigen or to a laboratory-purified autologous antigen. One of the special features of the humoral autoimmune response is that the autoantigens are highly conserved molecules, but, in the fine details, the conserved antigenic determinant is a complex epitope that consists of conformation-dependent discontinuous regions of the self-molecule. This autoepitope appears to be the functional site or the interactive binding region of the molecule. These findings are in striking contrast to the immune response to a foreign antigen. An important issue that needs to be resolved in the puzzle of autoimmunity is the elucidation of the mechanisms whereby the host regulates in such a specific manner its own immune response to a self-antigen.

In the design of antigen-specific immunotherapy, it would seem to be important to understand how the host with autoimmune disease has responded to its own self-antigens. In antigen-specific immunotherapy, it might be more appropriate to design peptides or fragments of the antigen that are the counterparts of the antigenic determinants recognized by the host. The host's immune system is informing us that it is capable of making an immune response to a specific region of the autoantigen and is unable or unwilling to make an immune response to other regions [21, 22]. Antigen-specific immunotherapy utilizing these precepts could be more promising. It is evident that this approach could also be used in designing immunotherapy targeting T cells, dendritic cells, and other immunocompetent cells playing roles in autoimmune disease.

Acknowledgment

This is publication #16947- MEM from The Scripps Research Institute, La Jolla, California. Supported in part by NIH Grant #CA56956.

References

1 R. M. Steinman and I. Melmann. Science 2004, 305, 197–200.

2 M. Feldman and R. N. Maini. Nat. Med. 2003 Oct; 9(10), 1245–1250.

3 A. Coles et al. Lancet 1999, 354, 1691–1695.

4 Steinman, L. Science 2004, 305, 212–216.

5 Z. Yu and N. P. Restifo. J. Clin. Invest. 2002, 110, 289–294.

6 E. C. Morris, G. M. Bendle and H. J. Stauss. Clin. Exp. Immunol. 2003, 131, 1–7.

7 E. M. Tan. Adv. Immunol. 1989, 44, 93–151.

8 E. K. L. Chan and E. M. Tan. J. Exp. Med. 1987, 166, 1627–1640.

9 K. Miyachi, M. J. Fritzler and E. M. Tan. J. Immunol. 1978, 121, 2228–2234.

10 G. Prolich, C.-K. Tan, M. Kostura et al. Nature 1987, 236, 517–520.

11 C.-K. Tan, K. Sullivan, X. Li, E. M. Tan, K. M. Downey and A. G. So. Nucl. Acids Res. 1987, 15, 9299–9308.

12 C. V. Dang, E. M. Tan and J. A. Traugh. FASEB J. 1988, 2, 2376–2379.

13 K. Ogata, Y. Ogata, Y. Takasaki and E. M. Tan. J. Immunol. 1987, 139, 2942–2946.

14 J. P. Huff, G. Roos, C. L. Peebles, R. Houghten, K. F. Sullivan and E. M. Tan. J. Exp. Med. 1990, 172, 419–429.

15 Y. Muro, W.-M. Tsai, R. Houghten and E. M. Tan. J. Biol. Chem. 1994, 269, 18529–18534.

16 W. G. Laver, G. M. Air, R. G. Webster and S. J. Smith-Gil. Cell 1990, 61, 553–556.

17 N. R. Parry, P. V. Barnett, E. J. Ouldridge, D. J. Rowlands and F. Brown. J. Gen. Virol. 1989, 70, 1493–1503.

18 J. M. Bidart, F. Troalen, P. Ghillani et al. Science 1990, 248, 736–739.

19 W. Richter, Y. Shi and S. Baekkeskov. Proc. Natl. Acad. Sci. USA 1993, 90, 2832–2836.

20 A. C. Powers, K. Bavik, J. Tremble, K. Daw, A. Scherbaum and J. P. Banga. Clin. Exp. Immunol. 1999, 118, 349–356.

21 E. M. Tan. J. Clin. Invest. 2001, 108, 1411–1415.

22 E. M. Tan and F.-D. Shi. Clin. Exp. Immunol. 2003, 134, 169–177.

Part 2
Autoimmunity

Autoantibodies and Autoimmunity: Molecular Mechanisms in Health and Disease. Edited by K. Michael Pollard
Copyright © 2006 WILEY-VCH Verlag GmbH & Co. KGaA, Weinheim
ISBN: 3-527-31141-6

3
Self/Non-self Recognition

Alan G. Baxter

3.1
Introduction

Tauber (1997), in his book *The Immune Self – Theory or Metaphor*, examined the origins and significance of the concept of self/non-self discrimination. In the process of asking whether immunological self constituted a theory or a metaphor, he drew parallels between the search for a guiding principle to immunoreactivity and the philosophical issue of identity. Tauber occupies much of the book discussing the contributions of Kant, Descartes, Hegel, and Fichte et al. to immunological theory. Macfarlane Burnet was responsible for introducing the term to immunology – although he used the phrase "self and not-self" – and it is clear from his writing that he did not see self as a deeply philosophical concept. His rationale for introducing the phrase was that the same biological processes involved in pathogen defenses appeared to be active in transplant rejection, ABO blood group incompatibilities, and the complications of fetal/maternal blood exchange during pregnancy. Thus, the activation of these processes had to involve a principle broader than just the recognition of infection (Burnet 1959) and these additional phenomena had to be incorporated into any concept of "what the immune system does." To him, self was neither a theory nor a metaphor, but an analogy.

3.2
Immunological Self

3.2.1
Burnet's Self-marker Hypothesis

Burnet published two editions of his monograph *The Production of Antibodies* (Burnet et al. 1941; Burnet and Fenner 1949). Both were concise but comprehensive summaries of the current findings pertaining to the character and regu-

Autoantibodies and Autoimmunity: Molecular Mechanisms in Health and Disease. Edited by K. Michael Pollard
Copyright © 2006 WILEY-VCH Verlag GmbH & Co. KGaA, Weinheim
ISBN: 3-527-31141-6

lation of immune responses and included attempts to draft general principles to explain these data. Two major changes in approach were made between the two editions. The first was that Burnet's original monograph built on the molecular (biochemical) understandings of immunological responses, while in the second edition he attempted to explain largely the same phenomena at a higher level of organization – the cellular level. The general form of this perspective was tentatively explored in a review in the December 1948 issue of *Heredity* (Burnet and Fenner 1948), which was published while they were still working on the revised version of *The Production of Antibodies*. Here, Burnet and Fenner combined clinical experience with experimental studies in forming this new perspective, which they justified by arguing (Burnet and Fenner 1948):

> ■ *Landsteiner's influence has been outstanding, and his ideas as developed by Marrack, Heidelburger, Pauling and others have given a strong bias towards interpretation of immunological phenomena in almost exclusively chemical terms... Nevertheless it must still be maintained that the phenomena of immunity are biological phenomena and are no more expressible simply in chemical terms than those of growth, bodily repair, or reproduction.*

The second major difference between the two editions, again tentatively raised in the *Heredity* manuscript, was the introduction of a principle to explain the immune system's congeniality to the body's own tissues. They cited examples of responses to infection, blood group incompatibility, and tissue transplantation and even foreshadowed the use of the term "not-self" to describe foreign molecules or particles subjected to immunogenic destruction within phagocytes.

Despite the similarity in approaches, it was not until the second edition of *The Production of Antibodies* that they persuasively argued for a biological principle of self/non-self discrimination. Again, working from a cellular perspective, they argued for a level of understanding broader than that of the chemists, writing that their monograph was "wholly concerned with... the processes of antibody formation and an attempt to interpret these findings in biological rather than chemic terms." It is clear, however, that they remained keen to incorporate the clues to mechanism provided by molecular studies. A significant proportion of the text deals with the chemical nature of antibody, and the basis of self/non-self discrimination is attributed to the ability of the cells of the immune system to recognize particular molecular "patterns" or "markers." Burnet and Fenner (1949) proposed that the immune system could react in two sharply different ways to body constituents on the one hand and foreign organic matter on the other:

> ■ *The hypothesis [is] put forward that differentiation is based on the existence of a small number of marker components in the expendable body cells... It is an obvious physiological necessity*

and a fact fully established by experiment that the body's
own cells should not provoke antibody formation... This is
not due to any intrinsic absence of antigenic components;
the same cells injected into a different species or even into
another unrelated animal of the same species may give rise to
active antibody production. The failure of antibody production
against autologous cells demands the postulation of an active
ability of the reticulo-endothelial cells to recognise "self"
pattern from "not-self" pattern in organic material taken
into their substance. The first requirement of an adequate
theory of antibody production is to account for this differen-
tiation of function by which the natural entry of foreign
micro-organisms or the artificial injection of foreign red cells
provokes an immunological reaction while the physically
similar autologous material is inert.

They proposed that the differentiation of self from non-self was achieved by
marking the body's own tissues with molecular tags unique to that individual
(or at least uncommonly shared with other organisms) (Burnet and Fenner 1948):

■ *We are driven to the conclusion that all body cells carry some*
or all of a relatively small number of marker components
whose specific character is determined by a correspondingly
small number of genes... On this view there is within each
phagocytic cell of the reticuloendothelial system a mechanism
tuned to respond to any "self-marker" in material which it
takes into its cytoplasm, by a non-immunological destructive
process. If organic material which contains none of the molec-
ular patterns characteristic of the self-markers enters the cell,
the latter responds by the development of the adaptive mech-
anism we have described, so initiating antibody production.

It was this hypothesis that Burnet and Fenner (1949) saw as the major intellectual contribution presented in the second edition, writing in the Preface:

■ *The absence of antigenicity of the body's own constituents*
and the failure of mammalian or avian embryos to produce
antibody are two aspects that have not previously been con-
sidered in relation to immunological theory. The introduction
of the "self-marker" hypothesis to bring these aspects into
the picture is the chief novelty of our presentation.

3.2.2
A Confusion of Level: Adaptive Enzymes

Paradoxically, their model was severely limited by Burnet's concept of "adaptive enzymes" as the source of antibody diversity. This was paradoxical since this mechanism operated at the molecular, rather than the cellular, level. Described originally in the first edition of *The Production of Antibodies* and essentially unchanged in the second edition, the concept was entirely based on the erroneous view that proteins could be self-replicating (see Fig. 3.1). It was proposed that they replicated not in the sense that we imagine prions can catalyze tertiary structural modifications, but in the sense that they were postulated to act as the template for the assembly of more of their own amino acid sequences (Burnet et al. 1941):

> ■ *If the protein by this enzyme activity reconstitutes itself in detail from amino acids or other protein fragments available, we have at once the pattern to which the new protein is built and at the same time the scaffolding on which it is constructed.*

In the early 1940s this view was not unconventional. By the end of the decade, it was a minority view preserved through a fundamental misappraisal of the available biological data. While geneticists were moving towards the view we now hold as Watson's "central dogma" of genetics, Burnet was clinging to an increasingly outdated biochemical model of protein production (Burnet and Fenner 1948):

> ■ *In practically every example that has been adequately studied, each antigenic pattern that is characteristic of the cells of some individuals and not others within a species, is inherited as if its character were controlled by a single gene. This has led to the suggestion, supported by Haldane, Sturtevant and others, that the molecular pattern responsible for antigenic specificity might be traced back to the gene itself... We feel that this may be an unduly sweeping generalization.*

In Burnet's view, proteins could be divided into living proteins – those enzymes capable of self-replication – and nonliving proteins, which equate to our current understanding of protein biochemistry. The production of antibodies was attributed to living proteins involved in the degradation of damaged autologous tissues. In response to foreign material, these enzymes underwent structural modification that allowed them to effectively bind to and eliminate the foreign template. Antibodies were postulated to be partial replicas of these enzymes (Burnet and Fenner 1948):

■ *[Antibodies] are synthesized within cells of the reticuloendothelial system by certain proteinase units of the cells. These liberate partial replicas of themselves (i.e. antibodies) ... eventually into the blood or lymph. These proteinases, in virtue of their enzymatic function, come into contact with any foreign antigens taken into the cell, and are lastingly modified by this contact.*

DIRECT TEMPLATE

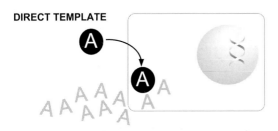

INDIRECT TEMPLATE

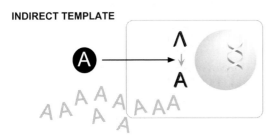

CLONAL SELECTION

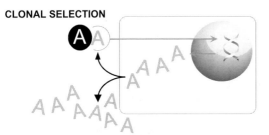

Fig. 3.1 Diagram illustrating the essential differences between the Haurowitz-Pauling direct template theory, the Burnet-Fenner indirect template theory, and the clonal selection theory. In the direct template theory, antigen itself enters the cell and stamps out a complementary pattern on each antibody molecule after it has been produced. In the indirect template theory, the antigen induces a structural change in the enzymatic machinery that generates antibodies, resulting in the production of complementary antibodies.

In the clonal selection theory, genetic machinery generates a soluble antibody and a cell-surface receptor with the same specificity. The binding of antigen to the surface receptor results in amplification of antibody production and clonal expansion of the cell bearing the appropriate specificity. The genetic machinery can be modified by somatic mutation and selection on the basis of the affinity of the surface receptor, thereby improving the affinity of the antibody produced. (After Burnet 1959, Fig. 6)

Similarly, from the second edition of *The Production of Antibodies* (Burnet and Fenner 1949):

> ■ Autologous material is dealt with by appropriate enzymatic
> systems without involving change from the existent status.
> Foreign material is dealt with by the same cells and processes
> but at some point in the mechanism a modification is neces-
> sary... An appropriate adaptive enzyme is produced which
> has the necessary configuration for effective adsorption to the
> unfamiliar substrate.

The refinements made to this model in the second edition were minor and were prompted mostly by new data on the requirements for antibody formation. For example, while antibody production was attributed to the reticuloendothelial cells in the first edition, in the second they stated that "it is immaterial...which histological cell type is responsible for the enzyme action involved..." Data on the effects of priming were incorporated thus (Burnet and Fenner 1949):

> ■ It seems highly probably that the function of first antigenic
> contact is to produce the adaptive modification while sub-
> sequent contacts stimulate its replication and eventual
> liberation of partial replicas into the blood stream.

The only retreat from the original concept was lexical (Burnet and Fenner 1949):

> ■ It is important not to press the analogy with known adaptive
> enzymes too closely... The essence of our hypothesis is that,
> irrespective of whether it is legitimate or not to call it an
> adaptive enzyme, a new self-replicating system is now present
> in the cell which can be caused to multiply by the appropriate
> stimulus.

The importance of Burnet's reliance on his "adaptive enzyme" hypothesis cannot be overstated. A direct consequence of it was that to the modern reader, five of the seven "General Aspects of Antibody Production" listed in the Summary and Conclusions chapter of the second edition of *The Production of Antibodies* would be regarded as being in error. This weakness was recognized by Burnet and Fenner (1949) at the time:

> ■ The weakness of such a formulation centres on the postulated
> intracellular enzymatic unit and its capacity to undergo adap-
> tive modification. This goes far beyond what is known of clas-
> sical enzyme chemistry.

3.2.3
The Boundaries of Self

Although barely mentioned, the concept of immunological self as introduced in the *Heredity* manuscript and presented in *The Production of Antibodies* had significant boundary problems. The brain and the anterior chamber of the eye are immunologically quiescent sites into which some foreign grafts can be transplanted without rejection (reviewed in Medawar 1948). Burnet excised these from the domain of the immune system, describing them as "nonexpendable organs" (Burnet and Fenner 1948):

> ■ *Both situations are morphologically and physiologically shielded from concern with significant, i.e. non-fatal, emergencies, and their tolerance of implanted foreign tissues is probably in some way related to this characteristic.*

Burnet's approach to biology was heavily influenced by evolutionary theory and it seems likely that evolutionary considerations motivated this decision. Presumably he felt – although this is not explicitly stated – that in evolutionary history severe infections of brain or eye led inevitably to greatly reduced reproductive fitness; thus, there was little evolutionary pressure to maintain effective immune defenses in these sites. Furthermore, as a robust immune response to a minor infection in brain or eye might do more damage than the infection itself, there may even have been a selective pressure against such responses.

A more confounding issue regarding these organs is the problem that both contain autologous tissues that are themselves immunogenic. This is acknowledged only in passing in the second edition of *The Production of Antibodies* (Burnet and Fenner 1949):

> ■ *Minor exceptions to this rule [that the body's own tissues do not provoke antibody responses] concern only tissues which are "unexpendable," parts of the central nervous system and the eye.*

This phenomenon has remained unexplained.

Ten percent of our dried body weight is, and 90% of all cells within our bodies are, microbial and not encoded in our own genome. Yet these appear, to all intents and purposes, to lie within the domain of "immunological self." The only attempt to deal with this problem was to introduce the requirement that for a macromolecular substance to be antigenic, it must not normally be present in the immunized animal.

3.2.4
Prenatal Tolerance: Testing the Model

Both the *Heredity* manuscript and second edition of *The Production of Antibodies* mentioned the lack of immunological responsiveness in embryonic and new-born individuals. In the *Heredity* manuscript, Burnet and Fenner (1948) described in passing the work of Ray Owen (1945), who had observed mutual tolerance of tissues from fraternal calf twins that had shared a placenta *in utero* (Burnet and Fenner 1948):

> ■ *Under circumstances where twins...have a common circula-tion, two types of red cell may be found in both twins for life. One corresponds genetically to its own cells, the other to its twin's. This finding seems to have been completely established and has the important implication that cells "foreign" to the host may be tolerated indefinitely provided they are implanted early in embryonic life.*

In *The Production of Antibodies*, an entire chapter is given over to the immuno-logical behavior of young animals, emphasizing the point that for a short time the young (at least of birds and mammals) are almost incapable of producing antibodies. They now cited the work of Owen (1945, 1946) more extensively (Burnet and Fenner 1949):

> ■ *Owen found that the common placental circulation of twin foetuses might .... result in two antigenic types of red blood cell being found in both twins for life... The important impli-cation of this work is that cells "foreign" to the host may be tolerated indefinitely providing they are implanted early in embryonic life... This raises the suggestion that the process by which self-pattern becomes recognizable takes place during the embryonic period or immediately post-embryonic stages.*

More significantly, they revisited the issue in their chapter on the theoretical as-pects of antibody production. After restating the observation that fetal mammals and chick embryos are incapable of generating antibodies and that the full capacity to do so develops only slowly in the young, Burnet and Fenner (1949) wrote:

> ■ *This raises the suggestion that the process by which self-pat-tern becomes recognizable takes place during the embryonic or immediately post-embryonic stages... If in embryonic life expendable cells from a genetically distinct race are implanted and established, no antibody response should develop against the foreign cell antigen when the animal takes on indepen-dent existence.*

They concluded:

> ■ **The self-marker concept seems to provide a number of sugges-**
> **tions for experimental work to substantiate or refute it.**
> **A virtually direct proof of its correctness could be obtained if**
> **experimental techniques could be developed to produce with a**
> **wider range of antigens introduced into embryos the persisting**
> **tolerance of foreign cells found by Owen in his studies on**
> **multiple births in cattle.**

At the time, Burnet and Fenner were in correspondence with Peter Medawar, a brilliant experimental biologist who had published extensively on immunological responses to allografts, especially skin allografts. Medawar's work had been motivated by the extreme difficulties in treating burn victims during the Second World War (discussed in Baxter 2000), and he became involved in clinical studies of human skin transplantation. He interpreted the finding that a second set of skin allografts from the same donor was rejected more rapidly than the first as evidence of an immunological process underlying the tissue destruction (Gibson and Medawar 1943). As he could not see any evidence of cellular infiltration into the grafts, he and Burnet corresponded on the results of experiments designed to test the hypothesis that antibodies were responsible for allograft rejection (Burnet and Fenner 1949).

In 1948, Medawar had offered to help Hugh Donald, a livestock geneticist, to distinguish between monozygotic and dizygotic twin cattle by skin transplantation, in the expectation that grafts between dizygotic twins would be rejected. The finding that this did not occur was inexplicable to him until he read of Owen's work in Burnet and Fenner's *The Production of Antibodies* (Medawar 1986; Baxter 2000). Owen's findings confirmed Medawar's own experience with other antigens. It was the theoretical underpinning of this work on Burnet and Fenner's self-marker concept, particularly as it pertained to prenatal tolerance, that spurred Medawar to directly test the hypothesis that the introduction of foreign cells into embryos would prevent the development of an immune response against them after birth.

Billingham et al. (1953) injected inbred CBA mouse embryos at 15–16 days of gestation with tissue fragments from albino A strain mice. Once the recipient mice reached eight weeks of age, rejection of A strain skin grafts was significantly inhibited and in some cases the grafts were tolerated indefinitely. Additional experiments demonstrated that the tolerance induced was donor-strain specific, did not affect rejection of third-party grafts, could be induced by injection of a wide variety of tissue types, and did not occur if injection was delayed until after birth. They concluded that the time of birth was a "critical point" in which the response to an antigenic challenge changed dramatically. Tolerance was a characteristic of the treated mouse, not the graft, since rejection could be induced by injection of syngeneic splenic cells from primed CBA mice, and the A skin grafts were capable of being rejected by new recipients if re-transplanted.

Seven years later, these findings led to the award of the Nobel Prize for Physiology or Medicine to Frank Macfarlane Burnet and Peter Brian Medawar "for the discovery of acquired immunological tolerance" (Brent 2003).

3.3
The Clonal Selection Theory

3.3.1
Immune Theories of Natural Selection

The contribution of the concept of natural selection to our understanding of self/non-self discrimination has been critical. Natural selection occurs in any system that undergoes replication, mutation, and selection. Darwin recognized that these processes were sufficient to account for evolution of species, but it took some time for the realization that natural selection was not limited to the production of well-adapted animals; it occurs to various degrees in any system in which these three processes operate. For example, Dawkins and Gould argued for many years whether natural section of organisms occurred at the level of the gene or of the individual (Dawkins 1998, 2003; Gould 1990). This argument had little merit (other than providing a vehicle for the discussion of interesting science) since both genes and individuals are subject to replication, mutation, and selection, and therefore both are potentially subject to natural selection.

The first person to attempt to incorporate natural selection into a theory of antibody production was Niels Jerne. He proposed that a broad range of specificities of antibodies were released into the blood spontaneously and that antibodies were subject to a replicative drive following their binding to antigen. In order to remain consistent with data indicating a cellular origin of antibody production, he postulated that on binding antigen, antibodies were shuttled to the appropriate cells for reproduction (see Fig. 3.1).

Jerne raised three interesting points in his manuscript. Firstly, his model provided an explanation for affinity maturation: "The reproduction [of antibody] need not be highly faithful; copying mistakes will be harmless, and may occasionally produce an improved fit" (Jerne 1955). Thus, as replication was likely to be prone to occasional copying mistakes, over the course of an immune response there would be a tendency for more avid antibodies to dominate, as they competed more effectively for antigen.

Secondly, the model introduced the requirement for some (presumably genetic) mechanism for generating a broad range of antibody specificities (Jerne 1955):

> ■ *Somewhere in the beginning... we have to postulate a spontaneous production of globulin molecules of a great variety of random specificities in order to start the process. Possibly a specialized lymphoid tissue, such as that of the thymus.... is engaged in this function.*

Thirdly, the model provided a potential mechanism for the induction of tolerance (Jerne 1955):

> ■ *If this small spontaneous production of globulin took place*
> *mainly in embryonic and early independent life... the early*
> *removal of a specific fraction of molecules might lead to the*
> *permanent disappearance of this type of specificity... The*
> *absence from the circulation of such antibodies would, in turn,*
> *prevent response to a later antigenic stimulus of this type.*

These three characteristics derive directly from the application of a natural selection model to immunity and immediately provided Jerne's theory with a great deal of credibility.

However, Jerne's theory had two major problems. He realized that a corollary of his theory was that the injection of an antibody specific for a particular antigen should boost subsequent elicited antibody responses to that antigen since increased numbers of antibody molecules would be available to undergo replication. Experimental results showed that in most cases, responses were suppressed. The second problem was one shared by Burnet's adaptive enzyme model, but by 1955 it was becoming a major sticking point: the great weight of evidence indicated that proteins did not act as replicative units but that their structure was encoded in a genomic template. Although Monod's work on transcription regulation was not fully developed until the early 1960s, by 1955 he had published extensively in French on the genetic control of enzyme biosynthesis, and a number of influential reviews had also been published in English. Burnet, at least, was aware of his work, since he cited it (Burnet 1956). Monod's model of enzyme induction was widely held and was incompatible with the ideas of proteins as templates or replicating units.

In 1956, Burnet published "a revision" of the Burnet and Fenner (1949) edition of *The Production of Antibodies*, entitled *Enzyme, Antigen and Virus* (Burnet 1956). This was extraordinarily bad timing as it was submitted in early September 1955, perhaps only one or two weeks before Jerne submitted a paper on his natural selection theory. The book contained an entirely new chapter on the biochemistry of protein synthesis and a revised mechanism for his adaptive enzyme hypothesis. The tide of opinion was now too strong to ignore (Burnet 1956):

> ■ *In view of the strong current opinion that, at least in the*
> *great majority of instances, adaptive enzymes are not pro-*
> *duced by self-replicating mechanism, special attention must*
> *be given to the question of the transmission of an antibody-*
> *producing capacity from a cell to its descendants.*

A significant part of the book then provided a biochemical model for an acquired heritable trait (antibody specificity) in a dividing population (lymphocytes); it was an RNA-based cytoplasmic process he called "genocopy." The book is a disappointment and leaves one with the feeling that a retreat further into biochemistry did not help his argument. It is likely that Burnet himself was unhappy with it, particularly in light of Jerne's paper, as he subsequently wrote that one of his reasons for discarding the indirect template hypothesis was that "several immunologists, including Jerne himself, have suggested that the self-marker theory is semi-mystical in character and generally unattractive" (Burnet 1959).

Early in 1957, Burnet received a preprint of a review entitled *Allergy and Immunology* by David Talmage (1957), then at the University of Chicago. Although much of the paper was devoted to issues specific to allergy, the paper summarized existing immunological theories and encapsulated a new model of antibody production. Despite couching his new model in tentative phrasing ("As a working hypothesis it is tempting to consider..."), his incisive dealing with the problems associated with previous models and the explanatory power of the model proposed betrayed a prodigious intellect and a great depth of thought on the subject. He borrowed from Burnet and Jerne, as well as from the model proposed by Ehrlich (1900) in which an antigen bound to specific cell-surface receptors and thereby triggered the cell to secrete soluble copies of antibodies with the same specificity as the particular receptor ligated (see Fig. 3.1). Talmage produced a hybrid model in which he proposed (1) that an initial range of antibodies were spontaneously produced and that an antigen selected those that bound with high affinity for expansion (like Jerne); (2) that this selection process occurred at the level of cell-bound antibody (like Ehrlich); and (3) that the unit responsible for expansion was the antibody-producing cell itself (his own contribution). For the first time, the replicating unit was shifted from proteins or hypothetical intracellular machinery to a unit known to be capable of replication – the cell. Furthermore, it was no longer necessary to postulate a protein template; instead, the model conformed to the generally accepted view that proteins were encoded by nucleic acids in the genome.

3.3.2
Clonal Selection

Burnet's response to receiving Talmage's paper was to write a "preliminary communication" titled "A Modification of Jerne's Theory of Antibody Production Using the Concept of Clonal Selection" (Burnet 1957). This paper cites Talmage, pays homage to his classification of previous theories, and explicitly acknowledges Talmage's priority in the idea that cells were the replicating elements responsible for the exponential expansion of antibody production. It claims priority for Burnet in viewing the processes involved from a clonal perspective. Burnet's reworking of Talmage's model can be presented in an abridged form (Burnet 1957):

■ *Among [antibodies] are molecules that can correspond prob-*
ably with varying degrees of precision to all, or virtually all,
the antigenic determinants that occur in biological material
other than that characteristic of the body itself. Each type of
pattern is a specific product of a clone of [lymphocytes] and
it is the essence of the hypothesis that each cell automatically
has available on its surface representative reactive sites
equivalent to those of the globulin they produce... It is
assumed that when an antigen enters the blood or tissue
fluids it will attach to the surface of any lymphocyte carrying
reactive sites which correspond to one of its antigenic determi-
nants... It is postulated that when antigen-[antibody] contact
takes place on the surface of a lymphocyte the cell is activated
to settle in an appropriate tissue... and there undergo prolif-
eration to produce a variety of descendents. In this way,
preferential proliferation will be initiated of all those clones
whose reactive sites correspond to the antigenic determinants
on the antigen used. The descendents will [be] capable of
active liberation of soluble antibody and lymphocytes which
can fulfil the same functions as the parental forms.

Burnet's preliminary communication was very brief – only two manuscript pages – but it rings with the excitement of a man who has suddenly gained a great insight. While Talmage presented the model as a logically sound solution to a much-pondered puzzle, Burnet's text is alive to the explanatory power and corollaries of such a hypothesis. In particular, he could see how the theory might explain the operation of neonatal tolerance, simply and elegantly (Burnet 1957):

■ *Its chief advantage over [the Burnet-Fenner theory] is its rele-*
vance to the nature of normal antibodies including the red
cell isoagglutanins (i.e. "natural antibodies," such as those in-
volved in ABO blood group antigen reactions) and the simpler
interpretation of tolerance to potential antigens experienced
in embryonic life... Despite the speculative character of much
of the detail of this modification of Jerne's theory – which
might be called the "clonal selection hypothesis" – it has so
many implications calling for experimental enquiry that it has
been thought justifiable to submit this preliminary account
for publication.

Burnet explored the full implications of the clonal selection theory to self/non-self discrimination the following year in a series of lectures presented at Vanderbilt University in Tennessee; these were subsequently published by Cambridge University Press (Burnet 1959) as *The Clonal Selection Theory of Acquired Immunity*. This book, like those he published in 1941, 1946, and 1949, provided a concise but comprehensive summary of current findings pertaining to the character and regulation of immunological responses. As in the past, he reviewed theories of antibody production, but in a broad outline borrowed from Talmage, he described the contributions by Ehrlich, Pauling, Jerne, and himself and Fenner. In his description of the clonal selection theory, he attributed contributions by Jerne, Ehlich, and Talmage (Burnet 1959):

> ■ *The great contribution of Jerne's theory was that it drew attention to the theoretical possibility that the recognition of self from not-self could be achieved in another fashion than by the recognition of "self markers." As Talmage points out, Ehrlich's side-chain theory was in many ways the logical equivalent of Jerne's concept ... [At the time] it seemed, and to most immunologists still seems, inconceivable that all types of antibody could be pre-existent in the normal complement of gamma globulins. Nevertheless, if Jerne is correct ... this would be an effective and much more elegant way of accounting for the differentiation of self from not-self.*
>
> *The outstanding difficulty in accepting Jerne's theory is the claim that when a given type of natural antibody is brought to a cell by antigen, the cell then proceeds to make more natural antibody molecules of the same type ... Talmage pointed out that it would be more satisfactory if the replicating elements essential to any such theory were cellular in character ...*

Burnet then presented his own perspective (Burnet 1959, underlined):

> ■ *Our own view is that any tenable form of Jerne's theory must involve the* existence of multiple clones of globulin-producing cells, *each responsible for one genetically determined type of antibody globulin ... Clearly it would simplify matters a great deal if the antigen were in a position to react with natural antibody or a pattern equivalent thereto on the surface of the cell which produced it. This is the crux of the clonal selection hypothesis ... Self-not-self recognition means simply that all those clones which would recognize (that is, produce antibodies against) a self component have been eliminated in embryonic life. All the rest are retained.*

Burnet (1959) described in detail how the clonal selection model could explain a broad range of immunological phenomena, including immunological memory (expanded clone), anamnestic responses ("original antigenic sin" – lower-affinity binding of expanded numbers of cells dominating a response to a new antigen), the effects of adjuvants (prolonged release of antigen from a depot allowing persistent expansion of a clone), mucosal immunity (preferential settling of clones in sites of stimulation), natural antibodies (all clones spontaneously make small amounts of antibody), and autoimmunity (somatic mutation of clones occasionally leading to acquisition of self-reactivity).

3.3.3
Corollaries of the Clonal Selection Theory

Perhaps of greater importance than the explanatory power of the clonal selection theory were the corollaries of the theory that related to the ontogeny of the immune system (including the "one cell–one antibody" hypothesis), affinity maturation, and the existence of peripheral tolerance mechanisms.

The one cell–one antibody hypothesis was an axiom of the theory. If a single lymphocyte, or a clone of lymphocytes, were able to make a variety of antibodies, then the specificity of antibody produced could not be used to select cells for expansion or destruction. Burnet regarded this axiom as so important that Joshua Lederberg, who was visiting the laboratory at the time, and his student Gustav Nossal were immediately set to address the question by assessing the specificity of antibody produced by individual plasma cells isolated from rats immunized with both *Salmonella typhi* and *Salmonella adelaide* (Nossal and Lederberg 1958).

A second axiom was that a vast array of specificities must be represented on the surfaces of various lymphocytes prior to antigen exposure. Since such a variety of specificities seemed unlikely to be encoded in the germ line, Burnet postulated that they be generated by an intense period of somatic mutation of the antibody-encoding genes within lymphocyte precursors early in ontogeny. This "phase of differentiation or randomization" had to be relatively short-lived, for in order for the development of tolerance by clonal deletion to be effective, the specificity of the developing lymphocytes had to be relatively stable at the time it occurred. The period immediately following tolerance induction, which was around the time of birth in mice, was proposed by Burnet to be the "critical point of Medawar". At this time, antigen exposure no longer caused tolerance, but did not yet result in immunization. This point was followed by maturation, with the liberation of natural antibodies and the potential of antigen-induced antibody production.

The concept of affinity maturation arose from Burnet's belief that all dividing cells are subject to replication errors. In the context of the clonal selection theory, this could result in a neutral, a beneficial, or a degenerative effect on the affinity of antibody binding. Those clones that by chance mutate to higher affinity should compete better for antigen and replication signals, eventually dominating the response (Burnet 1959):

> ■ *The combination of frequent minor mutation and a highly effective selective process would rapidly improve the accuracy of the complementary relationship [of antibody] to new antigenic determinant.*

> *If the right mutation occurs, the cell in question is, in the presence of the antigenic determinant, given a major advantage in the struggle to produce a larger clone of descendants than its congeners. If our general hypothesis is correct, there is no escape from the picture of (lymphocytes) as an evolving population as subject to mutation and selective survival as any large animal population in nature.*

The postulated existence of peripheral tolerance arose from a similar train of thought. Since replication errors were bound to occur at least occasionally in rapidly dividing clones of lymphocytes, a clone might mutate to a "forbidden" or deleted specificity. It was therefore necessary that a mechanism exist to inactivate such clones.

It should not escape the notice of the reader that each of these corollaries is testable. The general form of the model was easily adapted to incorporate the subsequent discovery of T cells (Miller 1961), MHC restriction (McDevitt 1968; Zinkernagel and Doherty 1974), the summing of activation signals (Forsdyke 1968; reviewed in Baxter and Hodgkin 2002), and the concept of active immunoregulation (Gershon et al. 1972). It seems that testing the relevance of Burnet's corollaries has occupied a significant proportion of experimental immunologists for much of the last 50 years.

3.4
Self Post-Burnet

In the 45 years since the clonal selection theory was proposed, almost every experimental finding in immunology either has been consistent with it or has confirmed it. There have been quibbles, of course. Silverstein and Rose (1997) point out that it is possible to induce tolerance in adults (although it is much easier to induce it prenatally) and that "there are no fundamental differences in mechanism between the acquisition of tolerance to autologous and heterologous antigens." It should be painfully obvious that Burnet was aware of this. It was this very fact that raised his awareness that a tolerance induction mechanism existed at all. But Silverstein and Rose (1997) go further. The main theme of their thesis is that "the immune system does not and cannot discriminate between intrinsically harmful and intrinsically harmless substances." This is an odd point of view. If we define "the immune system" as those organs, cells, and cell products involved in defense against infection[1], these components and their functions must be subject to evolutionary pressure – indeed, one would imagine that they are subject to considerable evolutionary pressure. As natural

---

1) Many published definitions of "immune system" define it in terms of self/non-self discrimination (e.g., *Stedman's Medical Dictionary*, *Merriam-Webster Medical Dictionary*, Langman and Cohn 1997). Such definitions were eschewed, as in this particular context the arguments by all participants would have become circular.

selection (Darwin's sort, not Burnet's) operates at the level of reproductive fitness and (from an evolutionary point of view) "harm" is something that reduces reproductive fitness, the ability of the immune system to differentiate "harm" from "harmless" would emerge sooner or later, even if it did not exist in the first place. In his criticism of the paper, Brent (1997) argued along similar lines.

Silverstein and Rose had a point to their piece, of course. They were provoked by the publication of three manuscripts (for an immediate reaction, see Silverstein 1996) announcing the possibility of inducing immune responses, rather than tolerance, by immunizing neonates (Ridge et al. 1996; Sarzotti et al. 1996; Forsthuber et al. 1996). It was not so much these papers themselves that wound them up, but a bizarrely gushing accompanying "news" piece by Elizabeth Pennisi, published in the same issue of the journal, which claimed the authors were "trying to topple one of immunology's seemingly most solid pillars" (Pennisi 1996). This interesting example of tabloid journalism prompted a spate of letters (and responses to the letters) as well as commentaries in other leading journals on the subject. All were critical, but all seem to have missed a critical point: Medawar did not publish a model of neonatal tolerance; he published a model of prenatal tolerance. His own findings support the possibility of immune competence of neonatal mice, depending on strain, antigen, and mode of administration. Burnet, who did not originally have the benefit of Medawar's data, covered his bets by claiming tolerance would be induced in the "embryonic period or immediately post-embryonic stages" (Burnet and Fenner 1949), but subsequently settled for "during the last stage of embryonic life" (Burnet 1956).

As Langman and Cohn (1997) pointed out, there is a period in embryonic life when self-antigens are present and antigen-specific lymphocytes are absent. As the first potential immune effectors develop, the effects of the induction of tolerance to antigens present in the primary lymphoid organs can be easily experimentally measured. Although, as with much of hematology, the processes clearly observed in ontogeny operate throughout productive life, Medawar's "critical point" remains critical because of the relative ease with which tolerance can be induced at an age when the periphery has not yet been seeded with potential effectors (Brent 1997).

3.4.1
The Immunologists' Dirty Little Secret

At the time the clonal selection theory was proposed, there were two main lines of evidence suggesting that it had significant problems. The first was the issue of adjuvants. Burnet attributed the action of adjuvants to their ability to provide "the prolonged maintenance of a depot of antigen" or "ensure that antigenic determinants are being made accessible at a more or less steady rate for a prolonged period of time" (Burnet 1959). He did not seem to fully appreciate the synergistic effects of adding bacteria or bacterial products, such as killed mycobacteria, to antigen/emulsion deposits (Freund et al. 1940). He appears to have attributed the ability of immunization with homologous brain extracts to induce anti-brain antibodies solely to a unique characteristic of the brain, rather than to the incorporation of heat-killed *Mycobacterium tuberculosis* into the inoculum of complete Freund's adjuvant (Kopeloff and Kopeloff 1944; Freund et al. 1947). Confronted with Witebsky et al.'s 1957 report that thyroiditis could be induced in rabbits by immunization with extracts of the rabbits' own thyroids in complete Freund's adjuvant, he assumed that thyroglobulin was also segregated from the immune system in some way (Burnet 1959). We now know that virtually any autologous tissue can be used to raise antibodies by immunization in the presence of killed bacteria; it is not the tissue that is special, it is the adjuvant.

Charles Janeway introduced the published proceedings of the 1989 Cold Spring Harbor Symposium on immune recognition with an article entitled *Approaching the Asymptote: Evolution and Revolution in Immunology* (Janeway 1989), writing:

> ■ *Immunologists have tended to use simple, well characterized proteins or hapten-proteins conjugates as their antigens... However, in order to obtain readily detectable responses to these antigens, they must be incorporated into a remarkable mixture termed complete Freund's adjuvant, heavily laced with killed Mycobacterium tuberculosis organisms or precipitated in alum and mixed with dead Bordetella pertussis organisms. I call this the immunologist's dirty little secret.*

The article raised the possibility that a major aspect of the immune system was being relatively overlooked (Janeway 1989):

> ■ *I believe that immunological recognition extends beyond antigen binding by the clonally distributed receptors... The Landsteinerian fallacy is the idea that the immune system has evolved to recognise equally all non-self substances... I contend that [it] has evolved specifically to recognise and respond to infectious organisms, and that this involves recognition not only of specific antigenic determinants, but also of certain characteristics or patterns common on infectious organisms but absent from the host.*

He later paraphrased this point as follows (Janeway 1998, my underlining):

> ■ *The implication of this article can best be summed up by the statement that the immune system does not just discriminate self from non-self, as Jerne, Talmage, Burnet, and many others believed, but rather that it could discriminate infectious non-self from non-infectious self.*

The second significant challenge to the clonal selection theory was related to the first and was recognized by Burnet (1959) himself:

> ■ **The most soundly based objections to a clonal selection theory of immunity will probably be derived from two sets of facts: (1) It has proved almost impossible to produce tolerance against bacterial antigens, (2) Yet bacteria and bacterial products are highly potent antigens...**

He commented that most experiments in which a failure to induce tolerance occurred had used gram-negative bacteria, and that the responses produced to such attempts at tolerance induction were similar to those induced by injecting the lipopolysaccharide (LPS) of gram-negative bacteria. LPS is a mitogen capable of activating and initiating the proliferation of most B lymphocytes but, in low concentrations, provides an adjuvant activity that can stimulate immune responses to antigens presented in otherwise non-immunogenic forms – for example, haptens conjugated to an autologous carrier (Schmidtke and Dixon 1972).

Three seemingly independent approaches were required to determine the mechanism of action of LPS. In the first, an LPS-binding protein (LPB) was purified from acute-phase reaction serum by rapid chilling and dialysis against a low ionic strength buffer at $4\,°C$; partial sequence was obtained (Tobias et al. 1986). LPB was subsequently found to be necessary to mediate the binding of LPS to a cell-surface receptor on macrophages (Wright et al. 1989) and this receptor was finally identified, by capping with monoclonal antibodies *in vitro*, to be CD14 (Wright et al. 1990). This method allowed a number of non-blocking anti-CD14 monoclonal antibodies to be screened. One such antibody was used to isolate CD14 from detergent lysates of macrophages and to demonstrate LPS binding to the purified molecule (Wright et al. 1990). Thus, LBP opsonizes LPS-bearing particles, such as gram-negative bacteria, and mediates their attachment via CD14 to macrophages and B cells. CD14 had been cloned and sequenced two years earlier and was found to be anchored to the cell membrane by a phosphatidylinositol linkage (Goyert et al. 1988; Haziot et al. 1988); therefore, an unidentified co-receptor was postulated to be responsible for signal transduction following LPS binding.

The second approach stemmed from the observation that the C3H/HeJ and C57BL/10ScCr mouse strains were unresponsive to LPS – in terms of both its mitogenic and adjuvant actions (Sultzer 1968; Watson and Riblet 1974; Coutinho et al. 1977). Linkage analyses in a backcross from C3H/HeJ to the CWB strain were consistent with the unresponsive state being encoded by a single dominant gene (Watson and Riblet 1974) that was subsequently mapped to mouse chromosome 4 in recombinant inbred strains (Watson et al. 1977) and a backcross to C57BL/6 mice (Watson et al. 1978).

The third approach was based on comparative genomics. Inspired by the observed sequence homology between the cytoplasmic domain of the *Drosophila melanogaster* Toll/Dorsal protein and that of the human IL-1 receptor (Gay and Keith 1991), Lemaitre and coworkers (1996) sought and found a major role for Toll in *Drosophila* immune defenses. This observation led Medzhitov et al. (1997) to perform an expressed sequence tag database search for other human sequences sharing sequence similarities to Toll. A clone was identified and sequenced and a fragment PCR was amplified for use as a probe to screen a human splenic cDNA library. A sequence that encoded a protein with significant homology throughout its entire length to *Drosophila* Toll was identified. Expression of a chimeric recombinant molecule with the human Toll cytoplasmic region and mouse CD4 external domains demonstrated that human Toll, like *Drosophila* Toll and mouse IL-1R, signaled through the NF-κB pathway (Medzhitov et al. 1997). Using similar methods, a family of Toll-like receptors (TLR) was independently identified and published, resulting in the homologue identified by Medzhitov et al. (1997) being named TLR4 (Rock et al. 1998).

These three independent strands of work were brought together by the positional cloning of the gene responsible for the defective LPS response in C3H/HeJ mice: *TLR4*. The sequencing of *TLR4* in the C3H/HeJ and C57BL/10ScCr mouse strains led to the extraordinary discovery that C57BL/10ScCr mice carry a null mutation and the C3H/HeJ allele contains a missense mutation in the third exon, producing a dominant negative effect on LPS-mediated immune activation (Poltorak et al. 1998). As TLR4 was already known to be capable of mediating proinflammatory signals, it became clear that it was the missing co-receptor responsible for LPS/LBP/CD14 signal transduction. Furthermore, TLR2, another member of the homologous family, was subsequently found to mediate the similar rapid immune activation induced by gram-positive bacteria (Yoshimura et al. 1999), including *Mycobacterium tuberculosis* (Means et al. 1999). Therefore, a common mechanism was responsible for both of the major problems identified with Burnet's clonal selection theory as it applied to self/non-self discrimination: the immune system handled products associated with pathogens differently. Specific receptors had evolved to recognize specific molecular patterns associated with bacterial, viral, and fungal structural elements, and these receptors, when triggered, were responsible for powerfully activating antigen-presenting cells, such as macrophages and B cells, providing a significant co-stimulus for anti-pathogen responses. This was the basis for the activity of adjuvants.

3.4.2
The Missing Self Hypothesis

Although the early understanding of the role of the MHC in tissue transplantation stemmed from tumor transplantation studies initiated by Snell (1948) (also discussed in Baxter 2000), this model provided far less predictable results than did skin grafting. For example, Furth et al. (1944) reported that while many lymphomas may behave similarly to other transplanted tissues, there were exceptions (Furth et al. 1944):

■ *The transplantation pattern of neoplastic cells arising in the same pure stock mice and their known hybrids varies greatly, while that of a normal tissue thus far studied follows a single pattern.*

The level of confusion generated was clearly very great, as Burnet largely avoided the subject in his writings at the time, and when he did try to interpret these results in terms of his self-marker concept, logic failed him (Burnet and Fenner 1949):

■ *It would be reasonable to assume that an essential require-ment for transplantability of tumour is a disappearance of the cell "markers" by a process of mutation.*

This comment was, of course, inconsistent with Burnet's own theory.

Part of the explanation for the variability in the survival of transplanted tu-mors was serendipitously identified by Snell (1958), when he found that some strain combinations, tumors from parental strains, could not be successfully transplanted into F_1 hybrids (Snell 1981):

■ *I came across this phenomenon (of hybrid resistance to trans-planted lymphomas) in the course of producing and analyzing the first two groups of congenic resistant lines. The phenome-non consists of a resistance of F_1 hybrids to tumours indige-nous to the parental strain, a resistance which, according to the accepted laws of transplantation, should not occur.*

Hybrid resistance was generalized to hemopoietic cells when Cudkowicz and Stimpfling (1964) found that irradiated F_1 recipients were also resistant to bone marrow transplants from either parent. Kiessling et al. (1975) described a popu-lation of splenic lymphocytes they termed "natural" killer (NK) cells, which were capable of rapidly lysing leukemia cells without the priming required by con-ventional lymphocytes. Finally, Harmon et al. (1977) and Kiessling et al. (1977) both proposed that NK cells were the mediators of hybrid resistance.

While the standard tumor line used to assay NK cell lytic activity was (and is still) the YAC-1 Moloney virus-induced lymphoma (Kiessling and Wigzell 1979), a number of other tumor lines highly susceptible to NK cell-mediated lysis were also identified; all were lacking or reduced in class MHC expression (e.g., Stern et al. 1980; Gidlund et al. 1981; Main et al. 1985). Karre et al. (1986) tested the hypothesis that NK cells were responding to the absence of MHC products on the tumor cell surfaces by selecting low MHC class I-expressing clones through selective depletion with alloserum and complement. While the native RBL-5 lymphoma was highly malignant in its syngeneic host (C57BL/6), the subline selected for loss of MHC expression (RMA) failed to grow. They commented:

> ■ *On the basis of our data, we suggest that natural killer cells are effector cells in a defence system geared to detect deleted or reduced expression of self-MHC... Such a system may ... have been fixed in mammals, despite the development of adaptive immunity. The selective pressures (of MHC-dependent T cell surveillance) would have required not only a back-up system eliminating aberrant (MHC-deficient) cells escaping detection by T lymphocytes, but also a rapid first-line defence with a certain selectivity.*

The hypothesis ran along natural selection lines. Since both viruses and tumors divide rapidly, undergo considerable mutation, and are under intense selection by the host's immune system, it is likely that at least some will mutate to avoid immune detection. As the adaptive immune system is dependent on T-cell recognition of MHC products, there should be a tendency for tumors or viruses to avoid immune surveillance by decreasing MHC expression. Ljunggren and Karre (1990) postulated that NK cells were responsible for providing a selective pressure against the downregulation of self-MHC antigens. This model was directly confirmed in 129 mice by the experimental targeted deletion of β2-microglobulin, which is essential for MHC class I surface expression. Although the resulting recombinant mice were tolerant of their own hemopoietic cells, irradiated syngeneic wild-type recipients rejected bone marrow transplants from the knockout mice (Bix et al. 1991).

3.5
Conclusions

In 1959, Burnet wrote:

> ■ *In some way there is a recognition of self components from "not self"; from the facts of immunological tolerance the recognition mechanism is laid down towards the end of embryonic life. Any such mechanism must differentiate between self and not self in one or both of two ways: Either (a) All significant antigenic patterns of the body are positively recognized by the antibody-producing mechanism. Foreign patterns, because they are not recognized, provoke an immune response; Or (b) All the possible types of foreign and antigenic determinant can be positively recognized as foreign and hence calling for an immune response.*

Burnet originally favored the first mechanism, and then settled for the second. We now know that, in a sense, both were correct.

Acknowledgments

The author is grateful for the influential views expressed in conversations and correspondence with Phil Hodgkin and Noel Rose. He is supported by funding from the Australian National Health and Medical Research Council.

References

Baxter AG (2000) *Germ warfare – break-throughs in immunology*. Allen and Unwin, Sydney.

Baxter AG, Hodgkin PD (2002) Activation rules: The two-signal theories of immune activation. *Nature Reviews Immunology* 2: 439–446.

Billingham RE, Brent L, Medawar PB (1953) Actively acquired tolerance of foreign cells. *Nature* 172: 603–606.

Bix M, Liao N-S, Zijlstra M, Loring J, Jaenisch R, Raulet D (1991) Rejection of class I MHC-deficient hemopoietic cells by irradiated NHC-matched mice. *Nature* 349: 329–331.

Brent L (1997) Commentary on Silverstein and Rose "On the mystique of the immunological self." *Immunol Rev* 159: 211–213.

Brent L (2003) The 50th anniversary of the discovery of immunologic tolerance. *N Eng J Med* 349: 1381–1383.

Burnet FM (1956) *Enzyme antigen and virus*. Cambridge University Press.

Burnet FM (1957) A modification of Jerne's theory of antibody production using the concept of clonal selection. *Aust J Sci* 20: 67–69.

Burnet FM (1959) *The clonal selection theory of acquired immunity*. Cambridge University Press.

Burnet FM, Fenner F (1948) *Genetics and Immunology*. *Heredity* 2: 289–324.

Burnet FM, Fenner F (1949) *The production of antibodies*. Macmillan London. Second edition.

Burnet FM, Freeman M, Jackson AV, Lush D (1941) *The production of antibodies*. Macmillan, Melbourne.

Coutinho A, Forni L, Melchers F, Watanabe T (1977) Genetic defect in responsiveness to the B cell mitogen lipopolysaccharide. *Eur J Immunol* 7: 325–328.

Cudkowicz G, Stimpfling JH (1964) Hybrid resistance to parental marrow grafts: association with the K region of H-2. *Science* 144: 1339–1340. See erratum *Science* 147: 1056.

Dawkins R (1998) *Unweaving the rainbow*. Penguin books, London.

Dawkins R (2003) *A devil's chaplain*. Weidenfeld and Nicolson, London.

Ehrlich P (1900) *Proc Royal Soc* (London) B 66: 424.

Forsdyke DR (1968) The liquid scintillation counter as an analogy for the distinction between self and not-self in immunological systems. *Lancet I*: 281–283.

Forsthuber T, Yip HC, Lehmann PV (1996) Induction of Th1 and Th2 immunity in neonatal mice. *Science* 271: 1728–1730.

Freund J, Casals-Ariet J, Genghof DS (1940) The synergistic effect of paraffin-oil combined with heat-killed tubercle bacilli. *J Immunol* 38: 67–79.

Freund J, Stern ER, Pisani TM (1947) Isoallergic encephalomyelitis and radiculitis in guinea pigs after one injection of brain and mycobacteria in water-in-oil emulsion. *J Immunol* 57: 179–194.

Furth J, Boon MA, Kaliss N (1944) On the genetic character of neoplastic cells as determined in transplantation experiments. *Cancer Research* 4: 1–10.

Gay NJ, Keith FJ (1991) Drosophila Toll and IL-1 receptor. *Nature* 351: 355–356.

Gershon RK, Cohen P, Hencin R, Liebhaber SA (1972) Suppressor T cells. *J Immunol* 108: 586–590.

Gibson T, Medawar PB (1943) The fate of skin homografts in man. *J Anat* 77: 299–310.

Gidlund M, Orn A, Pattengale PK, Jansson M, Wigzell H, Nilsson K (1981) Natural killer cells kill tumour cells at a given stage of differentiation. *Nature* 292: 848–850.

Gould SJ (1990) *An urchin in the storm.* Penguin books, London.

Goyert SM, Ferrero E, Rettig WJ, Yenamandra AK, Obata F, Le Beau MM (1988) The CD14 monocyte differentiation antigen maps to a region encoding growth factors and receptors. *Science* 239: 497–500.

Harmon RC, Clark EA, O'Toole C, Wicker LS (1977) Resistance and natural cytotoxicity to EL-4 are controlled by the H-2D-Hh-1 region. *Immunogenetics* 4: 601–607.

Haziot A, Chen S, Ferrero E, Low MG, Silber R, Goyert SM (1988) The monocyte differentiation antigen, CD14, is anchored to the cell membrane by a phosphatidylinositol linkage. *J Immunol* 141(2): 547–552.

Janeway CA (1998) Presential address to the American Association of Immunologists – A Road less travelled by; the role of innate immunity in the adaptive immune response. *J Immunol* 161: 539–544.

Janeway CA (1989) Approaching the asymptote? Evolution and revolution in immunology. *Cold Spring Harb Symp Quant Biol* 54: 1–13.

Jerne NK (1955) The natural-selection theory of antibody formation. Proceedings of the National Academy of Sciences USA 41: 849–857.

Karre K, Ljunggren HG, Piontek G, Kiessling R (1986) Selective rejection of H-2-deficient lymphoma variants suggests alternative immune defence strategy. *Nature* 319: 675–678.

Kiessling R, Hochmaan PS, Haller O, Shearer GM, Wigzell H, Cudkowicz G (1977) Evidence for a similar or common mechanism for natural killer cell activity and resistance to hemopoietic grafts. *Eur J Immunol* 7: 655–663.

Kiessling R, Klein E, Wigzell H (1975) Natural killer cells in the mouse: I. Cytotoxic cells with specificity for mouse Molony leukemia cells. Specificity and distribution according to genotype. *Eur J Immunol* 5: 112–117.

Kiessling R, Wigzell H (1979) An analysis of the murine NK cell as to structure, function and biological relevance. *Immunol Rev* 44: 165–208.

Kopeloff LM, Kopeloff N (1944) The production of antibrain antibodies in the monkey. *J Immunol* 48: 297–304.

Langman RE, Cohn M (1997) The essential self: a commentary on Silverstein and Rose "on the mystique of self." *Immunological Reviews* 159: 214–217.

Lemaitre B, Nicolas E, Michaut L, Reichhart JM, Hoffmann JA (1996) The dorsoventral regulatory gene cassette spätzle/toll/cactus controls the potent antifungal response in *Drosophila* adults. *Cell* 86: 973–983.

Ljunggren H-G, Karre K (1990) In search of the "missing self": MHC molecules and NK cell recognition. *Immunology Today* 11: 237–244.

Main EK, Lampson LA, Hart MK, Kornbluth J, Wilson DB (1985) Human neuroblastoma cell lines are susceptible to lysis by natural killer cells but not by cytotoxic T lymphocytes. *J Immunol* 135: 242–246.

McDevitt HO (1968) Genetic control of the antibody response in inbred mice: transfer of response by spleen cells and linkage to the major histocompatibility (H2) locus. *J Exp Med* 128: 1–11.

Means TK, Wang S, Lien E, Yoshimura A, Golenbock DT, Fenton MJ (1999) Human toll-like receptors mediate cellular activation by Mycobacterium tuberculosis. *J Immunol* 163: 3920–3927.

Medawar PB (1948) Immunity to homologous grafted skin, III The fate of skin homografts transplanted to the brain, to subcutaneous tissue, and to the anterior chamber of the eye. *Brit J Exp Pathol* 29: 58–69.

Medawar PB (1986) *Memoir of a thinking radish: an autobiography.* Oxford University Press, Oxford.

Medzhitov R, Preston-Hurlburt P, Janeway CA (1997) A human homologue of the *Drosophila* Toll protein signals activation of adaptive immunity. *Nature* 388: 394–397.

Miller JFAP (1961) Immunological function of the thymus. *Lancet II*: 748–749.

Nossal GJV, Lederberg J (1958) Antibody production by single cells. *Nature* 181: 1419–1420.

Owen RD (1945) Immunologic consequences of vascular anastomoses between bovine twins. *Science* 102: 400–401.

Owen RD (1946) Erythrocyte mosaics among bovine twins and quadruplets. *Genetics* 31: 227.

Pennisi E (1996) Teetering on the brink of danger. *Science* 271: 1665–1667.

Poltorak A, He X, Smirnova I, Liu MY, Van Huffel C, Du X, Birdwell D, Alejos E, Silva M, Galanos C, Freudenberg M, Ricciardi-Castagnoli P, Layton B, Beutler B (1998) Defective LPS signaling in C3H/HeJ and C57BL/10ScCr mice: mutations in Tlr4 gene. *Science* 282: 2085–2088.

Ridge JP, Fuchs EJ, Matzinger P (1996) Neonatal tolerance revisited: Turning on newborn T cells with dendritic cells. *Science* 271: 1723–1726.

Rock FL, Hardiman G, Timans JC, Kastelein RA, Bazan JF (1998) A family of human receptors structurally related to Drosophila Toll. *Proc Natl Acad Sci USA* 95: 588–593.

Sarzotti M, Robbins DS, Hoffman PM (1996) Induction of protective CTL responses in newborn mice by a murine retrovirus. *Science* 271: 1726–1728.

Schmidtke JR, Dixon FJ (1972) Immune response to a hapten coupled to a nonimmunogenic carrier. *J Exp Med* 136: 392–397.

Silverstein AM (1996) Immunological tolerance. *Science* 272: 1405–1406.

Silverstein AM, Rose NR (1997) On the mystique of the immunological self. *Immunological Reviews* 159: 197–206.

Snell GD (1948) Methods for the study of histocompatibility. *J Genet* 49: 87–108.

Snell GD (1981) Studies in histocompatibility. *Science* 213: 172–178.

Stern P, Gidlund M, Orn A, Wigzell H (1980) Natural killer cells mediate lysis of embryonal carcinoma cells lacking MHC. *Nature* 285: 341–342.

Sultzer BM (1968) Genetic control of leucocyte responses to endotoxin. *Nature* 219: 1253–1254.

Talmage DW (1957) Allergy and immunology. *Ann Rev Med* 8: 239–256.

Tauber AI (1997) *The immune self: theory or metaphor?* Cambridge University Press, UK.

Tobias PS, Soldau K, Elevitch RJ (1986) Isolation of a lipopolysaccharide-binding acute phase reactant from rabbit serum. *J Exp Med* 164: 777–793.

Watson J, Riblet R (1974) Genetic control of responses to bacterial lipopolysaccharides in mice. I Evidence for a single gene that influences mitogenic and immunogenic responses to lipopolysaccharides. *J Exo Med* 140: 1147–1161.

Watson J, Riblet R, Taylor BA (1977) The response of recombinant inbred strains of mice to bacterial lipopolysaccharides. *J Immunol* 118: 2088–2093.

Watson J, Kelly K, Largen M, Taylor BA (1978) The genetic mapping of a defective LPS response gene in C3H/HeJ mice. *J Immunol* 120: 422–424.

Witebsky E, Rose NR, Terplan K, Paine JR, Egan RW (1957) Chronic thyroiditis and autoimmunization. *JAMA* 164: 1439–1447.

Wright SD, Tobias PS, Ulevitch RJ, Ramos RA (1989) Lipopolysaccharide (LPS) binding protein oposonises LPS-bearing particles for recognition by a novel receptor on macrophages. *J Exp Med* 170: 1231–1241.

Wright SD, Ramos RA, Tobias PS, Ulevitch RJ, Mathison JC (1990) CD14, a receptor for complexes of lipopolysaccharide (LPS) and PLS binding protein. *Science* 249: 1431–1433.

Yoshimura A, Lien E, Ingalls RR, Tuomanen E, Dziarski R, Golenbock D (1999) Cutting edge: recognition of Gram-positive bacterial cell wall components by the innate immune system occurs via Toll-like receptor 2. *J Immunol* 163: 1–5.

Zinkernagel RM, Doherty PC (1974) Restriction of in vitro T cell-mediated cytotoxicity in lymphocytic choriomeningitis within a syngeneic or semiallogeneic system. *Nature* 248: 701–702.

4
Central and Peripheral Tolerance

Robert L. Rubin

4.1
Introduction

Immune self-tolerance within the bounds of normal existence (without medical intervention) refers to the failure to develop clinical autoimmune disease while maintaining the capacity to mount robust immune responses to infectious agents. This definition does not mean that a self-tolerant individual is free of autoreactive events, and there is a wealth of evidence that subclinical autoreactivities occur in a normally functioning immune system. Autoreactive events may be a reflection of imperfect tolerance, although it appears that weak self-reactivity is important in maintaining the vitality of immunocytes in a process called homeostatic proliferation [1]. Individuals who remain largely free of autoimmune disease have successfully developed immune tolerance mechanisms involving the central lymphoid organs and in the periphery where immunity is taking place.

The adaptive immune system, that part of protective immunity involving antigen-specific B and T cells, develops in the generative lymphoid organs through a fundamentally random process. Each of the two proteins comprising the receptors on B and T cells that confer antigen specificity is produced at the pre-lymphocyte stage by random recombination of either two (VJ) or three (VDJ) out of 50–100 genetic elements that, together with junctional diversity, has the potential to produce many more different receptor specificities than the total number of lymphocytes produced over an individual's lifetime. The immune system has evolved mechanisms to preferentially select and then expand clones that are either likely to be useful or proven to be useful as a result of their encounter with pathogens and to physically eliminate, suppress, or reduce the responsiveness of clones that are not useful or are potentially dangerous because of their capacity to react with self-antigens. These mechanisms are complex and redundant, and their relative importance for protective immunity and for minimizing autoimmunity is difficult to weigh. In addition, because of the fundamentally random origin of protective immunity and the imperfect nature of the machinery for selecting and controlling lymphocytes, deficiencies in protective immunity and opportunities for autoimmunity arise. It is not surprising, therefore, that antibiotics and vaccination with potential pathogens are often necessary to prevent infectious disease and that signs of autoimmunity can be readily detected and not infrequently lead to autoimmune disease.

This review will focus on autoimmunity with the perspective that the machinery invoked by the immune system to tolerate self while remaining vigilant to foreign threats cannot be readily distinguished. For example, failure to mount an adaptive immune response could be the result of immunological similarity between epitopes on the pathogen and those on self-molecules to which the organism is tolerant, resulting in risk of infection. Ironically, such a cross-reaction could also be considered as a risk for autoimmunity, because if an immune response is somehow elicited against the pathogen, it could initiate an autoimmune attack against a cross-reacting self-epitope in a process called molecular mimicry [2]. Whether tolerance to self can be "broken" by such a mechanism or whether tolerance to a foreign agent is preserved by its cross-reaction with self may depend on the robustness of the epitope-specific machinery of central and peripheral tolerance, the timing of antigen encounter, as well as qualitative and quantitative factors involved in antigen presentation.

4.2
Ignorance of Lymphocytes to Target Antigen

Many self-reactive B and T cells may exist indefinitely in the peripheral immune system in a naïve functional state. For B cells this "ignorance" condition is due to lack of T-cell help and/or access to sufficient antigen; T-cell ignorance refers to failure to encounter cognate antigen on professional antigen-presenting cells. With autoreactive lymphocytes recognizing organ- or tissue-specific antigens, ignorance is probably a common way for cells to avoid becoming activated because lymphocytes reside mainly in secondary lymphoid organs. However, autoreactive lymphocytes that can recognize systemic (non-organ-specific) antigens may be harder to hide. In addition, antigen can be readily presented remotely as a result of the transport of dendritic cells from an inflammatory site to the spleen or draining lymph node, where the antigen can be delivered to waiting, autoreactive lymphocytes in a process called indirect antigen presentation. For these reasons and because the immune system must be constructed to respond to pathogen intrusion wherever it occurs, ignorance is probably not a dependable means for cells to avoid activation. If simply avoiding activation were sufficient to prevent autoimmunity, there would be no need to evolve the complex tolerance machinery (Fig. 4.1).

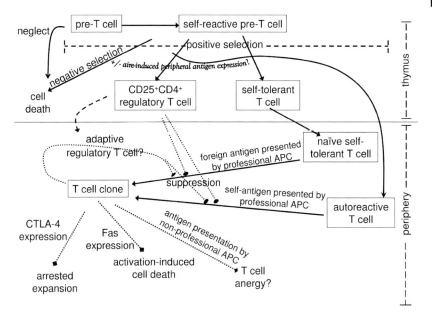

Fig. 4.1 Control of T-cell autoreactivity by tolerance machinery. In the thymus (upper panel), random rearrangement of genetic elements encoding the TCR produces pre-T cells that either die through neglect or are positively selected because their receptor has significant avidity for self-peptide bound to MHC. Maturation events transform thymocytes into self-tolerant T cells. During this process, if a thymocyte encounters peptide + MHC with high avidity for the TCR, it may either die through negative selection or mature into a CD25+CD4+ "natural" regulatory T cell (T_R). Expression of some peripheral antigens in the thymus driven by the Aire transcription factor promotes negative selection and/or T_R production. Some T cells may escape this central tolerance machinery and enter the periphery with autoreactive potential. In the periphery, if a naïve T cell encounters cognate peptide with high affinity for its TCR presented by professional APCs, it may become activated and multiply into a T-cell clone consisting of T cells with effector functions including T-helper activity. T_R may suppress this response by cell-cell contact. Other types of regulatory cells may be induced either through the action of T_R or in response to incomplete antigen presentation, and these adaptive regulatory T cells can blunt clonal expansion through inhibitory cytokine secretion. T-cell clones have inherent limitations on their expansion capacity due to upregulated expression of receptors such as CTLA-4, which creates inhibitory signaling, or Fas and its ligand, which cause cell death. It is also possible for a memory T cell to become functionally non-responsive or anergic if it encounters antigen on nonprofessional APCs. Fas-mediated AICD may be important in limiting inflammation or bystander activation of autoreactive lymphocytes and/or in preventing loss of the self-tolerant property acquired during positive selection.

4.3
Central T-cell Tolerance

After expressing CD4, CD8, and one of trillions of possible specificities of the T-cell receptor (TCR) on their cell surface, immature thymocytes must undergo positive selection to avoid death through neglect. In this process pre-T cells can proceed in development only if their TCRs productively interact with major histocompatibility complexes (MHC) on cortical thymic epithelial cells (cTECs) [3], resulting in signal transduction through the mitogen-activated protein kinase cascade [4]. In the absence of bound peptide, MHC molecules generally cannot correctly fold and are unstable on the cell surface. In the sterile *in vivo* environment of the thymus, the only peptides available for occupancy of the MHC would be derived from self-materials. Studies using mutants in the peptide-binding groove of the MHC [5–7] or of transporter-associated-with-antigen-processing knockout mice, which cannot load endogenous peptide into the MHC [8, 9], provide direct support for the view that a specific antigen is required for positive selection. This process restricts the repertoire of T cells to those with the capacity to recognize MHC plus peptide bearing a stereochemical, conformational, and/or electrostatic relationship to the selecting peptide. A structural relationship between the selecting and stimulating peptide(s) is often obscure because much higher affinity interactions between the peptide and the TCR are required for activation than for selection, as will be discussed below. Nevertheless, thymocytes that successfully proceed in development are intrinsically self-reactive because they require recognition of self-peptide/MHC complexes to avoid programmed cell death. Several processes have been proposed to explain why intrinsic autoreactivity is not normally manifested.

4.3.1
Tolerance Due to Negative T-cell Selection

Numerous laboratories (e.g., [10, 11]) have demonstrated deletion of potentially autoreactive T cells by active killing when $\alpha\beta$ TCRs on immature CD4$^+$CD8$^+$ thymocytes or semi-mature CD4$^+$ or CD8$^+$ (single-positive thymocytes characterized by elevated CD24) are engaged by MHC and peptide ligands of high affinity for the TCR. cTECs do not have the capacity to initiate this process of negative selection, probably because they lack costimulatory molecules such as B7-1, B7-2, and CD40L. Immature thymocytes must encounter other antigen-presenting cells, particularly those of hematopoietic origin such as dendritic cells or macrophages [12], or epithelial cells in the thymic medullary region [13, 14] to result in elimination. Estimates of the proportion of T cells that are deleted by high-affinity interactions with thymic antigen-presenting cells range from 5% [15] to over 50% [16] of T cells that had undergone positive selection in the thymic cortex. The process of clonal deletion of strongly self-reactive T cells that develop by chance in the thymus is widely believed to be the principal mechanism employed by the adaptive immune system to avoid production of autoreactive T cells.

Surprisingly, there is little direct support for the view that clonal deletion prevents autoimmunity. In fact, in most cases where the impact of negative selection was tested, there was little effect on autoimmunity. Instead, when negative selection was prevented or inhibited, potentially autoreactive cells appeared that were profoundly non-responsive. This was shown in a chimeric system in which viral superantigen-mediated deletion of T cells bearing the V6 element of the TCR β-chain was reduced by irradiation [17–19]; however, the Vβ6-bearing T cells that were positively selected were non-responsive to superantigen [18]. In another system, irradiated F$_1$ mice reconstituted with bone marrow cells from one of the parents showed partial deletion of Vβ11$^+$ T cells that normally occurs due to contact with I-E in the thymus, but Vβ11$^+$ thymocytes that developed in these chimeric mice were tolerant to host-type H-2 antigens based on mixed lymphocyte reaction and failure to reject skin grafts from the other parent [20]. In a different approach, partial inhibition of clonal deletion of monoclonal T cells reactive to the male H-Y antigen [21] or of Vβ17a-bearing thymocytes in an MHC I-E thymus [22] was brought about by cyclosporin treatment. This resulted in the appearance of potentially autoreactive T cells in the periphery, but these mice did not develop autoimmunity when cyclosporin was discontinued [21, 23]. Taken together, doubts can be raised about the general importance of deletion in preventing autoreactivity to the wide array of self-reactive T cells that could potentially arise during generation of the T-cell repertoire.

On the other hand, several studies have supported a role for negative selection in preventing autoimmunity. In mice capable of positive selection but not of deletion by the transgenic expression of MHC class II only on thymic cortical epithelium, autoreactivity of peripheral T cells was observed by a mixed lymphocyte reaction and cytotoxicity [15]. However, the specificity of these "autoreactive" T cells was not defined, and it was not excluded that the absence of medullary TECs in these transgenic mice resulted in failure to develop immunoregulatory T cells as discussed below. A more recent study by Gao et al. [24] succeeded in causing partial inhibition of negative selection by perinatal injection of anti-B7-1 + anti-B7-2 antibodies in mice transgenic for both the TCR and its cognate antigen, the P1A tumor antigen. Mononuclear cell infiltration occurred in the lung in male and female mice and in the kidney in females. The autoreactive cells that arose as a result of the presumed disruption of B7-CD28 signaling during negative selection were remarkably pathogenic, especially in lymphocyte transfer recipients made lymphopenic by irradiation. Autoimmunity was also observed after adoptive transfer of T cells that developed in anti-B7-treated non-transgenic mice as a result of inhibition of deletion of families of viral superantigen-reactive thymocytes or of other, undefined polyclonal T cells. While it has not been formally ruled out that transient blocking B7-1 and B7-2 had other effects such as inhibiting production of regulatory T cells, the study of Gao et al. [24] makes the strongest case to date that negative selection is important in preventing autoimmunity.

4.3.1.1 *Aire*-driven Peripheral Antigen Expression in Medullary Thymic Epithelial Cells

Certain proteins characteristic of differentiated cells or tissues in the periphery are also expressed in the thymus and may drive positive and negative selection [25, 26]. These findings helped address the question of how tolerance to tissue-specific antigens could be established; this dilemma had previously been relegated to peripheral tolerance mechanisms or to the hypothetical delivery of peripherally expressed proteins through the circulation and into the thymus. The possibility of ectopic or promiscuous gene expression of tissue-specific antigens in the thymus received a large boost from the report that a small population of medullary thymic epithelial cells (mTECs) expressed a diverse and seemingly unrelated array of proteins normally confined to peripheral tissues such as insulin (pancreas), C-reactive protein (liver), and myelin proteolipid protein (brain) [27]. It was subsequently shown that RNA transcripts of some 100–300 semi-tissue-specific proteins were expressed by mTECs in a phenomenon that depended on a functional gene called the autoimmune regulator (*Aire*) [28]. *Aire*-deficient mice and humans display a similar phenotype, characterized by T-cell infiltration and autoantibodies to skin, gastrointestinal tract, and certain endocrine organs (humans) [29] and ovary, stomach, eye, and salivary glands (mice) [28]. This finding suggests that Aire is a transcription factor that enhances the promiscuous expression of certain peripheral antigens in the thymus in order to force them to participate in deletion of the corresponding antigen-specific, autoreactive T cells. This idea was tested using double-transgenic mice expressing both a TCR specific to hen egg lysozyme (HEL) and HEL under the control of the insulin promoter. In this way HEL expression should be limited to the β-cells of the pancreas and, based on prior studies [28], the mTECs in the thymus. Deletion of transgenic T cells was efficient in wild-type mice but greatly reduced in $Aire^{-/-}$ mice, which did not have functional *Aire* and, therefore, would be presumed to not express HEL on mTECs in the thymus. These studies were considered to provide strong support for the view that tolerance to tissue-specific antigens occurred by negative selection of autoreactive T cells as a result of the promiscuous expression of these proteins on mTECs in the thymus [30].

While it is likely that thymocytes will be killed if a high-affinity antigen is presented on mTECs, it is not clear that this process is efficient enough or necessary to prevent autoimmunity. $Aire^{-/-}$ mice that failed to delete HEL-specific T cells were not reported to develop T-cell infiltration of the HEL$^+$ pancreas or other signs of autoimmunity [31], despite other studies using the same transgenic system that found that failure to delete HEL-specific T cells in non-obese diabetic (NOD) mice resulted in autoimmunity targeting β-cells that transgenically expressed HEL in the pancreas [32]. T cells developing on the NOD background are autoreactive for unknown reasons, while the same type of transgenic T cells developing in $Aire^{-/-}$ mice in a non-autoimmune-prone background such as B10.BR are tolerant; T-cell deletion efficiency does not distinguish these strains. Also, wild-type mice that were grafted with a thymus from mice incapable of producing the liver-specific protein serum amyloid P (SAP$^{-/-}$) were tolerant to immunization with SAP, indicating that SAP expression in mTECs is unnecessary to inhibit autoimmunity [27]. While SAP expression in the thymus alone, presumably in mTECs, was sufficient to induce tolerance to SAP [27], expression of other tissue-specific genes in the thymus was not necessarily *Aire*-dependent [28], and promiscuous expression was frequently detected in cTECs, hematopoietic cells, and/or testis [27]. Finally, it should be noted that the system used by Liston et al. [31] is favored to detect deletion by thymically expressed antigen because of the huge excess of transgenic T cells capable of undergoing deletion upon encountering high-affinity, cognate antigen in the thymus; in a normal environment any one specificity of an autoreactive T cell would be very rare. The probability is low that a thymocyte would encounter its cognate antigen on mTECs and be deleted based on calculations of MHC scanning rate, minimum number of peptide/MHC complexes needed to initiate negative selection, and residence time in the thymus [33]. Overall, the discovery of *Aire*-related expression of peripheral antigens in mTECs has not substantially strengthened the view that tolerance by negative selection is an effective mechanism for purging autoreactivity.

4.3.2
Self-tolerance Associated with Positive T-cell Selection

As mentioned above, immature thymocytes require self-peptide/MHC recognition through the TCR during positive selection to proceed in development, but thymocytes are normally not reactive with the selecting peptides. Tolerance to selecting self is presumed to reflect acquisition of a general increased resistance to agonist signals due to nonspecific maturational events such as signaling through the glucocorticoid receptor [34]. More specific hypotheses as to why thymocytes lose their responsiveness to the selecting antigens are based on the view that the pre-T cell undergoing development experiences partial or selective stimulation when encountering low-affinity antigens on cTECs, and this incomplete signaling increases the threshold needed for subsequent activation [35]. Multiple signaling events are required to activate mature T cells, and failure to fully engage at least one pathway during positive selection is the basis for several concepts to explain tolerance of the mature thymocyte to the selecting antigens. It has been proposed that incomplete signaling may be a consequence of the nature of the selecting antigens, the antigen-presenting cells, or the developing T cells themselves (reviewed in [36]). Selective signaling leaves the immature T cells permanently altered such that subsequent stimulation by the same antigens encountered in the periphery is largely ignored. Peptides could be functional agonists only if they happen to have adequate affinity and concentration to simultaneously engage a sufficient number of TCRs to overcome the higher activation threshold the T cell acquired during positive selection. Such peptides would normally be derived from foreign antigens but could also be derived from molecules expressed exclusively in the periphery.

The non-responsive state that thymocytes attain during positive selection is not absolute, its extent depending on the avidity of the selecting peptides it was exposed to. If the selecting self-peptides were of high affinity for the TCR, the threshold for activation of the resultant T cell would be set high. A peptide with deletional capacity could, therefore, produce cells by positive selection that would be unable to respond to the index peptide. These cells would probably be useless even without subsequent deletion by the negative selection machinery because it would be unlikely that any peptide exists that could overcome such a high activation threshold. While this phenomenon has not yet been formally demonstrated, and other tolerance mechanisms could be acting, failure to develop frank autoimmunity when negative selection was disrupted [17–23, 31] is consistent with the concept of a strong link between positive selection and central T-cell tolerance.

4.3.3
Self-tolerance Due to Thymus-derived Regulatory T Cells: Natural Regulatory T Cells

The past half-decade has seen a large upsurge of information on T cells that suppress the function of effector T cells. While such regulatory T cells (T_R) have come to be identified in different ways, a population of $CD4^+$ T cells that constitutively express CD25 (interleukin-2 receptor) initially described by Sakaguchi and coworkers (reviewed in [37, 38]) remains the most thoroughly studied. In a lymphopenic host these cells are necessary to prevent spontaneous autoimmunity to certain organs including testis, prostrate, ovaries, thyroid, pancreas, and stomach, depending on the mouse strain. $CD4^+CD25^+$ T_R comprise 5–10% of the peripheral T-cell pool and suppress the activation of $CD4^+$ and $CD8^+$ effector T cells by a process that requires cell-to-cell contact at a suppressor:effector cell ratio of 1:1 [39]. It is also possible that $CD4^+CD25^+$ T_R act on APCs to suppress T-cell activation, but inhibitory cytokines do not seem to be involved [37, 38]. Of particular relevance to central T-cell tolerance is the accumulated evidence that $CD4^+CD25^+$ T_R in the periphery have a direct lineage connection to $CD4^+CD25^+$ T cells in the thymus and are actively produced in the normal thymus. Using mice transgenic for both the influenza hemagglutinin and a TCR specific for a major determinant on this protein, Jordan et al. [40] demonstrated that $CD4^+CD25^+$ T cells are most efficiently produced upon high-affinity interaction between the TCR and its cognate antigen presented by radioresistant (non-hematopoietic-derived) thymic epithelium. Mice that transgenically expressed influenza hemagglutinin driven by another promoter displayed more complexity in the origin and phenotype of T_R [41], but this study, as well as that of Stephen and Ignaowicz [42] using a different approach, is consistent with the view that $CD4^+CD25^+$ T_R are dependent on high-affinity TCR-antigen interaction for their generation. What determines whether such interactions result in T_R production or in deletion by negative selection is unclear [43], as is whether mTECs or cTECS (or hematopoietic cells in one study [41]) are involved. Nevertheless, the generation of a population of T cells that do not respond to antigen after high-affinity interactions on thymic epithelium is reminiscent of the origin of self-tolerant T cells during positive selection, suggesting that cells selected on high-affinity antigens during positive selection have been salvaged by the immune system to create $CD4^+CD25^+$ T_R, thereby ensuring that highly autoreactive T cells produced during positive selection would have a T_R counterpart. Alternatively, stochastic events during negative selection on high-affinity antigens presented by mTECs initiate a commitment to a developmental program that results in survival rather than death of CD4$^+$ T cells; that such cells represent a genuinely distinct lineage is supported by the requirement for expression of the *Foxp3* gene, which encodes a transcription factor necessary for development of CD4$^+$CD25$^+$ T$_R$ [44]. It has been suggested [39] that T$_R$ generation is a component of negative rather than positive selection in part because of the requirement for B7-CD28 and CD40-CD40L interactions [45, 46], but interaction in the periphery of T$_R$ with immature dendritic cells expressing low levels of these costimulatory molecules may be necessary to sustain homeostatic proliferation of T$_R$ [47, 48].

The organ-specific autoimmune disease that develops when CD4$^+$CD25$^+$ T cells are removed from normal mice and the protection from autoimmunity by reconstituting mice with these cells strongly suggest that they directly suppress activation of constitutive autoreactive CD4$^+$(CD25$^-$) effector T cells. The need for this active form of tolerance suggests that tissue-specific autoreactive T cells frequently escape central T-cell tolerance. *Aire*-induced ectopic expression of peripheral antigens in the thymus may be more important in the production of T$_R$ than in forcing clonal deletion, and humans with the autoimmune polyendocrinopathy syndrome associated with *Aire* deficiency [29] may be deficient in T$_R$.

4.4
Peripheral T-cell Tolerance

It is generally believed that many T cells escape central tolerance, especially those with the capacity to react with self-antigens not expressed in the thymus. This view is consistent with the relative ease of inducing organ-specific autoimmunity by deliberate immunization with peripheral antigens. While tissue-specific, self-reactive T cells generally ignore their target antigen because it is inaccessible or not presented in an immunogenic form, organ-specific autoimmune diseases are common [49]. In order to minimize autoimmunity mediated by self-reactive T cells in the periphery, the immune system has apparently developed various peripheral tolerance mechanisms that can restrain, quell, or kill such cells. Peripheral tolerance is much more than a backup mechanism to prevent autoimmunity – it is an active process that is probably invoked to limit T-cell response to all antigens.

4.4.1
Self-tolerance Due to Regulatory T Cells Generated in the Periphery: Adaptive Regulatory T Cells

CD4$^+$ T cells with suppressive activity can be experimentally induced in the periphery, and these cells differ from CD4$^+$CD25$^+$ T$_R$ cells in phenotypic characteristics and various properties. They have been named T regulatory type 1 (Tr1) or

T-helper type 3 (Th3) ("Treg" for this discussion), and they act by a bystander mechanism to suppress antigen-specific responses of other cells through the production of inhibitory cytokines. Unlike T_R, Treg inhibitory activity did not depend on cell-to-cell contact and, where studied, generally involved release of inhibitory cytokines such as interleukin-10 (IL-10) or transforming growth factor-β (TGF-β). As with CD4$^+$CD25$^+$ T_R cells, Treg is typically anergic to a challenge with specific antigen but in co-culture suppresses the activation of naïve T cells by cognate antigen.

Treg cells have been induced by a variety of methods but tend to have in common procedures that cause partial T-cell activation. Treg has been induced by stimulating with specific antigen in the presence of blocking antibodies to the TCR, of the co-receptors CD4 or CD8, and of the costimulators CD40 or CD40L or when antigen is presented by immature or cytokine-treated dendritic cells that do not have good costimulation function (reviewed in [50]). It appears, therefore, that suppressive T cells are generated from the naïve T-cell repertoire when activation/expansion signals are created without the robust immune stimulation associated with professional APCs.

Protocols for generating Treg by stimulating naïve cells in the periphery are generally heroic or unnatural, and it is not certain that such cells are a normal and significant part of the T-cell repertoire. In addition, while the value of antigen-specific Treg in controlling autoimmune disease can be imagined, many of the experimental protocols used to reveal cells with Treg function could produce cells with the capacity to suppress T cells specific to foreign antigen as well as self-reactive T cells. It is unclear why there would be survival value in blunting or blocking adaptive immune responses by raising Tregs to foreign pathogens, although suppressing self-destructive inflammation or allergic responses might be desirable. One way the immune system could restrict adaptive Treg to preferentially inhibit autoreactive T cells would be if their development depended on natural T_R – either as direct precursors or by inducing CD4$^+$ autoreactive T cells undergoing antigen stimulation to deviate into suppressors secreting inhibitory cytokines as suggested [51, 52]. It has also been proposed that autoreactive T cells would become anergic (and suppressive?) as a consequence of the continuous presentation of low levels of self-peptide by immature dendritic cells [53]. Perhaps presentation of peptides from a pathogen in an inflammatory environment might have more abrupt kinetics and/or higher localized concentration, conditions not favoring the *de novo* production or function of Treg. Regardless of the real value of adaptive Tregs in controlling immune responses to foreign versus self-antigens, the existence of inhibitory machinery that can be tapped in conjunction with an adaptive immune response underscores the difficult problem that the immune system has taken on in remaining vigilant to foreign threats while tolerating self.

Some of the most interesting and suggestive observations for the existence of regulatory T cells (whether natural or adaptive) come from studies in humans. CD4$^+$CD25$^+$ T cells (presumably "natural" T_R) can be isolated from the circulation and transformed by sub-optimum stimulation with anti-CD3 into suppressor cells as measured by co-culture with CD4$^+$CD25$^-$ effector T cells; patients with multiple sclerosis who have autoimmune demyelinating disease had similar numbers but a threefold decrease in the functional activity in these cells [54]. Similarly, CD4$^+$CD25$^+$ T cells isolated from patients with asthma, an allergic disease associated with excessive Th2 effector cell activity, had reduced capacity to inhibit Th2 cell activation by allergen compared to Treg isolated from normal, non-atopic individuals [55]. Patients with ovarian cancer, a disease that could be considered a failure of immune surveillance of cancer-specific antigens, have Tregs that suppress tumor-specific immunity apparently by infiltrating the tumor due to its release of the chemoattractant CCL22 [56]. Mutations in the *FoxP3* gene are associated with the polyendocrinopathy, enteropathy, X-linked syndrome (IPEX), a fatal immune disorder with autoimmune features, and these patients are largely devoid of Treg [57]. Undoubtedly, the next few years will continue to see explosive growth in this area of research.

4.4.2
T-cell Anergy

A fundamental tenet of immunology is the requirement for dual receptor engagement of the T cell by an APC in order to achieve full activation. In addition to signaling through the TCR by peptide/MHC (signal 1), simultaneous ligation at a different site (signal 2), particularly CD28 on the T-cell membrane by the B7 family of ligands (CD80 and CD86), on the APC generally must occur. If costimulation does not occur, engagement of the TCR by a high-affinity ligand produces a long-lasting state of paralysis. Upon subsequent challenge with cognate antigen by "professional" APCs, i.e., cells expressing costimulatory molecules, T cells in this anergic state will not transcribe certain cytokines (most notably IL-2), will not respond to other T-cell growth factors, and will not proliferate [58]. Anergic T cells are deficient in helper activity for B cells but are not dead; they remain viable for an indefinite time and can be made to proliferate *in vitro* and provide helper activity with cognate antigen in the presence of high concentrations of IL-2 [59, 60]. Anergy is widely believed to be an important mechanism for peripheral T-cell tolerance because it is likely that autoreactive T cells could encounter their cognate antigen on nonprofessional APCs or immature dendritic cells that lack costimulatory function. In addition, various experimental protocols have been devised based on the concept of anergy in hopes of inducing tolerance to self-antigens and ameliorating autoimmune disease.

Unfortunately, T-cell anergy, as defined by non-responsiveness after signal 1-only, does not occur with naïve T cells. Prior studies on T-cell anergy have typically involved T-cell lines or clones, which are similar in phenotype to memory (antigen-experienced) T cells. Naïve T cells are insensitive to anergy induction *in vitro* and may even proliferate in response to signal 1-only, such as via anti-CD3 [61]. *In vivo*, transfer of naïve T cells from TCR transgenic mice into a host expressing the cognate antigen in a non-inflammatory environment [1, 28, 32] or on mature dendritic cells in the presence or absence of the costimulatory molecules B7-1 and B7-2 [48] or CD40 [62] initially results in activation and proliferation of the transgenic T cells, not anergy. Claims that naïve T cells can be anergized *in vitro* or *in vivo* typically involve experimental conditions in which the cells were forced to divide at least once or conditions in which a different form of T-cell tolerance was acting, such as T-cell adaptation to create Tregs, activation-induced cell death (see below), or engagement of cytotoxic T lymphocyte-antigen 4 (CTLA-4). It has been speculated that lipid rafts, which contain a variety of src-family kinases, must first be mobilized to the cell membrane in response to initial contact with antigen before the anergy-inducing machinery can function [63].

CTLA-4 is a ligand for B7 that is upregulated upon T-cell activation and that attenuates costimulation through CD28. Mice lacking functional CTLA-4 display massive lymphocyte activation and die of multi-organ lymphocyte infiltrates suggestive of systemic autoimmunity [64]. Blockage of B7 → CD28 signaling by therapeutic introduction of soluble CTLA-4-Ig prolongs allograft survival [65], inhibits disease progression and autoantibody load in murine lupus [66], and has been used successfully to treat psoriasis [67]. While upregulation and engagement of CTLA-4 are important mechanisms to terminate T-cell activation, these processes do not appear to cause permanent T-cell tolerance or to distinguish self from foreign antigen responses.

Overall, T-cell anergy in the periphery is not a dependable mechanism for preventing autoimmunity. Even if anergy could be induced in naïve autoreactive T cells, the first APC presenting the cognate self-antigen to a newly emerging T cell would have to be immature or nonprofessional without costimulatory molecules. However, there is no known compartmentalization of nascent, mature T cells in either the thymus, where professional APCs in the form of dendritic cells commonly coexist [12], or when they enter the circulation as naïve T cells and could potentially encounter any type of APC, including activated dendritic cells with full costimulation function (reviewed in [68]). A similar problem would be faced by an autoreactive T cell that was somehow activated and developed into a clone of memory T cells without causing disease and for some reason needed to be suppressed to avoid future pathology: while capable of being anergized, this process would require signaling through the TCR by a nonprofessional APC. The dilemma is that efficient presentation of antigen by professional APCs is an essential feature of a useful immune system, and functional APCs are constitutively available to endocytose and cross-present antigen whether from a foreign source or from shed self-material or dead cell debris. Discrimination between self and dangerous insults is greatly enhanced by the Toll-like receptors for "pathogen-associated recognition patterns" expressed on dendritic cells, resulting in maturation, cytokine and chemokine secretion, and enhanced survival of these APCs [69]. However, cross-presentation of self-antigens readily occurs, as demonstrated by adoptive transfer studies in which naïve TCR-transgenic T cells become activated when exposed to cognate antigen synthesized in non-lymphoid cells in a non-inflammatory environment [1, 28, 32, 62]. In a normal setting, central T-cell tolerance would avert such an autoimmune response. Although T-cell anergy is a very real phenomenon that can be manifested during positive selection in the thymus or experimentally by memory T cells in the periphery or by T-cell clones *in vitro*, there is considerable doubt about the physiological significance of peripheral anergy in preventing autoimmunity.

4.4.3
Activation-induced Cell Death

A remarkable feature of the T-cell response to antigen occurs after activation and clonal expansion. The bulk of these cells die by apoptosis due to cytokine depletion or to engagement by FasL of the death receptor Fas (APO-1 or CD95), a process called clonal contraction. Cytokine depletion after T-cell activation triggers the release of cytochrome c from the mitochondria, resulting in passive or programmed cell death, and may represent a failure to thrive rather than an active tolerance mechanism. However, Fas engagement by FasL, particularly on CD8 cells and on the Th1 subtype of T-helper cells, or engagement of the type I tumor necrosis factor receptor by TNF-a initiates the extrinsic pathway to apoptosis. These cell-surface molecules are upregulated upon T-cell activation, and their engagement leads to cell death through a complex series of signaling molecules and new gene transcription in a process called activation-induced cell death (AICD). While it is widely believed that AICD is a homeostatic mechanism to minimize tissue damage by proinflammatory cytokines or to avoid overloading the peripheral immune compartments with a limited T-cell repertoire, its only documented role is in preventing autoimmune reactions. In this sense, AICD is important for maintaining peripheral tolerance. Mice deficient in either Fas (*lpr/lpr* mice) or FasL (*gld/gld* mice) develop profound lymphoproliferation and autoantibodies after only a few months, and, when on the MRL background, by five months begin to die of autoimmune glomerulonephritis and other inflammatory abnormalities. Humans with defective *Fas* can develop an autoimmune lymphoproliferative syndrome (ALPS or Canale-Smith syndrome) [70]. Lymphadenopathy in mice and humans with Fas or FasL deficiency is not associated with increased risk of infection, raising doubts about the importance of AICD in "making space" for future immune needs. The autoimmune disease associated with the failure of this machinery is systemic rather than organ-specific autoimmunity, consistent with the view that AICD regulates uncontrolled proliferation of T cells (and B cells, as is discussed below) regardless of their specificity [71].

As mentioned in Section 4.1, antigen-specific T cells are created by a highly complex process in which intricate recombination events derive the a- and β-chain genes of the TCR from a reservoir of approximately 1.6 million base pairs of genomic DNA to produce the premier recognition entrée of the adaptive immune system, the TCR. After dedicating so much genetic resource to creating the T-cell repertoire, why would the immune system need to eliminate most of the progeny of an expanding clone? This paradox is especially manifested when some strains of lymphocytic choriomeningitis virus induce such a strong CD8 T-cell response that virus-specific cytotoxic lymphocytes become undetectable, presumably as a result of AICD, while virus and pathology persist [72]. Clonal contraction seems counterproductive to protective immunity. In addition, why, as a result of the failure of AICD, would continual clonal expansion of a T cell responding to a foreign antigen lead to autoreactivity?

A commonly repeated notion is that AICD is necessary to eliminate autoreactive T cells that escaped deletion in the thymus and happened to encounter their cognate self-antigen presented by professional APCs; AICD of T cells reacting with foreign antigens would be unavoidable in exchange for minimizing autoimmunity. Alternatively, limiting clonal expansion by AICD is a tradeoff to curtail the autoreactive potential that is intrinsic in all T cells. As previously discussed, T cells are positively selected in the thymus on self-antigen (+MHC); therefore, all T cells are potentially self-reactive. Negative regulators of T-cell activation are likely to accumulate during thymopoiesis, resulting in increased threshold requirements for signaling through the TCR and preventing mature T cells from responding to the selecting self-antigens. However, in the periphery, negative regulators might become increasingly diluted as a consequence of antigen-mediated clonal expansion. This loss would jeopardize tolerance to the selecting antigens, increasing the capacity of T cells to respond to low-affinity self-antigens in the periphery. This view places AICD as the companion of central T-cell tolerance associated with positive selection in that AICD eliminates the progeny of activated T cells before they can express their intrinsic self-reactivity.

While teleological arguments about the "purpose" of AICD can be defended to varying extents, discoveries in this field have made it difficult to support a unifying hypothesis. The lymphoproliferation in mice and humans deficient in Fas-mediated AICD is highly skewed to a normally rare lymphocyte that expresses the TCR but not the CD4 or CD8 coreceptor molecules. This "double negative" T cell, which also expresses the B-cell marker B220, appears to be derived from antigen-activated CD8$^+$ T cells [64]. The significance of the preferential expansion of this unusual type of T cell in the absence of AICD is unclear. Also, while FasL is primarily expressed by activated CD8$^+$ cytotoxic T cells as well as CD4$^+$ T cells comprising the Th0 and Th1 (helper) subsets, all T cells (and B cells) are susceptible to apoptosis by the extrinsic pathway. Perhaps FasL is released into the inflammatory milieu or expressed on non-lymphoid tissue [73], so that any activated lymphocytes in the immediate environment could be killed. Remarkably, the hypergammaglobulinemia and autoantibodies displayed by mice with defective Fas or FasL can be largely attributed to the failure to eliminate autoreactive B cells by Fas-mediated AICD rather than to failure of AICD in the T-cell compartment [74, 75], although humoral autoimmunity in MRL-*lpr/lpr* mice clearly requires T-cell help [76]. CD4$^+$ cytotoxic Th1 T cells and a portion of the cytotoxic activity of CD8$^+$ T cells employ FasL in their effector function to kill target cells expressing Fas, and CD4$^+$ Th cells may have co-opted this machinery to kill activated B cells [77]. Finally, it has been reported that tolerance to certain tissue-specific antigens in "immune-privileged sites" such as the testis, ovaries, brain, and eye is mediated by the constitutive expression of FasL in these tissues [73]. Overall, while Fas-mediated AICD is arguably the single most important peripheral tolerance mechanism, utilization of this machinery is complex, unpredictable, and probably overwhelmed in autoimmune disease.

4.5
B-cell Tolerance

B-cell maturation takes place in the fetal liver and in the bone marrow after birth. At the pre-B cell stage, somatic recombination of the V, D, and J genetic elements allows expression on the cell surface of the μ-chain of the immunoglobulin (Ig) receptor in association with an invariant, surrogate light chain. Because of the absence of a specific light chain, this pre-B cell receptor (BCR) does not possess the antigen specificity displayed by the mature BCR, although the heavy chain may have a dominant effect in determining specificity. Surprisingly, the pre-BCR is a completely assembled signaling complex that is required for further cell maturation, but there is no counterpart in pre-B cells to positive selection, which is necessary for continual survival of pre-T cells. Therefore, B cells are intrinsically less restricted than T cells to recognize antigen. At the immature B-cell stage, a rearranged, specific light chain replaces the surrogate light chain, and allelic exclusion is generally strictly enforced so that each B cell bears a single heavy and light chain. Three types of tolerance mechanisms have been described that are believed to minimize autoreactivity in B cells (Fig. 4.2).

4.5.1
Negative Selection of B Cells

Immature B cells that encounter antigen with high affinity for the BCR may die in the bone marrow by apoptosis. This process appears to be very effective for B cells specific to abundant, multivalent self-antigens displayed on cell surfaces, as has been shown for an MHC class I epitope [78] or for epitopes on erythrocytes [79], presumably resulting in extensive BCR cross-linkage. A concern of studies directly demonstrating deletion of Ig transgenic B cells is that these cells may not respond in a normal way to receptor engagement. However, comparisons in normal mice of the production of immature B cells in the bone marrow with B-cell emigration to the spleen indicate that only 15–20% [80] or 10% [81] of newly arising B cells reach the periphery, suggesting that the vast majority of newly formed B cells die in the bone marrow [81]. It is possible that many of these cells do not survive because they fail to produce functional BCR signaling machinery. However, Wardemann et al. [82] demonstrated that while 76% of pre-B cells or early immature B cells from human bone marrow are potentially self-reactive, this number drops to 40% in immature bone marrow

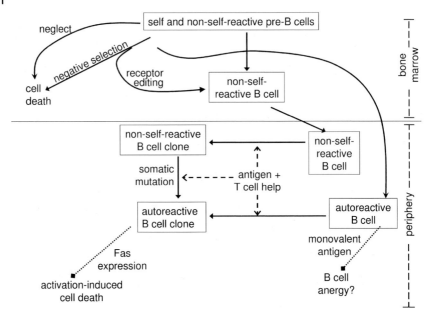

Fig. 4.2 B-cell tolerance and autoreactivity. In the bone marrow (upper panel), random rearrangement of genetic elements encoding the BCR produces pre-B cells that either die through neglect because of failure to assemble a functioning signaling complex or are tested for reactivity to multivalent self-antigens in their environment. Reactive cells either die through negative selection or engage the DNA recombinase machinery to produce an alternate light chain. Cells that replace their light chains by receptor editing to produce a BCR with low avidity for self emigrate to the periphery. Many B cells escape this central tolerance machinery and enter the periphery with autoreactive potential. Under some conditions, immature autoreactive B cells may become anergic by contact with antigen. In the periphery, if a B cell encounters antigen with high affinity for its BCR as well as specific T-cell help, it may become activated, multiply into a B-cell clone, and secrete antibody. Some B cells can be activated by multivalent antigens in the absence of T-cell help (not shown). Somatic mutation of the BCR driven by T-cell help can enhance the affinity of the BCR to produce an overtly autoreactive B cell. Upregulation of Fas limits expansion of the B-cell clone by initiating cell death upon encountering Fas ligand on activated T cells or as a soluble agonist in its environment. Other peripheral tolerance mechanisms have also been observed, including receptor editing, failure to develop proper germinal centers, and cytokine-mediated suppression.

B cells and 20% in mature, peripheral B cells, suggesting that most of the discrepancy between B-cell production in the bone marrow and B-cell immigrants in the periphery is due to negative selection of autoreactive cells. Nevertheless, the importance of this process in maintaining self-tolerance is unclear because it has not yet been shown that failure of or deficiency in negative selection of B cells results in autoimmunity.

4.5.2
B-cell Receptor Editing

After an immature B cell encounters multivalent self-antigen, there may be a one- to two-day delay before it dies by negative selection. During this time the recombinase-activating genes are transcribed, leading to additional light-chain V/J DNA rearrangement, and the newly formed light chain replaces the original light chain in the assembled Ig molecules. If this process of "receptor editing" produces a BCR that is not autoreactive, the cell can proceed in development. Autoantigen-induced secondary Ig gene rearrangement seems at odds with allelic exclusion, but apparently engagement of the BCR at the pre-B cell stage is a dominant signal to initiate receptor editing [83]. This phenomenon has been shown in several lines of mice transgenic for various Ig heavy and light chains in which the transgene-encoded antibody was bred into an environment that expressed the cognate antigen. Although peripheral B cells in these mice were abundant, a high percentage of them did not express the original transgenic light chain [84], suggesting that autoantigen-mediated receptor editing is a robust process to rescue B-cell precursors from death.

Receptor editing has also been observed in mice made transgenic for anti-DNA antibodies. Gay et al. [85] employed heavy and light chains that conferred anti-native (double-stranded) DNA activity in a hybridoma called 3H9, but the derivative transgenic mice had no anti-DNA activity as a result of the spontaneous swapping of transgenic light chains for endogenous light chains in the surviving B cells. When mice transgenic for just the heavy chain of 3H9 were studied, analysis of derived hybridomas revealed a skewed but diverse light-chain usage comprising 37 different V kappa genes [86]; none of these antibodies expressed anti-DNA activity. These results suggest that when pre-B cells encounter endogenous antigen, they are rescued from death by a second round or even multiple rounds of light-chain gene rearrangements. To minimize artifacts due to unnatural loci where Ig transgenes come to reside in the germ line, Pewzner-Jung et al. [87] constructed "knock-in" mice in which a rearranged anti-DNA heavy-chain gene was targeted to the heavy-chain locus, allowing Ig class switching and somatic mutations; the surviving B cells displayed highly skewed J kappa usage compared to bulk Ig, presumably to avoid acquiring anti-DNA activity. Silencing autoreactive properties of B cells by exchanging light chains seems to be a common mechanism for B-cell tolerance [88]. Taken together, these studies strongly suggest that B cells that happen to develop autoantigen-binding activity during early development and that are exposed to a multivalent form of the cognate antigen can be rescued from negative selection by reactivating their DNA recombination machinery and replacing the light chain in the BCR. The fact that receptor editing is so important in shaping the B-cell but not the T-cell repertoire may relate to the observation that autoreactive properties are such a predominant part of the pre-B-cell repertoire [82] that just allowing these cells to die would leave little for the humoral immune system to work with.

4.5.3
B-cell Anergy

Much of the description of B-cell anergy derives from a mouse model expressing transgenic heavy (μ) and light chains, which together encode an anti-hen egg lysozyme (HEL) antibody. These cells can be considered autoreactive when the mice are genetically crossed with, or when anti-HEL mature B cells are adoptively transferred into mice expressing lysozyme as a transgene. In contrast to the controls that spontaneously secreted IgM anti-HEL, antibody secretion in the double-transgenic mice was profoundly silenced [89]. HEL-specific B-cell precursors were still present but had downregulated approximately 95% of their surface IgM and were largely non-responsive to stimulation with antigen plus T cells in the appropriate host [89]. It was proposed that the functional tolerance or anergy that developed when B cells encountered high-affinity, monovalent antigen in the absence of T-cell help produced a critical level of BCR occupancy to initiate an anergy program rather than activation, ensuring that self-reactive B cells make the "correct response" to prevent autoimmunity [90].

It remains unclear how well these findings apply to B cells in a normal immune system where B cells can edit their receptor by swapping light chains at the pre-B cell stage, somatically mutate and isotype-switch in response to T-cell help, and traffic in an environment that is not overpopulated by a single clone. Two studies in which some of these shortcomings were overcome demonstrated that anergy of Ig-transgenic B cells specific for DNA due to encounter with endogenous antigen was readily broken by provision of T-cell help. In one study, adoptive transfer of hemagglutinin-specific T cells into a host expressing the T-cell target antigen and anergic transgenic B cells specific to DNA induced anti-DNA antibodies [91]. Another study used a different transgenic Ig heavy chain that conferred single-stranded DNA binding activity; when these mice received allogeneic T cells, the strong T-cell help associated with the subsequent graft-versus-host reaction resulted in the appearance of anti-DNA-secreting B cells [92], in large part due to secondary rearrangement of the heavy chain driven by endogenous antigen (receptor editing in the periphery) [93]. In contrast to the behavior of anti-DNA-specific B cells, anti-HEL-specific B cells were preferentially excluded from the spleen and lymph node follicles after exposure to soluble HEL [94] or triggered to undergo Fas-mediated AICD when provided with T-cell help [77]. The seemingly opposite results between the HEL/anti-HEL systems and the anti-DNA systems cannot be readily reconciled. However, the use of receptor-transgenic mice to delineate fundamentals of immune regulation runs the risk of misleading observations because of the abnormal loci in which the transgenes come to reside and the possible anomalous *in vivo* behavior of a large population of monoclonal lymphocytes.

4.6
Breaking Tolerance

For each putative tolerance mechanism, there have been numerous descriptions of its breakdown that could lead to autoimmunity. Genetic alterations in intracellular signaling pathways are prime candidates because enhanced signaling through the antigen receptor, reduced signaling through inhibitory receptors, or abnormalities in intracellular negative regulators of lymphocyte activation could readily contribute to autoreactivity (reviewed in [95]). Also, extracellular factors that could influence tolerance and contribute to autoimmunity have been invoked, such as viral- or bacterial-derived antigens that cross-react with the BCR or TCR (reviewed in [96]), coincidental signaling through Toll-like receptors to enhance APC function by pathogens (reviewed in [97]), or even self-materials [98] or increased self-antigen load due to a deficiency in antigen clearance machinery [99]. However, of primary importance in the productive activation of B cells is the availability of T-cell help, because somatic mutation to produce the high-affinity antibodies that characterize protective immunity and of autoantibodies that can arise spontaneously in autoimmune disease generally requires the action of CD4$^+$ T-helper cells (see Chapter 5).

Even in autoimmune mouse strains where B-cell defects have been described, T cells are necessary for full expression of autoimmune disease (reviewed in [100]). Of all the B-cell tolerance mechanisms, only deletion, the ultimate form of tolerance, can resist strong T-cell drive. However, there is no shortage of newly emerging autoreactive B cells that escape negative selection and receptor editing; in a recent study 4% of the normal, mature B-cell repertoire had autoreactivity to native DNA [82], the prototypic target of autoantibodies in systemic lupus erythematosus (see Chapter 11). Furthermore, somatic mutation driven by Th and self-antigen could readily convert weakly autoreactive B cells to produce high-affinity autoantibodies [101]. Taken together, it is difficult to escape the conclusion that the onus for control of immune tolerance is the predominate purview of the T-cell repertoire.

4.7
Concluding Remarks

Intolerance to infectious agents and tolerance to self would seem to be the aim of an ideal immune system, and elaborate machinery to protect against foreign intrusions while avoiding pathogenic self-reactivity has been assembled by the immune system. However, it is a messy arrangement involving a patchwork of mechanisms in which various processes for minimizing autoreactivity have been cobbled together during the evolution of the adaptive immune system, filling loopholes or gaps in the tolerance machinery that resulted in failure to thrive or to survive long enough to reproduce. The adaptive immune system presumably preserved the most effective features of this sporadically acquired tolerance machinery. However, the way these processes are currently defined is at least in part an intellectual construct that tries to make sense of phenomena that probably arose over the course of 200 million years. Gradual improvements during the evolution of the adaptive immune system may not readily conceptualize into coherent mechanisms. As a result, some of our current ideas about immune tolerance will prove to be wrong or at least their importance overemphasized; others have yet to be discovered. The challenges inherent in having an adaptive immune system are surpassed only by the challenges in explaining it and in exploiting opportunities for enhancing immunity to pathogens and subverting its tendency to autoreactivity.

Acknowledgments

I thank Bryce Chackerian, Ph.D., for critical reading of the manuscript. This work was supported in part by NIH Grant ES06334.

References

1 B. Rocha, A. Grandien, A. A. Freitas, *J. Exp. Med.* **1995**, 181, 993–1003.
2 C. Benoist, D. Mathis, *Nat. Immunol.* **2001**, 2, 797–801.
3 H. von Boehmer, *Cell* **1994**, 76, 219–228.
4 J. Alberola-Ila, K. A. Forbush, R. Seger, E. G. Krebs, R. G. Perlmutter, *Nature* **1995**, 373, 620–623.
5 W. C. Sha et al., *Proc. Natl. Acad. Sci. USA* **1990**, 87, 6186–6190.
6 J. Nikolic-Zugic, M. J. Bevan, *Nature* **1990**, 344, 65–67.
7 H. Jacobs, H. von Boehmer, C. J. M. Melief, A. Berns, *Eur. J. Immunol.* **1990**, 20, 2333–2337.
8 P. G. Ashton-Rickardt et al., *Cell* **1994**, 76, 651–663.
9 E. Sebzda et al., *Science* **1994**, 263, 1615–1618.
10 J. W. Kappler, N. Roehm, P. C. Marrack, *Cell* **1987**, 149, 273–280.
11 P. Kisielow, H. Blüthmann, U. D. Staerz, M. Steinmetz, H. von Boehmer, *Nature* **1988**, 333, 742–746.
12 D. Lo, J. Sprent, *Nature* **1986**, 319, 672–675.
13 L. C. Burkly et al., *J. Immunol.* **1993**, 151, 3954–3960.
14 S. Degermann, C. D. Surh, L. H. Glimcher, J. Sprent, D. Lo, *J. Immunol.* **1994**, 152, 3254–3263.
15 T. M. Laufer, J. DeKoning, J. S. Markowitz, D. Lo, L. H. Glimcher, *Nature* **1996**, 383, 81–85.
16 J. P. M. van Meerwijk et al., *J. Exp. Med.* **1997**, 185, 377–383.
17 F. Ramsdell, T. Lantz, B. J. Fowlkes, *Science* **1989**, 246, 1038–1041.
18 J. L. Roberts, S. O. Sharrow, A. Singer, *J. Exp. Med.* **1990**, 171, 935–940.
19 D. E. Speiser, Y. Chvatchko, R. M. Zinkernagel, H. R. MacDonald, *J. Exp. Med.* **1990**, 172, 1305–1314.
20 E.-K. Gao, D. Lo, J. Sprent, *J. Exp. Med.* **1990**, 171, 1101–1121.
21 K. B. Urdahl, D. M. Pardoll, M. K. Jenkins, *Int. Immunol.* **1992**, 4, 1341–1349.
22 M. K. Jenkins, R. H. Schwartz, D. M. Pardoll, *Science* **1988**, 241, 1655–1658.
23 G. J. Prud'homme, R. Sander, N. A. Parfey, H. Ste-Croix, *J. Autoimmun.* **1991**, 4, 357–368.
24 J. X. Gao et al., *J. Exp. Med.* **2002**, 195, 959–971.
25 A. Khan, Y. Tomita, M. Sykes, *Transplantation* **1996**, 62, 380–387.

26 L. Klein, B. Kyewski, *Curr. Opin. Immunol.* **2000**, 12, 179–186.

27 J. Derbinski, A. Schulte, B. Kyewski, L. Klein, *Nat. Immunol.* **2001**, 2, 1032–1039.

28 M. S. Anderson et al., *Science* **2002**, 298, 1395–1401.

29 K. Nagamine et al., *Nat. Genet.* **1997**, 17, 393–398.

30 J. Sprent, C. D. Surh, *Nat. Immunol.* **2003**, 4, 303–304.

31 A. Liston, S. Lesage, J. Wilson, L. Peltonen, C. C. Goodnow, *Nat. Immunol.* **2003**, 4, 350–354.

32 S. Lesage et al., *J. Exp. Med.* **2002**, 196, 1175–1188.

33 V. Muller, S. Bonhoeffer, *Trends Immunol.* **2003**, 24, 132–135.

34 G. L. Stephens, J. D. Ashwell, L. Ignatowicz, *Int. Immunol.* **2003**, 15, 623–632.

35 P. S. Ohashi, *Curr. Opinion Immunol.* **1996**, 8, 808–814.

36 R. L. Rubin, A. Kretz-Rommel, *Crit. Rev. Immunol.* **1999**, 19, 199–218.

37 S. Sakaguchi et al., *Immunol. Rev.* **2001**, 182, 18–32.

38 E. M. Shevach, *Annu. Rev. Immunol.* **2000**, 18, 423–449.

39 Z. Fehervari, S. Sakaguchi, *Curr. Opin. Immunol.* **2004**, 16, 203–208.

40 M. S. Jordan et al., *Nat. Immunol.* **2001**, 2, 301–306.

41 I. Apostolou, A. Sarukhan, L. Klein, H. von Boehmer, *Nat. Immunol.* **2002**, 3, 756–763.

42 G. L. Stephens, L. Ignatowicz, *Eur. J. Immunol.* **2003**, 33, 1282–1291.

43 K. Kawahata et al., *J. Immunol.* **2002**, 168, 4399–4405.

44 S. Hori, T. Nomura, S. Sakaguchi, *Science* **2003**, 299, 1057–1061.

45 A. Kumanogoh et al., *J. Immunol.* **2001**, 166, 353–360.

46 B. Salomon et al., *Immunity* **2000**, 12, 431–440.

47 J. A. Bluestone, A. K. Abbas, *Nat. Rev. Immunol.* **2003**, 3, 253–257.

48 J. Lohr, B. Knoechel, E. C. Kahn, A. K. Abbas, *J. Immunol.* **2004**, 173, 5028–5035.

49 D. L. Jacobson, A. N. Ganges, N. R. Rose, N. M. H. Graham, *Clin. Immunol. Immunopathol.* **1997**, 84, 223–243.

50 M. A. Curotto de Lafaille, J. J. Lafaille, *Curr. Opin. Immunol.* **2002**, 14, 771–778.

51 D. Dieckmann, C. H. Bruett, H. Ploettner, M. B. Lutz, G. Schuler, *J. Exp. Med.* **2002**, 196, 247–253.

52 H. Jonuleit et al., *J. Exp. Med.* **2002**, 196, 255–260.

53 K. Kawahata et al., *J. Immunol.* **2002**, 168, 1103–1112.

54 V. Viglietta, C. Baecher-Allan, H. L. Weiner, D. A. Hafler, *J. Exp. Med.* **2004**, 199, 971–979.

55 E. M. Ling et al., *Lancet* **2004**, 363, 608–615.

56 T. J. Curiel et al., *Nat. Med.* **2004**, 10, 942–949.

57 C. L. Bennett et al., *Nat. Genet.* **2001**, 27, 20–21.

58 R. H. Schwartz, *Science* **1990**, 248, 1349–1356.

59 D. G. Telander, D. L. Mueller, *J. Immunol.* **1997**, 158, 4704–4713.

60 M. K. Jenkins, C. Chen, G. Jung, D. L. Mueller, R. H. Schwartz, *J. Immunol.* **1990**, 144, 16–22.

61 F. Andris, S. Denanglaire, F. de Mattia, J. Urbain, O. Leo, *J. Immunol.* **2004**, 173, 3201–3208.

62 S. K. Lathrop et al., *J. Immunol.* **2004**, 172, 6735–6743.

63 R. H. Schwartz, *Annu. Rev. Immunol.* **2003**, 21, 305–334.

64 D. H. Kono, A. N. Theofilopoulos, The genetics of murine lupus erythematosus in *Dubois' Lupus Erythematosus*, 6th edition, D. J. Wallace, B. H. Hahn (Eds.) Lippincott, Williams and Wilkins, 2002, 121–143.

65 C. P. Larsen et al., *Nature* **1996**, 381, 434–438.

66 B. K. Finck, P. S. Linsley, D. Wofsy, *Science* **1994**, 265, 1225–1227.

67 J. R. Abrams et al., *J. Clin. Invest.* **1999**, 103, 1243–1252.

68 J. Westermann, R. Pabst, *Immunol. Today* **1996**, 17, 278–282.

69 Reis e Sousa, *Curr. Opin. Immunol.* **2004**, 16, 21–25.

70 F. Rieux-Laucat et al., *Blood* **1999**, 94, 2575–2582.

71 E. Dondi, G. Roue, V. J. Yuste, S. A. Susin, S. Pellegrini, *J. Immunol.* **2004**, 173, 3740–3747.

72 D. Moskophidis, F. Lechner, H. Pircher, R. M. Zinkernagel, *Nature* **1993**, 362, 758–761.

73 E. Bonfoco et al., *Immunity* **1998**, 9, 711–720.

74 E. A. Reap, D. Leslie, M. Abrahams, R. A. Eisenberg, P. L. Cohen, *J. Immunol.* **1995**, 154, 936–943.

75 E. S. Sobel et al., *J. Exp. Med.* **1991**, 173, 1441–1449.

76 A. D. Steinberg, J. B. Roths, E. D. Murphy, R. T. Steinberg, E. S. Raveche, *J. Immunol.* **1980**, 125, 871–873.

77 J. C. Rathmell et al., *Nature* **1995**, 376, 181–183.

78 D. A. Nemazee, K. Burki, *Nature* **1989**, 337, 562–566.

79 M. Okamoto et al., *J. Exp. Med.* **1992**, 175, 71–79.

80 D. M. Allman, S. E. Ferguson, V. M. Lentz, M. P. Cancro, *J. Immunol.* **1993**, 151, 4431–4444.

81 A. G. Rolink, J. Andersson, F. Melchers, *Eur. J. Immunol.* **1998**, 28, 3738–3748.

82 H. Wardemann et al., *Science* **2003**, 301, 1374–1377.

83 D. Nemazee, *Adv. Immunol.* **2000**, 74, 89–126.

84 S. L. Tiegs, D. M. Russell, D. Nemazee, *J. Exp. Med.* **1993**, 177, 1009–1020.

85 D. Gay, T. Saunders, S. Camper, M. Weigert, *J. Exp. Med.* **1993**, 177, 999–1008.

86 M. Z. Radic, J. Erikson, S. Litwin, M. Weigert, *J. Exp. Med.* **1993**, 177, 1165–1173.

87 Y. Pewzner-Jung et al., *J. Immunol.* **1998**, 161, 4634–4645.

88 H. Wardemann, J. Hammersen, M. C. Nussenzweig, *J. Exp. Med.* **2004**, 200, 191–199.

89 C. C. Goodnow, J. Crosbie, H. Jorgensen, R. A. Brink, A. Basten, *Nature* **1989**, 342, 385–391.

90 C. C. Goodnow, S. Adelstein, A. Basten, *Science* **2004**, 248, 1373–1379.

91 S. J. Seo et al., *Immunity* **2002**, 16, 535–546.

92 D. R. Sekiguchi et al., *J. Immunol.* **2002**, 168, 4142–4153.

93 D. R. Sekiguchi, R. A. Eisenberg, M. Weigert, *J. Exp. Med.* **2003**, 197, 27–39.

94 J. G. Cyster, S. B. Hartley, C. C. Goodnow, *Nature* **1994**, 371, 389–395.

95 P. S. Ohashi, A. L. DeFranco, *Curr. Opin. Immunol.* **2002**, 14, 744–759.

96 C. L. Vanderlugt, S. D. Miller, *Nat. Rev Immunol.* **2002**, 2, 85–95.

97 B. Beutler, *Nature* **2004**, 430, 257–263.

98 E. A. Leadbetter et al., *Nature* **2002**, 416, 603–607.

99 U. S. Gaipl et al., *Arthritis Rheum.* **2004**, 50, 640–649.

100 A. N. Theofilopoulos, Murine models of lupus in *Systemic lupus erythematosus,* 2nd edition, R. G. Lahita (Ed.) Churchill Livingstone, New York, 1992, 121–194.

101 S. K. Ray, C. Putterman, B. Diamond, *Proc. Natl. Acad. Sci. USA* **1996**, 93, 2019–2024.

5
T-B Cell Interactions in Autoimmunity

Barbara Schraml and Stanford L. Peng

5.1
Introduction

Although to some degree all autoimmune diseases likely represent systemic hyperactivation of both T and B cells, only the autoantibody-mediated syndromes – such as systemic lupus erythematosus (SLE) or myasthenia gravis (MG) – are hallmarked by and clearly require B-cell effector functions (e.g., antibody secretion), produced with the assistance of T-cell help, to mediate disease [1–3]. SLE has remained the prototype of such diseases, and evidence for the importance of T-B interactions in autoimmunity at multiple levels has largely accumulated from studies in both animal models and patients with SLE. This chapter discusses the current understanding of collaborative interactions between T and B cells in autoimmunity, focusing primarily on insight gained from studies of SLE, MG, and other autoantibody-mediated diseases.

5.2
Direct T-B Cell Interactions: Receptor-mediated Contacts

During normal immune responses involving T-dependent antibody production, T cells are primed with antigen by antigen-presenting cells (APC), such as dendritic cells, in the T-cell zone of the secondary lymphoid organs [4] (Fig. 5.1). These activated T cells migrate to the follicular border where they interact, via MHC class II as well as costimulatory molecules such as CD28 and CD40, with activated B cells that have also encountered antigen, leading to B-cell activation, follicular entry, and germinal center (GC) formation. These transient structures foster somatic hypermutation and immunoglobulin isotype class switching, allowing the generation of high-affinity antibodies.

In model animal systems, self-reactive B cells are usually excluded from the follicular microenvironment due to (1) the lack of activated self-reactive T cells; (2) death via CD95-induced apoptosis; and/or (3) the lack of costimulatory mole-

Autoantibodies and Autoimmunity: Molecular Mechanisms in Health and Disease. Edited by K. Michael Pollard
Copyright © 2006 WILEY-VCH Verlag GmbH & Co. KGaA, Weinheim
ISBN: 3-527-31141-6

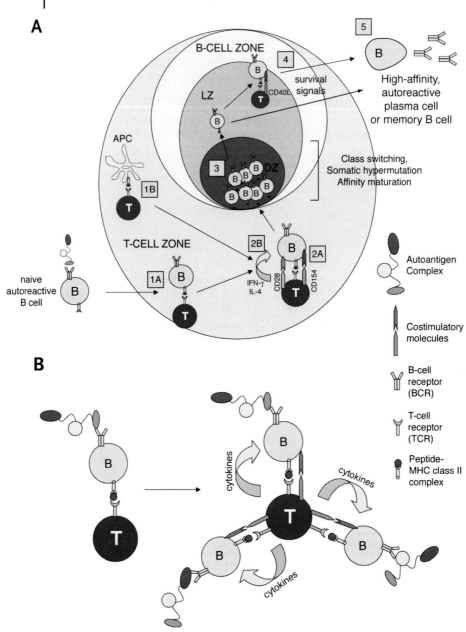

Fig. 5.1 (legend see page 87)

cule-mediated survival signals [5–7]. In autoimmune diseases, the activation and maturation of autoreactive B cells presumably reflect the loss of such control mechanisms. Autoantibodies in autoimmune diseases characteristically are iso-type-switched and display high affinity for autoantigen, implicating somatic hypermutation and affinity maturation in T-dependent germinal centers [8–10]. In addition, abnormal spontaneous germinal center formation has been observed in lupus-prone mice, including (NZB×NZW) F_1, MRL/+, MRL/*lpr*, and BXSB [11]. Consequently, many studies have investigated the role of costimula-tory molecules in disease pathogenesis, particularly in terms of their role in germinal center formation.

5.2.1
CD40-CD154

The tumor necrosis factor receptor (TNFR) superfamily member CD40 is consti-tutively expressed on B cells, while its ligand CD154 (CD40 ligand, CD40L, gp39) is expressed on activated T and B cells. Mice deficient in CD40 or CD154 fail to develop functional germinal centers and display impaired class switching in response to T-dependent antigens [12, 13]. These phenotypes presumably re-flect defective T-cell activation, although some studies suggest that activated B cells may express functional CD154 and therefore promote bystander autoreac-tive B-cell activation independent of T-cell help [14, 15]. Interestingly, CD40-

◄─────────────────────────────────────

Fig. 5.1 T cell-dependent induction of auto-immune reactions in B cell-mediated auto-immune diseases. (A) Initiation of autoreac-tive B- and T-cell activation. Autoreactive T cells are activated when autoreactive B cells encounter antigen in the periphery, travel to lymphoid organs, and act as antigen-presenting cells (APC, 1A), or when profes-sional APCs process and present autoanti-gens and/or other T-cell epitopes in the T-cell zone (1B). These activated T cells can then in turn activate the same or other auto-reactive B cells via costimulatory molecules such as CD154 and/or CD28 (2A), or by se-creting cytokines such as IFN-γ and/or IL-4 (2B), which promote and/or augment B-cell activation and class switching. Activated autoreactive B cells then travel to the B-cell zone where they form germinal centers and undergo class switching, somatic hypermu-tation, and affinity maturation in the dark zone (DZ, 3). They escape apoptosis by receiving survival signals in the light zone (LZ, 4), either from activated T cells (CD154, cytokines, etc.) or other APCs (BAFF, etc.), eventually exiting the follicular reaction as autoantibody-secreting plasma cells or memory B cells (5). Effective thera-peutic manipulations in T-B interactions have involved both costimulatory and cyto-kine blockade, which presumably disrupt steps (2) and/or (4). (B) Amplification and epitope spreading of autoimmunity. Once activated, an autoreactive B cell specific for a determinant in an autoantigenic complex internalizes the antigens, processes them, and can present any epitope derived from this complex via MHC class II. T cells recog-nizing such an epitope become activated, upregulate costimulatory molecules and secrete cytokines, and can interact with and activate other B cells displaying the proper T-cell epitope on their surface, even though their BCRs recognize different B-cell epi-topes. As such, autoantigenic determinants expand and amplify during autoimmune inflammation.

Table 5.1 Costimulatory interventions in systemic lupus erythematosus[a)].

System/ Intervention	Model	Anti-DNA	Glomerulonephritis	Ref.
CD40/CD154				
Anti-CD154	(SWR×NZW) F_1	↓↓	↓↓	17
Anti-CD154	(NZB×NZW) F_1	↓↓	↓↓	24, 200
Anti-CD154	Human SLE	↓	↓	25
CD154 −/−	MRL/*lpr*	↓↓	↓↓	22, 23
CD28				
CD28 −/−	MRL/*lpr*	↓↓	↓↓	46
Anti-CD80	MRL/*lpr*	→	→	49
Anti-CD86	MRL/*lpr*	↓	→	49
Anti-CD80/CD86	MRL/*lpr*	↓↓	↓↓	49
Anti-CD80	(NZB×NZW) F_1	→	→	52
Anti-CD86	(NZB×NZW) F_1	↓↓	↓↓	52
CD80 −/−	MRL/*lpr*	→	↑	49
CD86 −/−	MRL/*lpr*	→	↓	49
CD80/CD86 −/−	MRL/*lpr*	↓↓	↓↓	48
Anti-B7H	(NZB×NZW) F_1	↓↓	↓↓	50
CTLA4Ig	MRL/*lpr*	↓↓	↓↓	47
CTLA4Ig	(NZB×NZW) F_1	↓↓	↓↓	51, 201
CD137				
Anti-CD137	MRL/*lpr*	↓↓	↓↓	58
Anti-CD137	(NZB×NZW) F_1	↓↓	↓↓	59

a) Effect of blocking antibodies or genetic deficiencies on the autoimmune syndromes of humans and mice with lupus. Significant versus mild reductions in the indicated disease parameters are indicated by ↓↓ and ↓, respectively; significant versus mild exacerbations in the indicated disease parameters are indicated by ↑↑ and ↑, respectively; no significant difference in a disease parameter is indicated by →.

CD154 interactions may also be required at least in part for the maintenance of T-cell tolerance [16].

Nonetheless, the dominant importance of CD40-CD154 in the pathogenic arm of autoimmune diseases has been repeatedly demonstrated in multiple studies (Tables 5.1 to 5.3). Several investigations have demonstrated abnormal expression of CD154 by both B and T cells in humans and mice with autoimmune diseases such as SLE [17–20], perhaps reflecting a primary defect in signaling molecules [21]. In addition, CD154-deficient MRL/*lpr* mice are generally protected from the development of IgG hypergammaglobulinemia, anti-DNA autoantibodies, and renal disease [22, 23], and anti-CD154 antibody treatment significantly delayed the development of anti-DNA antibodies and glomerulonephritis in both lupus-prone (NZB×SWR) F_1 and (NZB×NZW) F_1 mice [17, 24], as well as in humans with SLE [25]. Similarly, intervention in the CD40-CD154 system protects against autoantibody and other autoimmune manifestations in

Table 5.2 Costimulatory interventions in myasthenia gravis [a].

System/ Intervention	Model[b]	Anti-AchR[b]	Myopathy	Ref.
CD40/CD154				
Anti-CD154	Rat-EAMG	↓↓	↓↓	27
CD154 −/−	B6-EAMG	↓↓	↓↓	26
CD28				
CD28 −/−	B6-EAMG	↓	↓	26
Anti-CD80	B6-EAMG	↓	↓	54
Anti-CD86	B6-EAMG	↓↓	↓↓	54
CD80 −/−	B6-EAMG	↓↓	↓↓	54
CD80/CD86 −/−	B6-EAMG	↓↓	↓↓	54
CTLA4Ig	Rat-EAMG	↓↓	↓↓	53

a) Effect of blocking antibodies or genetic deficiencies on the autoimmune syndromes of rodents with experimental myasthenia gravis. Significant versus mild reductions in the indicated disease parameters are indicated by ↓↓ and ↓, respectively.

b) AchR = acetylcholine receptor; B6 = C57BL/6; EAMG = experimental autoimmune myasthenia gravis.

Table 5.3 CD40/CD154 interventions in other autoimmune diseases [a].

System/ Intervention	Model/ Background[b]	Autoantibodies	End-organ disease	Ref.
Anti-CD154	AO-ZP	↓↓	↓↓	28
Anti-CD154	AO-TX	↓↓	↓↓	29
Anti-CD154	Grave-scid	↓↓	→	30
Anti-CD154	Hg	↓↓	↓↓	31
Anti-CD154	KRN	↓↓	↓↓	32
Anti-CD154	GVHD	↓↓	↓↓	33
Anti-CD154	Human SSc (*in vitro*)	↓↓	ND	34
CD154 Tg	C57BL/6	↑↑	↑↑	35, 37
CD154-L929	C3H	↑↑	↑↑	36

a) Effect of blocking antibodies or other genetic alterations within the CD40/ CD154 system on various autoimmune syndromes. Significant versus mild reductions in the indicated disease parameters are indicated by ↓↓ and ↓, respectively; significant versus mild exacerbations in the indicated disease parameters are indicated by ↑↑ and ↑, respectively; no significant difference in a disease parameter is indicated by →.

b) AO-ZP = autoimmune oophoritis induced by zona pellucida peptides; AO-TX = autoimmune oophoritis induced by day-3 neonatal thymectomy; Grave-scid = Graves' thyroid tissue xenografted upon severe combined immunodeficient mice; GVHD = graft-versus-host disease; Hg = mercury-induced autoimmunity; KRN = K/B×N transgenic spontaneous arthritis mouse; SSc = systemic sclerosis (scleroderma); ND = not determined.

experimental autoimmune myasthenia gravis (EAMG) [26, 27], autoimmune oo-phoritis [28, 29], autoimmune thyroid disease [30], mercury-induced autoimmu-nity [31], the K/B×N immune-complex arthritis model [32], graft-versus-host disease [33], and systemic sclerosis [34]. Conversely, ectopic expression and/or prolonged exposure to CD154 signals can result in pathogenic autoantibody production and end-organ disease [35–37]. Thus, the CD40-CD154 system has emerged as a dominant target system in the pathogenesis and therapy of multi-ple autoimmune syndromes.

5.2.2
CD28 System

The CD28 system includes a growing family of stimulatory (e.g., CD28) and in-hibitory (CD152/CTLA4) receptors and B7 ligands (CD80/B7.1, CD86/B7.2, B7-H, B7-H1, etc.). CD28 and CD152 are expressed on T cells, while the ligands are expressed on antigen-presenting cells, including B cells. Non-autoimmune mice deficient in CD28, CD80, or CD86 exhibit impaired antibody class switch-ing and somatic hypermutation, attributed to defective germinal center forma-tion [38, 39]. Since these molecules also provide essential costimulatory signals to T cells during the interaction of their TCR with peptide-MHC complexes, their role in GC development likely reflects their critical role in T-cell activation.

Several clinical observations have strongly implicated a pathogenic role for the CD28-related molecules in autoantibody-mediated diseases: abnormal ex-pression of CD28 and related molecules have been demonstrated in autoanti-body-mediated diseases such as MG and SLE [40, 41], and genetic polymorph-isms in CD152 have been found in association with autoimmune thyroid disease and MG [42, 43]. In addition, B7-reactive autoantibodies present in patients' sera may promote autoreactivity by costimulating autoreactive lymph-ocytes [44]. On the other hand, as for CD40-CD154, some studies have sug-gested a tolerogenic role for the B7 molecules [45].

Still, interventions upon the CD28 system have consistently revealed an im-portant role of these molecules in the pathogenesis of autoimmunity (Tables 5.1, 5.2, and 5.4): lupus-prone MRL/*lpr* mice deficient in CD28 or in both CD80 and CD86 develop significantly lower autoantibody titers, associated with dimin-ished renal disease and mortality [46–48]. Interestingly, blockade of both CD80 and CD86 interactions, and/or B7-H, appears to be required for disease protec-tion in this model, since antibody blockade of either one is insufficient to confer protection [49, 50]. In contrast, although the CD28 system is also important in the (NZB×NZW) F$_1$ lupus model [51], CD86 blockade alone is sufficient to sup-press autoantibody production and renal disease [52]. In EAMG, blockade of the CD28 system is effective in reducing autoantibodies and disease and can be achieved with deficiency in either CD80 or CD86 alone [26, 53, 54]. Similarly successful findings have been reported with CD28 system intervention in graft-versus-host disease [55], mercury-induced autoimmunity [31], experimental oo-phoritis [28], collagen-induced arthritis [56], and an anti-glomerular basement

Table 5.4 CD28 system interventions in other autoimmune diseases[a].

System/ Intervention	Model/ Background[b]	Autoantibodies	End-organ disease	Ref.
CTLA4Ig	AO-ZP	↓↓	↓↓	28
CTLA4Ig	CIA	↓↓	↓↓	56
CTLA4Ig	EAG	↓↓	↓↓	57
CTLA4Ig	GVHD	↓↓	↓↓	55
CTLA4Ig	Hg	↓↓	↓↓	31
Anti-CTLA4	CIA	→	→	56

a) Effect of blocking antibodies or other genetic alterations within the CD28 system on various autoimmune syndromes. Significant versus mild reductions in the indicated disease parameters are indicated by ↓↓ and ↓, respectively; no significant difference in a disease parameter is indicated by →.

b) AO-ZP = autoimmune oophoritis induced by zona pellucida peptides; CIA = collagen-induced arthritis; EAG = experimental autoimmune glomerulonephritis; GVHD = graft-versus-host disease; Hg = mercury-induced autoimmunity.

membrane model of glomerulonephritis [57]. Thus, although the relative roles and importance of the various B7 molecules likely differ between different disease subsets, the CD28 system overall clearly plays a critical role in the generation of affinity-matured, class-switched pathogenic autoantibodies.

5.2.3
Other Costimulatory Systems

Although accumulating studies have demonstrated the importance of other costimulatory systems in antibody production during conventional immune responses, relatively few have directly addressed their roles in autoreactive T-B interactions. For example, CD137 (4-1BB) antibodies inhibit autoantibody production in both MRL/*lpr* and (NZB×NZW) F$_1$ lupus-prone mice [58, 59], as well as in graft-versus-host disease models [60], but may exert an indirect effect via CD8 cells, rather than upon the interaction between helper T cells and autoreactive B cells. In addition, several studies have demonstrated abnormal expression of CD134 (OX40 ligand) in SLE [61] and MG [62], as well as of CD30 in SLE [63], autoimmune thyroid disease [64], systemic sclerosis [65], pemphigoid [66], and primary biliary cirrhosis [67]. Other studies have suggested both inhibitory and costimulatory functions for tumor necrosis factor–related apoptosis-inducing ligand (TRAIL) [68, 69], and PD-1 deficiency can cause a lupus-like arthritis and glomerulonephritis, as well as an autoantibody-mediated cardiomyopathy [70, 71]. Thus, multiple additional costimulatory systems may modulate the interactions between T and B cells, possibly in both protective and pathogenic fashions.

5.2.4
Cell Death

In addition to activation, T-B cell interactions may also result in cell death or apoptosis, generally of the B cell [72]. Such interactions typically involve death receptors such as CD95 (Fas), TNFR1 (TNF receptor-1), and the TRAIL receptors DR4 and DR5, whose dysfunction may lead to autoimmune manifestations, in part due to the inability to exclude autoreactive B cells from the lymphoid follicle and germinal center reaction [5, 73, 74]. However, a detailed description of cell death and apoptosis in autoimmunity is beyond the scope of this chapter, and the reader is directed to other sections of this book for further details (e.g., see Chapters 4 and 6).

5.3
Indirect T-B Cell Interactions: Soluble Mediators

5.3.1
Th1 versus Th2 Cytokines in Humoral Autoimmunity

During immune responses, all helper CD4+ T (Th) cells produce interleukin-3 (IL-3) and granulocyte-macrophage colony-stimulating factor (GM-CSF), but differences in environmental stimulation skews them broadly towards two subtypes bearing distinct patterns of cytokine production: (1) Th1 cells, which produce predominantly IL-2, interferon-γ (IFN-γ), lymphotoxin (LT), and tumor necrosis factor-a (TNF-a); and (2) Th2 cells, which produce IL-4, IL-5, IL-6, IL-9, IL-10, and IL-13 [75–77]. This dichotomy has become less clear as recent studies have further detailed the increasingly complex environments of natural immune responses [78, 79], but nevertheless it has remained of great utility because Th1 cytokines have consistently been associated with cellular immune functions, such as delayed-type hypersensitivity and macrophage activation, while Th2 cytokines have been associated with B cell–dependent antibody responses, such as allergy [76, 80]. As such, humoral autoimmune diseases were initially predicted to be Th2 response-dominated [81, 82]; however, continued investigation has revealed a Th1-predominance in several autoantibody-mediated diseases, including SLE [83–86], MG [87, 88], and autoimmune gastritis [89]. Still, Th2 predominance is seen in syndromes such as pemphigus vulgaris [90, 91] and even in some facets of Th1-predominant diseases, such as the intrarenal T cells in SLE [92]. Other diseases fail to demonstrate any particular Th1/Th2 skewing, such as primary biliary cirrhosis [93]. As such, while T cell–derived cytokines clearly promote humoral autoimmunity, the relative importance and distinction between the Th1- versus Th2-related types of response may not apply absolutely to these diseases. Nonetheless, several cytokines clearly propagate the autoimmune collaboration between T and B cells (Tables 5.5 to 5.7 and Figure 5.1).

Table 5.5 Cytokine interventions in systemic lupus erythematosus[a)].

Cytokine/ Intervention	Model[b)]	Anti-DNA	Glomerulo-nephritis	Ref.
IFN-γ				
rIFN-γ	(NZB×NZW) F$_1$	↑↑	↑↑	96
Anti-IFN-γ	MRL/*lpr*	ND	→	202
Anti-IFN-γ	(NZB×NZW) F$_1$	↓↓	↓	97
IFN-γ −/−	MRL/*lpr*	↓↓	↓↓	99-102
IFN-γR −/−	(NZB×NZW) F$_1$	↓↓	↓↓	98
IL-4				
Anti-IL-4	(NZB×NZW) F$_1$	↓↓	↓↓	111
IL-4 −/−	MRL/*lpr*	→	↓	100
IL-4 −/−	BALB/c-peptide	↑	↓	112
IL-4 −/−	BXSB	→	→	113
IL-4 Tg	(NZW×B6.Yaa) F$_1$	↓	↓↓	114
IL-6				
Anti-IL-6	(NZB×NZW) F$_1$	↓↓	↓↓	141
IL-6 −/−	BALB/c-pristane	↓↓	↓↓	142
IL-10				
rIL-10	(NZB×NZW) F$_1$	↑↑	↑↑	157
Anti-IL-10	(NZB× NZW) F$_1$	↓↓	↓↓	157
Anti-IL-10	Human SLE	↓↓	ND	158–160
IL-10 −/−	MRL/*lpr*	↑↑	↑↑	165

a) Effect of cytokine modulations in systemic lupus erythematosus. Significant versus mild reductions in the indicated disease parameters are indicated by ↓↓ and ↓, respectively; significant versus mild exacerbations in the indicated disease parameters are indicated by ↑↑ and ↑, respectively; no significant difference in a disease parameter is indicated by →.

b) BALB/c-peptide=DWEYSVWLSN-induced lupus in BALB/c mice. ND=not determined.

5.3.2
IFN-γ

IFN-γ, the prototypical Th1 cytokine, exerts pleiotropic effects upon B cells, up-regulating MHC class II and promoting class switching to IgG2a and possibly IgG3 [94, 95]. Treatment of lupus-prone (NZB×NZW) F$_1$ mice with IFN-γ exacerbated autoantibody production and mortality [96], while treatment with neutralizing antibody to IFN-γ or IFN-γ receptor deficiency significantly delayed the development of anti-DNA antibodies and renal disease [97, 98]. Similar results have been described with IFN-γ or IFN-γ receptor deficiency on the lupus-prone MRL/*lpr* background [99–102], as well as in EAMG [103–107]. These results have been largely attributed to the importance of IFN-γ in the promotion in B cells of "Th1-like" IgG isotypes, particularly IgG2a and IgG3, which are likely particularly pathogenic in autoantibody-mediated, immune-complex diseases

5.3.4
IL-6

IL-6, produced by both B and T cells, regulates B-cell proliferation and differentiation, particularly of terminally differentiated plasma cells [124–126]. Given the importance of plasma cells in antibody secretion in humoral autoimmune diseases [10, 127–132], IL-6 has remained an attractive pathogenic and therapeutic target in humoral autoimmunity. Indeed, IL-6 levels are often elevated in human and murine SLE [133–136], where constitutive expression of the IL-6 receptor has also been demonstrated [137]. In addition, thymic cells from patients with MG and thyroiditis often overproduce IL-6 [138–140].

However, definitive evidence for IL-6 in these diseases remains largely scant, albeit encouraging. Neutralizing anti-IL-6 treatment of $(NZB \times NZW)$ F_1 mice reduced anti-dsDNA titers, delaying the onset of kidney disease and prolonging survival [141], while IL-6 deficiency abrogated anti-DNA, but not anti-snRNP, autoantibody production in the pristane model of experimental SLE [142]. In one study with EAMG, IL-6 deficiency also prevented significant autoantibody formation and end-organ disease [143], and, at least *in vitro*, IL-6 may be important in the production of anti-topoisomerase I autoantibodies in systemic sclerosis [144]. These effects may relate to a role for IL-6 in B-cell activation, perhaps in the promotion of germinal center formation and/or plasma cell differentiation [145].

5.3.5
IL-10

As a promoter of B-cell growth and differentiation, IL-10, produced by T cells, B cells, and macrophages, has been proposed as a pathogenic agent in humoral autoimmunity [146, 147]. However, it also exerts inhibitory effects, particularly on T cells, likely via its role in regulatory T cells [147]. Nonetheless, evidence of elevated IL-10 activity has often been found in these diseases, including SLE [148–150] and rheumatoid arthritis [151]. Furthermore, genetic polymorphisms in the IL-10 promoter are associated with autoantibody production and disease in SLE [152–155] and RA [156], suggesting that IL-10 may play a truly etiologic role in disease.

In SLE, continuous administration of IL-10 to $(NZB \times NZW)$ F_1 mice accelerates the development of autoantibodies and renal disease, whereas neutralizing anti-IL-10 treatment significantly reduces autoantibody production, nephritis, and mortality [157]. Neutralization of IL-10, both *in vivo* and *in vitro*, appears to abrogate the hyperactivity of human SLE lymphocytes and improve disease parameters [158–160]. Similarly, in an animal model of autoimmune hemolytic anemia, IL-10 administration exacerbated anti-RBC antibodies and anemia [161], while anti-IL-10 therapy largely prevented autoantibody production and anemia [162]. In EAMG, overexpression of IL-10 promotes autoantibody production and disease [163, 164]. Thus, in several settings IL-10 plays a clear pathogenic role.

However, IL-10-deficient lupus-prone MRL/*lpr* mice develop exacerbated anti-DNA autoantibody production and end-organ disease, associated with accentuated Th1 responses [165], and in at least some cases of human SLE, IL-10 promotes CD95-mediated activation-induced cell death [166], supporting an important role for this cytokine in immunoregulation. Indeed, in diabetes-prone NOD mice, adenoviral vector–mediated delivery of IL-10 attenuates anti-insulin antibodies and diabetes [167]; in a passive transfer model of pemphigus vulgaris, IL-10 suppresses, while IL-10 deficiency exacerbates, disease [168]; and in EAT, IL-10 administration improves thyroiditis in association with increasing the IgG1/IgG2a autoantibody isotype ratio [169, 170]. Thus, like other cytokines, IL-10 likely possesses both pathogenic and protective roles, with different relative importance in different diseases.

5.3.6
Other Cytokines

Several other T cell- or B cell-derived cytokines may also participate in the pathogenesis of humoral autoimmune diseases. For example, IL-5, produced by T cells, has been demonstrated to exacerbate autoantibodies in a murine model of AIHA [161] as well as in the (NZB × NZW) F_1 murine lupus model [81]. Prior studies have implicated IL-12 – which is primarily produced by macrophages but is also produced by B cells [171] – in the pathogenesis of EAT [172], EAMG [106, 173], (NZB×NZW) F_1, and MRL/*lpr* lupus [111, 174], as well as in collagen-induced arthritis [175]. But other studies have suggested that it may be protective, at least in mercury-induced autoimmunity [176] and GVHD [177, 178]. However, given the recent discovery of multiple members of the IL-12 family that share common active subunits, such as IL-23 and IL-27, these findings are likely confounded and thus require revisitation [179]. Finally, soluble forms of surface receptors, such as soluble CD154 [180, 181], have been described in these diseases. Thus, pathological contexts for many additional soluble mediators remain to be defined.

5.4
The Nature of T-B Interactions in Autoimmunity: Ongoing Issues

The majority of interactions between T and B cells in autoimmunity are presumed to involve the active provision of helper functions by T cells upon autoreactive B cells to secrete autoantibodies (Figure 5.1) [2]. In such a model, autoreactive T cells, activated via the cognate recognition of autoantigenic peptide complexed with MHC on the surface of an activated APC, subsequently activate autoreactive B cells, which present the same autoantigenic peptide-MHC complex to the T cell. Such interactions promote subsequent B-cell activation and autoantibody secretion via these aforementioned costimulatory molecules and cytokines.

The initial T-cell help given to B cells, however, need not be self-reactive, or even autoantigen-specific. For instance, DNA-peptide complexes can induce pathogenic anti-DNA responses in mice in a hapten-carrier-like fashion, where DNA is the hapten [182], and viral proteins may complex with self-antigens like DNA, eliciting viral peptide-driven autoreactive responses [183]. Indeed, T cells are not required for the generation of autoantibodies per se, but autoantibodies that arise in the absence of T cells lack the high-affinity, class-switched characteristics of pathogenic autoantibodies [184, 185]. Accordingly, non-autoantigen-specific T cells [186], or T cells of limited repertoire [187], are capable of augmenting autoantibody production by B cells but still are unable to promote the production of high-affinity, class-switched autoantibodies. Thus, autoantigen-specific T cells are not required for the initiation of autoreactive B-cell responses, but some autoantigen specificity by T cells is necessary to propagate and/or mature such responses to acquire fully pathogenic characteristics.

Such true autoantigen-specific T cells respond to classically predictable components of the autoantigens themselves; for example, in lupus these may include histone-derived [188–190] or interestingly autoantibody immunoglobulin-derived [191] peptides. Such observations suggest that B cells themselves may participate in the activation of pathogenic T cells: for example, anti-histone (DNA) B cells could take up autoantigens via B-cell receptor-mediated endocytosis and then process and present either autoantigenic or Ig peptides to T cells. These B cells could be of autoantigen specificities different from that of the responding T cell(s), leading to epitope spreading and diversification of the activated autoimmune repertoire [192]. Such a concept is supported by studies in murine lupus, where B-cell deficiency abrogates T cell–mediated cellular autoimmunity independent of an effect on autoantibody secretion [193, 194]. Thus, in addition to their role in autoantibody secretion, autoimmune B cells may also trigger autoimmunity by acting as the initial antigen presenting cells to autoreactive T cells. Similarly, potentially critical APC functions for B cells may also be required for diabetes [195–197] and possibly for multiple sclerosis [198]; however, this effect may reflect a requirement for B cells to secrete autoantibodies, which themselves may induce end-organ injury and prime T cells [199].

In this sense, the spectrum of interactions between T and B cells in autoimmunity likely extends far beyond the simple provision of antibody-producing help by autoreactive T cells to autoreactive B cells via costimulatory molecules and cytokines. Continued further investigation will hopefully provide further insight into the immunoregulatory network in these autoimmune conditions, not only in terms of the factors and conditions that mediate and/or foster T-cell help to autoreactive B cells, but also in terms of the cognate antigen specificity of the T- and B-cell responses, as well as the reciprocal synergistic interactions that arise between these two populations.

References

1 B. L. Kotzin, *Cell* **1996**, *85*, 303–306.
2 M. J. Shlomchik, J. E. Craft, and M. J. Mamula, *Nature Rev. Immunol.* **2001**, *1*, 147–153.
3 M. Milani, N. Ostlie, W. Wang, and B. M. Conti-Fine, *Ann. NY Acad. Sci.* **2003**, *998*, 284–307.
4 T. Manser, *J. Immunol.* **2004**, *172*, 3369–3375.
5 J. G. Cyster, *Immunol. Rev.* **1997**, *156*, 87–101.
6 B. Pulendran, R. van Driel, and G. J. Nossal, *Immunol. Today* **1997**, *18*, 27–32.
7 M. van Eijk, T. Defrance, A. Hennino, and C. de Groot, *Trends Immunol.* **2001**, *22*, 677–682.
8 M. J. Shlomchik, A. Marshak-Rothstein, C. B. Wolfowicz, T. L. Rothstein, M. G. Weigert, *Nature* **1987**, *328*, 805–811.
9 E. Bonifacio, M. Scirpoli, K. Kredel, M. Fuchtenbusch, and A. G. Ziegler, *J. Immunol.* **1999**, *163*, 525–532.
10 G. P. Sims, H. Shiono, N. Willcox, and D. I. Stott, *J. Immunol.* **2001**, *167*, 1935–1944.
11 I. G. Luzina, S. P. Atamas, C. E. Storrer, L. C. daSilva, G. Kelsoe, J. C. Papadimitriou, and B. S. Handwerger, *J. Leukoc. Biol.* **2001**, *70*, 578–584.
12 J. Xu, T. M. Foy, J. D. Laman, E. A. Elliott, J. J. Dunn, T. J. Waldschmidt, J. Elsemore, R. J. Noelle, and R. A. Flavell, *Immunity* **1994**, *1*, 423–431.
13 E. Castigli, F. W. Alt, L. Davidson, A. Bottaro, E. Mizoguchi, A. K. Bhan, and R. S. Geha, *Proc. Natl. Acad. Sci. USA* **1994**, *91*, 12135–12139.
14 A. C. Grammer, M. C. Bergman, Y. Miura, K. Fujita, L. S. Davis, and P. E. Lipsky, *J. Immunol.* **1995**, *154*, 4996–5010.
15 S. Blossom, E. B. Chu, W. O. Weigle, and K. M. Gilbert, *J. Immunol.* **1997**, *159*, 4580–4586.
16 A. Kumanogoh, X. Wang, I. Lee, C. Watanabe, M. Kamanaka, W. Shi, K. Yoshida, T. Sato, S. Habu, M. Itoh, N. Sakaguchi, S. Sakaguchi, and H. Kikutani, *J. Immunol.* **2001**, *166*, 353–360.
17 C. Mohan, Y. Shi, J. D. Laman, and S. K. Datta, *J. Immunol.* **1995**, *154*, 1470–1480.
18 A. Desai-Mehta, L. Lu, R. Ramsey-Goldman, and S. K. Datta, *J. Clin. Invest.* **1996**, *97*, 2063–2073.
19 M. Koshy, D. Berger, and M. K. Crow, *J. Clin. Invest.* **1996**, *98*, 826–837.
20 H. Lettesjo, G. P. Burd, and R. A. Mageed, *J. Immunol.* **2000**, *165*, 4095–4104.
21 Y. Yi, M. McNerney, and S. K. Datta, *J. Immunol.* **2000**, *165*, 6627–6634.
22 J. Ma, J. Xu, M. P. Madaio, Q. Peng, J. Zhang, I. S. Grewal, R. A. Flavell, and J. Craft, *J. Immunol.* **1996**, *157*, 417–426.
23 S. L. Peng, J. M. McNiff, M. P. Madaio, J. Ma, M. J. Owen, R. A. Flavell, A. C. Hayday, and J. Craft, *J. Immunol.* **1997**, *158*, 2464–2470.
24 G. S. Early, W. Zhao, and C. M. Burns, *J. Immunol.* **1996**, *157*, 3159–3164.
25 A. C. Grammer, R. Slota, R. Fischer, H. Gur, H. Girschick, C. Yarboro, G. G. Illei, and P. E. Lipsky, *J. Clin. Invest.* **2003**, *112*, 1506–1520.
26 F. D. Shi, B. He, H. Li, D. Matusevicius, H. Link, and H. G. Ljunggren, *Eur. J. Immunol.* **1998**, *28*, 3587–3593.
27 S. H. Im, D. Barchan, P. K. Maiti, S. Fuchs, and M. C. Souroujon, *J. Immunol.* **2001**, *166*, 6893–6898.
28 N. D. Griggs, S. S. Agersborg, R. J. Noelle, J. A. Ledbetter, P. S. Linsley, and K. S. Tung, *J. Exp. Med.* **1996**, *183*, 801–810.
29 C. Sharp, C. Thompson, E. T. Samy, R. Noelle, and K. S. Tung, *J. Immunol.* **2003**, *170*, 1667–1674.
30 E. Resetkova, K. Kawai, T. Enomoto, G. Arreaza, R. Togun, T. M. Foy, R. J. Noelle, and R. Volpe, *Thyroid* **1996**, *6*, 267–273.
31 L. Biancone, G. Andres, H. Ahn, A. Lim, C. Dai, R. Noelle, H. Yagita, C. De Martino, and I. Stamenkovic, *J. Exp. Med.* **1996**, *183*, 1473–1481.
32 D. Kyburz, D. A. Carson, and M. Corr, *Arthritis Rheum.* **2000**, *43*, 2571–2577.
33 F. H. Durie, A. Aruffo, J. Ledbetter, K. M. Crassi, W. R. Green, L. D. Fast, and R. J. Noelle, *J. Clin. Invest.* **1994**, *94*, 1333–1338.
34 M. Kuwana, T. A. Medsger, Jr., and T. M. Wright, *J. Immunol.* **1995**, *155*, 2703–2714.

35 A. Mehling, K. Loser, G. Varga, D. Metze, T. A. Luger, T. Schwarz, S. Grabbe, and S. Beissert, *J. Exp. Med.* **2001**, *194*, 615–628.

36 L. Santos-Argumedo, I. Alvarez-Maya, H. Romero-Ramirez, and L. Flores-Romo, *Eur. J. Immunol.* **2001**, *31*, 3484–3492.

37 T. Higuchi, Y. Aiba, T. Nomura, J. Matsuda, K. Mochida, M. Suzuki, H. Kikutani, T. Honjo, K. Nishioka, and T. Tsubata, *J. Immunol.* **2002**, *168*, 9–12.

38 S. E. Ferguson, S. Han, G. Kelsoe, and C. B. Thompson, *J. Immunol.* **1996**, *156*, 4576–4581.

39 F. Borriello, M. P. Sethna, S. D. Boyd, A. N. Schweitzer, E. A. Tivol, D. Jacoby, T. B. Strom, E. M. Simpson, G. J. Freeman, and A. H. Sharpe, *Immunity* **1997**, *6*, 303–313.

40 N. Teleshova, D. Matusevicius, P. Kivisakk, M. Mustafa, M. Pirskanen, and H. Link, *Muscle Nerve* **2000**, *23*, 946–953.

41 M. Bijl, G. Horst, P. C. Limburg, and C. G. Kallenberg, *Ann. Rheum. Dis.* **2001**, *60*, 523–526.

42 Y. Tomer, D. A. Greenberg, G. Barbesino, E. Concepcion, and T. F. Davies, *J. Clin. Endocrinol. Metab.* **2001**, *86*, 1687–1693.

43 X. B. Wang, M. Kakoulidou, Q. Qiu, R. Giscombe, D. Huang, R. Pirskanen, and A. K. Lefvert, *Genes Immun.* **2002**, *3*, 46–49.

44 H. Dong, S. E. Strome, E. L. Matteson, K. G. Moder, D. B. Flies, G. Zhu, H. Tamura, C. L. Driscoll, and L. Chen, *J. Clin. Invest.* **2003**, *111*, 363–370.

45 W. K. Suh, B. U. Gajewska, H. Okada, M. A. Gronski, E. M. Bertram, W. Dawicki, G. S. Duncan, J. Bukczynski, S. Plyte, A. Elia, A. Wakeham, A. Itie, S. Chung, J. Da Costa, S. Arya, T. Horan, P. Campbell, K. Gaida, P. S. Ohashi, T. H. Watts, S. K. Yoshinaga, M. R. Bray, M. Jordana, and T. W. Mak, *Nature Immunol.* **2003**, *4*, 899–906.

46 Y. Tada, K. Nagasawa, A. Ho, F. Morito, S. Koarada, O. Ushiyama, N. Suzuki, A. Ohta, and T. W. Mak, *J. Immunol.* **1999**, *163*, 3153–3159.

47 M. Takiguchi, M. Murakami, I. Nakagawa, A. Yamada, S. Chikuma, Y. Kawaguchi, A. Hashimoto, and T. Uede, *Lab. Invest.* **1999**, *79*, 317–326.

48 K. Kinoshita, G. Tesch, A. Schwarting, R. Maron, A. H. Sharpe, and V. R. Kelley, *J. Immunol.* **2000**, *164*, 6046–6056.

49 B. Liang, R. J. Gee, M. J. Kashgarian, A. H. Sharpe, and M. J. Mamula, *J. Immunol.* **1999**, *163*, 2322–2329.

50 H. Iwai, M. Abe, S. Hirose, F. Tsushima, K. Tezuka, H. Akiba, H. Yagita, K. Okumura, H. Kohsaka, N. Miyasaka, and M. Azuma, *J. Immunol.* **2003**, *171*, 2848–2854.

51 B. K. Finck, P. S. Linsley, and D. Wofsy, *Science* **1994**, *265*, 1225–1227.

52 A. Nakajima, M. Azuma, S. Kodera, S. Nuriya, A. Terashi, M. Abe, S. Hirose, T. Shirai, H. Yagita, and K. Okumura, *Eur. J. Immunol.* **1995**, *25*, 3060–3069.

53 K. R. McIntosh, P. S. Linsley, and D. B. Drachman, *Cell. Immunol.* **1995**, *166*, 103–112.

54 M. A. Poussin, E. Tuzun, E. Goluszko, B. G. Scott, H. Yang, J. U. Franco, and P. Christadoss, *J. Immunol.* **2003**, *170*, 4389–4396.

55 C. S. Via, V. Rus, P. Nguyen, P. Linsley, and W. C. Gause, *J. Immunol.* **1996**, *157*, 4258–4267.

56 E. Quattrocchi, M. J. Dallman, and M. Feldmann, *Arthritis Rheum.* **2000**, *43*, 1688–1697.

57 J. Reynolds, F. W. Tam, A. Chandraker, J. Smith, A. M. Karkar, J. Cross, R. Peach, M. H. Sayegh, and C. D. Pusey, *J. Clin. Invest.* **2000**, *105*, 643–651.

58 Y. Sun, H. M. Chen, S. K. Subudhi, J. Chen, R. Koka, L. Chen, and Y. X. Fu, *Nat. Med.* **2002**, *8*, 1405–1413.

59 J. Foell, S. Strahotin, S. P. O'Neil, M. M. McCausland, C. Suwyn, M. Haber, P. N. Chander, A. S. Bapat, X. J. Yan, N. Chiorazzi, M. K. Hoffmann, and R. S. Mittler, *J. Clin. Invest.* **2003**, *111*, 1505–1518.

60 K. Nozawa, J. Ohata, J. Sakurai, H. Hashimoto, H. Miyajima, H. Yagita, K. Okumura, and M. Azuma, *J. Immunol.* **2001**, *167*, 4981–4986.

61 J. Aten, A. Roos, N. Claessen, E. J. Schilder Tol, I. J. Ten Berge, and J. J. Weening, *J. Amer. Soc. Nephrol.* **2000**, *11*, 1426–1438.

62 J. Onodera, T. Nagata, K. Fujihara, M. Ohuchi, N. Ishii, K. Sugamura, and

Y. Itoyama, *Acta Neurol. Scand.* **2000**, *102*, 236–243.

63 F. Caligaris-Cappio, M.T. Bertero, M. Converso, A. Stacchini, F. Vinante, S. Romagnani, and G. Pizzolo, *Clin. Exp. Rheumatol.* **1995**, *13*, 339–343.

64 M. Okumura, Y. Hidaka, S. Kuroda, K. Takeoka, H. Tada, and N. Amino, *J. Clin. Endocrinol. Metab.* **1997**, *82*, 1757–1760.

65 C. Mavalia, C. Scaletti, P. Romagnani, A.M. Carossino, A. Pignone, L. Emmi, C. Pupilli, G. Pizzolo, E. Maggi, and S. Romagnani, *Am. J. Pathol.* **1997**, *151*, 1751–1758.

66 O. De Pita, A. Frezzolini, G. Cianchini, M. Ruffelli, P. Teofoli, and P. Puddu, *Arch. Dermatol. Res.* **1997**, *289*, 667–670.

67 S.M. Krams, S. Cao, M. Hayashi, J.C. Villanueva, and O.M. Martinez, *Clin. Immunol. Immunopathol.* **1996**, *80*, 311–320.

68 K. Song, Y. Chen, R. Goke, A. Wilmen, C. Seidel, A. Goke, and B. Hilliard, *J. Exp. Med.* **2000**, *191*, 1095–1104.

69 H.F. Tsai, J.J. Lai, A.H. Chou, T.F. Wang, C.S. Wu, and P.N. Hsu, *Arthritis Rheum.* **2004**, *50*, 629–639.

70 H. Nishimura, M. Nose, H. Hiai, N. Minato, and T. Honjo, *Immunity* **1999**, *11*, 141–151.

71 T. Okazaki, Y. Tanaka, R. Nishio, T. Mitsuiye, A. Mizoguchi, J. Wang, M. Ishida, H. Hiai, A. Matsumori, N. Minato, and T. Honjo, *Nat. Med.* **2003**, *9*, 1477–1483.

72 A. Ashkenazi, and V.M. Dixit, *Science* **1998**, *281*, 1305–1308.

73 J.G. Cyster, S.B. Hartley, and C.C. Goodnow, *Nature* **1994**, *371*, 389–395.

74 S.J. Seo, M.L. Fields, J.L. Buckler, A.J. Reed, L. Mandik-Nayak, S.A. Nish, R.J. Noelle, L.A. Turka, F.D. Finkelman, A.J. Caton, and J. Erikson, *Immunity* **2002**, *16*, 535–546.

75 T.R. Mosmann, H. Cherwinski, M.W. Bond, M.A. Giedlin, and R.L. Coffman, *J. Immunol.* **1986**, *136*, 2348–2357.

76 T.R. Mosmann, and S. Sad, *Immunol. Today* **1996**, *17*, 138–146.

77 D.F. Fiorentino, M.W. Bond, and T.R. Mosmann, *J. Exp. Med.* **1989**, *170*, 2081–2095.

78 J.E. Allen, and R.M. Maizels, *Immunol. Today* **1997**, *18*, 387–392.

79 S.L. Constant, and K. Bottomly, *Ann. Rev. Immunol.* **1997**, *15*, 297–322.

80 S.L. Swain, *Curr. Opin. Immunol.* **1999**, *11*, 180–185.

81 L.R. Herron, R.L. Coffman, M.W. Bond, and B.L. Kotzin, *J. Immunol.* **1988**, *141*, 842–848.

82 D. Asthana, Y. Fujii, G.E. Huston, and J. Lindstrom, *Clin. Immunol. Immunopathol.* **1993**, *67*, 240–248.

83 S. Takahashi, L. Fossati, M. Iwamoto, R. Merino, R. Motta, T. Kobayakawa, and S. Izui, *J. Clin. Invest.* **1996**, *97*, 1597–1604.

84 M. Akahoshi, H. Nakashima, Y. Tanaka, T. Kohsaka, S. Nagano, E. Ohgami, Y. Arinobu, K. Yamaoka, H. Niiro, M. Shinozaki, H. Hirakata, T. Horiuchi, T. Otsuka, and Y. Niho, *Arthritis Rheum.* **1999**, *42*, 1644–1648.

85 K. Masutani, M. Akahoshi, K. Tsuruya, M. Tokumoto, T. Ninomiya, T. Kohsaka, K. Fukuda, H. Kanai, H. Nakashima, T. Otsuka, and H. Hirakata, *Arthritis Rheum.* **2001**, *44*, 2097–2106.

86 R.W. Chan, L.S. Tam, E.K. Li, F.M. Lai, K.M. Chow, K.B. Lai, P.K. Li, and C.C. Szeto, *Arthritis Rheum.* **2003**, *48*, 1326–1331.

87 L. Moiola, M.P. Protti, D. McCormick, J.F. Howard, and B.M. Conti-Tronconi, *J. Immunol.* **1994**, *152*, 4686–4698.

88 Q. Yi, and A.K. Lefvert, *J. Immunol.* **1994**, *153*, 3353–3359.

89 T. Katakai, T. Hara, M. Sugai, H. Gonda, and A. Shimizu, *J. Immunol.* **2003**, *171*, 4359–4368.

90 M.S. Lin, S.J. Swartz, A. Lopez, X. Ding, M.A. Fernandez-Vina, P. Stastny, J.A. Fairley, and L.A. Diaz, *J. Clin. Invest.* **1997**, *99*, 31–40.

91 C. Veldman, A. Stauber, R. Wassmuth, W. Uter, G. Schuler, and M. Hertl, *J. Immunol.* **2003**, *170*, 635–642.

92 H. Murata, R. Matsumura, A. Koyama, T. Sugiyama, M. Sueishi, K. Shibuya, A. Tsutsumi, and T. Sumida, *Arthritis Rheum.* **2002**, *46*, 2141–2147.

93 J. Van de Water, A. Ansari, T. Prindiville, R.L. Coppel, N. Ricalton, B.L. Kotzin, S. Liu, T.E. Roche, S.M. Krams, and S. Munoz, *J. Exp. Med.* **1995**, *181*, 723–733.

94 C.M. Snapper, and W.E. Paul, *Science* **1987**, *236*, 944–947.

95 C.M. Snapper, T.M. McIntyre, R. Mandler, L.M. Pecanha, F.D. Finkelman, A. Lees, and J.J. Mond, *J. Exp. Med.* **1992**, *175*, 1367–1371.

96 H. Heremans, A. Billiau, A. Colombatti, J. Hilgers, and P. de Somer, *Infect. Immun.* **1978**, *21*, 925–930.

97 C.O. Jacob, P.H. van der Meide, and H.O. McDevitt, *J. Exp. Med.* **1987**, *166*, 798–803.

98 C. Haas, B. Ryffel, and M. Le Hir, *J. Immunol.* **1998**, *160*, 3713–3718.

99 C. Haas, B. Ryffel, and M. Le Hir, *J. Immunol.* **1997**, *158*, 5484–5491.

100 S.L. Peng, J. Moslehi, and J. Craft, *J. Clin. Invest.* **1997**, *99*, 1936–1946.

101 D. Balomenos, R. Rumold, and A.N. Theofilopoulos, *J. Clin. Invest.* **1998**, *101*, 364–371.

102 A. Schwarting, T. Wada, K. Kinoshita, G. Tesch, and V.R. Kelley, *J. Immunol.* **1998**, *161*, 494–503.

103 B. Balasa, C. Deng, J. Lee, L.M. Bradley, D.K. Dalton, P. Christadoss, and N. Sarvetnick, *J. Exp. Med.* **1997**, *186*, 385–391.

104 D. Gu, L. Wogensen, N.A. Calcutt, C. Xia, S. Zhu, J.P. Merlie, H.S. Fox, J. Lindstrom, H.C. Powell, and N. Sarvetnick, *J. Exp. Med.* **1995**, *181*, 547–557.

105 G.X. Zhang, B.G. Xiao, X.F. Bai, P.H. van der Meide, A. Orn, and H. Link, *J. Immunol.* **1999**, *162*, 3775–3781.

106 P.I. Karachunski, N.S. Ostlie, C. Monfardini, and B.M. Conti-Fine, *J. Immunol.* **2000**, *164*, 5236–5244.

107 H.B. Wang, F.D. Shi, H. Li, P.H. van der Meide, H.G. Ljunggren, and H. Link, *Clin. Immunol.* **2000**, *95*, 156–162.

108 H. Tang, G.C. Sharp, K.P. Peterson, and H. Braley-Mullen, *J. Immunol.* **1998**, *160*, 5105–5112.

109 T. Hamaoka, and S. Ono, *Ann. Rev. Immunol.* **1986**, *4*, 167–204.

110 R.R. Singh, *Clin. Immunol.* **2003**, *108*, 73–79.

111 A. Nakajima, S. Hirose, H. Yagita, and K. Okumura, *J. Immunol.* **1997**, *158*, 1466–1472.

112 B. Deocharan, P. Marambio, M. Edelman, and C. Putterman, *Clin. Immunol.* **2003**, *108*, 80–88.

113 D.H. Kono, D. Balomenos, M.S. Park, and A.N. Theofilopoulos, *J. Immunol.* **2000**, *164*, 38–42.

114 M.L. Santiago, L. Fossati, C. Jacquet, W. Muller, S. Izui, and L. Reininger, *J. Exp. Med.* **1997**, *185*, 65–70.

115 M. Ochel, H.W. Vohr, C. Pfeiffer, and E. Gleichmann, *J. Immunol.* **1991**, *146*, 3006–3011.

116 B. Balasa, C. Deng, J. Lee, P. Christadoss, and N. Sarvetnick, *J. Immunol.* **1998**, *161*, 2856–2862.

117 P.I. Karachunski, N.S. Ostlie, D.K. Okita, and B.M. Conti-Fine, *J. Neuroimmunol.* **1999**, *95*, 73–84.

118 N. Ostlie, M. Milani, W. Wang, D. Okita, and B.M. Conti-Fine, *J. Immunol.* **2003**, *170*, 604–612.

119 R.N. Dogan, C. Vasu, M.J. Holterman, and B.S. Prabhakar, *J. Immunol.* **2003**, *170*, 2195–2204.

120 Y. Nagayama, H. Mizuguchi, T. Hayakawa, M. Niwa, S.M. McLachlan, and B. Rapoport, *J. Immunol.* **2003**, *170*, 3522–3527.

121 B.M. Ruger, K.J. Erb, K. He, J.M. Lane, P.F. Davis, and Q. Hasan, *Eur. J. Immunol.* **2000**, *30*, 2698–2703.

122 S.C. Morris, N.L. Dragula, and F.D. Finkelman, *J. Immunol.* **2002**, *169*, 1696–1704.

123 H. Trebeden-Negre, B. Weill, C. Fournier, and F. Batteux, *Eur. J. Immunol.* **2003**, *33*, 1603–1612.

124 A. Muraguchi, T. Hirano, B. Tang, T. Matsuda, Y. Horii, K. Nakajima, and T. Kishimoto, *J. Exp. Med.* **1988**, *167*, 332–344.

125 T. Kishimoto, and T. Hirano, *Ann. Rev. Immunol.* **1988**, *6*, 485–512.

126 J.T. Cross, and H.P. Benton, *Inflamm. Res.* **1999**, *48*, 255–261.

127 A.C. Grammer, and P.E. Lipsky, *Arthritis Rheum.* **2002**, *46*, 1417–1429.

128 G. Cassese, S. Lindenau, B. de Boer, S. Arce, A. Hauser, G. Riemekasten, C. Berek, F. Hiepe, V. Krenn, A. Radbruch, and R.A. Manz, *Eur. J. Immunol.* **2001**, *31*, 2726–2732.

129 E. Arce, D.G. Jackson, M.A. Gill, L.B. Bennett, J. Banchereau, and V. Pascual, *J. Immunol.* **2001**, *167*, 2361–2369.

130 G. J. Goldenberg, F. Paraskevas, and L. G. Israels, *Arthritis Rheum.* **1969**, *12*, 569–579.

131 J. Dechanet, P. Merville, I. Durand, J. Banchereau, and P. Miossec, *J. Clin. Invest.* **1995**, *95*, 456–463.

132 A. M. Jacobi, M. Odendahl, K. Reiter, A. Bruns, G. R. Burmester, A. Radbruch, G. Valet, P. E. Lipsky, and T. Dorner, *Arthritis Rheum.* **2003**, *48*, 1332–1342.

133 Y. Tanaka, K. Saito, F. Shirakawa, T. Ota, H. Suzuki, S. Eto, and U. Yamashita, *J. Immunol.* **1988**, *141*, 3043–3049.

134 M. Linker-Israeli, R. J. Deans, D. J. Wallace, J. Prehn, T. Ozeri-Chen, and J. R. Klinenberg, *J. Immunol.* **1991**, *147*, 117–123.

135 A. Kitani, M. Hara, T. Hirose, M. Harigai, K. Suzuki, M. Kawakami, Y. Kawaguchi, T. Hidaka, M. Kawagoe, and H. Nakamura, *Clin. Exp. Immunol.* **1992**, *88*, 75–83.

136 R. W. McMurray, R. W. Hoffman, W. Nelson, and S. E. Walker, *Clin. Immunol. Immunopathol.* **1997**, *84*, 260–268.

137 H. Nagafuchi, N. Suzuki, Y. Mizushima, and T. Sakane, *J. Immunol.* **1993**, *151*, 6525–6534.

138 K. Bendtzen, K. Buschard, M. Diamant, T. Horn, and M. Svenson, *Lymphokine Res.* **1989**, *8*, 335–340.

139 D. Emilie, M. C. Crevon, S. Cohen-Kaminsky, M. Peuchmaur, O. Devergne, S. Berrih-Aknin, and P. Galanaud, *Hum. Pathol.* **1991**, *22*, 461–468.

140 S. Cohen-Kaminsky, O. Devergne, R. M. Delattre, I. Klingel-Schmitt, D. Emilie, P. Galanaud, and S. Berrih-Aknin, *Eur. Cytokine Network* **1993**, *4*, 121–132.

141 B. K. Finck, B. Chan, and D. Wofsy, *J. Clin. Invest.* **1994**, *94*, 585–591.

142 H. B. Richards, M. Satoh, M. Shaw, C. Libert, V. Poli, and W. H. Reeves, *J. Exp. Med.* **1998**, *188*, 985–990.

143 C. Deng, E. Goluszko, E. Tuzun, H. Yang, and P. Christadoss, *J. Immunol.* **2002**, *169*, 1077–1083.

144 M. Kuwana, T. A. Medsger, Jr., and T. M. Wright, *J. Immunol.* **2000**, *164*, 6138–6146.

145 P. C. Heinrich, I. Behrmann, S. Haan, H. M. Hermanns, G. Muller-Newen, and F. Schaper, *Biochem. J.* **2003**, *374*, 1–20.

146 F. Rousset, E. Garcia, T. Defrance, C. Peronne, N. Vezzio, D. H. Hsu, R. Kastelein, K. W. Moore, and J. Banchereau, *Proc. Natl. Acad. Sci. USA* **1992**, *89*, 1890–1893.

147 K. W. Moore, R. de Waal Malefyt, R. L. Coffman, and A. O'Garra, *Ann. Rev. Immunol.* **2001**, *19*, 683–765.

148 E. Hagiwara, M. F. Gourley, S. Lee, and D. K. Klinman, *Arthritis Rheum.* **1996**, *39*, 379–385.

149 L. Llorente, Y. Richaud-Patin, J. Couderc, D. Alarcon-Segovia, J. Ruiz-Soto, N. Alcocer-Castillejos, J. Alcocer-Varela, J. Granados, S. Bahena, P. Galanaud, and D. Emilie, *Arthritis Rheum.* **1997**, *40*, 1429–1435.

150 G. Grondal, H. Kristjansdottir, B. Gunnlaugsdottir, A. Arnason, I. Lundberg, L. Klareskog, and K. Steinsson, *Arthritis Rheum.* **1999**, *42*, 1649–1654.

151 L. Llorente, Y. Richaud-Patin, R. Fior, J. Alcocer-Varela, J. Wijdenes, B. M. Fourrier, P. Galanaud, and D. Emilie, *Arthritis Rheum.* **1994**, *37*, 1647–1655.

152 C. C. Mok, J. S. Lanchbury, D. W. Chan, and C. S. Lau, *Arthritis Rheum.* **1998**, *41*, 1090–1095.

153 R. Mehrian, F. P. Quismorio, Jr., G. Strassmann, M. M. Stimmler, D. A. Horwitz, R. C. Kitridou, W. J. Gauderman, J. Morrison, C. Brautbar, and C. O. Jacob, *Arthritis Rheum.* **1998**, *41*, 596–602.

154 S. D'Alfonso, M. Rampi, D. Bocchio, G. Colombo, R. Scorza-Smeraldi, and P. Momigliano-Richardi, *Arthritis Rheum.* **2000**, *43*, 120–128.

155 A. W. Gibson, J. C. Edberg, J. Wu, R. G. Westendorp, T. W. Huizinga, and R. P. Kimberly, *J. Immunol.* **2001**, *166*, 3915–3922.

156 L. R. Lard, F. A. van Gaalen, J. J. Schonkeren, E. J. Pieterman, G. Stoeken, K. Vos, R. G. Nelissen, R. G. Westendorp, R. C. Hoeben, F. C. Breedveld, R. E. Toes, and T. W. Huizinga, *Arthritis Rheum.* **2003**, *48*, 1841–1848.

157 H. Ishida, T. Muchamuel, S. Sakaguchi, S. Andrade, S. Menon, and M. Howard, *J. Exp. Med.* **1994**, *179*, 305–310.

158 L. Llorente, W. Zou, Y. Levy, Y. Richaud-Patin, J. Wijdenes, J. Alcocer-Varela, B. Morel-Fourrier, J.C. Brouet, D. Alarcon-Segovia, P. Galanaud, and et al., *J. Exp. Med.* **1995**, *181*, 839–844.

159 B.R. Lauwerys, N. Garot, J.C. Renauld, and F.A. Houssiau, *Arthritis Rheum.* **2000**, *43*, 1976–1981.

160 L. Llorente, Y. Richaud-Patin, C. Garcia-Padilla, E. Claret, J. Jakez-Ocampo, M.H. Cardiel, J. Alcocer-Varela, L. Grangeot-Keros, D. Alarcon-Segovia, J. Wijdenes, P. Galanaud, and D. Emilie, *Arthritis Rheum.* **2000**, *43*, 1790–1800.

161 S. Nisitani, T. Tsubata, M. Murakami, and T. Honjo, *Eur. J. Immunol.* **1995**, *25*, 3047–3052.

162 N. Watanabe, K. Ikuta, S. Nisitani, T. Chiba, and T. Honjo, *J. Exp. Med.* **2002**, *196*, 141–146.

163 N.S. Ostlie, P.I. Karachunski, W. Wang, C. Monfardini, M. Kronenberg, and B.M. Conti-Fine, *J. Immunol.* **2001**, *166*, 4853–4862.

164 G.X. Zhang, B.G. Xiao, L.Y. Yu, P.H. van der Meide, and H. Link, *J. Neuroimmunol.* **2001**, *113*, 10–18.

165 Z. Yin, G. Bahtiyar, N. Zhang, L. Liu, P. Zhu, M.E. Robert, J. McNiff, M.P. Madaio, and J. Craft, *J. Immunol.* **2002**, *169*, 2148–2155.

166 L. Georgescu, R.K. Vakkalanka, K.B. Elkon, and M.K. Crow, *J. Clin. Invest.* **1997**, *100*, 2622–2633.

167 K. Goudy, S. Song, C. Wasserfall, Y.C. Zhang, M. Kapturczak, A. Muir, M. Powers, M. Scott-Jorgensen, M. Campbell-Thompson, J.M. Crawford, T.M. Ellis, T.R. Flotte, and M.A. Atkinson, *Proc. Natl. Acad. Sci. USA* **2001**, *98*, 13913–13918.

168 P. Toto, C. Feliciani, P. Amerio, H. Suzuki, B. Wang, G.M. Shivji, D. Woodley, and D.N. Sauder, *J. Immunol.* **2000**, *164*, 522–529.

169 K. Mignon-Godefroy, O. Rott, M.P. Brazillet, and J. Charreire, *J. Immunol.* **1995**, *154*, 6634–6643.

170 F. Batteux, H. Trebeden, J. Charreire, and G. Chiocchia, *Eur. J. Immunol.* **1999**, *29*, 958–963.

171 W.T. Watford, M. Moriguchi, A. Morinobu, and J.J. O'Shea, *Cytokine Growth Factor Rev.* **2003**, *14*, 361–368.

172 P. Zaccone, P. Hutchings, F. Nicoletti, G. Penna, L. Adorini, and A. Cooke, *Eur. J. Immunol.* **1999**, *29*, 1933–1942.

173 L. Moiola, F. Galbiati, G. Martino, S. Amadio, E. Brambilla, G. Comi, A. Vincent, L.M. Grimaldi, and L. Adorini, *Eur. J. Immunol.* **1998**, *28*, 2487–2497.

174 E. Kikawada, D.M. Lenda, and V.R. Kelley, *J. Immunol.* **2003**, *170*, 3915–3925.

175 P. Matthys, K. Vermeire, T. Mitera, H. Heremans, S. Huang, and A. Billiau, *Eur. J. Immunol.* **1998**, *28*, 2143–2151.

176 L.M. Bagenstose, P. Salgame, and M. Monestier, *J. Immunol.* **1998**, *160*, 1612–1617.

177 B.R. Lauwerys, J.C. Renauld, and F.A. Houssiau, *Eur. J. Immunol.* **1998**, *28*, 2017–2024.

178 T. Okubo, E. Hagiwara, S. Ohno, T. Tsuji, A. Ihata, A. Ueda, A. Shirai, I. Aoki, K. Okuda, J. Miyazaki, and Y. Ishigatsubo, *J. Immunol.* **1999**, *162*, 4013–4017.

179 G. Trinchieri, S. Pflanz, R.A. Kastelein, *Immunity* **2003**, *19*, 641–644.

180 K. Kato, E. Santana-Sahagun, L.Z. Rassenti, M.H. Weisman, N. Tamura, S. Kobayashi, H. Hashimoto, and T.J. Kipps, *J. Clin. Invest.* **1999**, *104*, 947–955.

181 R.K. Vakkalanka, C. Woo, K.A. Kirou, M. Koshy, D. Berger, and M.K. Crow, *Arthritis Rheum.* **1999**, *42*, 871–881.

182 D.D. Desai, and T.N. Marion, *Int. Immunol.* **2000**, *12*, 1569–1578.

183 U. Moens, O.M. Seternes, A.W. Hey, Y. Silsand, T. Traavik, B. Johansen, and O.P. Rekvig, *Proc. Natl. Acad. Sci. USA* **1995**, *92*, 12393–12397.

184 S.L. Peng, M.P. Madaio, D.P. Hughes, I.N. Crispe, M.J. Owen, L. Wen, A.C. Hayday, and J. Craft, *J. Immunol.* **1996**, *156*, 4041–4049.

185 S. L. Peng, M. P. Madaio, A. C. Hayday, and J. Craft, *J. Immunol.* **1996**, *157*, 5689–5698.

186 S. L. Peng, S. Fatenejad, and J. Craft, *J. Immunol.* **1996**, *157*, 5225–5230.

187 B. W. Busser, B. S. Adair, J. Erikson, and T. M. Laufer, *J. Clin. Invest.* **2003**, *112*, 1361–1371.

188 J. P. Portanova, J. C. Cheronis, J. K. Blodgett, and B. L. Kotzin, *J. Immunol.* **1990**, *144*, 4633–4640.

189 S. Adams, P. Leblanc, and S. K. Datta, *Proc. Natl. Acad. Sci. USA* **1991**, *88*, 11271–11275.

190 A. Kaliyaperumal, C. Mohan, W. Wu, and S. K. Datta, *J. Exp. Med.* **1996**, *183*, 2459–2469.

191 R. R. Singh, B. H. Hahn, B. P. Tsao, and F. M. Ebling, *J. Clin. Invest.* **1998**, *102*, 1841–1849.

192 F. Monneaux, and S. Muller, *Arthritis Rheum.* **2002**, *46*, 1430–1438.

193 M. J. Shlomchik, M. P. Madaio, D. Ni, M. Trounstein, and D. Huszar, *J. Exp. Med.* **1994**, *180*, 1295–1306.

194 O. T. Chan, L. G. Hannum, A. M. Haberman, M. P. Madaio, and M. J. Shlomchik, *J. Exp. Med.* **1999**, *189*, 1639–1648.

195 T. Akashi, S. Nagafuchi, K. Anzai, S. Kondo, D. Kitamura, S. Wakana, J. Ono, M. Kikuchi, Y. Niho, and T. Watanabe, *Int. Immunol.* **1997**, *9*, 1159–1164.

196 M. Falcone, J. Lee, G. Patstone, B. Yeung, and N. Sarvetnick, *J. Immunol.* **1998**, *161*, 1163–1168.

197 H. Noorchashm, Y. K. Lieu, N. Noorchashm, S. Y. Rostami, S. A. Greeley, A. Schlachterman, H. K. Song, L. E. Noto, A. M. Jevnikar, C. F. Barker, and A. Naji, *J. Immunol.* **1999**, *163*, 743–750.

198 J. A. Lyons, M. San, M. P. Happ, and A. H. Cross, *Eur. J. Immunol.* **1999**, *29*, 3432–3439.

199 S. A. Greeley, M. Katsumata, L. Yu, G. S. Eisenbarth, D. J. Moore, H. Goodarzi, C. F. Barker, A. Naji, and H. Noorchashm, *Nat. Med.* **2002**, *8*, 399–402.

200 X. Wang, W. Huang, M. Mihara, J. Sinha, and A. Davidson, *J. Immunol.* **2002**, *168*, 2046–2053.

201 M. Mihara, I. Tan, Y. Chuzhin, B. Reddy, L. Budhai, A. Holzer, Y. Gu, and A. Davidson, *J. Clin. Invest.* **2000**, *106*, 91–101.

202 F. Nicoletti, P. Meroni, R. Di Marco, W. Barcellini, M. O. Borghi, M. Gariglio, A. Mattina, S. Grasso, and S. Landolfo, *Immunopharmacology* **1992**, *24*, 11–16.

6
Cell Death and Autoimmunity

Carlos A. Casiano and Fabio J. Pacheco

6.1
Introduction

The survival of multicellular organisms depends on their ability to maintain the delicate balance between the rate of cell death and the rate of cell proliferation. It has been recognized that alteration of this balance, leading to either too much or too little cell death, underlies the etiology of the majority of human diseases, including systemic autoimmunity, osteoarthritis, cancer, heart disease, diabetes, liver disease, and neurodegenerative disorders [1–7]. Cell death has been traditionally considered as a process that occurs via two morphologically distinct mechanisms, apoptosis and necrosis [8, 9]. This dual classification relies mainly on the observation that apoptosis and necrosis are the major types of cell death associated with most physiological and pathological processes. Although recent studies have provided evidence for the existence of novel forms of cell demise with features that either do not fit into the classical apoptotic or necrotic morphologies or are shared by both modalities [10–15], most of our knowledge of cell death has derived from the analysis of molecular and biochemical mechanisms underlying apoptosis and necrosis.

A central question in the study of autoimmune diseases is how immune tolerance to self-antigens that are associated with essential cellular or organ functions is broken, thereby turning these antigens into malicious immunogens capable of inciting and maintaining vigorous and prolonged humoral and cellular immune responses. Numerous mechanisms have been proposed to explain this phenomenon, including molecular mimicry and structural modifications of self-antigens caused by mutations or exposure to xenobiotics and infectious agents [16–19]. Compelling evidence has accumulated during the past decade to support the general hypothesis that dysfunctional cell death plays a pivotal role in the induction of autoimmunity, both systemic and organ-specific [20–23]. This hypothesis is supported by several major lines of evidence, derived from studies with animal models of autoimmune diseases and patients with autoimmune disorders, as well as from *in vitro* model systems. These include (1) the identifi-

Autoantibodies and Autoimmunity: Molecular Mechanisms in Health and Disease. Edited by K. Michael Pollard
Copyright © 2006 WILEY-VCH Verlag GmbH & Co. KGaA, Weinheim
ISBN: 3-527-31141-6

cation of defects in genes involved in the regulation of the activation of T and B lymphocytes and the deletion of autoreactive lymphocytes [23–25]; (2) the detection of excessive cell death induced by autoreactive cytotoxic T cells (CTLs) in target organs in certain organ-specific autoimmune diseases [4, 26]; (3) the link between systemic autoimmunity and deficiencies in genes involved in the clearance of immune complexes and dying cells [27–30]; and (4) the observation that many intracellular autoantigens undergo structural modifications during cell death (both apoptotic and necrotic) that might reveal potentially immunostimulatory cryptic epitopes under a proinflammatory context [31–34].

While the contribution of dysfunctional apoptosis to autoimmunity has attracted considerable attention, the contribution of necrosis has been largely ignored. This is due in part to the emphasis on the molecular dissection of apoptotic pathways and their contribution to human disease, combined with the generalized perception that necrosis is an accidental mode of cell death that is not mechanistically driven. In recent years, however, there has been an increased interest in the analysis of biochemical mechanisms underlying necrosis and the potential contribution of this mode of cell death to the generation of autoimmune responses, particularly within the context of systemic autoimmunity. In this chapter, we provide a general overview of the two major modes of cell death and the evidence supporting their role in autoimmunity.

6.2
Apoptosis

Apoptosis is a genetically programmed cell-demise process that facilitates the elimination of damaged or unwanted cells in various circumstances, including organ and tissue development during embryogenesis, immune system development and function, normal tissue homeostasis, and tissue healing [35, 36]. Under normal conditions, humans lose millions of cells every day via apoptosis, a process that is balanced by the generation of new cells. Apoptosis can be induced by a large number of internal or external stimuli, including UV irradiation [37], oxidative stress [38], hypoxia [39], cytokines such as tumor necrosis factor (TNF) and Fas ligand (FasL) [40], DNA-damaging drugs [41], drugs of abuse such as cocaine and heroin [42, 43], complement attack [44], nitric oxide [45], inhibitors of survival proteins [46], and natural substances such as lycopene and resveratrol [47, 48].

Apoptotic cells can be distinguished from necrotic cells by their distinctive morphological features (Fig. 6.1), which include general shrinkage, cytoskeleton disruption, cytoplasmic membrane blebbing, nuclear membrane solubilization, and chromatin margination and fragmentation [9, 35, 36]. A hallmark feature of apoptosis is the fragmentation of the dying cell into numerous blebs or apoptotic bodies, which in the early stages of the death process remain surrounded by a relatively impermeable cytoplasmic membrane. Retention of cytoplasmic membrane integrity is important for the exposure of membrane signals such as

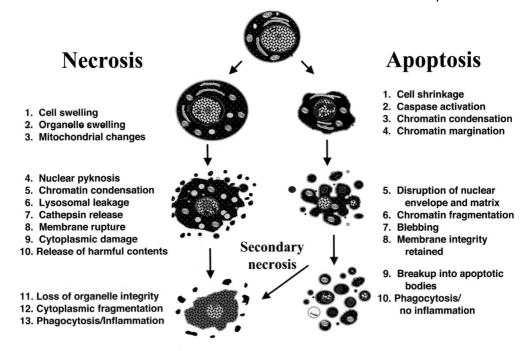

Necrosis

1. Cell swelling
2. Organelle swelling
3. Mitochondrial changes

4. Nuclear pyknosis
5. Chromatin condensation
6. Lysosomal leakage
7. Cathepsin release
8. Membrane rupture
9. Cytoplasmic damage
10. Release of harmful contents

11. Loss of organelle integrity
12. Cytoplasmic fragmentation
13. Phagocytosis/Inflammation

Apoptosis

1. Cell shrinkage
2. Caspase activation
3. Chromatin condensation
4. Chromatin margination

5. Disruption of nuclear envelope and matrix
6. Chromatin fragmentation
7. Blebbing
8. Membrane integrity retained

9. Breakup into apoptotic bodies
10. Phagocytosis/ no inflammation

Secondary necrosis

Fig. 6.1 Key events associated with the progression of apoptosis and necrosis.

the externalization of phosphatidylserine, which in essence sends a message to phagocytic cells to "eat me now or else" [49]. These signals are essential for facilitating recognition and processing of dying cells by phagocytes. This recognition process normally occurs swiftly; otherwise, apoptotic cells or bodies that linger for too long will eventually lose their cytoplasmic membrane integrity and develop secondary necrosis [49]. Secondary necrosis in turn leads to the release of noxious intracellular contents, such as proteases, nucleases, and proinflammatory "danger" signals, that could not only damage the surrounding tissue but also provoke a localized inflammatory response [50]. The efficient clearance of apoptotic cells is therefore a protective mechanism operating in higher organisms to prevent unnecessary inflammatory responses.

6.2.1
Mechanistic Events in Apoptosis

The central effector mechanism in apoptosis is the activation of cysteine proteases of the caspase (cysteine aspartic acid-specific proteases) family [51–53]. While approximately 14 mammalian caspases have been identified, only about half of them actively participate in apoptosis. The apoptotic caspases are classified as initiators (caspase-2, -8, -9, -10, and -12) or executioners (caspase-3, -6, and -7) of the apoptotic process. The non-apoptotic caspases (caspase-1, -4, -5,

-11, -13, and -14) are involved in cytokine activation during inflammation or in cell differentiation. Caspases are found in the cell as proenzymes with low catalytic activity and are activated at the onset of apoptosis by an autoaggregation process mediated by adaptor proteins that promotes the autocatalytic processing of the initiator caspases. Typically, activation of the initiation caspases leads to a cascade of events that converge in the activation of the executioner or effector caspases, particularly caspase-3.

The activation of initiator caspases can occur through several pathways. The extrinsic pathway of apoptosis involves the engagement of death receptors, such as Fas, tumor necrosis factor receptor 1 (TNF-R1), and DR4/DR5 by their respective ligands FasL, TNF, and TNF-related apoptosis-inducing ligand (TRAIL) [40, 54]. The death-receptor pathway leads mainly to activation of caspase-8, although caspase-2 and -10 are also activated in this pathway depending on the cell type and the death-inducing ligand [54]. The intrinsic pathway of apoptosis involves the permeabilization of the outer membrane of the mitochondria, leading to the release of a wide variety of apoptosis effector proteins normally residing in the mitochondria [55–57]. Some of these proteins, such as cytochrome *c*, promote the activation of initiator caspase-9, whereas others, such as apoptosis-inducing factor (AIF) and endonuclease G, contribute to nuclear DNA-damage in a caspase-independent manner. The intrinsic pathway of apoptosis is regulated by members of the Bcl-2 family of proteins, which include both anti-apoptotic and pro-apoptotic proteins [58]. A third pathway of caspase-activation is that triggered during CTL-mediated cell death associated with inflammatory responses [59, 60]. CTLs can induce apoptosis in their target cells either by activating the Fas-mediated pathway or by delivering granule proteases such as granzyme B (GrB) into the target cells through perforin, a protein that forms pores in the cytoplasmic membrane [61]. GrB induces apoptosis by directly activating caspases or by cleaving Bid, a cytoplasmic protein that, upon truncation by caspases or GrB, translocates to the mitochondria and promotes the release of mitochondrial apoptotic effector proteins, consequently resulting in caspase activation [62]. More recently, a novel apoptosis pathway apparently mediated by a combined effort of the endoplasmic reticulum (ER) and the mitochondria in response to ER stress, and involving the activation of caspase-12, was identified [63].

Once activated, initiator caspases cleave and process the executioner caspases, which in turn cleave a limited number of proteins, including specific nuclear and cytoplasmic autoantigens targeted in systemic autoimmune diseases [31, 51–53, 64]. The effector caspases disrupt the normal cellular architecture and impair virtually all pathways of macromolecular synthesis through cleavage of key proteins after specific aspartic acid residues. These cleavages constitute the pivotal event of apoptosis, leading to the characteristic morphology associated with this cell-death process. It was reported that the effector caspases, particularly caspase-3, cleave more than 280 different cellular proteins and that the great majority of these cleavages either inactivate the function of the substrate protein or generate active cleavage fragments that are required to amplify the apoptotic signal [64]. There is compelling evidence indicating that caspase-3 cleaves specific proteins involved in signal transduction and survival pathways, generating fragments with dominant interfering functions that either amplify the apoptosis process or sensitize cells to die in response to specific stress or apoptotic insults [64]. These fragments often lack regulatory or inhibitory sequences and behave as pro-apoptotic proteins. The conversion of anti-apoptotic into pro-apoptotic regulators now constitutes a well-documented positive feedback loop in apoptosis, removing proteins that antagonize the apoptotic process and promoting caspase activation [64].

While caspases appear to be the primary effector proteases in apoptosis, there is growing evidence that other proteases (intrinsic to the cell or derived from infectious agents) play an important role in the execution of the apoptotic program. These proteases include lysosomal cathepsins, calpains, gingipains, granzymes, and serine proteases [62, 65–68]. Of these proteases, the lysosomal cathepsins have attracted considerable attention recently. Lysosomes appear to function as integrators of death signals in certain types of apoptosis by releasing in a controlled manner the cathepsins, particularly B, D, and L [66, 69]. These cathepsins mediate specific early events of the apoptotic program through cleavage of substrates such as Bid and Brm and activation of caspases [70, 71]. Knockdown of the activity or expression of specific cathepsins with protease inhibitors, small interfering RNA (siRNA), or genetic methods has been shown to inhibit or delay caspase-dependent and -independent apoptosis [72, 73], suggesting that these proteases play a key role in cell death.

6.3
Necrosis

Morphologically, necrosis is very different from apoptosis (Fig. 6.1). Unlike the cell shrinking that occurs early in apoptosis, early stages of necrosis are characterized by "oncosis" or swelling [9]. The typical blebbing into multiple bodies observed during apoptosis is not observed in necrotic cells. Necrotic cell swelling is associated with organelle enlargement and rupture, which eventually leads to cytoplasmic destruction and nuclear shrinkage [8, 9]. In fact, a key feature that distinguishes necrosis from apoptosis is the rapid and early loss of cytoplasmic membrane integrity, concomitant with extensive cytoplasmic damage. These events are likely to be mediated by the enzymatic activity of lysosomal proteases such as the cathepsins, which are released upon lysosomal rupture [74]. Loss of cytoplasmic membrane integrity facilitates the release into the surrounding medium of intracellular proteases and other dangerous intracellular contents, including proinflammatory signals [49, 50]. Interestingly, the nuclear membrane stays relatively intact during the early stages of necrosis [8, 9, 75], which could be associated with the preservation of lamin B integrity during this cell death process [33, 34, 75]. Lamin B is important for maintaining nuclear membrane integrity, and its cleavage early during apoptosis facilitates nuclear fragmentation [76]. Chromatin fragmentation occurs in necrotic cells but does not appear to lead to the nucleosomal ladder typically observed in apoptotic cells [77]. There is evidence, however, that serum nucleases such as DNAse I can penetrate necrotic cells and induce nucleosomal laddering [78].

Traditionally necrosis has been considered a non-programmed, accidental mode of cell death associated mainly with pathological conditions and that develops in response to acute cell injury caused by ischemia, extreme heat, severe bacterial and viral infections, and exposure to high levels of chemicals or toxins [8, 9, 65, 79]. There is, however, growing evidence to support the notion that there might be two types of necrosis, one that is physiological and involved in programmed cell death (PCD) and another that is mainly associated with pathological conditions [11, 12, 77, 80]. Physiological necrosis, considered a type of necrosis-like PCD, has been implicated in development-associated interdigital cell death [81], development-associated regression of the human tail [82], follicular maturation during oogenesis [83, 84], normal renewal of small and large intestines [85, 86], natural killer cell–mediated cytotoxicity [87, 88], complement-mediated cell killing [89], and activation-induced cell death of T lymphocytes [90].

In both pathological and experimental conditions, necrosis often coexists with apoptosis, arising either independently or as a secondary event following apoptosis [8, 9, 65, 79, 91–96]. Under certain pathological conditions such as ischemia, extensive necrosis in the affected area within a tissue may trigger secondary damage in surrounding areas, usually occurring through apoptosis [65, 97, 98]. It has been recognized that necrosis and apoptosis can be induced by the same insults, but the intensity of these insults, the biochemical environment, and the cell type determine which mode of cell death predominates [99].

Caspases may play a key role in guarding the cell against unwanted necrotic death [77]. This notion is supported by the observation that a caspase-independent mode of cell death with necrotic morphology usually ensues when specific cell types are exposed to apoptosis inducers in the presence of broad caspase inhibitors such as benzyloxycarbonyl-Val-Ala-Asp-fluoromethyl ketone (z-VAD-fmk) [100]. This type of cell death could be considered as a backup cellular defense system that ensures the cell's demise in the event that the caspase activation program is rendered nonfunctional, e.g., during a viral infection. Viruses are known to modulate host cell apoptosis by producing proteins that antagonize caspases and perhaps other components of the apoptotic program [101]. Agents that can induce caspase-independent cell death with necrotic morphology in the presence of caspase inhibitors include cancer drugs [102, 103], death receptor ligands [104, 105], oncogenes [106], anti-CD2 antibodies [107], staurosporine (STS) [107], and viral proteins [108].

It is likely that in the presence of cell-death stimuli, caspase-independent necrotic cell death is activated as a background pathway that runs concurrently with apoptosis, leading eventually to the secondary necrosis that follows apoptosis in the absence of phagocytosis. This background pathway might be activated by death-enhancing factors – such as reactive oxygen species (ROS) or cytochrome c – that are generated or released by mitochondria [77, 109, 110]. In the event the caspase activation program is impaired, this pathway might then be revealed or enhanced. Alternatively, caspase-independent necrotic cell death may be activated only after the cell senses that caspases are not able to respond to a specific death signal. For instance, LCC human carcinoma cells deficient in caspases die via necrosis in the presence of a zinc chelator, whereas cells expressing caspases respond to the same insult by activating the apoptosis pathway [111]. Inhibition of effector caspases by exogenous nitric oxide is also known to switch apoptosis to necrosis [112]. Moreover, necrotic cell death plays an important role in driving the development of mouse embryos in which caspases were inhibited or genetically deleted [12, 81, 113]. It should be noted that not all caspase-independent cell-death processes display necrotic morphology, since some display the morphological features of apoptosis [10, 11].

6.3.1
Mechanistic Events in Necrosis

Evidence is accumulating to support the notion that necrosis, like apoptosis, is a mechanistic cell-death process. For instance, necrosis can also be induced by death ligands such as TNF and Fas, redox signaling pathways involving ROS generation, stress-activated protein kinases such as JNK and p38, and release of mitochondrial factors [77, 100, 104, 105]. Anti-apoptotic members of the Bcl-2 family such as Bcl-2 and Bcl-xL delay or protect against necrosis induced by a variety of insults in different cell lines [77]. Recent studies conducted in our laboratory indicate that the transcription co-activator and stress-regulated protein lens epithelium–derived growth factor p75 (LEDGF/p75) protects cultured mammalian cells from necrosis induced by *tert*-butyl hydroperoxide (unpublished observations). This protection appears to be mediated by transcriptional upregulation of antioxidant proteins.

As in apoptosis, proteases also play a major role in the execution of necrosis. While the role of caspases in apoptosis is well established, it was not until recently that the morphological changes associated with necrosis have been linked to the activation of non-caspase proteases such as the calcium-dependent calpains and the lysosomal cathepsins [65, 74]. The elevation of intracellular free calcium during certain pathological processes leads to activation of calpains, phospholipases, and endonucleases; alteration of membrane protein and lipid; generation of toxic ROS; and mitochondrial disruption [65]. Excessive activation of calpains has been associated with lysosomal membrane disruption, leading to the release of cathepsins into the cytoplasm with the resultant cell autolysis [65].

Important insights into biochemical mechanisms associated with necrotic cell death have been obtained using the murine L929 fibrosarcoma cell line. Upon exposure to TNF, L929 cells die preferentially via a slow necrotic process [100]. This necrosis is dependent on the death domain of TNFR-55 [114]. Treatment with TNF in the presence of broad caspase inhibitors such as Z-VAD-fmk or inhibitors of caspase-8 and caspase-3 dramatically sensitizes these cells to necrotic cell death [100, 115]. These inhibitors also sensitize L929 cells overexpressing the human Fas receptor to necrosis, although less dramatically, if these cells are treated with agonistic anti-Fas antibody [115]. Anti-Fas antibody and forced multimerization of the adaptor protein FADD (Fas-associated protein with death domain), which is required for initiating the caspase-8-mediated apoptotic pathway, have also been shown to induce necrosis in a caspase-8-deficient subline (JB6) of Jurkat T cells [114–117]. While there is no evidence that caspase-8 activation is required for death receptor–induced caspase-independent cell death with a necrotic phenotype, it appears that inactivation of caspase-8 or deficiency of this caspase does favor this death process [114–118]. Whether inactivation of other initiator caspases favors death receptor–induced necrosis remains to be established, although inhibition of the effector caspase-3 has been implicated in this process [100]. Other apoptosis-inducing ligands such as TRAIL have also been shown to cause necrosis [90]. Death receptor–induced necrosis is mediated by the RIP kinase, which is thought to phosphorylate and regulate a yet unidentified key factor involved in the necrotic process [11, 90].

Death receptor–induced necrotic cell death under caspase-inhibition conditions appears to be mediated by the generation of ROS in the mitochondria because it can be partially inhibited by antioxidants [77, 110]. Although the mechanisms by which caspase inhibition potentiates the death receptor signaling in L929 cells are not entirely clear, various studies have demonstrated that poly (ADP-ribose) polymerase (PARP) acts as a molecular switch between apoptosis and necrosis in these cells [119, 120]. According to these studies, excessive ROS generation leads to profound DNA damage, which in turn leads to excessive PARP activation and increased poly-ADP-ribosylation. The use of ATP for the synthesis of the PARP substrate NAD^+ then leads to a dramatic depletion of intracellular ATP, which results in necrotic cell death [120]. It should be noted that PARP is unable to respond in a similar fashion to DNA damage caused by apoptotic stimuli because it is cleaved and inactivated by effector caspases very early on in the apoptotic process, which prevents ATP depletion and ensures a well-controlled, non-inflammatory cell demise [121, 122].

How do the events mentioned above lead to lysosomal rupture, which appears to be the critical event for triggering the typical necrotic morphology? Recent studies show that under persistent oxidative stress conditions, intralysosomal labile iron catalyzes Fenton reactions, which result in rupture of lysosomal membranes and subsequent efflux of iron and cathepsins into the cytoplasm [123, 124]. From there, cathepsins can relocate to the cytoplasm and nucleus where they cause proteolysis of limited substrates, leading to cytoplasmic destruction and plasma membrane permeabilization. Consistent with this, Ono et al. [74] demonstrated that TNF induces rupture of lysosomes in L929 cells, leading to plasma membrane disruption. The rupture of lysosomes that precedes the appearance of the necrotic morphology is a molecular event that can be regulated. A recent study demonstrated that heat shock protein 70 (HSP70), a stress protein that is known to inhibit apoptosis, also inhibits necrotic cell death by concentrating in lysosomes and preventing their rupture through interactions with components of lysosomal membranes [125]. Taken together, these observations indicate that apoptosis and necrosis share some biochemical mechanisms and strengthen the notion that the capability of the cell to die via these pathways and their variants is essential to ensure its elimination when absolutely necessary.

6.4
Impaired Lymphocyte Cell Death and Autoimmunity

Apoptosis and necrosis can contribute to autoimmunity, both organ-specific and systemic, in many different ways. For instance, defects in genes involved in the regulation of lymphocyte activation and the deletion of autoreactive lymphocytes may lead to ineffective removal of unwanted lymphocytes during negative selection or after lymphocyte activation. Evidence for this mechanism derived from studies involving mouse models of systemic autoimmunity and patients with lymphoproliferative disorders [23–25]. In *lpr/lpr* mice, considered as a mouse model of lupus-like disease, a spontaneous mutation in the death receptor Fas interferes with the elimination of autoreactive lymphocytes both centrally and in the periphery, leading to lymphoproliferation, splenomegaly, and systemic autoimmunity [126]. Similar symptoms are observed in *gld/gld* mice, which carry a point mutation in the intracellular apoptotic domain of FasL [127]. The discovery of these mutations led to a search for similar mutations in patients with SLE, but the results were disappointing. FasL mutations were found only in a rare form of lupus [128]. However, humans with Canale-Smith syndrome, also called human autoimmune lymphoproliferative syndrome, carry mutations in Fas, FasL, and caspase genes [25]. This hereditary syndrome, which is usually diagnosed early in life, presents lymphoproliferation characterized by large numbers of double-negative CD4-CD8 lymphocytes, splenomegaly, antinuclear autoantibody production, rheumatoid factor production, thrombocytopenia, glomerulonephritis, arthritis, and vasculitis [23–25]. Lymphocytes from these patients are resistant to FasL-induced apoptosis [25].

More recent evidence for the hypothesis that impaired T-cell death promotes autoimmunity derives from studies with mice deficient in the T cell–specific adapter protein (TSAd). This protein is expressed in thymocytes and in activated mature T cells and is involved in signal transduction [129]. TSAd-deficient mice display defective T-cell death *in vivo* and develop lupus-like autoimmunity, suggesting that TSAd is a critical regulator of T-cell death whose absence or inactivation promotes systemic autoimmunity [129]. The requirement of T-cell apoptosis for the suppression of autoimmunity was also illustrated recently by studies using BXSB lupus-prone mice deficient in the cyclin kinase inhibitor p21, a regulator of cell death and proliferation [130]. Absence of p21 in these mice resulted in enhanced Fas/FasL-mediated activation-induced T-cell death and increased B-cell apoptosis. Consequently, the development of systemic autoimmunity was inhibited in these mice.

Failure of the immune system to eliminate autoreactive lymphocytes may lead to excessive cell death induced by autoreactive T cells in target organs in certain organ-specific autoimmune diseases. For instance, insulin-dependent diabetes mellitus (IDDM) is characterized by T cell–mediated selective destruction of the insulin-producing β-cells of the Langerhans islets of the pancreas [20]. In the non-obese diabetic (NOD) mouse model, both autoreactive CD4$^+$ and CD8$^+$ T cells are involved in β-cell destruction via recognition of presented peptides derived from self-antigens such as insulin, GAD65/67, and HSP70 [20]. CD4$^+$ T cells can directly induce β-cell apoptosis through FasL-Fas interactions or promote the effector functions of cytotoxic CD8$^+$ T lymphocytes (CTL) and natural killer (NK) cells, which involve perforin-dependent delivery of cytotoxic granules. Lymphocyte-mediated cytotoxicity has been also proposed to explain the destruction of oligodendrocytes in multiple sclerosis as well as thyroid cells in Hashimoto's thyroiditis [20].

6.5
Cell Death-associated Autoantigen Proteolysis and Autoimmunity

6.5.1
Autoantigen Proteolysis During Apoptosis

In the early 1990s the Rosens and colleagues elegantly demonstrated that specific SLE-associated autoantigens relocalize to surface blebs in cultured cells induced to die by apoptosis upon exposure to UV irradiation [131]. Following this observation, these investigators reported that the nuclear autoantigens PARP and U1-70 kDa (70-kDa protein of the U1 ribonucleoprotein particle) were proteolytically cleaved by caspases during apoptosis [132, 133]. These observations led to the hypothesis that apoptotic cells are reservoirs of structurally modified forms of autoantigens that could initiate autoantibody responses in patients with systemic autoimmune diseases such as SLE and scleroderma. The development of this hypothesis triggered a search for modified forms of autoantigen that are generated in different types of cell death. Autoantigen modifications found to be associated with cell death included, but were not limited to, proteolysis, changes in the phosphorylation state, and citrullination [32]. Of these modifications, the most extensively studied has been proteolysis. This is due to the fact that the discovery of autoantigen cleavage during apoptosis coincided with the discovery of caspases and the elucidation of the main apoptotic pathways. Autoantibodies to intracellular autoantigens obtained from patients with systemic autoimmune diseases turned out to be highly valuable in these studies because of their reactivity with multiple epitopes within a given autoantigen, which facilitated the identification of cleavage fragments that otherwise may escape detection when using sequence-specific, experimentally induced antibodies.

In their initial systematic study on the cleavage of autoantigens during cell death, Rosen and colleagues [133] reported that a subset of intracellular autoantigens targeted in systemic autoimmune diseases was specifically cleaved in various systems of apoptosis. This subset included PARP, U1-70 kDa, the catalytic subunit of DNA-dependent protein kinase (DNA-PKcs), the nuclear mitotic apparatus protein (NuMA), lamins A and B, and several other unidentified autoantigens. In a subsequent study, our group reported that a subset (7 of 33) of intracellular autoantigens was cleaved during Fas-mediated T-cell apoptosis [134]. This subset included PARP, lamin B, U1-70 kDa, topoisomerase I and II (topo I and II), NuMA, and the upstream binding factor of RNA polymerase I (UBF/NOR-90). Subsequent studies by various groups reported the apoptotic cleavage of additional intracellular autoantigens [31, 135, 136].

Originally, it was hypothesized that cleavage of intracellular autoantigens during aberrant apoptosis may reveal previously immunocryptic epitopes in individuals with the appropriate class II MHC molecules and trigger autoantibody responses to intracellularly sequestered autoantigens [32, 132, 133]. However, it soon became obvious that this hypothesis had limitations for three main reasons. First, a large number of intracellular autoantigens frequently targeted by autoantibodies in systemic autoimmune diseases were not found to be cleaved by caspases or modified during classical apoptosis, which suggested that susceptibility to post-translational modifications may not be a generalized property of these autoantigens [132, 134]. Second, evidence accumulated to support the notion that apoptosis, being a physiological death process that occurs constantly in the human body, is essential for tolerizing the immune system against intracellular antigens [30, 137, 138]. This notion is supported by the fact that systemic autoimmunity is absent in most individuals, in spite of the constant exposure of their immune system to self-antigens (modified or not) derived from cells dying under a myriad of physiological situations (e.g., regulation of immune responses, infections, aging, homeostasis, tissue turnover and remodeling, etc.). Third, apoptotic cells are not highly immunogenic, are relatively inefficient by themselves in inducing maturation of dendritic cells (DCs), and appear to release anti-inflammatory signals [139–144]. A concept that is currently gaining wide acceptance is that exposure to the immune system of intracellular antigens and their modified forms derived from apoptotic cells plays a tolerogenic role under normal conditions and that this exposure may not be sufficient to incite and sustain autoantibody responses unless it occurs in conjunction with other dangerous conditions, such as defective clearance of dying cells, a proinflammatory environment, and breakdown of self-tolerance [27, 30, 49].

6.5.2
Autoantigen Proteolysis During Granzyme B-mediated Cytotoxicity

More recently, Rosen and colleagues demonstrated that the majority of autoantigens targeted in human systemic autoimmune diseases are efficiently cleaved by granzyme B *in vitro* and during CTL-induced cell death, generating unique fragments not observed during apoptosis [145, 146]. Interestingly, GrB cleaved several autoantigens previously reported as not susceptible to cleavage during cell death, such as Ku-70, Jo-1, CENP-B, and PM-Scl, but failed to cleave other protease-resistant autoantigens, including SSA/Ro, Ku-80, ribosomal P proteins, histones, and the Sm proteins [145, 146]. *In vivo* killing of target cells by CTLs generated low amounts of the unique autoantigen fragments produced by GrB *in vitro* but favored the production of fragments corresponding to those generated by caspases during apoptosis, indicating that caspase-mediated proteolysis is the predominant pathway used during GrB-mediated apoptosis. However, the production of GrB-specific fragments was enhanced in the presence of the caspase-specific inhibitor AC-DEVD-CHO, suggesting that GrB may facilitate cell death independent of caspase-activation by directly cleaving intracellular substrates. This implies that under conditions where caspase activation is blocked by either viral proteins or endogenous inhibitors, GrB may generate modified forms of autoantigens that might be immunostimulatory in a proinflammatory context.

In a recent study, Rosen's group demonstrated that the nucleolar autoantigen B23 was efficiently cleaved by GrB *in vitro* but was highly resistant to cleavage by GrB during CTL-induced cell death of many different types, with the exception of differentiated vascular smooth muscle cells, suggesting that the cleavage of this autoantigen is dependent upon cell type [147]. Given that B23 is associated with pulmonary vascular phenotype in scleroderma, it was concluded that GrB-mediated proteolytic modification of autoantigens may occur selectively in the target tissue and may play a role in shaping the phenotype-specific autoimmune response. According to this hypothesis, the immunizing microenvironment might play a central role in determining autoantibody responses in human systemic autoimmunity. To further test this hypothesis, it would be important to determine whether other autoantigens targeted *in vitro* by GrB (e.g., topo I, fibrillarin, CENP-B, PARP, and NuMA) are susceptible to GrB-mediated cleavage specifically in the tissues that are most affected in the autoimmune disease associated with these autoantigens. More importantly, it would be necessary to use mouse models deficient in GrB in order to determine whether the presence of GrB is required for the generation of autoantibodies to intracellular autoantigens.

6.5.3
Autoantigen Cleavage During Necrosis

It should be emphasized that the proteolytic modification of intracellular autoantigens is not limited to classical apoptosis or GrB-dependent cytotoxicity. In previous studies we reported the selective cleavage of autoantigens during primary necrosis, secondary necrosis, and caspase-independent cell death with necrotic morphology of a variety of cell lines exposed to high levels of mercury, ethanol, hydrogen peroxide, heat, cytotoxic drugs, or apoptotic stimuli in the presence of Z-VAD-fmk [33, 34]. Autoantigens found to be cleaved into fragments that are distinct from those generated during apoptosis included topo I, LEDGF/p75, NuMA, PARP, UBF/NOR-90, and U1-70 kDa (see Fig. 6.2 for examples). Interestingly, all of the autoantigens that we had previously observed

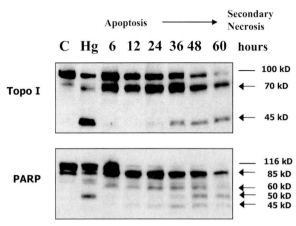

Fig. 6.2 Proteolytic fragmentation of topo I and PARP during the progression of apoptosis to secondary necrosis. Immunoblots were carried out using total protein from Jurkat T cells treated in culture with 150 μM etoposide for up to 60 h. Note that topo I and PARP are cleaved into their signature apoptotic fragments, 70 kDa and 85 kDa, respectively, during the first 24 h of treatment. After 24 h, these autoantigens undergo further cleavage into well-defined fragments as cells enter secondary necrosis. Some of these late-appearing fragments are also present in cells undergoing primary necrosis induced by treatment with 40 μM mercuric chloride for 6 h (Hg). C = control untreated cells. Protein bands were detected using highly specific human autoantibodies. Intact proteins are indicated by lines, whereas proteolytic fragments are indicated by arrows.

cleaved in apoptosis, with the exception of lamin B, were also cleaved during necrosis, albeit into distinct fragments. Worth noticing is that autoantigens such as Jo-1, Ku, PCNA, p80 coilin, rRNP, Sm, and SSA/Ro, which had been reported previously as resistant to proteolysis during caspase-dependent apoptosis [34, 133], also appeared to be resistant to cleavage during necrosis. This suggested that specific caspase substrates might be highly susceptible to proteolysis during forms of cell death other than apoptosis. This has been confirmed by other studies showing that certain caspase substrates also undergo cleavage during necrosis [75, 148]. It cannot be ruled out that some autoantigens that are resistant to proteolysis during necrosis may sustain in this cell-death process other modifications or limited proteolysis into fragments that are not detectable by immunoblotting. This would be consistent with the observation of Pollard et al. [149] that fibrillarin undergoes limited cleavage during mercury-induced necrosis into a 19-kDa fragment that is detected only by immunoprecipitation.

There is increasing evidence indicating that lysosomal cathepsins, but not caspases, are involved in the cleavage of autoantigens during necrotic cell death. It has been demonstrated that these cleavages are not dependent on caspase activation because they cannot be blocked by caspase inhibitors [33, 75]. This would be in agreement with the generalized view that caspase activation is not an integral component of the proteolytic machinery operating in necrosis. Consistent with this view, we have not observed proteolytic processing of caspases or caspase activation during primary necrosis induced by mercury in Jurkat T cells or in L929 cells exposed to TNF in the presence of Z-VAD-fmk (unpublished observations). The involvement of cathepsins in autoantigen cleavage during necrosis was first reported by Gobeil et al. [150], who demonstrated that lysosomal-rich fractions from Jurkat T cells promoted *in vitro* the cleavage of purified PARP into fragments identical to those found in lysates from Jurkat cells undergoing necrosis. These investigators also showed that purified cathepsins B and G, but not D, were able to generate *in vitro* the necrotic PARP fragments.

6.5.4
Topo I, a Model to Study Mechanisms of Cathepsin-mediated Autoantigen Cleavage During Necrosis

Anti–topo I autoantibodies are associated with diffuse cutaneous involvement and pulmonary fibrosis in patients with systemic sclerosis (SSc), and their serum levels correlate positively with disease severity and activity [151, 152]. The original molecular target of these autoantibodies was designated Scl-70 (scleroderma-associated autoantigen of 70 kDa) because of its migration as a 70-kDa band on SDS-PAGE [153, 154]. Subsequent studies demonstrated that this 70-kDa band was a proteolytic fragment corresponding to the catalytic C-terminal domain of topo I [155, 156]. A recent study demonstrated that anti–topo I autoantibodies from SSc patients recognize epitopes in the central and C-terminal portions of the protein, but not in the N-terminus, suggesting that the 70-kDa fragment is processed by antigen-presenting cells (APCs) to initiate an immune response to topo I *in vivo* [151]. Consistent with this, fragmented topo I presented by DCs elicited a vigorous T-cell response *in vitro* more efficiently than full-length topo I [157]. These observations strongly suggest that cryptic epitopes generated by *in vivo* proteolytic fragmentation of topo I might drive the generation of anti–topo I responses in SSc.

Our group has demonstrated conclusively in two independent studies that during apoptosis topo I is cleaved into a fragment of approximately 70 kDa, whereas in necrosis or caspase-independent cell death, the protein is cleaved into fragments of 70 kDa and 45 kDa [33, 34]. The 45-kDa fragment appears to be specifically associated with necrotic cell death since it has been observed only in cells undergoing primary necrosis, secondary necrosis, and caspase-independent cell death with necrotic morphology. We have proposed that the presence of this fragment can be used to distinguish apoptosis from necrosis by immunoblotting analysis of dying cells. By contrast, the 70-kDa fragment appears in most types of cell death. Samejima et al. [158] showed that during apoptosis caspase-3 and caspase-6 cleave topo I to generate C-terminal fragments ranging from 70 kDa to 80 kDa that are recognized by autoantibodies from SSc patients and are catalytically active. Topo I fragments of 70–75 kDa are also produced by GrB both *in vivo* and *in vitro* during CTL-induced cell death [117, 118].

In a recent study, we hypothesized that cathepsins, which were previously implicated in PARP cleavage and are released from lysosomes during necrosis

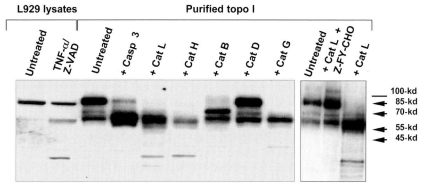

Fig. 6.3 Immunoblots showing *in vitro* cleavage of topo I by individual cathepsins. Approximately 200 ng of purified human topo I was incubated for 1 h at 37 °C with 1.5 mU of various cathepsins. Lysates from untreated L929 cells and cells treated with TNF/Z-VAD-fmk for 6 h were included as controls for topo I cleavage during necrosis. Caspase-3 was also included as a control for *in vitro* cleavage of topo I into the 70-kDa signature apoptotic fragment. Cathepsins L and H generated the 45-kDa cleavage product observed in necrotic cells. Cleavage of topo I by cathepsin L was blocked by the specific cathepsin L inhibitor Z-FY-CHO (left panel). Cathepsin G generated the 70-kDa fragment and other minor fragments. Cathepsin B generated a product of 75–80 kDa not normally observed during cell death. Cathepsin D did not cleave topo I. Bands corresponding to intact topo I are indicated by lines, whereas major proteolytic fragments are indicated by arrows.

[159], might be involved in the cleavage of topo I during necrosis. We demonstrated that this autoantigen is cleaved by cathepsins into its signature 70-kDa and 45-kDa necrotic fragments in L929 cells undergoing necrosis induced by TNF/Z-VAD-fmk. *In vitro*, cathepsins L and H produced both fragments, whereas cathepsin G produced only the 70-kDa fragment (Fig. 6.3). In that study, we observed that during L929 necrosis, cathepsin L activity leaks out of lysosomes and into the cytoplasm and nucleus, whereas a portion of topo I relocalizes in the cytoplasm, suggesting that the two proteins can encounter each other in each compartment. We also observed that Z-FY-CHO, a specific inhibitor of cathepsin L, delays necrosis and topo I cleavage by interfering with cathepsin L processing and lysosomal disruption, suggesting that active cathepsin L contributes to the progression of necrosis. It should be noted that preliminary studies conducted in our laboratory using cathepsin L–deficient cell lines failed to reveal that cathepsin L is essential for topo I cleavage and progression of necrosis (Pacheco and Casiano, unpublished observations). This would support the view that cathepsins may play redundant roles in the cytoplasmic destruction that is characteristic of necrotic cell death.

It is interesting to note that topo I fragments of approximately 70–75 kDa are generated by caspases, GrB, and cathepsins [33, 34, 117, 118, 158, 159]. Because these proteases cleave at different sites, it is unlikely that some of these cleavage fragments are identical. It is possible, however, that topo I has a protease-sensitive region that includes recognition sites for various proteases. The susceptibility of topo I to proteolytic cleavage during classical apoptosis, GrB-mediated cytotoxicity, primary and secondary necrosis, and caspase-independent cell death with necrotic morphology raises the possibility that cell death–associated fragmentation of topo I could trigger the production of autoantibodies against this protein in certain patients with systemic sclerosis. Although it is expected that the immune system should be tolerized against topo I cleavage fragments generated during physiological apoptosis, it is unclear whether cleavage fragments generated during primary or secondary necrosis would be tolerogenic. These necrotic fragments are likely to be immunogenic because they might be taken up and processed by DCs in the presence of "danger signals" released from necrotic cells, leading to DC maturation and activation [160]. We have also observed that cleavage of topo I into 70-kDa and 45-kDa fragments can occur in cultured endothelial cells undergoing necrotic cell death and that the fragments are recognized by the majority of SSc sera containing anti–topo I antibodies [159]. Because endothelial cell death appears to play an important role in the pathogenesis of SSc [161], it is possible that dying endothelial cells could serve as reservoirs of potentially immunogenic fragments of topo I in SSc patients, as long as these fragments are presented to autoreactive lymphocytes in a proinflammatory context.

Our group is currently conducting additional studies to determine whether other scleroderma-associated autoantigens are also susceptible to cathepsin-mediated fragmentation. An issue that remains to be investigated, using cathepsin-deficient mouse models of autoimmunity, is whether the presence of specific cathepsins *in vivo* is essential for the generation of autoantibodies to topo I, PARP, or other cathepsin substrates. Whether autoantigen fragments that are produced during necrosis are immunogenic and capable of triggering autoantibody responses also remains to be fully investigated in animal models. Preliminary evidence for this comes from studies by Pollard et al. [149] demonstrating that a 19-kDa fragment of the scleroderma-associated autoantigen fibrillarin uniquely generated during mercury-induced necrotic cell death was capable of inducing an anti-fibrillarin autoantibody response similar to that observed during mercury-induced autoimmunity in B10.S (H-2^s) mice. These results, combined with the previous observation by the same group that mercury modifies the structure of fibrillarin [18], suggested that an autoimmunity-inducing xenobiotic such as mercury might generate unique immunostimulatory fragments from a self-antigen, most likely by a combination of chemical modification and necrosis-associated proteolysis. An interesting study by Duthoit et al. [162] revealed that oxidative stress–induced necrosis generates an immunoreactive thyroglobulin (Tg) fragment of 40 kDa that contains the immunodominant region recognized by anti-Tg antibodies in patients with autoimmune thyroid diseases. This suggested that the necrotic fragmentation of Tg is associated with the development of anti-Tg autoantibodies in these diseases.

6.6
Defective Clearance of Apoptotic Cells and Autoimmunity

The role of impaired phagocytosis of apoptotic cells in the development of auto-antibodies in systemic autoimmunity has attracted considerable attention in recent years. Under normal circumstances, apoptotic bodies are recognized and engulfed by phagocytic cells. Professional phagocytic cells such as macrophages and DCs clear apoptotic cells swiftly, whereas nonprofessional phagocytes appear to take up apoptotic cells when they reach the later stages of the dying process [163]. This clearance process is facilitated by the presence of "eat me" signals exposed in apoptotic cells (e.g., phosphatidylserine), apoptotic cell recognition receptors in phagocytic cells (e.g., phosphatidylserine receptor, $\beta2$-glycoprotein 1 receptor, vitronectin receptor, complement receptors, and tyrosine kinase Mer receptor), and serum proteins (e.g., complement cascade components such as C1q, C-reactive protein (CRP), and serum amyloid protein) [164]. It is widely accepted that the efficient clearance of apoptotic cells controls inflammatory responses by preventing the release of danger signals from dying cells and by suppressing proinflammatory cytokines, such as TNF, that may be expressed by macrophages [27, 28, 30, 49, 164]. This suppression is mediated by the production of anti-inflammatory mediators such as TGF-β, prostaglandin E, and IL-10 [164].

The efficient clearance of apoptotic cells is crucial for the avoidance of auto-immune responses to intracellular antigens [27, 28, 30, 34, 49, 164, 165]. This clearance results in the exposure of intracellular self-antigens to the immune system under non-inflammatory conditions, leading to tolerization of these antigens, regardless of whether or not they are modified by caspases. It has been proposed that under these conditions circulating DC precursors take up apoptotic cells that they encounter in the various tissues and travel to lymphoid organs, where they present self-antigens from apoptotic cells to T cells in the absence of costimulatory molecules [137, 138, 166]. However, under certain circumstances these intracellular self-antigens could be processed and presented to the immune system under proinflammatory conditions, potentially leading to a pathogenic autoimmune response. These circumstances may include increased secondary necrosis due to inefficient clearance of apoptotic cells, enhanced apoptosis rates, infections causing cell death (both apoptotic and necrotic), or the presence of proinflammatory molecules in the environment in which cell death and clearance occurs [20, 21, 27–30, 163, 165].

Apoptotic cells that are not removed efficiently by phagocytosis ultimately lose their cytoplasmic membrane integrity and undergo secondary necrosis (also referred to as late apoptotic stage, post-apoptotic necrosis, or post-apoptotic cell lysis) [34, 165]. Secondary necrosis occurs as a consequence of the disruption of mitochondrial function, ATP depletion, and the activation of lysosomal enzymes. It is becoming evident that deficiencies in proteins involved in the phagocytic clearance of dying cells and immune complexes, including C1q, C-reactive protein, serum amyloid P (SAP), and the Mer tyrosine kinase, may lead to impairment of phagocytic function, with resulting excessive accumulation of cells in different stages of the cell death continuum, particularly in secondary necrosis [167–172].

The accumulation of cells in secondary necrosis would facilitate the release of proinflammatory signals that induce DC maturation and presentation of modified self-antigens from the dying cells. Evidence for this comes from studies by Manfredi and colleagues [173, 174], who demonstrated *in vitro* that excessive apoptosis or delayed apoptosis leading to secondary necrosis, mimicking a failure of their *in vivo* clearance, was sufficient to trigger DC maturation and presentation of intracellular antigens. This could skew the outcome of cross-presentation of intracellular antigens to autoimmunity if intracellular antigens, proteins, and nucleic acids are presented to autoreactive lymphocytes under the appropriate cytokine environment. As mentioned previously, we have reported that the transition from apoptosis to secondary necrosis is associated with proteolysis of specific autoantigens [34]. In these studies, various cell lines were exposed for up to 60 hours to specific apoptosis inducers. Under these conditions, cells underwent a rapid apoptosis that gradually progressed to secondary necrosis. This progression coincided with the loss of cytoplasmic membrane integrity, as assessed by trypan blue exclusion, and irregular cellular fragmentation characteristic of late necrotic cell death. Immunoblotting analysis indicated that the progression to secondary necrosis was associated with a second wave of proteolysis of specific intracellular autoantigens that are cleaved during apoptosis, including LEDGF/p75, PARP, SSB/La, topo I, and U1-70 kDa. Interestingly, although some of the cleavage fragments produced during secondary necrosis were also detected in primary necrosis, identical cleavage patterns were not observed in these pathways for all the autoantigens tested. This could be attributed to differential compartmentalization of the proteases mediating these cleavages during upstream events leading to primary and secondary necrosis.

6.7
Immunostimulatory Properties of Dying Cells

There is compelling evidence indicating that both apoptotic and necrotic cells are capable of stimulating immune responses [139–144]. However, signals derived from necrotic cells appear to make these cells more efficient than apoptotic cells in eliciting immune responses. This concept was initially highlighted by Gallucci et al. [160], who reported that DCs undergo maturation *in vitro* and present antigens in a pro-immune manner *in vivo* upon stimulation by signals from stressed, virally infected, or necrotic cells, but not from healthy or apoptotic cells. They proposed that signals derived from necrotic but not apoptotic cells act as potent natural adjuvants. Along the same line, Sauter et al. [144] demonstrated that immature DCs efficiently ingest apoptotic and necrotic tumor cells, but only the latter provide maturation signals. Remarkably, in these studies only tumor cell lines, and not primary cell lines, induced maturation of DCs, suggesting that signals specifically associated with tumor cells may enhance the induction of DC maturation factors. These authors also observed that the cellular damage associated with necrosis has to be extensive enough to facilitate the release of those maturation factors. It was also demonstrated that macrophages exposed to necrotic, but not apoptotic, cells expressed increased levels of costimulatory molecules and stimulated specific T-cell responses [142–143]. More recently, two different studies provided evidence that DCs internalize both early apoptotic cells and late apoptotic cells (secondary necrosis) with similar efficiency, but DCs that had taken up cells in secondary necrosis acquired the mature DC phenotype and had a higher capacity to stimulate T-cell responses [175, 176].

In contrast to these findings, several studies have shown that, like necrotic cells, apoptotic cells are also capable of inducing maturation of DCs and stimulating immune responses *in vivo* [140, 141, 177]. Furthermore, it was demonstrated that DC uptake of apoptotic or necrotic cells alone does not shift the immune response from tolerance to autoimmunity in systemic autoimmune conditions [178]. Moreover, a recent report indicated that phagocytosis of apoptotic or necrotic cells by macrophages does not lead to induction of expression of proinflammatory cytokines in the macrophages clearing the dying cells [179]. However, these investigators also found that the clearance of necrotic cells (primary or secondary) is significantly less efficient than the clearance of apoptotic cells, which could lead to macrophages remaining at the injury site longer, thus increasing the likelihood of a proinflammatory state to develop. They also suggested that the proinflammatory environment produced by necrotic cells might be due to the release of factors or proinflammatory cytokines from the necrotic cells themselves.

What determines, then, whether apoptotic or necrotic cells become immunostimulatory? Based on the studies of Bondanza et al. [180], it seems that a two-hit signal, composed of (1) autoantigens derived from dying cells (apoptotic or necrotic) and (2) environmental signals or adjuvants at the site of the clearance of death cells that induce DC maturation and immune responses, shapes the features and severity of autoimmune disease. The nature of these "danger signals" is not entirely clear, but there is compelling evidence, as suggested by Brouckaert et al. [179], that some of them are released from dying cells, particularly cells that have acquired the necrotic phenotype. Factors released from dying cells that have been positively identified as potential "danger signals" that trigger the production of inflammatory cytokines include the high-mobility group 1 (HMGB1) protein [181–183], immune complexes containing nucleic acids [184], uric acid [185], and heat shock protein 70 [186–189]. It is not clear at the present time whether all these signals are released from both primary necrotic and secondary necrotic cells. Scaffidi et al. [181] reported that HMGB1 is released by necrotic cells but retained by apoptotic cells and cells undergoing secondary necrosis and that this represents a safeguard against confusing necrotic from apoptotic cells.

An additional source of danger signals provided by necrotic cells could be complexes between self-antigens and antigens derived from infectious agents.

For instance, the induction of massive apoptosis by a viral infection *in vitro* was found to be associated with DC-mediated activation of virus-specific CTLs [190]. Consistent with this observation, Salio et al. [191] reported that the capacity of necrotic or apoptotic cells to induce DC maturation *in vitro* was dependent on the presence of a mycoplasma infection, suggesting that cell death in the presence of an infectious agent provides the necessary proinflammatory signals for stimulating a DC-mediated immune response. Green and Beere [192] argued that extensive necrosis associated with an infection would induce an inflammatory response, leading the nearby DCs, which engulf both necrotic cells and infected apoptotic cells, to display costimulatory molecules and self-peptides derived from the dying cells, as well as foreign peptides from the infectious agent.

Given the mounting evidence suggesting that necrotic cells are a source of danger signals that could trigger a proinflammatory context and DC-mediated, antigen-specific immune responses, it would seem plausible that post-translational modifications of autoantigens associated with necrotic cell death, such as cathepsin-mediated autoantigen proteolysis, may also give rise to potentially immunostimulatory forms of intracellular or membrane-associated autoantigens. Under a proinflammatory cytokine environment, these modified autoantigens, which may also expose cryptic epitopes, might be processed by mature DCs and presented to either naïve T cells that have not been tolerized against the cryptic epitopes or to autoreactive CD4$^+$ and CD8$^+$ T cells that escaped deletion due to defects in T-cell apoptosis. Subsequently, the autoreactive CD4$^+$ T cells may stimulate autoreactive B cells to produce pathogenic autoantibodies, whereas CD8$^+$ T cells may attack tissues expressing the autoantigens, leading to organ damage. Figure 6.4 shows a schematic diagram summarizing the various factors and dangers encountered on the road leading from cell death to autoimmunity.

6.8
Conclusions

The progress achieved during the past decade in our understanding of biochemical mechanisms associated with cell death has significantly impacted the field of autoimmunity. It is now evident that cell death has many different faces, each of which may contribute to autoimmunity through diverse mechanisms. These mechanisms include defects in genes involved in the regulation of the activation of T and B lymphocytes and the deletion of autoreactive lymphocytes, excessive cell death induced by autoreactive CTL in target organs, modifications in intracellular self-antigens that increase their immunogenicity, defective clearance of immune complexes and dying cells, and release of danger signals from dying cells leading to a proinflammatory environment. As knowledge derived from the molecular dissection of different variants of cell death *in vitro* and in animal models of autoimmunity continues to accumulate, the potential role of these variants in the generation of autoimmunity will become more evident. This knowledge will facilitate the development of novel therapeutic strategies

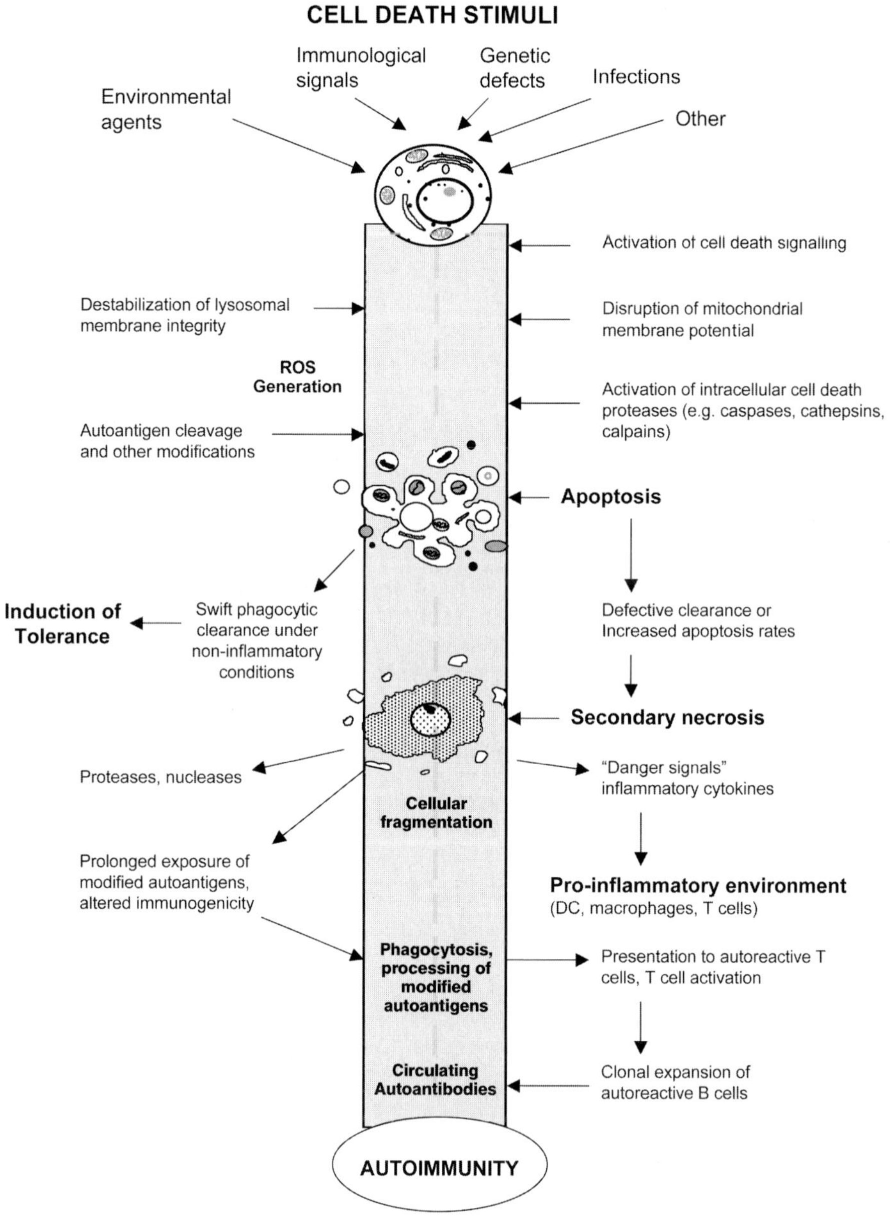

Fig. 6.4 The road to perdition: summary of events implicated in the path leading from cell death to autoimmunity.

aimed at modulating the delicate balance between cell death and survival in autoimmune diseases.

Acknowledgments

The authors are grateful to the members of the Center for Molecular Biology and Gene Therapy at the Loma Linda University School of Medicine for their valuable suggestions and input on this work. F.J. Pacheco was supported by the Federal University of Sao Paulo and the Adventist University of Sao Paulo in Brazil. This work was supported by NIH-NIAID Grant AI44088 to C.A. Casiano and by basic science grants from the Loma Linda University School of Medicine.

References

1 Grodzicky T, Elkon KB. Apoptosis: a case where too much or too little can lead to autoimmunity. Mt Sinai J Med. 2002; 69:208–219.

2 D'Andrea MR. Evidence linking neuronal cell death to autoimmunity in Alzheimer's disease. Brain Res. 2003; 982: 19–30.

3 Okada H, Mak TW. Pathways of apoptotic and non-apoptotic death in tumour cells. Nat Rev Cancer. 2004; 4:592–603.

4 Hui H, Dotta F, Di Mario U, Perfetti R. Role of caspases in the regulation of apoptotic pancreatic islet beta-cells death. J Cell Physiol. 2004; 200:177–200.

5 Chen QM, Tu VC. Apoptosis and heart failure: mechanisms and therapeutic implications. Am J Cardiovasc Drugs. 2002; 2:43–57.

6 Aigner T, Kim HA. Apoptosis and cellular vitality: issues in osteoarthritic cartilage degeneration. Arthritis Rheum. 2002; 46:1986–1996.

7 Rust C, Gores GJ. Apoptosis and liver disease. Am J Med. 2000; 108:567–574.

8 Buja LM, Eigenbrodt ML, Eigenbrodt EH. Apoptosis and necrosis: basic types and mechanisms of cell death. Arch Pathol Lab Med. 1993; 117:1208–1214.

9 Majno G, Joris I. Apoptosis, oncosis, and necrosis: an overview of cell death. Amer J Pathol. 1995; 146:3–15.

10 Guimaraes CA, Linden R. Programmed cell deaths. Apoptosis and alternative deathstyles. Eur J Biochem. 2004; 271:1638–1650.

11 Jaattela M, Tschopp J. Caspase-independent cell death in T lymphocytes. Nat Immunol. 2003; 4:416–423.

12 Zeiss CJ. The apoptosis-necrosis continuum: insights from genetically altered mice. Vet Pathol. 2003; 40:481–495.

13 Nicotera P. Apoptosis and age-related disorders: role of caspase-dependent and caspase-independent pathways. Toxicol Lett. 2002; 127:189–195.

14 Lockshin RA, Zakeri Z. Caspase-independent cell deaths. Curr Opin Cell Biol. 2002; 14:727–733.

15 Adams JM. Ways of dying: multiple pathways to apoptosis. Genes Dev. 2003; 17:2481–2495.

16 Kohm AP, Fuller KG, Miller SD. Mimicking the way to autoimmunity: an evolving theory of sequence and structural homology. Trends Microbiol. 2003; 11:101–105.

17 Turk MJ, Wolchok JD, Guevara-Patino JA, Goldberg SM, Houghton AN. Multiple pathways to tumor immunity and concomitant autoimmunity. Immunol Rev. 2002; 188:122–135.

18 Pollard KM, Lee DK, Casiano CA, Blüthner M, Johnston MM, Tan EM. The autoimmunity-inducing xenobiotic mercury interacts with the autoantigen fibrillarin and modifies its molecular and

antigenic properties. J. Immunol. 1997; 158:3521–3528.

19 Rosen A, Casciola-Rosen L, Ahearn J. Novel packages of viral and self-antigens are generated during apoptosis. J Exp Med. 1995; 181:1557–1561.

20 Todaro M, Zeuner A, Stassi G. Role of apoptosis in autoimmunity. J Clin Immunol. 2004; 24:1–11.

21 Mevorach D. The role of death-associated molecular patterns in the pathogenesis of systemic lupus erythematosus. Rheum Dis Clin North Am. 2004; 30:487–504.

22 Stuart L, Hughes J. Apoptosis and autoimmunity. Nephrol Dial Transplant. 2002; 17:697–700.

23 Kuhtreiber WM, Hayashi T, Dale EA, Faustman DL. Central role of defective apoptosis in autoimmunity. J Mol Endocrinol. 2003; 31:373–399.

24 Rieux-Laucat F, Le Deist F, Fischer A. Autoimmune lymphoproliferative syndromes: genetic defects of apoptosis pathways. Cell Death Differ. 2003; 10:124–133.

25 Dianzani U, Chiocchetti A, Ramenghi U. Role of inherited defects decreasing Fas function in autoimmunity. Life Sci. 2003; 72:2803–2824.

26 Baker JR Jr. The nature of apoptosis in the thyroid and the role it may play in autoimmune thyroid disease. Thyroid. 2001; 11:245–247.

27 Pittoni V, Valesini G. The clearance of apoptotic cells: implications for autoimmunity. Autoimmun Rev. 2002; 1:154–161.

28 Rovere-Querini P, Dumitriu IE. Corpse disposal after apoptosis. Apoptosis. 2003; 8:469–479.

29 Botto M. Links between complement deficiency and apoptosis. Arthritis Res. 2001; 3:207–210.

30 Navratil JS, Sabatine JM, Ahearn JM. Apoptosis and immune responses to self. Rheum Dis Clin North Am. 2004; 30:193–212.

31 Hall JC, Casciola-Rosen L, Rosen A. Altered structure of autoantigens during apoptosis. Rheum Dis Clin North Am. 2004; 30:455–471.

32 Utz PJ, Anderson P. Posttranslational protein modifications, apoptosis, and the bypass of tolerance to autoantigens. Arthritis Rheum. 1998; 41:1152–1160.

33 Casiano CA, Ochs RL, Tan EM. Distinct cleavage products of nuclear proteins in apoptosis and necrosis revealed by autoantibody probes. Cell Death Differ. 1998; 5:183–190.

34 Wu X, Molinaro C, Johnson N, Casiano CA. Secondary necrosis is a source of proteolytically modified forms of specific intracellular autoantigens: implications for systemic autoimmunity. Arthritis Rheum. 2001; 44:2642–2652.

35 Wyllie AH, Kerr JFR, Currie AC. Cell death: the significance of apoptosis. Int Rev Cytol 1980; 68:251–305.

36 Ellis RE, Yuan J, Horvitz HR. Mechanisms and function of cell death. Annu Rev Cell Biol. 1991; 7:663–698.

37 Casciola-Rosen L, Rosen A. Ultraviolet light-induced keratinocyte apoptosis: a potential mechanism for the induction of skin lesions and autoantibody production in LE. Lupus 1997; 6:175–180.

38 Simon HU, Haj-Yehia A, Levi-Schaffer F. Role of reactive oxygen species (ROS) in apoptosis induction. Apoptosis. 2000; 5:415–418.

39 Greijer AE, van der Wall E. The role of hypoxia inducible factor 1 (HIF-1) in hypoxia induced apoptosis. J Clin Pathol. 2004; 57:1009–1014.

40 Krammer PH. CD95(APO-1/Fas)-mediated apoptosis: live and let die. Adv Immunol. 1999; 71:163–210.

41 Kawanishi S, Hiraku Y. Amplification of anticancer drug-induced DNA damage and apoptosis by DNA-binding compounds. Curr Med Chem Anti-Canc Agents. 2004; 4:415–419.

42 He J, Xiao Y, Casiano CA, Zhang L. Role of mitochondrial cytochrome c in cocaine-induced apoptosis in coronary artery endothelial cells. J Pharmacol Exp Ther. 2000; 295:896–903.

43 Oliveira MT, Rego AC, Macedo TR, Oliveira CR. Drugs of abuse induce apoptotic features in PC12 cells. Ann NY Acad Sci. 2003; 1010:667–670.

44 Bohana-Kashtan O, Ziporen L, Donin N, Kraus S, Fishelson Z. Cell signals trans-

duced by complement. Mol Immunol. 2004; 41:583–597.

45 Andreka P, Tran T, Webster KA, Bishopric NH. Nitric oxide and promotion of cardiac myocyte apoptosis. Mol Cell Biochem. 2004; 263:35–53.

46 de Graaf AO, de Witte T, Jansen JH. Inhibitor of apoptosis proteins: new therapeutic targets in hematological cancer? Leukemia. 2004; 18:1751–1759.

47 Hwang ES, Bowen PE. Cell cycle arrest and induction of apoptosis by lycopene in LNCaP human prostate cancer cells. J Med Food. 2004; 7:284–289.

48 Kang JH, Park YH, Choi SW, Yang EK, Lee WJ. Resveratrol derivatives potently induce apoptosis in human promyelocytic leukemia cells. Exp Mol Med. 2003; 35:467–474.

49 Gaipl US, Brunner J, Beyer TD, Voll RE, Kalden JR, Herrmann M. Disposal of dying cells: a balancing act between infection and autoimmunity. Arthritis Rheum. 2003; 48:6–11.

50 Savill J, Fadok V. Corpse clearance defines the meaning of cell death. Nature. 2000; 407:784–788.

51 Chang HY, Yang X. Proteases for cell suicide: functions and regulation of caspases. Microbiol Mol Biol Rev. 2000; 64:821–846.

52 Earnshaw WC, Martins LM, Kaufmann SH. Mammalian caspases: structure, activation, substrates, and functions during apoptosis. Annu Rev Biochem. 1999; 68:383–424.

53 Denault JB, Salvesen GS. Caspases: keys in the ignition of cell death. Chem Rev. 2002; 102:4489–4500.

54 Bhardwaj A, Aggarwal BB. Receptor-mediated choreography of life and death. J Clin Immunol. 2003; 23:317–332.

55 Ravagnan L, Roumier T, Kroemer G. Mitochondria, the killer organelles and their weapons. J Cell Physiol. 2002; 192:131–137.

56 Cande C, Cohen I, Daugas E, Ravagnan L, Larochette N, Zamzami N, Kroemer G. Apoptosis-inducing factor (AIF): a novel caspase-independent death effector released from mitochondria. Biochimie. 2002; 84:215–222.

57 Lorenzo HK, Susin SA. Mitochondrial effectors in caspase-independent cell death. FEBS Lett. 2004; 557:14–20.

58 Tsujimoto Y. Cell death regulation by the Bcl-2 protein family in the mitochondria. J Cell Physiol. 2003; 195:158–167.

59 Sarin A, Williams MS, Alexander-Miller MA, Berzofsky JA, Zacharchuk CM, Henkart PA. Target cell lysis by CTL granule exocytosis is independent of ICE/Ced-3 family proteases. Immunity. 1997; 6:209–215.

60 Trapani JA, Jans DA, Jans PJ, Smyth MJ, Browne KA, Sutton VR. Efficient nuclear targeting of granzyme B and the nuclear consequences of apoptosis induced by granzyme B and perforin are caspase-dependent, but cell death is caspase-independent. J Biol Chem. 1998; 273:27934–27938.

61 Trapani JA, Davis J, Sutton VR, Smyth MJ. Proapoptotic functions of cytotoxic lymphocyte granule constituents in vitro and in vivo. Curr Opin Immunol. 2000; 12:323–329.

62 Waterhouse NJ, Sedelies KA, Brown KA, Wowk ME, Newbold A, Sutton VR, Clarke CJ, Oliaro J, Lindemann RK, Bird PI, Johnstone RW, Trapani JA. A central role for Bid in granzyme B-induced apoptosis. J Biol Chem. 2004; 280:4476–4482.

63 Breckenridge DG, Germain M, Mathai JP, Nguyen M, Shore GC. Regulation of apoptosis by endoplasmic reticulum pathways. Oncogene. 2003; 22:8608–8618.

64 Fischer U, Janicke RU, Schulze-Osthoff K. Many cuts to ruin: a comprehensive update of caspase substrates. Cell Death Differ. 2003; 10:76–100.

65 Yamashima T. Implication of cysteine proteases calpain, cathepsin and caspase in ischemic neuronal death of primates. Prog Neurobiol. 2000; 62:273–295.

66 Turk B, Stoka V, Rozman-Pungercar J, Cirman T, Droga-Mazovec G, Oresic K, Turk V. Apoptotic pathways: involvement of lysosomal proteases. Biol Chem. 2002; 383:1035–1044.

67 Stenson-Cox C, FitzGerald U, Samali A. In the cut and thrust of apoptosis, serine proteases come of age. Biochem Pharmacol. 2003; 66:1469–1474.

68 Chen Z, Casiano CA, Fletcher HM. Protease-active extracellular protein preparations from Porphyromonas gingivalis W83 induce N-cadherin proteolysis, loss of cell adhesion, and apoptosis in human epithelial cells. J Periodontol. 2001; 72:641–650.

69 Jaattela M, Cande C, Kroemer G. Lysosomes and mitochondria in the commitment to apoptosis: a potential role for cathepsin D and AIF. Cell Death Differ. 2004; 11:135–136.

70 Biggs JR, Yang J, Gullberg U, Muchardt C, Yaniv M, Kraft AS. The human brm protein is cleaved during apoptosis: the role of cathepsin G. Proc Natl Acad Sci USA. 2001; 98:3814–3819.

71 Stoka V, Turk B, Schendel SL, Kim TH, Cirman T, Snipas SJ, Ellerby LM, Bredesen D, Freeze H, Abrahamson M, Bromme D, Krajewski S, Reed JC, Yin XM, Turk V, Salvesen GS. Lysosomal protease pathways to apoptosis. Cleavage of bid, not pro-caspases, is the most likely route. J Biol Chem. 2001; 276:3149–3157.

72 Gan L, Ye S, Chu A, Anton K, Yi S, Vincent VA, von Schack D, Chin D, Murray J, Lohr S, Patthy L, Gonzalez-Zulueta M, Nikolich K, Urfer R. Identification of cathepsin B as a mediator of neuronal death induced by Abeta-activated microglial cells using a functional genomics approach. J Biol Chem. 2004; 279:5565–5572.

73 Bidere N, Lorenzo HK, Carmona S, Laforge M, Harper F, Dumont C, Senik A. Cathepsin D triggers Bax activation, resulting in selective apoptosis-inducing factor (AIF) relocation in T lymphocytes entering the early commitment phase to apoptosis. J Biol Chem. 2003; 278:31401–31411.

74 Ono K, Kim SO, Han J. Susceptibility of lysosomes to rupture is a determinant for plasma membrane disruption in tumor necrosis factor alpha-induced cell death. Mol Cell Biol. 2003; 23:665–676.

75 Bortul R, Zweyer M, Billi AM, Tabellini G, Ochs RL, Bareggi R, Cocco L, Martelli AM. Nuclear changes in necrotic HL-60 cells. J Cell Biochem. 2001; 36:19–31.

76 Rao L, Perez D, White E. Lamin proteolysis facilitates nuclear events during apoptosis. J Cell Biol. 1996; 135:1441–1455.

77 Proskuryakov SY, Konoplyannikov AG, Gabai VL. Necrosis: a specific form of programmed cell death? Exp Cell Res. 2003; 283:1–16.

78 Napirei M, Wulf S, Mannherz HG. Chromatin breakdown during necrosis by serum Dnase1 and the plasminogen system. Arthritis Rheum. 2004; 50:1873–1883.

79 Kaplowitz N. Mechanisms of liver cell injury. Hepatol. 2000; 32:39–47.

80 Leist M, Jaattela M. Four deaths and a funeral: from caspases to alternative mechanisms. Nat Rev Mol Cell Biol. 2001; 2:589–598.

81 Chautan M, Chazal G, Cecconi F, Gruss P, Golstein P. Interdigital cell death can occur through a necrotic and caspase-independent pathway. Curr Biol. 1999; 9:967–970.

82 Sapunar D, Vilovic K, England M, Saraga-Babic M. Morphological diversity of dying cells during regression of the human tail. Ann Anat. 2001; 183:217–222.

83 Kaneko T, Iida H, Bedford JM, Mori T. Spermatozoa of the shrew, Suncus murinus, undergo the acrosome reaction and then selectively kill cells in penetrating the cumulus oophorus. Biol Reprod. 2001; 65:544–553.

84 Murdoch WJ, Wilken C, Young DA. Sequence of apoptosis and inflammatory necrosis within the formative ovulatory site of sheep follicles. J Reprod Fertil. 1999;117:325–329.

85 Mayhew TM, Myklebust R, Whybrow A, Jenkins R. Epithelial integrity, cell death and cell loss in mammalian small intestine. Histol Histopathol. 1999; 14:257–267.

86 Barkla DH, Gibson PR. The fate of epithelial cells in the human large intestine. Pathology. 1999; 31:230–238.

87 Blom WM, De Bont HJ, Meijerman I, Kuppen PJ, Mulder GJ, Nagelkerke JF. Interleukin–2-activated natural killer cells can induce both apoptosis and necrosis in rat hepatocytes. Hepatology. 1999; 29:785–792.

88 Gardiner CM, Reen DJ. Differential cytokine regulation of natural killer cell-mediated necrotic and apoptotic cytotoxicity. Immunology. 1998; 93:511–517.

89 Shimizu A, Masuda Y, Kitamura H, Ishizaki M, Ohashi R, Sugisaki Y, Yamanaka N. Complement-mediated killing of mesangial cells in experimental glomerulonephritis: cell death by a combination of apoptosis and necrosis. Nephron. 2000; 86:152–160.

90 Holler N, Zaru R, Micheau O, Thome M, Attinger A, Valitutti S, Bodmer JL, Schneider P, Seed B, Tschopp J. Fas triggers an alternative, caspase-8-independent cell death pathway using the kinase RIP as effector molecule. Nat Immunol. 2000; 1:489–495.

91 Gukovskaya AS, Pandol SJ. Cell death pathways in pancreatitis and pancreatic cancer. Pancreatology. 2004; 4:567–586.

92 Columbano A. Cell death: current difficulties in discriminating apoptosis from necrosis in the context of pathological processes in vivo. J. Cell. Biochem. 1995; 58:181–190.

93 Nicotera P, Leist M, Ferrando-May E. Apoptosis and necrosis: different execution of the same death. Biochem Soc Symp. 1999; 66:69–73.

94 Watson AJM. Necrosis and apoptosis in the gastrointestinal tract. Gut 1995; 37:165–167.

95 Snider BJ, Gottron FJ, Choi DW. Apoptosis and necrosis in cerebrovascular disease. Ann NY Acad Sci. 1999; 893:243–253.

96 Kelly L, Reid L, Walker NI. Massive acinar cell apoptosis with secondary necrosis, origin of ducts in atrophic lobules and failure to regenerate in cyanohydroxybutene pancreatopathy in rats. Int J Exp Pathol. 1999; 80:217–226.

97 Roy M, Sapolsky R. Neuronal apoptosis in acute necrotic insults: why is this subject such a mess? Trends Neurosci. 1999; 22:419–422.

98 Zeng YS, Xu ZC. Co-existence of necrosis and apoptosis in rat hippocampus following transient forebrain ischemia. Neurosci Res. 2000; 37:113–125.

99 Leist M, Nicotera P. The shape of cell death. Biochem Biophys Res Comm. 1997; 236:1–9.

100 Vercammen D, Beyaert R, Denecker G, Goossens V, Van Loo G, Declercq W, Grooten J, Fiers W, Vandenabeele P. Inhibition of caspases increases the sensitivity of L929 cells to necrosis mediated by tumor necrosis factor. J Exp Med. 1998; 187:1477–1485.

101 Michaelis M, Kotchetkov R, Vogel JU, Doerr HW, Cinatl J Jr. Cytomegalovirus infection blocks apoptosis in cancer cells. Cell Mol Life Sci. 2004; 61:1307–1316.

102 Sane AT, Bertrand R. Caspase inhibition in camptothecin-treated U-937 cells is coupled with a shift from apoptosis to transient G1 arrest followed by necrotic cell death. Cancer Res. 1999; 59:3565–3569.

103 Amarante-Mendes GP, Finucane DM, Martin SJ, Cotter TG, Salvesen GS, Green DR. Anti-apoptotic oncogenes prevent caspase-dependent and independent commitment for cell death. Cell Death Differ. 1998; 5:298–306.

104 Kawahara A, Ohsawa Y, Matsumura H, Uchiyama Y, Nagata S. Caspase-independent cell killing by Fas-associated protein with death domain. J Cell Biol. 1998; 143:1353–1360.

105 Denecker G, Vercammen D, Steemans M, Vanden Berghe T, Brouckaert G, Van Loo G, Zhivotovsky B, Fiers W, Grooten J, Declercq W, Vandenabeele P. Death receptor-induced apoptotic and necrotic cell death: differential role of caspases and mitochondria. Cell Death Differ. 2001; 8:829–840.

106 McCarthy NJ, Whyte MK, Gilbert CS, Evan GI. Inhibition of Ced-3/ICE-related proteases does not prevent cell death induced by oncogenes, DNA damage, or the Bcl-2 homologue Bak. J Cell Biol. 1997; 136:215–227.

107 Deas O, Dumont C, MacFarlane M, Rouleau M, Hebib C, Harper F, Hirsch F, Charpentier B, Cohen GM, Senik A. Caspase-independent cell death induced by anti-CD2 or staurosporine in activated human peripheral T lymphocytes. J Immunol. 1998; 161:3375–3383.

108 Liu Y, Tergaonkar V, Krishna S, Androphy EJ. Human papillomavirus type 16

E6-enhanced susceptibility of L929 cells to tumor necrosis factor alpha correlates with increased accumulation of reactive oxygen species. J Biol Chem. 1999; 274:24819–24827.

109 Kitanaka C, Kuchino Y. Caspase-independent programmed cell death with necrotic morphology. Cell Death Differ. 1999; 6:508–515.

110 Fiers W, Beyaert R, Declercq W, Vandenabeele P. More than one way to die: apoptosis, necrosis and reactive oxygen damage. Oncogene. 1999; 18:7719–7730.

111 Kolenko V, Uzzo RG, Bukowski R, Bander NH, Novick AC, Hsi ED, Finke JH. Dead or dying: necrosis versus apoptosis in caspase-deficient human renal cell carcinoma. Cancer Res. 1999; 59:2838–2842.

112 Melino G, Catani MV, Corazzari M, Guerrieri P, Bernassola F. Nitric oxide can inhibit apoptosis or switch it into necrosis. Cell Mol Life Sci. 2000; 57:612–622.

113 Smith KG, Strasser A, Vaux DL. CrmA expression in T lymphocytes of transgenic mice inhibits CD95 (Fas/APO–1)-transduced apoptosis, but does not cause lymphadenopathy or autoimmune disease. EMBO J. 1996; 15:5167–5176.

114 Boone E, Vanden Berghe T, Van Loo G, De Wilde G, De Wael N, Vercammen D, Fiers W, Haegeman G, Vandenabeele P. Structure/Function analysis of p55 tumor necrosis factor receptor and fas-associated death domain. Effect on necrosis in L929sA cells. J Biol Chem. 2000; 275:37596–375603.

115 Vercammen D, Brouckaert G, Denecker G, Van de Craen M, Declercq W, Fiers W, Vandenabeele P. Dual signaling of the Fas receptor: Initiation of both apoptotic and necrotic cell death pathways. J Exp Med. 1998; 188:919–930.

116 Matsumura H, Shimizu Y, Ohsawa Y, Kawahara A, Uchiyama Y, Nagata S. Necrotic death pathway in Fas receptor signaling. J Cell Biol. 2000; 151:1247–1256.

117 Khwaja A, Tatton L. Resistance to the cytotoxic effects of tumor necrosis factor alpha can be overcome by inhibition of a FADD/caspase-dependent signaling pathway. J Biol Chem. 1999; 274:36817–36823.

118 Jones BE, Lo CR, Liu H, Srinivasan A, Streetz K, Valentino KL, Czaja MJ. Hepatocytes sensitized to tumor necrosis factor-alpha cytotoxicity undergo apoptosis through caspase-dependent and caspase-independent pathways. J Biol Chem. 2000; 275:705–712.

119 Los M, Mozoluk M, Ferrari D, Stepczynska A, Stroh C, Renz A, Herceg Z, Wang ZQ, Schulze-Osthoff K. Activation and caspase-mediated inhibition of PARP: a molecular switch between fibroblast necrosis and apoptosis in death receptor signaling. Mol Biol Cell. 2002; 13:978–988.

120 Ha HC, Snyder SH. Poly(ADP-ribose) polymerase is a mediator of necrotic cell death by ATP depletion. Proc Natl Acad Sci U S A. 1999; 96:13978–13982.

121 Herceg Z, Wang ZQ. Failure of poly-(ADP-ribose) polymerase cleavage by caspases leads to induction of necrosis and enhanced apoptosis. Mol Cell Biol. 1999; 19:5124–5133.

122 Walisser JA, Thies RL. Poly (ADP-ribose) polymerase inhibition in oxidant-stressed endothelial cells prevents oncosis and permits caspase activation and apoptosis. Exp Cell Res. 1999; 251:401–413.

123 Zhao M, Antunes F, Eaton JW, Brunk UT. Lysosomal enzymes promote mitochondrial oxidant production, cytochrome *c* release and apoptosis. Eur J Biochem 2003; 270:3778–3786.

124 Kurz T, Leake A, von Zglinicki T, Brunk UT. Lysosomal redox-active iron is important for oxidative stress-induced DNA damage. Ann NY Acad Sci. 2004; 1019:285–288.

125 Nylandsted J, Gyrd-Hansen M, Danielewicz A, Fehrenbacher N, Lademann U, Hoyer-Hansen M, Weber E, Multhoff G, Rohde M, Jaattela M. Heat shock protein 70 promotes cell survival by inhibiting lysosomal membrane permeabilization. J Exp Med. 2004; 200:425–435.

126 Watanabe-Fukunaga R, Brannan CI, Copeland NG, Jenkins NA, Nagata S. Lymphoproliferation disorder in mice explained by defects in Fas antigen that mediates apoptosis. Nature. 1992; 356:314–317.

127 Takahashi T, Tanaka M, Brannan CI, Jenkins NA, Copeland NG, Suda T, Nagata S. Generalized lymphoproliferative disease in mice, caused by a point mutation in the FasLigand. Cell. 1994; 76:969–976.

128 Wu J, Wilson J, He J, Xiang L, Schur PH, Mountz JD. FasLigand mutation in a patient with systemic lupus erythematosus and lymphoproliferative disease.J Clin Invest. 1996; 98:1107–1113.

129 Drappa J, Kamen LA, Chan E, Georgiev M, Ashany D, Marti F, King PD. Impaired T cell death and lupus-like autoimmunity in T cell-specific adapter protein-deficient mice. J Exp Med. 2003; 198:809–821.

130 Lawson BR, Baccala R, Song J, Croft M, Kono DH, Theofilopoulos AN. Text Deficiency of the cyclin kinase inhibitor p21(WAF-1/CIP-1) promotes apoptosis of activated/memory T cells and inhibits spontaneous systemic autoimmunity. J Exp Med. 2004; 199:547–557.

131 Casciola-Rosen LA, Anhalt G, Rosen A. Autoantigens targeted in systemic lupus erythematosus are clustered in two populations of surface structures on apoptotic keratinocytes. J Exp Med. 1994; 179:1317–1330.

132 Casciola-Rosen LA, Miller DK, Anhalt G, Rosen A. Specific cleavage of the 70-kD protein component of the U1 small nuclear ribonucleoprotein is a characteristic biochemical feature of apoptotic cell death. J Biol Chem. 1994; 269:30757–30760.

133 Casciola-Rosen LA, Anhalt G, Rosen A. DNA-dependent protein kinase is one of a subset of autoantigens specifically cleaved early during apoptosis. J Exp Med. 1995; 182:1625–1634.

134 Casiano CA Martin SJ, Green DR, Tan EM. Selective cleavage of nuclear autoantigens during CD95 (Fas/APO-1)-mediated T cell apoptosis. J Exp Med. 1996; 184:765–770.

135 Kaplan MJ. Apoptosis in systemic lupus erythematosus. Clin Immunol. 2004; 112:210–218.

136 Rosen A, Casciola-Rosen L. Autoantigens as substrates for apoptotic proteases: implications for the pathogenesis of systemic autoimmune disease. Cell Death Differ. 1999; 6:6–12.

137 Steinman RM, Nussenzweig MC. Avoiding horror autotoxicus: the importance of dendritic cells in peripheral T cell tolerance. Proc Natl Acad Sci USA. 2002; 99:351–358.

138 Turley SJ. Dendritic cells: inciting and inhibiting autoimmunity. Curr Opin Immunol. 2002; 14:765–770.

139 Mevorach D, Zhou JL, Song X, Elkon KB. Systemic exposure to irradiated apoptotic cells induces autoantibody production. J Exp Med. 1998; 188: 387–392.

140 Gensler TJ, Hottelet M, Zhang C, Schlossman S, Anderson P, Utz PJ. Monoclonal antibodies derived from BALB/c mice immunized with apoptotic Jurkat T cells recognize known autoantigens. J Autoimmun. 2001; 16:59–69.

141 Ronchetti A, Rovere P, Iezzi G, Galati G, Heltai S, Protti MP, Garancini MP, Manfredi AA, Rugarli C, Bellone M. Immunogenicity of apoptotic cells in vivo: role of antigen load, antigen-presenting cells, and cytokines. J Immunol. 1999; 163:130–136.

142 Reiter I, Krammer B, Schwamberger G. Cutting edge: differential effect of apoptotic versus necrotic tumor cells on macrophage antitumor activities. J Immunol. 1999; 163:1730–1732.

143 Barker RN, Erwig L, Pearce WP, Devine A, Rees AJ. Differential effects of necrotic or apoptotic cell uptake on antigen presentation by macrophages. Pathobiology. 1999; 67:302–305.

144 Sauter B, Albert ML, Francisco L, Larsson M, Somersan S, Bhardwaj N. Consequences of cell death: exposure to necrotic tumor cells, but not primary tissue cells or apoptotic cells, induces the maturation of immunostimulatory dendritic cells. J Exp Med. 2000; 191:423–434.

145 Andrade F, Roy S, Nicholson D, Thornberry N, Rosen A, Casciola-Rosen L. Granzyme B directly and efficiently cleaves several downstream caspase substrates: implications for CTL-induced apoptosis. Immunity. 1998; 8:451–460.

146 Casciola-Rosen L, Andrade F, Ulanet D, Wong WB, Rosen A. Cleavage by granzyme B is strongly predictive of autoantigen status: implications for initiation of autoimmunity. J Exp Med. 1999; 190:815–826.

147 Ulanet DB, Flavahan NA, Casciola-Rosen L, Rosen A. Selective cleavage of nucleolar autoantigen B23 by granzyme B in differentiated vascular smooth muscle cells: insights into the association of specific autoantibodies with distinct disease phenotypes. Arthritis Rheum. 2004; 50:233–241.

148 Nozawa K, Casiano CA, Hamel JC, Molinaro C, Fritzler MJ, Chan EK. Fragmentation of Golgi complex and Golgi autoantigens during apoptosis and necrosis. Arthritis Res. 2002; 4(4):R3. (electronic publication)

149 Pollard KM, Pearson DL, Blüthner M, Tan EM. Proteolytic cleavage of a self-antigen following xenobiotic-induced cell death produces a fragment with novel immunogenic properties. J Immunol. 2000; 165: 2263–2270.

150 Gobeil S, Boucher CC, Nadeau D, Poirier GG. Characterization of the necrotic cleavage of poly (ADP-ribose) polymerase (PARP-1): implication of lysosomal proteases. Cell Death Differ. 2001; 8:588–594.

151 Hu QP, Fertig N, Medsger TAJ, Wright TM. Molecular recognition patterns of serum anti-DNA topoisomerase I antibody in systemic sclerosis. J Immunol 2004; 173:2834–2841.

152 Hu QP, Fertig N, Medsger TAJ, Wright TM. Correlation of serum anti-DNA topoisomerase I antibody levels with disease severity and activity in systemic sclerosis. Arthritis Rheum 2003; 48:1363–73.

153 Douvas AS, Achten M, Tan EM. Identification of a nuclear protein (Scl–70) as a unique target of human antinuclear antibodies in scleroderma. J Biol Chem. 1979; 254:10514–10522.

154 Guldner HH, Szostecki C, Vosberg HP, Lakomek HJ, Penner E, Bautz FA. Scl 70 autoantibodies from scleroderma patients recognize a 95-kDa protein identified as DNA topoisomerase I. Chromosoma. 1986; 94:132–138.

155 Shero JH, Bordwell B, Rothfield NF, Earnshaw WC. High titers of autoantibodies to topoisomerase I (Scl–70) in sera from scleroderma patients. Science. 1986; 23:737–740.

156 D'Arpa P, Machlin PS, Ratrie H, Rothfield NF, Cleveland DW, Earnshaw WC. cDNA cloning of human DNA topoisomerase I: Catalytic activity of a 67.7-kDa carboxyl-terminal fragment. Proc Natl Acad Sci 1988; 85:2543–2547.

157 Oriss TB, Hu PQ, Wright TM. Distinct autoreactive T cell responses to native and fragmented DNA topoisomerase I: influence of APC type and IL–2. J Immunol. 2001; 166:5456–5463.

158 Samejima K, Svingen PA, Basi GS, Kottke T, Mesner PWJ, Stewart L, Durrieu F, Poirier GG, Alnemri ES, Champoux JJ, Kaufmann SH, Earnshaw WC. Caspase-mediated cleavage of DNA topoisomerase I at unconventional sites during apoptosis. J Biol Chem 1999; 274:4335–4340.

159 Pacheco FJ, Servin JA, Dang D, Kim J, Molinaro C, Daniels T, Brown-Bryan TA, and Casiano CA Involvement of cathepsins in the cleavage of topoisomerase I during necrosis. Arthritis Rheum. 2005; 52:2133–2145.

160 Gallucci S, Lolkema M, Matzinger P. Natural adjuvants: endogenous activators of dendritic cells. Nat Med. 1999; 5:1249–1255.

161 Jun JB, Kuechle M, Harlan JM, Elkon KB. Fibroblast and endothelial apoptosis in systemic sclerosis. Curr Opin Rheumatol. 2003; 15:756–760.

162 Duthoit C, Estienne V, Giraud A, Durand-Gorde JM, Rasmussen AK, Feldt-Rasmussen U, Carayon P, Ruf J. Hydrogen peroxide-induced production of a 40 kDa immunoreactive thyroglobulin fragment in human thyroid cells:

the onset of thyroid autoimmunity? Biochem J. 2001; 360:557–562.

163 Parnaik R, Raff MC, Scholes J. Differences between the clearance of apoptotic cells by professional and non-professional phagocytes. Curr Biol. 2000; 10:857–860.

164 Liu H, Pope RM. Phagocytes: mechanisms of inflammation and tissue destruction. Rheum Dis Clin North Am. 2004; 30:19–39.

165 Ren Y, Savill J. Apoptosis: the importance of being eaten. Cell Death Differ. 1998; 5:563–568.

166 Steinman RM, Turley S, Mellman I, Inaba K. The induction of tolerance by dendritic cells that have captured apoptotic cells. J Exp Med. 2000; 191:411–416.

167 Botto M, Dell'Agnola C, Bygrave AE, Thompson EM, Cook HT, Petry F, Loos M, Pandolfi PP, Walport MJ. Homozygous C1q deficiency causes glomerulonephritis associated with multiple apoptotic bodies. Nat Genet. 1998; 19:596–599.

168 Mitchell DA, Taylor PR, Cook HT, Moss J, Bygrave AE, Walport MJ, Botto M. Cutting edge: C1q protects against the development of glomerulonephritis independently of C3 activation. J Immunol. 1999; 162:5676–5679.

169 Taylor PR, Carugati A, Fadok VA, Cook HT, Andrews M, Carroll MC, Savill JS, Henson PM, Botto M, Walport MJ. A hierarchical role for classical pathway complement proteins in the clearance of apoptotic cells in vivo. J Exp Med. 2000; 192:359–366.

170 Gershov D, Kim S, Brot N, Elkon KB. C-Reactive protein binds to apoptotic cells, protects the cells from assembly of the terminal complement components, sustains an antiinflammatory innate immune response. Implications for systemic autoimmunity. J Exp Med. 2000; 192:1353–1364.

171 Bickerstaff MC, Botto M, Hutchinson WL, Herbert J, Tennent GA, Bybee A, Mitchell DA, Cook HT, Butler PJ, Walport MJ, Pepys MB. Serum amyloid P component controls chromatin degradation and prevents antinuclear

autoimmunity. Nat Med. 1999; 5:694–697.

172 Scott RS, McMahon EJ, Pop SM, Reap EA, Caricchio R, Cohen PL, Earp HS, Matsushima GK. Phagocytosis and clearance of apoptotic cells is mediated by MER. Nature. 2001; 411:207–211.

173 Rovere P, Vallinoto C, Bondanza A, Crosti MC, Rescigno M, Ricciardi-Castagnoli P, Rugarli C, Manfredi AA. Bystander apoptosis triggers dendritic cell maturation and antigen-presenting function. J Immunol. 1998; 161:4467–4471.

174 Rovere P, Sabbadini MG, Vallinoto C, Fascio U, Zimmermann VS, Bondanza A, Ricciardi-Castagnoli P, Manfredi AA. Delayed clearance of apoptotic lymphoma cells allows cross-presentation of intracellular antigens by mature dendritic cells. J Leukoc Biol. 1999; 66:345–349.

175 Ip WK, Lau YL. Distinct maturation of, but not migration between, human monocyte-derived dendritic cells upon ingestion of apoptotic cells of early or late phases. J Immunol. 2004; 173:189–196.

176 Buttiglieri S, Galetto A, Forno S, De Andrea M, Matera L. Influence of drug-induced apoptotic death on processing and presentation of tumor antigens by dendritic cells. Int J Cancer. 2003; 106:516–520.

177 Kotera Y, Shimizu K, Mule JJ. Comparative analysis of necrotic and apoptotic tumor cells as a source of antigen(s) in dendritic cell-based immunization. Cancer Res. 2001; 61:8105–8109.

178 Clayton AR, Prue RL, Harper L, Drayson MT, Savage CO. Dendritic cell uptake of human apoptotic and necrotic neutrophils inhibits CD40, CD80, and CD86 expression and reduces allogeneic T cell responses: relevance to systemic vasculitis. Arthritis Rheum. 2003; 48:2362–2374.

179 Brouckaert G, Kalai M, Krysko DV, Saelens X, Vercammen D, Ndlovu', Haegeman G, D'Herde K, Vandenabeele P. Phagocytosis of necrotic cells

by macrophages is phosphatidylserine dependent and does not induce inflammatory cytokine production. Mol Biol Cell. 2004; 15:1089–1100.

180 Bondanza A, Zimmermann VS, Dell'Antonio G, Cin ED, Balestrieri G, Tincani A, Amoura Z, Piette JC, Sabbadini MG, Rovere-Querini P, Manfredi AA. Requirement of dying cells and environmental adjuvants for the induction of autoimmunity. Arthritis Rheum. 2004; 50:1549–1560.

181 Scaffidi P, Misteli T, Bianchi ME. Release of chromatin protein HMGB1 by necrotic cells triggers inflammation. Nature. 2002; 418:191–195.

182 Andersson U, Tracey KJ. HMGB1 as a mediator of necrosis-induced inflammation and a therapeutic target in arthritis. Rheum Dis Clin North Am. 2004; 30:627–637.

183 Bianchi ME, Manfredi A. Chromatin and cell death. Biochim Biophys Acta. 2004; 1677:181–186.

184 Lovgren T, Eloranta ML, Bave U, Alm GV, Ronnblom L. Induction of interferon-alpha production in plasmacytoid dendritic cells by immune complexes containing nucleic acid released by necrotic or late apoptotic cells and lupus IgG. Arthritis Rheum. 2004; 50:1861–1872.

185 Shi Y, Evans JE, Rock KL. Molecular identification of a danger signal that alerts the immune system to dying cells. Nature. 2003; 425:516–521.

186 Millar DG, Garza KM, Odermatt B, Elford AR, Ono N, Li Z, Ohashi PS. Hsp70 promotes antigen-presenting cell function and converts T-cell tolerance to autoimmunity in vivo. Nat Med. 2003; 9:1469–1476.

187 Melcher A, Todryk S, Hardwick N, Ford M, Jacobson M, Vile RG. Tumor immunogenicity is determined by the mechanism of cell death via induction of heat shock protein expression. Nat Med. 1998; 4:581–587.

188 Todryk S, Melcher AA, Hardwick N, Linardakis E, Bateman A, Colombo MP, Stoppacciaro A, Vile RG. Heat shock protein 70 induced during tumor cell killing induces Th1 cytokines and targets immature dendritic cell precursors to enhance antigen uptake. J Immunol. 1999; 163:1398–1408.

189 Todryk SM, Melcher AA, Dalgleish AG, Vile RG. Heat shock proteins refine the danger theory. Immunology. 2000; 99:334–337.

190 Albert ML, Sauter B, Bhardwaj N. Dendritic cells acquire antigen from apoptotic cells and induce class I-restricted CTLs. Nature. 1998; 392:86–89.

191 Salio M, Cerundolo V, Lanzavecchia A. Dendritic cell maturation is induced by mycoplasma infection but not by necrotic cells. Eur J Immunol. 2000; 30:705–708.

192 Green DR, Beere HM. Apoptosis. Gone but not forgotten. Nature. 2000; 405:28–29.

7
Self-antigen Modification and Autoimmunity

Stuart M. Levine, Livia Casciola-Rosen, and Antony Rosen

7.1
Introduction

One of the hallmarks of the systemic autoimmune diseases is the striking association between clinical phenotype and the specific targeting of ubiquitously expressed cellular "housekeeping" proteins [1, 2]. These associations are so predictable that autoantibody tests are frequently used to confirm clinical diagnoses and guide therapy. Specific examples of these associations include the targeting of nucleosomal and splicing ribonuclear protein (snRNP) components in systemic lupus erythematosus (SLE), topoisomerase I in the diffuse form of scleroderma, centromere proteins in the limited form of scleroderma, and several components of the translational machinery in the autoimmune inflammatory myopathies. The molecules targeted by the immune system share seemingly little in common; they have diverse sizes, structures, functions and cellular localizations, and yet all become specifically targeted in the systemic autoimmune diseases.

These associations of autoantibody response and phenotype are all the more striking in light of several studies over the past decade that have demonstrated that the immune responses to autoantigens in both animals and humans are antigen- and T-cell driven. Autoantibodies have features of adaptive immune responses, as they undergo clonal expansion, class switching, and affinity maturation and demonstrate immunologic memory [3–5]. These findings have focused attention on the circumstances during which autoantigens might have satisfied the stringent criteria necessary for the initiation and propagation of a T cell–dependent immune response. These criteria include the presence of novel, non-tolerized structure at suprathreshold concentrations in a pro-immune (i.e., inflammatory) environment. Of these, the most important criterion for initiation of a primary T-cell response is that the molecule targeted has not been previously presented in that form and therefore failed to induce T-cell tolerance. This chapter will focus on some of the mechanisms and circumstances in which autoantigens might become modified to generate novel, non-tolerized

Autoantibodies and Autoimmunity: Molecular Mechanisms in Health and Disease. Edited by K. Michael Pollard
Copyright © 2006 WILEY-VCH Verlag GmbH & Co. KGaA, Weinheim
ISBN: 3-527-31141-6

structure, with a special focus on the contributions that proteolytic cleavage during certain forms of cell death have on this process.

7.2
Learning to Ignore the "Self": Immunologic Dominance and Crypticity

Over the past two decades, studies on various model antigens have made it clear that an antigen's macromolecular structure may influence its subsequent processing and presentation by MHC class II molecules [6–10]. Eli Sercarz has shown that not all determinants on an intact protein antigen are equally immunogenic; due to certain structural features of the antigen itself, specific determinants are preferentially and reproducibly presented to T cells [11–13]. For a given antigen conformation, the processing pathway has constant and predictable output, with few determinants effectively loaded onto MHC class II molecules (dominant epitopes). Developing T cells that recognize dominant epitopes of self-antigens in the thymus are thereby deleted. In contrast, cryptic epitopes are not presented in significant amounts on MHC class II molecules, and potentially autoreactive T cells recognizing such epitopes are therefore not deleted and persist. Since the products of antigen processing are constant under homeostatic conditions, these cryptic epitopes are not generated under most circumstances and autoreactive T cells remain ignorant. However, were cryptic epitopes to be generated during some unusual antigen-processing event, autoreactive T cells recognizing these epitopes could conceivably be activated and drive autoimmune responses to self-molecules [13].

Several factors contribute to the selection of a molecule's immunodominant epitope, including (1) its intrinsic affinity for MHC class II proteins; (2) the properties of neighboring structural determinants that may influence the binding of this peptide to the binding groove; and (3) the sequence of unfolding and specific cleavage along the endosome/lysosome pathway. Understanding how the structure and processing of self-antigens might be altered during different physiologic and pathologic states is therefore of significant relevance. Of particular importance are early proteolytic events and the effects of high-affinity binding of antibody or other molecules on subsequent antigen processing.

Experiments using tetanus toxin C fragment as a model antigen have demonstrated that a hierarchy of antigen-processing events exists that regulates the loading of particular peptides onto an MHC class II molecule [14, 15]. First, it has been shown that processing of tetanus toxin is initiated upon cleavage by a lysosomal enzyme, asparaginyl endopeptidase (AEP), at a single defined site. There is an absolute requirement for this cleavage event to generate the dominant T-cell epitope, as elimination of the AEP cleavage site by mutagenesis dramatically alters the efficiency of immunodominant peptide presentation to an antigen-specific T-cell clone *in vitro*. Second, it has been demonstrated that a single conservative mutation at the enzyme cleavage site leads to the generation of novel epitopes during antigen processing. Third, inhibiting the AEP protease also alters processing of the whole antigen, resulting in different peptides being loaded onto MHC class II [15]. Thus, in this example, antigen processing occurs in a stepwise manner, with cleavage by a single, initial protease being necessary for the subsequent processing steps that generate the dominant T-cell epitopes. Subtle changes in antigen structure that alter such key upstream processing sites can dramatically alter processing of the intact antigen. Where such changes cause the revelation of epitopes not normally seen by the immune system, the subsequent development of an autoimmune response is enabled [16].

Is there any evidence that such altered processing may contribute to the development of autoimmunity to previously non-tolerized epitopes *in vivo*? Indeed, several experimental systems have demonstrated that immunization with cryptic epitopes can lead to the activation of autoreactive T cells. For example, immunization of mice with unprocessed mouse cytochrome *c* fails to induce an immune response. However, immunization with non-immunodominant peptides derived from mouse cytochrome *c* activates T cells specific for these epitopes [9], thereby establishing that challenging with "cryptic" peptides not generated during the natural processing of cytochrome *c* can activate specific T-cell responses directed against the cryptic sequence.

Similar findings have been made using snRNPs as model antigens, where an immune response against previously tolerized intact molecules could be initiated by immunizing mice with cryptic peptides derived from these molecules. Once the initial peptide-specific immune response is generated, many components of the snRNP complex are subsequently targeted [17]. This phenomenon of "epitope spreading" has been described in anti-snRNP autoimmunity in humans as well [18]. Therefore, in the context of human autoimmune disease, it is possible that novel or impaired proteolysis could generate previously non-tolerized peptides that serve as the antigen source for initiating and propagating an autoreactive T-cell response, and, by extension, an autoimmune humoral response as well.

Cryptic epitopes may also be generated *in vivo* via specific protease activity that more efficiently destroys a dominant epitope in the thymus than in the periphery, preventing the deletion of autoreactive cells in the thymus and increasing the chances that antigen-processing events in the periphery could stimulate these cells and contribute to tissue damage in a pro-immune context. This has been demonstrated in the murine experimental autoimmune encephalomyelitis (EAE) model of multiple sclerosis. In this model, the efficient cleavage of a myelin basic protein (MBP) epitope by AEP destroys the dominant T-cell epitope recognized by encephalitogenic T-cell clones [19]. In the presence of AEP inhibitors in antigen-presenting cells, presentation of the epitope is enhanced. The authors propose that since AEP is highly expressed in thymic antigen-presenting cells, destructive processing by this enzyme limits presentation of this epitope in the thymus and allows encephalitogenic T-cell clones to escape to the periphery, where they contribute to tissue damage and disease.

This paradigm of dominance and crypticity raises two key questions to consider for the study of autoantigens: (1) whether a set of circumstances exists *in vivo* that could reproducibly lead to the altered processing of self-antigens during initiation of an autoimmune response; and (2) whether such conditions are ubiquitous across the spectrum of the autoimmune diseases, or whether disease- and/or tissue-specific mechanisms might be important in modulating these processing steps. Approximately a decade ago, and with these questions in mind, we observed that autoantigens targeted in systemic autoimmune diseases, though sharing seemingly little else in common, are unified by their clustering and concentration within surface blebs on apoptotic cells. We proposed that such molecules were unified by their propensity to undergo structural modifications during some forms of cell death, generating novel structures not previously tolerized by the host [20]. Accumulating experimental evidence indicates that most autoantigens are indeed unified by their susceptibility to structural modification during cell death [21–23], including striking susceptibility to cleavage by apoptotic proteases to generate novel fragments during this process.

Although this chapter focuses primarily on apoptosis-specific proteolysis as a primary mechanism of structural change during cell death, other post-translational changes occur frequently during various death processes and may profoundly affect antigen processing and presentation [21, 24]. Examples of cell death-associated autoantigen modifications include:

- proteolytic cleavage,
- phosphorylation/dephosphorylation,
- isoaspartyl modification,
- transglutamination,
- deimination,
- altered glycosylation, and
- altered subcellular localization.

Autoantigens may undergo novel proteolytic modifications during necrotic death that are distinct from those observed during apoptosis. Further, reactive oxygen species (ROS) can also generate unique proteolytic fragments under certain circumstances, as demonstrated for the scleroderma autoantigen topoisomerase I and the large subunit of RNA polymerase II, which undergo unique proteolysis following metal-catalyzed reactions [25, 26] such as that which may occur during ischemia-reperfusion-type injury. Novel proteolysis also occurs in the setting of mercury-associated cell death. Pollard and colleagues have shown that unique antigenic fibrillarin fragments not seen during other forms of apoptotic and non-apoptotic cell death are generated following mercury treatment both *in vitro* and *in vivo* [27, 28].

Other non-apoptotic proteases have been implicated in generating autoimmune responses as well. Among the best-studied examples of this phenomenon is the proteolytic degradation of the bullous pemphigoid autoantigen BP180 (collagen XVII) by matrix metalloproteinase 9 (MMP9) and neutrophil elastase (NE). The role for MMP-9/NE-mediated proteolysis in the pathogenesis of BP is illustrated by the following observations: (1) MMP9- and NE-deficient mice are resistant to the subepidermal blistering seen in wild-type animals upon treatment with anti-BP180 antibodies [29]; (2) MMP9 is released from tissue-infiltrating eosinophils at the sites of blister formation and is highly expressed in blister fluid [30]; (3) NE cleaves BP180 both *in vitro* and *in vivo* to induce blister formation [31]; and (4) MMP9 inactivates the serpin inhibitor of NE (a-1 proteinase inhibitor), resulting in increased NE levels and subsequent increases in cleaved BP180 at the dermal-epidermal junction [32].

7.3
Proteolytic Cleavage of Autoantigens During Apoptosis

Apoptosis, or "programmed cell death" (reviewed extensively in [33]), is a sequence of morphological and biochemical changes characterized by nuclear condensation and membrane blebbing [34]. During the apoptotic process, cleavage and activation of a series of cysteine proteases called caspases result in the activation of a proteolytic cascade that cleaves downstream molecules that function in pathways essential to cell survival [35, 36]. Cells that die via this pathway do so in an orderly and predictable fashion and are thereafter cleared by macrophages in a non-inflammatory way, with prominent secretion of TGF-β and IL-10.

The caspases, a family of cysteine proteases with an absolute requirement for cleavage after aspartic acid, constitute the most prominent apoptotic protease family [35]. In initial studies looking for modification of autoantigen structure in apoptotic cells, we and others noted that although caspases cleave only a limited number of substrates during the apoptotic process (perhaps a few hundred at maximum), autoantigens are highly represented among these molecules [37–43]. In a minority of cases (e.g., NuMA, CENP-C), the cleaved form of the antigen is better recognized by patient autoantibodies than is the intact protein, suggesting that cleavage may improve accessibility to the relevant epitopes [44]. There are also reports that some U1-70-kDa autoantibodies specifically recognize the apoptotically modified form of this molecule, and that such antibodies are associated with distinct clinical features [45, 46]. In contrast, there are many more examples of autoantigens (e.g., PARP, Mi-2) that are cleaved by caspases, in which no effect of cleavage on recognition by autoantibodies is discernable.

While there is significant data demonstrating the effects of caspase cleavage on autoantibody recognition of self-antigens, less is known about the effects that such cleavage events have on T-cell recognition of these antigens. Recent studies of patient T-cell responses to the U1-70-kDa antigen have demonstrated that autoreactive T-cell clones specifically recognize a highly restricted set of epitopes that are located upstream of both the caspase and granzyme B cleavage sites [47]. Such autoreactive clones were not found in any of the healthy HLA-matched controls in this study. These data suggest that proteolytic cleavage events may indeed be critical in generating autoreactive T-cell epitopes under certain circumstances. Experiments addressing the effects of caspase cleavage on T-cell recognition of other naturally selected autoantigens have not yet been performed, and although they are complex, they are of high priority.

The striking association of caspase-mediated cleavage and autoantigen status is of significant interest but remains of uncertain mechanistic relevance. It remains unclear whether this association reflects events occurring during development of central or peripheral tolerance or events occurring during subsequent immunization peripherally with self-antigens. Similarly, it is not known whether the association requires cleavage by caspases, or whether the presence and structural features of the cleavage site might influence antigen processing and epitope selection. In terms of the first set of possibilities, the following observations are relevant:

1. Apoptotic cell death occurs throughout development and during tissue homeostasis; in these circumstances, the immune consequences are predominantly non-inflammatory and tolerance-inducing [48–51].
2. Apoptosis occurs with great frequency during lymphocyte development and education in the thymus and bone marrow [52].
3. Significant experimental evidence indicates that apoptotic cells themselves constitute a prominent source of toleragen in these settings [53, 54].
4. A role of apoptotic cells in the establishment and maintenance of tolerance to peripheral tissues has also been established [55–60], providing the immune system with the appropriate forms of autoantigens that will likely be encountered during homeostatic cell death of self-tissues.

Since caspase-mediated cleavages typify this form of tolerance-inducing cell death, it is likely but still unproven that caspase fragments of autoantigens are actively tolerized. Consequently, abnormalities in the processes regulating clearance of, and tolerance induction by, apoptotic cells may play important roles in rendering individuals susceptible to initiation of systemic autoimmunity. The phenomenon of decreased apoptotic clearance associated with systemic autoimmunity is seen in both human disease (as in patients with C1q deficiency) and in animal models [61–63].

In addition to abnormalities in processes regulating clearance and tolerance induction by apoptotic cells, recent studies have stressed the possibility that certain forms of apoptotic death may be pro-immune, particularly those occurring occur during virus infection or killing of transformed cells. The associations among (1) viral infection and initiation and flare-ups of autoimmune diseases; (2) cancer and autoimmunity; and (3) the alterations in autoantigen expression, structure, and conformation that are known to occur in such settings are highly relevant in this regard. For example, viral infection may directly alter the structure of self-antigens. The structural changes that autoantigens undergo during these forms of non-tolerance-inducing cell death may be particularly relevant in selecting the molecular targets of such autoimmunity.

7.4
Cytotoxic Lymphocyte Granule–induced Death Pathways

Cytotoxic lymphocytes induce target cell death through several different pathways, including ligation of the Fas receptor on the surface of the target cell, as well as release of proteases (called granzymes) contained in lytic granules within the cytotoxic cell [64]. Transduction of the Fas signal occurs through multiple protein-protein interactions that activate the caspase cascade by inducing processing of caspase-8 and -10 [65]. Cytolysis induced via the Fas pathway is thought to be predominantly associated with immune regulatory processes [66, 67]. Granule pathway–mediated killing utilizes several granule components with unique activities and is thought to be predominantly involved in more pro-immune death processes such as those that occur during clearance of virally infected or transformed cells.

The most abundant cytotoxic granule components are perforin (a pore-forming protein) and a family of serine proteases termed granzymes [68]. Perforin has long been considered crucial for the entry of granzymes into the target cell, but the mechanisms underlying its activity still remain controversial [69]. Following release into the cytosol with the help of perforin, granzyme B (GrB), a rapidly acting apoptotic enzyme, catalyzes the cleavage and activation of several downstream substrates, inducing apoptotic changes in the target cell (Fig. 7.1). Prominent among the upstream mediators of the GrB effect are Bid and several procaspases, which are directly cleaved by GrB to generate their active forms. Thus, through the early cleavage and activation of Bid, GrB rapidly recruits the mitochondrial amplification loop of caspase activation [70, 71]. GrB similarly cleaves and activates effector caspases that further amplify the apoptotic proteolytic cascade, resulting in cleavage of multiple downstream substrates and generation of the apoptotic phenotype. GrB can also directly cleave several downstream signature death substrates, constituting an important caspase-independent death pathway that can lead to cell death even in the absence of caspase activity [72, 73]. For example, GrB directly cleaves and activates the apoptotic nuclease DFF45/ICAD; such cleavage is required for optimal granzyme-induced target cell death [74]. In an analogous fashion to that described above for the caspases, autoantigens targeted in human autoimmune diseases are highly represented among these GrB substrates [37, 73, 75–80].

The most abundant serine protease in cytotoxic lymphocyte granules is granzyme A, whose mechanisms of action have recently been defined. GrA induces a caspase-independent form of cell death, with several overall similarities to that induced by caspases and GrB. For example, following entry into the cell and translocation to the nucleus, GrA induces single-stranded DNA nicking by cleaving the nuclear assembly protein SET, also known as the inhibitor of GrA-activated DNAse, or IGAAD, to release the nucleoside diphosphate kinase NM23-H1 (the GrA-activated DNAse, GAAD). This process of inactivating a DNAse inhibitor to induce DNA breakdown is similar to that seen in caspase and GrB-mediated apoptosis, where ICAD (inhibitor of caspase-activated DNAse) is

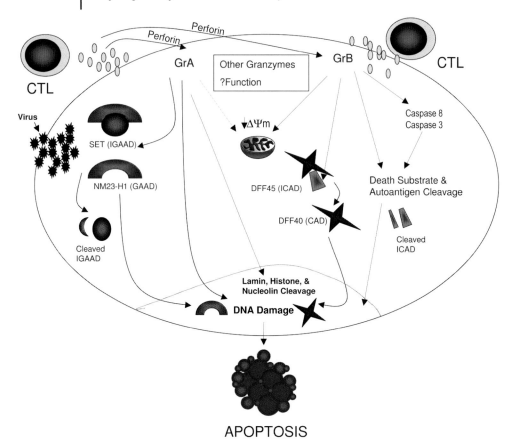

APOPTOSIS

Fig. 7.1 Mechanisms of granule-mediated cytotoxicity. Following cytotoxic T lymphocyte (CTL) recognition of a virally infected or transformed cell, granules containing perforin and granzymes are released into the target cell. After gaining entry into the cell, the two major granzymes, A and B, can cause cell death by apoptosis via several mechanisms. GrB can (1) cleave procaspase-3 and -8, leading to downstream caspase activation and cleavage of downstream substrates including autoantigens; (2) cleave DFF45 (inhibitor of caspase-associated DNAse, ICAD) to liberate DFF40 (caspase-associated DNAse, CAD), which migrates to the nucleus and causes DNA fragmentation; (3) activate the mitochondrial apoptotic pathway directly; and (4) directly cleave downstream death substrates independent of caspase activation. GrA induces caspase-independent cell death via cleavage of SET (inhibitor of granzyme A–associated DNAse, IGAAD) to liberate NM23-H1 (granzyme A-associated DNAse, GAAD), which translocates to the nucleus, resulting in DNA nicking and fragmentation. It can also directly cleave nuclear targets such as lamins, nucleolin, and histones. The coordinated function of these enzymes leads to apoptosis of the target cell.

cleaved to release CAD (caspase-activated DNAse) [81, 82]. Interestingly, both SET and NM23-H1 have been implicated in oncogenesis, although the mechanism for this link remains unclear.

Further, both GrB and GrA have been shown to alter mitochondrial transmembrane potential and function, although release of classic mitochondrial mediators (i.e., cytochrome c, endonuclease G, apoptosis-inducing factor) is not seen after GrA treatment [82], suggesting alternate mechanisms for GrA-mediated mitochondrial disruption. GrA also cleaves lamins, histones, and the nuclear phosphoprotein nucleolin, which are all known autoantigens in systemic autoimmune diseases [83–85]. Whether GrA cleaves other autoantigens, and the immunological relevance of such cleavages, remains unknown at this time but is of significant interest.

Finally, although CTL granules are replete with additional granzyme activities (particularly in mice), the substrate specificity of these "orphan" granzymes remains unclear. Although this chapter focuses predominantly on GrB as a cytotoxic lymphocyte protease that may modify the structure of self-antigens, it is important to note that this principle may be equally applicable to other granule proteases.

7.5
Many Autoantigens Are Specifically Cleaved by GrB, Generating Fragments Not Observed During Other Forms of Cell Death

The number of autoantigens that are cleaved by GrB is steadily growing (Table 7.1). The observation that many autoantigens targeted across the spectrum of human autoimmune diseases are directly and efficiently cleaved by GrB is remarkable for several reasons:

1. Susceptibility to cleavage by GrB is a highly specific feature of autoantigens, and non-autoantigens are not similarly susceptible to cleavage by GrB at sites not cleaved by caspases [73].
2. A very similar group of autoantigens is cleaved by caspases and GrB, although at distinct sites, thus generating different fragments [72].
3. The cleavage sites in autoantigens are uniquely suited to cleavage by GrB and are resistant to cleavage by the upstream activating caspases (caspase-8 and -9) due to the enrichment of residues in the P2 and P3 substrate positions that are preferred by GrB but not tolerated by caspases [73].
4. GrB activation of caspases leads to significant amplification of caspase cleavages, and when efficiency of cleavage of a substrate by caspases and GrB is similar, products of caspase cleavage generally predominate.

Generation of GrB fragments is thus enhanced by inhibition of the caspase pathway [72, 73]. Also of particular note is that GrB and other components of the lytic granule pathway are not expressed in the thymus [86], and cleavage

Table 7.1 Autoantigens as granzyme B substrates.

Nuclear proteins	Cytoplasmic proteins	Other
NuMa	Histidyl tRNA synthetase	PDC-E2 (mitochondria)
U1-70-kDa	Alanyl tRNA synthetase	GluR3B (neuronal surface receptor)
Topoisomerase I	Isoleucyl tRNA synthetase	Golgin-160 (Golgi apparatus)
DNA-PKcs	UFD2	M3 acetylcholine receptor
Ku 70	SRP 72	
XRCC4	Fodrin	
B23		
PMS1		
La		
Mi-2		
NOR 90		
CENP B		
CENP C		
PMScl		
RNA polymerases I & II		
Ki 67		
PARP		
Lamin B		
Fibrillarin		

products generated by such proteases are therefore unlikely to have been tolerized during development.

The striking association between susceptibility of a substrate to cleavage by GrB and autoantigen status strongly suggests that these properties are mechanistically related. As noted for the caspases above, it remains unknown whether it is the properties of the cleavage site or cleavage itself that plays a role in selecting molecules against which autoimmune responses are generated. If cleavage is the important parameter, the reciprocal relationship between caspase activity and generation of granzyme-specific autoantigen fragments suggests that initial immunization occurs in a setting in which caspases are under endogenous (e.g., IAP proteins) or exogenous inhibition (e.g., viral caspase inhibitors) [87–91].

The effect of autoantigen cleavage on recognition by autoantibodies has been addressed in part using an immunoblotting approach; however, there is as yet no common feature that unifies all the antigens in terms of antibody recognition. Indeed, it is striking that GrB cleavage can have various effects on recognition of different molecules by autoantibodies. Although infrequently observed, GrB-generated fragments of autoantigens may be recognized better by autoantibodies than the intact molecule (e.g., the scleroderma autoantigen CENP-C [44], enriched in patients with scleroderma and ischemic digital loss). There are also clear examples where GrB cleavage of an autoantigen greatly inhibits recognition by autoantibodies. For example, Gershwin and colleagues [92] demonstrated that autoantibodies recognizing the intact pyruvate dehydrogenase E2 subunit (PDC-E2) fail to recognize the GrB cleaved form of PDC-E2. Similar findings have also been made for XRCC4, a member of the DNA-PK/Ku complex of autoantigens [93]. However, for most autoantigens studied, cleavage by GrB has no effect on recognition by autoantibodies.

The fact that cleavage can enhance or destroy recognition of some molecules by autoantibodies demonstrates that the GrB cleavage site can either enhance or suppress accessibility of epitopes, occasionally at the level of the autoantibody, but potentially more generally at the level of the T cell. Although autoantibodies are excellent probes of the targets of the autoimmune response, they are less well suited to defining the particular conformation of the antigen that initiated the T-cell response. Interestingly, studies by Mamula and colleagues examining the generation of autoimmune responses to an isoaspartyl-containing Sm-D or cytochrome *c* peptide have demonstrated that T cells recognize only the iso-aspartyl form of the antigen, while autoantibodies bind both modified and un-modified forms [94]. Defining the effects of the intact GrB cleavage site, and its destruction after proteolysis, on the processing and presentation of antigens to T cells therefore remains a major priority.

7.6
GrB-induced Cleavage of Tissue-specific Autoantigens

Structural changes of autoantigens induced by post-translational modification can alter the processing of self-antigens and influence the ability to generate an immune response against self. For example, recent studies have shown that the neuronal glutamate receptor subunit 3 is an autoantigen in patients with a se-vere form of pediatric epilepsy, Rasmussen's encephalitis [95]. Autoantibodies tend to be of low affinity, and many recognize a well-defined extracellular epi-tope residing in the receptor-activating epitope that is aligned on the surface of the folded protein [96]. Of note, the GrB cleavage site contains an asparagine that is normally *N*-glycosylated and is found within a major epitope that is rec-ognized by autoantibodies in Rasmussen's encephalitis [80]. Interestingly, Ghar-ing and colleagues showed that deglycosylated GluR3 is susceptible to cleavage by GrB, whereas the glycosylated form of this receptor is poorly cleaved, possi-bly because the N-linked sugar sterically hinders the ability of GrB to bind to its substrate. The authors postulate that inflammatory events may inhibit the glyco-sylation of GluR3, thus rendering it susceptible to cleavage by GrB, and poten-tially to initiation of GluR3-directed autoimmunity.

7.7
Novel Conformation of Phenotype-specific Autoantigens

In spite of the fact that many autoantigens in systemic autoimmune diseases are ubiquitously expressed, there is nevertheless a striking association of specific antibody responses with unique clinical phenotypes. One potential explanation for this observation is that changes in autoantigen structure may be limited to the relevant disease microenvironment and may contribute to initiation of an autoimmune response. As several autoantigens that are targeted in systemic autoimmune diseases can also be targeted in patients with hepatocellular carcinoma (HCC), we have sought to define microenvironment-specific changes in autoantigens in liver tissue of patients with HCC as a model system in which to investigate the link between autoantigen expression and cancer. Interestingly, the nucleolar HCC autoantigen B23 (nucleophosmin) exists in a truncated form in HCC liver, lacking six amino acids at the N-terminus. While full-length B23 (expressed in all other tissues) is very resistant to cleavage by GrB, HCC B23 is strikingly sensitive to such cleavage [97].

B23 has also been found to be a scleroderma autoantigen associated with the development of pulmonary hypertension [98] and, in an analogous fashion to HCC B23, is also uniquely cleaved by GrB in differentiated smooth muscle cells [99]. Whether this selective cleavage in vascular smooth muscle cells reflects expression of cleavable B23 in areas of hyperplasia that is characteristic of pulmonary hypertension is unknown, but the association is tantalizing nonetheless. The striking restriction of a novel B23 conformation to the likely sites of immunization may indicate that distinct autoantigen conformations responsible for specific cellular functions (e.g., cell growth) are present during disease initiation and/or propagation. It is possible that such pathways of autoantigen expression and conformation may become therapeutically tractable in the autoimmune diseases.

7.8
Conclusion: A Model of Antigen Selection During Cell Death

The clustering and concentration of autoantigens at the surface of apoptotic cells, in combination with the striking tolerance-inducing function of apoptotic cells, have focused attention on abnormalities in apoptotic cell execution and clearance as potential susceptibility and initiating factors in systemic autoimmunity. The susceptibility of the majority of autoantigens across the spectrum of human autoimmune diseases to cleavage by aspartic acid–specific apoptotic proteases is a major unifying feature of this apparently unrelated group of molecules. We propose that caspase-cleaved autoantigens are the major form of the molecule tolerized during development and homeostasis, and that where apoptotic cell clearance is normal, tolerance to such fragments is fully established. Abnormalities in clearance of apoptotic cells and tolerance induction may allow autoreactive T cells recognizing caspase-cleaved antigens to persist and potentially to be activated by a large load of apoptotic cells containing caspase-induced fragments. We further propose that certain pro-immune circumstances (e.g., viral infection, early tumorigenesis) in which the cytotoxic lymphocyte granule pathway is active, and the caspase pathway potentially inhibited, allow preferential activity of the granzyme pathway, generating novel autoantigen fragments not previously tolerized by the host. Such fragments may allow the generation of cryptic epitopes during antigen processing, and autoreactive T cells recognizing cryptic epitopes may become activated. Alternate modifications of autoantigen structure occurring during cell damage or death (e.g., other proteolytic cleavages, deimination, oxidation, isoaspartyl formation, glycosylation) may similarly be important in modifying the processing and presentation of self-antigens and thus in initiation of autoimmunity. Direct demonstration of the differential immunogenicity of different forms of proteins in dying cells remains a major priority.

References

1 von Muhlen CA, Tan EM. Autoantibodies in the diagnosis of systemic rheumatic diseases. Semin Arthitis Rheum 1995; 24:323–358.

2 Hall JC, Casciola-Rosen L, Rosen A. Altered structure of autoantigens during apoptosis. Rheum Dis Clin North Am 2004; 30(3):455–471.

3 Burlingame RW, Rubin RL, Balderas RS, Theofilopoulos AN. Genesis and evolution of antichromatin autoantibodies in murine lupus implicates T-dependent immunization with self-antigen. J Clin Invest 1993; 91:1687–1696.

4 Diamond B, Katz JB, Paul E, Aranow C, Lustgarten D, Scharff MD. The role of somatic mutation in the pathogenic anti-DNA response. Ann Rev Immunol 1992; 10:731–757.

5 Radic MZ, Weigert M. Origins of Anti-DNA antibodies and their implications for B-Cell tolerance. Ann NY Acad Sci 1995; 764:384–396.

6 Schneider SC, Ohmen J, Fosdick L, Gladstone B, Guo J, Ametani A et al. Cutting edge: introduction of an endopeptidase cleavage motif into a determinant flanking region of hen egg lysozyme results in enhanced T cell determinant display. J Immunol 2000; 165(1):20–23.

7 Lipham WJ, Redmond TM, Takahashi H, Berzofsky JA, Wiggert B, Chader GJ et al. Recognition of peptides that are immunogenic but cryptic: Mechanisms that allow lymphocytes sensitized against cryptic peptides to initiate pathogenic autoimmune processes. J Immunol 1991; 146:3757–3762.

8 Streicher HZ, Berkower IJ, Busch M, Gurd FRN, Berzofsky JA. Antigen conformation determines processing requirements for T cell activation. Proc Natl Acad Sci USA 1984; 81:6831–6835.

9 Mamula MJ. The inability to process a self-peptide allows autoreactive T cells to escape tolerance. J Exp Med 1993; 177:567–571.

10 Mamula MJ, Lin R-H, Janeway CAJr, Hardin JA. Breaking T cell tolerance with foreign and self co-immunogens. A study of autoimmune B and T cell epitopes of cytochrome c. J Immunol 1992; 149:789–795.

11 Sercarz EE. Processing creates the self. Nat Immunol 2002; 3(2):110–112.

12 Sercarz EE, Lehmann PV, Ametani A, Benichou G, Miller A, Moudgil K. Dominance and crypticity of T cell antigenic determinants. Ann Rev Immunol 1993; 11:729–766.

13 Lanzavecchia A. How can cryptic epitopes trigger autoimmunity? J Exp Med 1995; 181:1945–1948.

14 Manoury B, Hewitt EW, Morrice N, Dando PM, Barrett AJ, Watts C. An asparaginyl endopeptidase processes a microbial antigen for class II MHC presentation. Nature 1998; 396(6712):695–699.

15 Antoniou AN, Blackwood SL, Mazzeo D, Watts C. Control of antigen presentation by a single protease cleavage site. Immunity 2000; 12(4):391–398.

16 Moudgil KD, Sercarz EE. Dominant determinants in hen eggwhite lysozyme correspond to the cryptic determinants within its self-homologue, mouse lysozyme: Implications in shaping of the T cell repertoire and autoimmunity. J Exp Med 1993; 178:2131–2138.

17 Bockenstedt LK, Gee RJ, Mamula MJ. Self-peptides in the initiation of lupus autoimmunity. J Immunol 1995; 154:3516–3524.

18 James JA, Gross T, Scofield RH, Harley JB. Immunoglobulin epitope spreading and autoimmune disease after peptide immunization: Sm B/B'-derived PPPGMRPP and PPPGIRGP induce spliceosome autoimmunity. J Exp Med 1995; 181(2):453–461.

19 Manoury B, Mazzeo D, Fugger L, Viner N, Ponsford M, Streeter H et al. Destructive processing by asparagine endopeptidase limits presentation of a dominant T cell epitope in MBP. Nat Immunol 2002; 3(2):169–174.

20 Casciola-Rosen LA, Anhalt G, Rosen A. Autoantigens targeted in systemic lupus erythematosus are clustered in two populations of surface structures on apoptotic keratinocytes. J Exp Med 1994; 179:1317–1330.

21 Doyle HA, Mamula MJ. Posttranslational protein modifications: new flavors in the menu of autoantigens. Curr Opin Rheumatol 2002; 14(3):244–249.

22 Rosen A, Casciola-Rosen L. Autoantigens as substrates for apoptotic proteases: Implications for the pathogenesis of systemic autoimmune disease. Cell Death Differ 1999; 6:6–12.

23 Utz PJ, Anderson P. Posttranslational protein modifications, apoptosis, and the bypass of tolerance to autoantigens. Arthritis Rheum 1998; 41(7):1152–1160.

24 Utz PJ, Gensler TJ, Anderson P. Death, autoantigen modifications, and tolerance. Arthritis Res 2000; 2(2):101–114.

25 Casciola-Rosen L, Wigley F, Rosen A. Scleroderma autoantigens are uniquely fragmented by metal-catalyzed oxidation reactions: implications for pathogenesis. J Exp Med 1997; 185(1):71–79.

26 Rosen A, Casciola-Rosen L, Wigley FM. Early pathogenesis of scleroderma: Role of metal-catalyzed oxidation reactions. Curr Opin Rheumatol 1997; 9:538–543.

27 Pollard KM, Lee DK, Casiano CA, Bluther M, Johnston MM, Tan EM. The autoimmunity-inducing xenobiotic mercury interacts with the autoantigen fibrillarin and modifies its molecular and antigenic properties. J Immunol 1997; 158:3521–3528.

28 Pollard KM, Pearson DL, Bluthner M, Tan EM. Proteolytic cleavage of a self-antigen following xenobiotic-induced cell death produces a fragment with novel immunogenic properties. J Immunol 2000; 165(4):2263–2270.

29 Liu Z, Shipley JM, Vu TH, Zhou X, Diaz LA, Werb Z et al. Gelatinase B-deficient mice are resistant to experimental bullous pemphigoid. J Exp Med 1998; 188(3):475–482.

30 Stahle-Backdahl M, Inoue M, Guidice GJ, Parks WC. 92-kD gelatinase is produced by eosinophils at the site of blister formation in bullous pemphigoid and cleaves the extracellular domain of recombinant 180-kD bullous pemphigoid autoantigen. J Clin Invest 1994; 93(5):2022–2030.

31 Verraes S, Hornebeck W, Polette M, Borradori L, Bernard P. Respective Contribution of Neutrophil Elastase and Matrix Metalloproteinase 9 in the Degradation of BP180 (Type XVII Collagen) in Human Bullous Pemphigoid. Journal of Investigative Dermatology 2001; 117(5):1091–1096.

32 Liu Z, Zhou X, Shapiro SD, Shipley JM, Twining SS, Diaz LA et al. The serpin alpha1-proteinase inhibitor is a critical substrate for gelatinase B/MMP-9 in vivo. Cell 2000; 102(5):647–655.

33 Hengartner MO. The biochemistry of apoptosis. Nature 2000; 407(6805):770–776.

34 Kerr JFR, Wyllie AH, Currie AR. Apoptosis: a basic biological phenomenon with wide-ranging implications in tissue kinetics. Br J Cancer 1972; 26:239–257.

35 Thornberry NA, Lazebnik Y. Caspases: Enemies within. Science 1998; 281(5381):1312–1316.

36 Green DR, Kroemer G. The pathophysiology of mitochondrial cell death. Science 2004; 305(5684):626–629.

37 Casciola-Rosen LA, Miller DK, Anhalt GJ, Roscn A. Specific cleavage of the 70-kDa protein component of the U1 small nuclear ribonucleoprotein is a characteristic biochemical feature of apoptotic cell death. J Biol Chem 1994; 269:30757–30760.

38 Utz PJ, Hottelet M, Le TM, Kim SJ, Geiger ME, van Venrooij WJ et al. The 72-kDa component of signal recognition particle is cleaved during apoptosis. J Biol Chem 1998; 273:35362–35370.

39 Malmegrim de Farias KC, Saelens X, Pruijn GJ, Vandenabeele P, van Venrooij WJ. Caspase-mediated cleavage of the UsnRNP-associated Sm-F protein during apoptosis. Cell Death Differ 2003; 10(5):570–579.

40 Casiano CA, Martin SJ, Green DR, Tan EM. Selective cleavage of nuclear autoantigens during CD95 (Fas/APO-1)-mediated T cell apoptosis. J Exp Med 1996; 184:765–770.

41 Rutjes SA, Utz PJ, van der Heijden A, Broekhuis C, van Venrooij WJ, Pruijn GJ. The La (SS-B) autoantigen, a key protein in RNA biogenesis, is dephosphorylated and cleaved early during apoptosis. Cell Death Differ 1999; 6(10):976–986.

42 Ayukawa K, Taniguchi S, Masumoto J, Hashimoto S, Sarvotham H, Hara A et al. La Autoantigen Is Cleaved in the COOH Terminus and Loses the Nuclear Localization Signal during Apoptosis. J Biol Chem 2000; 275(44):34465–34470.

43 Casciola-Rosen LA, Anhalt GJ, Rosen A. DNA-dependent protein kinase is one of a subset of autoantigens specifically cleaved early during apoptosis. J Exp Med 1995; 182:1625–1634.

44 Schachna L, Wigley FM, Morris S, Gelber AC, Rosen A, Casciola-Rosen L. Recognition of Granzyme B-generated autoantigen fragments in scleroderma patients with ischemic digital loss. Arthritis Rheum 2002; 46(7):1873–1884.

45 Greidinger EL, Foecking MF, Magee J, Wilson L, Ranatunga S, Ortmann RA et al. A major B cell epitope present on the apoptotic but not the intact form of the U1-70-kDa ribonucleoprotein autoantigen. J Immunol 2004; 172(1):709–716.

46 Greidinger EL, Casciola-Rosen L, Morris SM, Hoffman RW, Rosen A. Autoantibody recognition of distinctly modified forms of the U1-70-kd antigen is associated with different clinical disease manifestations. Arthritis Rheum 2000; 43(4):881–888.

47 Greidinger EL, Foecking MF, Schafermeyer KR, Bailey CW, Primm SL, Lee DR et al. T Cell Immunity in Connective Tissue Disease Patients Targets the RNA Binding Domain of the U1-70kDa Small Nuclear Ribonucleoprotein. J Immunol 2002; 169(6):3429–3437.

48 Huynh ML, Fadok VA, Henson PM. Phosphatidylserine-dependent ingestion of apoptotic cells promotes TGF-beta1 secretion and the resolution of inflammation. J Clin Invest 2002; 109(1):41–50.

49 Fadok VA, Bratton DL, Konowal A, Freed PW, Westcott JY, Henson PM. Macrophages that have ingested apoptotic cells in vitro inhibit proinflammatory cytokine production through autocrine/paracrine mechanisms involving TGF-β, PGE2, and PAF. J Clin Invest 1998; 101(4):890–898.

50 Voll RE, Herrmann M, Roth EA, Stach C, Kalden JR, Girkontaite I. Immunosuppressive effects of apoptotic cells. Nature 1997; 390(6658):350–351.

51 Gershov D, Kim S, Brot N, Elkon KB. C-Reactive protein binds to apoptotic cells, protects the cells from assembly of the terminal complement components, and sustains an antiinflammatory innate immune response: implications for systemic autoimmunity. J Exp Med 2000; 192(9):1353–1364.

52 Surh CD, Sprent J. T-cell apoptosis detected *in situ* during positive and negative selection in the thymus. Nature 1994; 372:100–103.

53 Li H, Jiang Y, Cao H, Radic M, Prak EL, Weigert M. Regulation of anti-phosphatidylserine antibodies. Immunity 2003; 18(2):185–192.

54 Cocca BA, Seal SN, D'Agnillo P, Mueller YM, Katsikis PD, Rauch J et al. Structural basis for autoantibody recognition of phosphatidylserine-beta 2 glycoprotein I and apoptotic cells. Proc Natl Acad Sci USA 2001; 20;98(24):13826–13831.

55 Liu K, Iyoda T, Saternus M, Kimura Y, Inaba K, Steinman RM. Immune tolerance after delivery of dying cells to dendritic cells in situ. J Exp Med 2002; 196(8):1091–1097.

56 Steinman RM, Nussenzweig MC. Avoiding horror autotoxicus: the importance of dendritic cells in peripheral T cell tolerance. Proc Natl Acad Sci USA 2002; 99(1):351–358.

57 Miller JF, Kurts C, Allison J, Kosaka H, Carbone F, Heath WR. Induction of peripheral CD8+ T-cell tolerance by cross-presentation of self antigens. Immunol Rev 1998; 165:267–277.

58 Belz GT, Behrens GM, Smith CM, Miller JF, Jones C, Lejon K et al. The CD8alpha(+) dendritic cell is responsible for inducing peripheral self-tolerance to tissue-associated antigens. J Exp Med 2002; 196(8):1099–1104.

59 Hugues S, Mougneau E, Ferlin W, Jeske D, Hofman P, Homann D et al. Tolerance to islet antigens and prevention from diabetes induced by limited apoptosis of pancreatic beta cells. Immunity 2002; 16(2):169–181.

60 Huang FP, Platt N, Wykes M, Major JR, Powell TJ, Jenkins CD et al. A discrete subpopulation of dendritic cells transports apoptotic intestinal epithelial cells to T cell areas of mesenteric lymph nodes. J Exp Med 2000; 191(3):435–444.

61 Cohen PL, Caricchio R, Abraham V, Camenisch TD, Jennette JC, Roubey RA et al. Delayed apoptotic cell clearance and lupus-like autoimmunity in mice lacking the c-mer membrane tyrosine kinase. J Exp Med 2002; 196(1):135–140.

62 Walport MJ, Davies KA, Morley BJ, Botto M. Complement deficiency and autoimmunity. Ann NY Acad Sci 1997; 815: 267–281.

63 Scott RS, McMahon EJ, Pop SM, Reap EA, Caricchio R, Cohen PL et al. Phagocytosis and clearance of apoptotic cells is mediated by MER. Nature 2001; 411(6834):207–211.

64 Andrade F, Casciola-Rosen LA, Rosen A. Granzyme B-induced cell death. Acta Haematol 2004; 111(1–2):28–41.

65 Siegel RM, Chan FK, Chun HJ, Lenardo MJ. The multifaceted role of Fas signaling in immune cell homeostasis and autoimmunity. Nat Immunol 2000; 1(6):469–474.

66 Lenardo MJ. Molecular regulation of T lymphocyte homeostasis in the healthy and diseased immune system. Immunol Res 2003; 27(2–3):387–398.

67 Tibbetts MD, Zheng L, Lenardo MJ. The death effector domain protein family: regulators of cellular homeostasis. Nat Immunol 2003; 4(5):404–409.

68 Henkart PA. Lymphocyte-mediated cytotoxicity: Two pathways and multiple effector molecules. Immunity 1994; 1:343–346.

69 Russell JH, Ley TJ. Lymphocyte-mediated cytotoxicity. Annu Rev Immunol 2002; 20:323–370.

70 Sutton VR, Wowk ME, Cancilla M, Trapani JA. Caspase activation by granzyme B is indirect, and caspase autoprocessing requires the release of proapoptotic mitochondrial factors. Immunity 2003; 18(3):319–329.

71 Sutton VR, Davis JE, Cancilla M, Johnstone RW, Ruefli AA, Sedelies K et al. Initiation of apoptosis by granzyme B requires direct cleavage of bid, but not direct granzyme B-mediated caspase activation. J Exp Med 2000; 192(10):1403–1414.

72 Andrade F, Roy S, Nicholson D, Thornberry N, Rosen A, Casciola-Rosen L. Granzyme B directly and efficiently cleaves several downstream caspase substrates: Implications for CTL-induced apoptosis. Immunity 1998; 8(4):451–460.

73 Casciola-Rosen L, Andrade F, Ulanet D, Wong WB, Rosen A. Cleavage by granzyme B is strongly predictive of autoantigen status: Implications for initiation of autoimmunity. J Exp Med 1999; 190(6):815–825.

74 Thomas DA, Du C, Xu M, Wang X, Ley TJ. DFF45/ICAD can be directly processed by granzyme B during the induction of apoptosis. Immunity 2000; 12(6):621–632.

75 Casciola-Rosen L, Nicholson DW, Chong T, Rowan KR, Thornberry NA, Miller DK et al. Apopain/CPP32 cleaves proteins that are essential for cellular repair: a fundamental principle of apoptotic death. J Exp Med 1996; 183(5):1957–1964.

76 Mancini M, Machamer CE, Roy S, Nicholson DW, Thornberry NA, Casciola-Rosen LA et al. Caspase-2 is localized at the Golgi complex and cleaves golgin-160 during apoptosis. J Cell Biol 2000; 149(3):603–612.

77 Nagaraju K, Cox A, Casciola-Rosen L, Rosen A. Novel fragments of the Sjogren's syndrome autoantigens alpha-fodrin and type 3 muscarinic acetylcholine receptor are generated during cytotoxic lymphocyte granule-induced cell death. Arthritis Rheum 2001; 44:2376–2386.

78 Casciola-Rosen L, Pluta AF, Plotz PH, Cox AE, Morris S, Wigley FM et al. The DNA mismatch repair enzyme PMS1 is a myositis-specific autoantigen. Arthritis & Rheumatism 2001; 44:389–396.

79 Mahoney JA, Odin JA, White SM, Shaffer D, Koff A, Casciola-Rosen L et al. The human homologue of the yeast polyubiquitination factor Ufd2p is cleaved by caspase 6 and granzyme B during apoptosis. Biochem J 2002; 361(Pt 3):587–595.

80 Gahring L, Carlson NG, Meyer EL, Rogers SW. Granzyme B proteolysis of a neuronal glutamate receptor generates an autoantigen and is modulated by glycosylation. J Immunol 2001; 166(3):1433–1438.

81 Fan Z, Beresford PJ, Zhang D, Lieberman J. HMG2 Interacts with the Nucleosome Assembly Protein SET and Is a Target of the Cytotoxic T-Lymphocyte Protease Granzyme A. Mol Cell Biol 2002; 22(8):2810–2820.

82 Lieberman J, Fan Z. Nuclear war: the granzyme A-bomb. Curr Opin Immunol 2003; 15(5):553–559.

83 Zhang D, Beresford PJ, Greenberg AH, Lieberman J. Granzymes A and B directly cleave lamins and disrupt the nuclear lamina during granule-mediated cytolysis. PNAS 2001; 98(10):5746–5751.

84 Pasternack MS, Bleier KJ, McInerney TN. Granzyme A binding to target cell proteins. Granzyme A binds to and cleaves nucleolin in vitro. J Biol Chem 1991; 266(22):14703–14708.

85 Hirata D, Iwamoto M, Yoshio T, Okazaki H, Masuyama Ji, Mimori A et al. Nucleolin as the Earliest Target Molecule of Autoantibodies Produced in MRL/lpr Lupus-Prone Mice. Clinical Immunology 2000; 97(1):50–58.

86 Shresta S, Heusel JW, MacIvor DM, Wesselschmidt RL, Russell JH, Ley TJ. Granzyme B plays a critical role in cytotoxic lymphocyte-induced apoptosis. Immunol Rev 1995; 146:211–221.

87 Roy N, Deveraux QL, Takahashi R, Salvesen GS, Reed JC. The c-IAP-1 and c-IAP-2 proteins are direct inhibitors of specific caspases. EMBO J 1997; 16(23):6914–6925.

88 Li F, Ambrosini G, Chu EY, Plescia J, Tognin S, Marchisio PC et al. Control of apoptosis and mitotic spindle checkpoint by survivin. Nature 1998; 396(6711):580–584.

89 Deveraux QL, Roy N, Stennicke HR, Van Arsdale T, Zhou Q, Srinivasula SM et al. IAPs block apoptotic events induced by caspase-8 and cytochrome *c* by direct inhibition of distinct caspases. EMBO J 1998; 17(8):2215–2223.

90 Deveraux QL, Takahashi R, Salvesen GS, Reed JC. X-linked IAP is a direct inhibitor of cell-death proteases. Nature 1997; 388(6639):300–304.

91 Kobzik L, Reid MB, Bredt DS, Stamler JS. Nitric oxide in skeletal muscle. Nature 1994; 372(6506):546–548.

92 Matsumura S, Van De Water J, Kita H, Coppel RL, Tsuji T, Yamamoto K et al. Contribution to antimitochondrial antibody production: cleavage of pyruvate dehydrogenase complex-E2 by apoptosis-related proteases. Hepatology 2002; 35(1):14–22.

93 Lee KJ, Dong X, Wang J, Takeda Y, Dynan WS. Identification of Human Autoantibodies to the DNA Ligase IV/XRCC4

Complex and Mapping of an Autoimmune Epitope to a Potential Regulatory Region. J Immunol 2002; 169(6):3413–3421.

94 Mamula MJ, Gee RJ, Elliott JI, Sette A, Southwood S, Jones PJ et al. Isoaspartyl post-translational modification triggers autoimmune responses to self-proteins. J Biol Chem 1999; 274(32):22321–22327.

95 Rogers SW, Andrews PI, Gahring LC, Whisenand T, Cauley K, Crain B et al. Autoantibodies to glutamate receptor GluR3 in Rasmussen's encephalitis. Science 1994; 265(5172):648–651.

96 Twyman RE, Gahring LC, Spiess J, Rogers SW. Glutamate receptor antibodies activate a subset of receptors and reveal an agonist binding site. Neuron 1995; 14(4):755–762.

97 Ulanet DB, Torbenson M, Dang CV, Casciola-Rosen L, Rosen A. Unique conformation of cancer autoantigen B23 in hepatoma: a mechanism for specificity in the autoimmune response. Proc Natl Acad Sci USA 2003; 100(21):12361–12366.

98 Ulanet DB, Wigley FM, Gelber AC, Rosen A. Autoantibodies against B23, a nucleolar phosphoprotein, occur in scleroderma and are associated with pulmonary hypertension. Arthritis Rheum 2003; 49(1):85–92.

99 Ulanet DB, Flavahan NA, Casciola-Rosen L, Rosen A. Selective cleavage of nucleolar autoantigen B23 by granzyme B in differentiated vascular smooth muscle cells: insights into the association of specific autoantibodies with distinct disease phenotypes. Arthritis Rheum 2004; 50(1):233–241.

Part 3
Autoantibodies as Diagnostic Markers

Autoantibodies and Autoimmunity: Molecular Mechanisms
in Health and Disease. Edited by K. Michael Pollard
Copyright © 2006 WILEY-VCH Verlag GmbH & Co. KGaA, Weinheim
ISBN: 3-527-31141-6

Indirect immunofluorescence

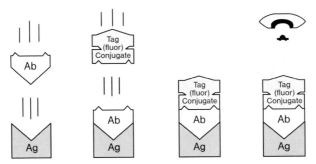

Fig. 8.1 Illustration of the steps performed in IIF tests. First the antibody interacts with the antigen (left panel). After washing the slide, a detecting antibody that is conjugated to a fluorescent tag is added. The detecting antibody will bind to any patient antibody that is bound to the antigen. The detecting antibody can be visualized in a fluorescent microscope (right panel).

There are two disadvantages of the IIF technique in large clinical laboratories. First, a relatively high amount of skilled labor is required to perform the test. Addition of sample and detecting reagent, and wash steps, can be easily automated. However, a trained technologist must read and interpret the slide by examining it under a fluorescent microscope and must manually enter the resulting data into the laboratory's information system. Second, there is significant variation between laboratories performing IIF tests. Part of the variation is caused by the subjective interpretation of the fluorescent pattern by the person examining the slide. Other factors leading to high inter-laboratory variation are the differences between microscopes, different detecting reagents used by different manufacturers of the same test, and the dilution of the patient sample that is chosen for use by a laboratory. Even with these problems, IIF is still the best technique to use for detecting some autoantibodies (see below) and is the only technique available for detecting others.

Ouchterlony immunodiffusion is a powerful technique in many ways [2]. The assay is simple to perform and yields very high specificity, and no special equipment is needed. It requires only a crude soluble extract for the antigen, and the labor to perform the test is very low. Serum is put in one well in an agar plate and a soluble extract from spleen, thymus, or tissue culture is put into another well in the plate and allowed to incubate over one or two days. If there is a precipitating reaction between antibodies and antigens, a visible precipitin line will form between the well containing the serum and the well with extract (Fig. 8.2). Reactivity to any precipitating antigen in the extract can be detected. A control serum with known reactivity must be included next to the sample in order to identify the specific reaction that occurs. If precipitin lines from two adjacent wells meet, they contain the same autoantibody. If the precipitin lines cross, the antibodies are different, whereas if they form a "T" there is partial identity.

Immunodiffusion reactions

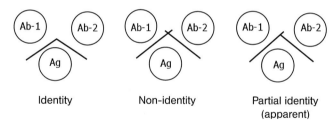

Identity   Non-identity   Partial identity
                                     (apparent)

Fig. 8.2 Illustration of the three types of positive results that occur in Ouchterlony immunodiffusion. When antibodies from two different sources are the same, the precipitin lines will curve and come together, forming a line of identity (left panel). If the antibodies in the two sources are different, their precipitin lines will remain straight and will cross each other (center panel). If one source has two precipitating antibodies and the other source contains just one of them, the precipitin lines will meet, but there will also be a spur that protrudes from the sample that has two reactivities (right panel). Sometimes two separate lines form in samples that have two reactivities.

While the test is simple and specific, there are also serious limitations to this technique. The antibody-antigen complex must form a visible precipitin line. This means that the amounts of both antibody and antigen must be optimized. Only certain antibody-antigen pairs will form precipitin lines since there must be multiple reactive epitopes on the antigen to allow cross-linking and precipitation of the antibody-antigen complex. Thus, antibodies that do not precipitate an antigen, and antibodies to antigens that are insoluble, cannot be detected by Ouchterlony immunodiffusion. Additionally, each positive reaction needs to be tested next to a positive control, which requires large amounts of control sera, and reading the Ouchterlony plate requires time and skill. This technique is excellent when a small number of samples need to be tested, but it is difficult to use on a large number of samples.

Most large laboratories use ELISA to detect a wide variety of autoantibodies [3]. In this technique purified antigen is coated onto the wells of a 96-well microtiter plate. The antigen binds extremely tightly to the plastic in the ELISA plate because the plastic is naturally reactive or has been activated by radiation. Once the antigen has bound to the plate, it will not come off in low or high pH, detergent, sheer stress, or chaotropic agents. The vast majority of proteins and protein-nucleic acid complexes bind directly to the ELISA plate, as does denatured DNA. Native DNA will not bind to the plate directly and binds instead to a positively charged substrate that must be added to the ELISA plate first. A wide variety of antigens saturate an ELISA plate at concentration between 2 µg mL^{-1} and 4 µg mL^{-1}. Interestingly, it is easy to add six to eight different antigens to an ELISA plate at near-saturating concentrations of each, and little or no inhibition of antigen binding to the ELISA plate is detected. One interpretation of this finding is that there are a wide variety of microenvironments on the

ELISA plate, and each antigen is preferentially binding to a different microenvironment. Inhibition of binding among most antigens is noticed after eight to 10 different antigens are added to the plate at the same time. Occasionally an antigen binds to the ELISA plate so well that other antigens never inhibit its binding, while another antigen may be out-competed at a relatively low concentration of other antigens.

After the antigen is bound to the plate and any free binding sites are blocked, the plate is ready for use. Diluted patient serum is added to the well and incubated, and the well is washed. At this step any specific autoantibody that reacts with the antigen on the plate will stay bound to the antigen, while all other antibodies will be washed away. After washing, a detecting anti-human antibody conjugated with an enzyme is added to the well and incubated. If antibody from the patient is bound to the antigen, the conjugated detecting antibody binds to the patient antibody. If no patient antibody is bound to the antigen, all the detecting antibody will be washed away. After the wells are washed, the bound conjugate is detected by adding a substrate that changes color in the presence of the enzyme on the detecting antibody.

The detecting antibody is typically goat anti-human IgG that is conjugated to horseradish peroxidase. This is detected by a dye, such as TMB (3,3',5,5'-tetramethylbenzidine) or ABTS (2,2'-azino-di-[3-ethylbenzthiazolinsulfonate]), that changes color in the presence of the enzyme and hydrogen peroxide. The change in color is quantified on a spectrophotometer and is proportional to the amount of enzyme in the well, which is in turn proportional to the amount of autoantibody bound to the antigen on the plate. Other specificities of the detecting antibody such as anti-IgM, anti-IgA, or anti-polyvalent are used when appropriate. Different enzyme-substrate pairs or chemiluminescent reactions can also be used to detect the bound autoantibodies.

ELISA is an extremely robust and flexible technique. Many tens of thousands of samples are tested by ELISA every day in clinical labs around the world. In both clinical and research laboratories, hundreds of different antigens have been used as substrates. There are many attractive features of ELISA compared to other techniques used to detect autoantibodies. It can be a sensitive and specific test. It can be performed manually with just some pipettes and an inexpensive plate reader, or the process can be completely automated on a large machine that can perform ELISAs on four to eight plates simultaneously. All steps from making dilutions of patient sera to reporting the results of the ELISA to the central computer can be automated on such a machine. Also, the results from ELISA are objective. If a standard curve is used and there is an international standard for quantitation, such as the World Health Organization standard for DNA, the results can be reported in international units and the test is considered quantitative. If a single point calibrator is used and there is no international standard, the results are reported in arbitrary units and are considered semi-quantitative.

Another advantage of ELISA is that usually there is only one antigen on the plate, so there is no interference from other antibodies in a serum. Most

ELISAs can be performed in two to five hours total time, so it is easy to do one or two runs per shift in a clinical or research laboratory. In the early days of ELISA plate manufacturing, the plates were not always uniform and it was necessary to run controls and samples in duplicate. Today, the ELISA plates are extremely uniform and samples can safely be run in singleton. Depending on the number of calibrators and controls run on a plate, this means that over 90 samples can be run on one plate, lowering the cost per test. ELISAs show good within-run variation, usually between 5% and 10%, as well as good between-run variation, usually 10% to 15%. Careful manufacturing procedures for both the ELISA plates and the components in the kits mean that there is good lot-to-lot reproducibility. All of the above reasons contribute to the fact that ELISAs are the main technique used to detect specific autoantibodies in clinical laboratories throughout the world today.

One large impetus for the development of new ELISAs is to replace IIF assays. The latter tests require experienced laboratory technicians to run them, and their interpretation is subjective. In contrast, ELISAs can be automated and are objective. There has been limited success so far replacing the HEp-2 IIF test with an ANA ELISA because of the multiplicity of antigens needed for a good screening test. However, there has been good success when only one antigen is needed to replace an IIF assay. Tissue transglutaminase (tTG) was recently discovered to be the endomysial antigen from primate esophagus [4]. Additionally, the antigen in two different IIF assays, anti-keratin and perinuclear factor, was identified as citrullinated filaggrin [5]. The smooth muscle pattern of IIF on sections of stomach that is found in people with autoimmune hepatitis is caused by autoantibodies to f-actin [6]. These discoveries led to the development of ELISAs that allowed for more widespread testing than was possible using IIF. There has been a dramatic increase in testing for anti-tTG to help diagnose celiac disease and an even more dramatic increase in testing for anti-citrullinated proteins to help diagnose rheumatoid arthritis (RA). It is not practical to screen large numbers of people by IIF techniques, while it is relatively easy to do so using ELISA.

Another driving force behind new ELISAs is the discovery of new diagnostically important autoantibodies. In some cases these replace a test using another technology such as IIF, but sometimes these are completely new tests. Examples of the latter are ELISAs for GP210 and Sp100 to help diagnose primary biliary cirrhosis (PBC) [7], for soluble liver antigen to help diagnose autoimmune hepatitis [8], and for anti-*Saccharomyces cerevisiae* mannan antibodies to help diagnose Crohn's disease [9].

ELISAs have a number of limitations as well. For some purposes other techniques are better. As mentioned below, IIF on HEp-2 cells is a more sensitive screening test for autoantibodies found in connective tissue diseases, rheumatoid factor (RF) is usually detected by agglutination assays, and Ouchterlony immunodiffusion may be more appropriate to detect extractable nuclear antigens (ENAs) in small laboratories. Milligram quantities of pure, immunoreactive antigen are required to manufacture ELISAs. Some antigens are difficult to isolate in milligram amounts or in immunoreactive form. For some tests, such as atypical or X-ANCA (anti-neutrophil cytoplasmic antibody), lupus anticoagulant, and some patterns on HEp-2 cells, the reactive antigen is not known and thus it is impossible to make a corresponding ELISA.

Many other techniques are used to detect autoantibodies in clinical and research laboratories. These include counter-immunoelectrophoresis, Western blot, and agglutination assays. Because they are not as common in clinical laboratories as the three techniques mentioned above, they will not be covered in this chapter. Entire chapters of books have been written about all of these techniques [10–12].

8.2
Comparison of Common Tests

The most commonly performed test to measure autoantibodies in clinical laboratories is IIF to screen for the presence of ANAs [1] (Fig. 8.3). Almost all patients with systemic lupus erythematosus (SLE) are ANA positive, so a negative result on this test virtually rules out SLE [13]. Patients with many other systemic autoimmune diseases, as well as some healthy individuals, are also positive for ANAs [14]. Thus, a positive result is suggestive that the person has an autoimmune disease, but it is not diagnostic. Originally, the ANA IIF test was performed on thin sections of tissue such as mouse kidney. Because of the relatively small size and random orientation of the cells, only a few staining patterns could be observed on this substrate. Also, antibodies to one of the more common autoantigens, SS-A/Ro, were not detected on mouse kidney slides [15]. A significant improvement to screening for ANAs occurred when cells that grow in a monolayer in culture, like HEp-2 cells, were used as the substrate instead of mouse kidney sections. HEp-2 is a human cell line that grows on the surface of the slide and has a relatively large nucleus. The cells are present in all stages of the cell cycle and contain antigens not present in rodent cells, including SS-A/Ro, proliferating cell nuclear antigen that is present at the S phase of the cell cycle [16], and other cell cycle–related antigens. In addition, certain autoantibody specificities, such as anti-centromere, yield clearly identifiable patterns using IIF on HEp-2 cells because of the pattern seen in mitotic cells [17]. While centromere staining is detected in rodent tissues, it is not specifically identifiable, as it requires mitotic-phase cells for confirmation. Other fluorescent patterns in the nucleus include homogeneous, fine-speckled, coarse-speckled, and nucleolar. Several different antibody specificities can yield the same pattern on HEp-2 cells; therefore, it is necessary to perform follow-up testing in order to identify the specificity of the antibody (see below). There are also several structures in the cytoplasm of the cell that react with autoantibodies, particularly mitochondria, Golgi, tRNA synthetases, ribosomes, and GW bodies. Some of these autoantibodies are useful for diagnosing autoimmune diseases [18].

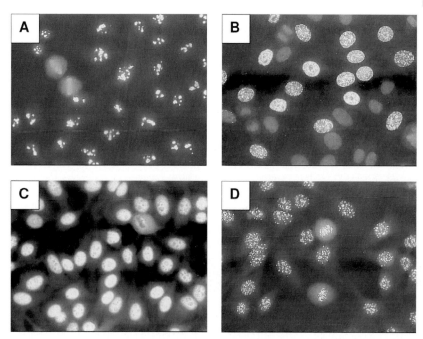

Fig. 8.3 Patterns of immunofluorescence on HEp-2 cells. (A) Antibodies to fibrillarin stain the nucleolus of most cells and decorate the mitotic chromosomes in cells undergoing mitosis. (B) Antibodies to PCNA show various levels of staining in cells that are in S phase but do not stain cells in other phases of the cell cycle. (C) Antibodies to SS-A/Ro yield a fine-speckled pattern. (D) Antibodies to centromere proteins yield small dots in all cells. In cells that are in mitosis, the dots are aligned with the mitotic chromosomes.

The IIF test for ANA on HEp-2 cells is powerful because it can detect any autoantibody that binds to structures inside the cell. Antibodies with both known and unknown specificities, giving a wide variety of patterns, are seen. However, as mentioned above, there are a number of problems associated with this test in the clinical lab. It requires a trained technologist to read the slide and thus is labor intensive. There is large lab-to-lab variation in reporting results of IIF on HEp-2 cells due to differences in microscopes such as the power of the objectives and the strength of the fluorescent light, differences in technicians' interpretation of the IIF patterns, differences in the conjugates used to detect the bound autoantibodies (IgG-specific compared to IgG-, IgA-, IgM-, or polyspecific), and differences of the starting dilution of serum (1:40, 1:80, 1:160) among laboratories [14]. More subtle variation is caused by differences in the ways that HEp-2 cells are fixed by various manufacturers [19]. Nonetheless, IIF on HEp-2 cells is the gold standard for screening for ANAs. International standards for identifying many patterns and determining the cutoff between negative and positive are available for ANA screening by IIF on HEp-2 cells [20]. Clinical laboratories could use these standards so that more uniform results can be obtained among laboratories.

Recently, several ELISAs to screen for ANAs were developed [21, 22]. They have gained some popularity because they are easy to automate to reduce labor, the results are objective rather than subjective, and there is not much variation among results performed on ANA ELISAs from the same manufacturer in different laboratories. Notwithstanding these improvements over IIF on HEp-2 cells, the ANA ELISA has many drawbacks. The differences between the ANA ELISAs produced by different manufacturers are much greater than the differences between various HEp-2 cell preparations. Additionally, no ANA ELISA detects all of the autoantibodies detected by HEp-2 cells or all the autoantibodies made by people with diagnosed disease. Thus, some SLE patients are negative on an ANA ELISA but positive by IIF on HEp-2 cells. This defeats the main purpose of the traditional ANA screening test, because a negative result on the ANA ELISA does not rule out SLE. Thus, a negative result on an ANA ELISA is not as useful diagnostically as a negative HEp-2 reading. However, since the best ANA ELISAs will detect the majority of diagnostically important autoantibodies but not many autoantibodies of unknown clinical relevance, a positive result by an ANA ELISA may be more indicative that a person has an autoimmune disease than a positive result by IIF on HEp-2 cells. To a large extent this depends on the cutoff used between positive and negative, since a low cutoff can yield many positive results on an ANA ELISA even in the normal population. The rheumatologist should know what type of ANA screen is used in the laboratory where he sends his patients for testing.

A large number of autoantibodies besides ANAs are detected by IIF on various substrates. Three of the most common and diagnostically important IIF tests are anti-DNA on *Crithidia luciliae* substrate, ANCA on neutrophils, and anti-endomysial antibody on primate esophagus. These same autoantibodies are identified by other techniques as well. Certain advantages and pitfalls in measuring these antibodies are common to all IIF tests, while others are specific for each type of test.

Because the presence of anti-native DNA antibodies is one of the criteria for diagnosing SLE [13], these autoantibodies have more clinical utility than most. The technique for measuring anti-DNA autoantibodies that has the greatest clinical utility is immunoprecipitation of radiolabeled DNA, commonly called the Farr assay [23]. Patient serum is mixed with radiolabeled DNA, and immune complexes are precipitated with ammonium sulfate. The amount of precipitated radioactivity compared to the radioactivity left in solution determines the amount of anti-DNA autoantibodies present. This technique is quite sensitive and specific, and for many years it was the most common method used in laboratories to measure anti-DNA antibodies. However, it is labor-intensive and uses radioactivity, so it is not as commonly performed today. Either anti-DNA ELISAs [24] or IIF on *Crithidia luciliae* [25] has largely replaced it. *Crithidia luciliae* has DNA in both the nucleus and the kinetoplast. Depending on the method of fixation and the fine specificity of the anti-DNA autoantibodies, an anti-DNA–positive sample stains both the nucleus and the kinetoplast or just the kinetoplast.

Numerous studies have compared these three different types of assays [26, 27]. Virtually all of the studies show that the Farr assay has the best clinical sensitivity and specificity to help diagnose patients with SLE. The DNA ELISA is also sensitive, but it is not as specific for SLE patients as the Farr assay. In addition, DNA ELISAs made by different manufacturers vary widely from each other. This is mostly caused by the way that the DNA is bound to the ELISA plate, but is also influenced by the cutoff between positive and negative supplied with the kit and the isotype specificity of the detecting reagent (IgG or polyspecific). IIF on *Crithidia luciliae* is the least sensitive of these methods. The general interpretation that ELISA measures both high- and low-affinity antibodies while the Farr assay measures only high-affinity antibodies and IIF measures a subset of anti-DNA antibodies cannot be correct. If this interpretation were right, the ELISA would measure all anti-DNA antibodies, the Farr assay would detect most of those detected by ELISA but not others, and IIF would detect just some of those. This is not what is found. There is usually an 80–90% overlap of reactivity between the techniques, with each technique measuring antibodies that are not detected by the other techniques and not detecting some that are measured by one or both of the other techniques [26, 27]. Thus, there must be complicated interactions between anti-DNA antibodies and the various forms of DNA used to detect the antibodies. Briefly, the Farr assay measures all classes of antibodies that can bind to soluble DNA in high salt and may also measure histone-containing immune complexes that can bind to DNA and cause it to precipitate in high salt [28]. High salt increases the strength of hydrophobic interactions, decreases the strength of ionic interactions, and does not affect van der Waals interactions, the three main forces used in antibody-antigen binding. The DNA in both ELISA and *Crithidia luciliae* is not soluble but is bound to a solid phase and is thus constrained compared to the DNA in the Farr assay. The kinetoplast DNA in *Crithidia luciliae* is thought to be supercoiled, while the DNA in most anti-DNA ELISAs is not. Furthermore, even subtle differences in the positively charged substrate used to bind DNA to the ELISA plate can cause large differences in the anti-DNA antibodies detected. The amount of single-stranded DNA in the double-stranded DNA preparation is also important because many people without SLE make anti-single-stranded DNA antibodies. Finally, the specificity of the conjugate (IgG- or polyreactive) that is used to detect the anti-DNA autoantibodies in the ELISA and *Crithidia luciliae* assay is a strong variable. The subtle differences in the results from these three techniques are not as clinically important as might be expected because the diagnosis of SLE requires that a number of symptoms and laboratory results be positive in a given patient [13, 26].

Positive ANCA results by IIF on ethanol-fixed neutrophils aid in the diagnosis of Wegener's granulomatosis – a rare, life-threatening inflammation of the arteries – and some other types of small-vessel vasculitis. Three specific patterns on ANCA IIF tests are diagnostically important. The c-ANCA pattern, which has a coarse-speckled cytoplasmic stain with interlobular accentuation, indicates that the patient has Wegener's granulomatosis. A perinuclear pattern called p-ANCA is sometimes found in patients with Wegener's granulomatosis but is more common in people with microscopic polyangiitis. [29]. The p-ANCA can be confirmed on formalin-fixed neutrophils by the conversion of the perinuclear pattern to a c-ANCA. Follow-up testing by ELISA for two specific autoantibodies, anti-myeloperoxidase (MPO) for p-ANCA and anti-proteinase-3 for c-ANCA, can confirm the IIF results [30]. Patients with anti-PR3 reactivity often have more severe disease than those with anti-MPO antibodies [31]. A few patients with Wegener's granulomatosis are positive on ANCA IIF but not on anti-MPO or PR3 ELISAs, so the ANCA IIF should not be replaced with the ELISAs.

The third important pattern is called X-ANCA or atypical ANCA. This is a perinuclear pattern that is different from p-ANCA and is found primarily in patients with inflammatory bowel disease [32]. The atypical ANCA on ethanol-fixed neutrophils becomes negative on formalin-fixed neutrophils. Any pattern other than the three described above should be called "negative" or "indeterminate." Sometimes the presence of another antibody can mask a c-ANCA or p-ANCA pattern. For example, a strong homogeneous pattern of the nucleus of the neutrophil is not a positive ANCA result because it is not perinuclear. Obviously, it requires a well-trained technician to correctly read ANCA slides.

For many years the gold standard to diagnose people with celiac disease was a characteristic finding on biopsy of the small intestine. Additionally, virtually all of these patients showed an endomysial pattern by IIF on primate esophagus that was from IgA autoantibodies. Recently it was found that autoantibodies to tTG cause the IIF pattern typical of patients with celiac disease [4]. Originally, guinea pig tTG was used as the substrate in ELISA, but it was less sensitive and specific than IIF on primate esophagus. Now that human rather than guinea pig antigen is used, the ELISAs are as good as or better than IIF [33], because antibodies that interfere with IIF do not affect ELISA results. Celiac disease is caused by an immunologic reaction to gluten in wheat and other grains and is typically diagnosed in children who have a failure to thrive and in some other people with stomach ailments. The cure is for the patient to go on a gluten-free diet, which is safe and simple but not easy because wheat is present in so many foods.

With the availability of the tTG ELISA, more immunologic screening for celiac disease has been performed in the last few years than ever before. The disease has been found to be more prevalent than previously expected. When an adolescent population in Switzerland was screened for anti-tTG autoantibodies, this reactivity was found in about 1 in 150 people [34]. Because some people with subclinical celiac disease have symptoms that are not usually associated with the disease, such as headache, muscle ache, or general fatigue, the ability to perform widespread screening will be very useful [35]. The symptoms of many people with subclinical celiac disease improve on a gluten-free diet. This is an example where an improvement in technology allowed wider testing of the general population and new insights into the frequency and manifestations of a disease. There is also some discussion among gastroenterologists that a biopsy does not need to be performed to diagnose celiac disease when a person has a positive anti-tTG test, in conjunction with improvement on a gluten-free diet. If this becomes standard, a serologic test will replace an invasive diagnostic procedure.

There are many more clinically useful IIF tests to detect autoantibodies found in both systemic and organ-specific autoimmune diseases. All IIF tests require a large amount of skilled labor to read and interpret the slide. For a number of autoantibodies, alternative tests are available in a format like ELISA that is less labor intensive and less subjective. Sometimes the ELISA performs as well as or better than the IIF test, while in other cases the ELISA is different enough from the IIF test that it yields different clinical sensitivity and specificity. Each auto-antibody-antigen system needs to be examined individually.

The first three autoantibodies detected were rheumatoid factor (RF), the false-positive VDRL (Venereal Disease Research Laboratory) result, and lupus erythe-matosus (LE) cell factor. Interestingly, at the time these tests were developed no one knew that they were measuring an autoantibody-antigen reaction. Aggluti-nation of sheep red blood cells coated with rabbit IgG was used to detect RF, usually found in patients with RA [36]. Flocculation seen under a microscope of the reagent from the VDRL was used to detect reagin, which is found in people with syphilis and in some people with SLE. The SLE patients were usually neg-ative on a separate test to detect anti-syphilis reactivity and thus were considered false positive on the VDRL test [37]. Phagocytosis of nuclei by segmented neu-trophils seen in a stained blood smear was used to detect LE cell factor [38]. In one form or another, these autoantibodies are still commonly measured today and the techniques used to detect them have evolved over the years.

RFs are autoantibodies that recognize the Fc portion of IgG. Most RFs are IgM class, but may also be IgG or IgA. RFs are found in 50–90% of rheumatoid arthritis patients. RFs are sometimes present even before symptoms of disease develop but become positive in a higher percentage of RA patients as their dis-ease progresses [39]. Even with the large technological advances over the last 50 years, RFs are still often measured by agglutination tests. Some labs still use IgG-coated red blood cells or latex beads, but more often the test is performed in a nephelometer or related machine so that the test is completely automated. Because they are pentamers, IgM antibodies are detected with approximately 10 times more sensitivity than IgG antibodies in agglutination tests. Therefore, any agglutination test is biased to detect IgM isotypes.

ELISAs that detect RFs use IgG-, IgM-, and IgA-specific detecting reagents to detect RFs of each immunoglobulin class. RFs are increased in people with acute infections, some chronic infections such as hepatitis C virus, certain auto-immune diseases such as Sjögren's syndrome, and rarely in healthy individuals [40]. Thus, they are not specific for rheumatoid arthritis. A new diagnostic test to help identify people with rheumatoid arthritis has recently been discovered. The antigen in two IIF tests that were used to help diagnose RA, the anti-kera-tin test on rat stomach and the perinuclear factor test on buccal cells, was iden-tified as citrullinated filaggrin [5]. An ELISA that contains a peptide with the modified amino acid citrulline was developed [41]. At this time the best-accepted test is to a cyclic citrullinated peptide (CCP) that mimics a citrullinated epitope on filaggrin. Anti-CCP antibodies are found in about 65% of RA patients and are rarely found in people with infections or other autoimmune diseases [42]. Anti-CCP antibodies are found early in the course of disease, often when RFs are not present. About 80% of RF-positive RA patients are also positive for anti-CCP antibodies. Importantly, about 40% of RF-negative RA patients are positive for anti-CCP. There is clinical utility in measuring both RF and anti-CCP. Someone who is positive for both autoantibodies is very likely to have RA. Because some RA patients are positive for only one or the other autoantibody, measuring both autoantibodies detects a greater percentage of RA patients than does measuring one autoantibody alone.

Flocculation of VDRL was generally used as a test for syphilis. When more specific tests for anti-treponema antibodies were developed, it was shown that some people with SLE yielded false-positive results on the VDRL test. Today, the VDRL reagent has been replaced by tests that are more specific for anti-treponema antibodies. An anti-cardiolipin ELISA is used to screen for the type of autoantibodies that yielded the false-positive VDRL results in patients with SLE. The false-positive VDRL test is one of the criteria to diagnose SLE [13]. Recently, it was suggested that this criterion be changed to a positive anti-cardiolipin result [43]. However, an anti-cardiolipin test and a false-positive VDRL test do not measure the same antibodies [44].

Besides people with SLE, anti-cardiolipin autoantibodies are found in people with antiphospholipid syndrome, a condition in which the chances of thrombosis, stroke, and recurrent fetal loss are increased. Patients with syphilis make true anti-cardiolipin antibodies. However, the majority of diagnostically important autoantibodies measured by the anti-cardiolipin ELISA actually react with beta 2-glycoprotein 1 (β2-GP1), a positively charged serum protein that binds to the negatively charged cardiolipin on the ELISA plate [45, 46]. The β2-GP1 originates in bovine serum added to the blocking solution for the cardiolipin ELISA plate or the sample diluent or from the patient's serum itself. Once β2-GP1 binds to cardiolipin, it becomes reactive with the autoantibodies in sera. β2-GP1 can also bind directly onto an ELISA plate in an immunologically active form. The titers of anti-cardiolipin and anti-β2-GP1 antibodies have a relatively strong correlation with each other. The data so far suggest that some "anti-cardiolipin" autoantibodies bind epitopes on β2-GP1 alone and that some bind an epitope comprised of both cardiolipin and β2-GP1, but virtually none of them bind to cardiolipin by itself. Because of historic precedence, the terms "antiphospholipid syndrome" and "anti-cardiolipin" antibodies are still used, even though they are technically incorrect.

Another assay that measures autoantibodies that are correlated to an autoimmune coagulation disorder is the lupus anticoagulant test [47]. This test is performed on plasma that has been treated with calcium and phospholipid. A positive result is a prolonged clotting time, which is ironic because people with this activity are at risk for increased clotting *in vivo*. There is only a modest correlation between anti-cardiolipin, anti-β2-GP1, and the presence of lupus anticoagulant. Finding an ELISA that matches the lupus anticoagulant test is an active area of research because the lupus anticoagulant test is clinically correlated with clotting problems in SLE patients, some of whom are anti-β2-GP1 negative. Because the lupus anticoagulant has not been identified, it is possible that it is not an autoantibody, while it also might be a set of autoantibodies.

For many years the LE cell test to help diagnose people with SLE was routinely performed in many laboratories throughout the world. In its most typical form, clotted blood was passed through a strainer to break open some lymphocytes, and allowed to incubate for several hours. A drop was smeared on a slide, stained, and examined under a microscope. LE cells were formed when a segmented neutrophil engulfed nuclear material [38]. This occurred in the presence of three things: autoantibodies that bound the nuclear material, active complement, and viable cells. LE cell reactivity was found predominantly in people with SLE, but also in people with drug-induced lupus and lupoid hepatitis. Numerous studies in the 1950s through the 1970s found that adsorption with chromatin (called deoxyribonucleoprotein at that time), but not its individual components, i.e., DNA-free histone or histone-free DNA, could remove LE cell reactivity from sera [48, 49]. Thus, it was concluded that anti-chromatin, but not anti-DNA or anti-histone, autoantibodies accounted for LE cell reactivity. Recently, some papers have suggested that antibodies to histone H1 account for the LE cell reactivity [50]. There is no explanation for many other researchers finding the opposite result.

The LE cell test is very labor-intensive, is difficult to reproduce, and requires fresh blood. It is rarely performed in the U.S. today but is still performed in other countries. It has largely been replaced or supplemented by anti-DNA testing for these technical reasons. However, the LE cell factor was generally found in a higher percentage of SLE patients than were anti-DNA autoantibodies, so it would be clinically useful if there were an ELISA to replace it [13]. The anti-chromatin ELISA has many of the same properties as the LE cell test. Anti-chromatin autoantibodies are more common than anti-DNA in SLE patients, and they are found in people with SLE, drug-induced lupus, and lupoid hepatitis but not other diseases [51]. Additionally, numerous studies from labs around the world found that anti-chromatin autoantibodies are a sensitive and specific marker for SLE and correlate with kidney disorders or active disease [52]. These are similar to correlations with the LE cell assay.

Autoantibodies to ENAs such as SS-A/Ro, SS-B/La, Sm, RNP, and Scl-70 are common in people with systemic connective tissue diseases such as SLE, Sjögren's syndrome (SS), and systemic sclerosis (SSc) [53]. Jo-1 is an extractable cytoplasmic antigen and antibodies to it are helpful in diagnosing people with polymyositis or dermatomyositis (PM/DM) [54]. Originally, all these antibodies were detected by the Ouchterlony immunodiffusion technique. This is still the technique used in hundreds of small laboratories and some large ones. Once the above antigens were purified, these tests could all be performed by ELISA. This was the method of choice for large laboratories for several years. Because autoantibodies to the ENAs are typically measured in all people suspected of having one of the autoimmune connective tissue diseases, they were the first autoantibodies detected by the three multiplex technologies described in the last section.

8.3
Comparison of Antigens, Conjugates, and Cutoff Values

By far the most important parameter in an ELISA, or in any test that measures a specific autoantibody, is the antigen. Each antigen has to be optimized to detect the clinically important autoantibody it was designed to measure. Very often a native antigen produced in a human or closely related mammal works better than a cloned antigen or an antigen from a source far removed from humans on the evolutionary tree. The interpretation generally given for this finding is that most autoantibodies are produced by an immune response against the antigen in the host. So even though the immune response is abnormal in the sense that the person is reacting against something in their own body, it is a typical antibody response because the autoantibodies are exquisitely tuned to recognize the antigen that stimulated them in the first place.

Native antigens may work best for a number of reasons. Some autoantibodies recognize epitopes that are expressed in a macromolecular complex comprised of two or more separate macromolecules. There are diagnostically important antibodies in SLE and drug-induced lupus patients that recognize chromatin but not isolated DNA-free histones or histone-free DNA [55, 56]. Similarly, antibodies recognizing the native RNP particle, but not the individual proteins or RNA moiety, are found in patients with SLE and mixed connective tissue disease [57]. In some cases autoantibodies recognize parts of proteins that are changed by post-translational modifications. The best example of this is the recently discovered autoantibody reactivity in RA patients that recognize only proteins whose arginines have been changed to citrulline [5]. Finally, there are numerous examples of autoantibodies that recognize conformational epitopes that are present on the native form of the protein but not on the denatured protein [58].

For the above reasons, cloned proteins expressed in bacteria or insect cells, and synthesized peptides, rarely work as well as native antigen to detect autoantibodies. Some exceptions to the above statement are autoantibodies against ribosomal P proteins that react with a 23-amino-acid peptide [59] and autoantibodies to SS-A/Ro-52 that react with the denatured protein better than the native [60].

The most important feature in the conjugate is the class of immunoglobulin that it recognizes. The main choices are the class-specific antibodies that recognize the heavy chains of IgG, IgM, or IgA and the polyspecific conjugates that react with all the heavy chains. Antibodies that recognize the kappa and lambda light chains are also polyspecific because all classes of immunoglobulins have the same light chains. For some tests, such as IgM RF, IgA anti-tTG, and IgG anti-CCP, there is no debate about the most important class of immunoglobulin to measure. However, for many other very common tests there is no consensus. This is particularly true for IIF on HEp-2 cells, anti-DNA by both ELISA and IIF, anti-histone, and anti-MPO and anti-PR3. Some manufacturers make kits with IgG-specific conjugates, while others are made with polyspecific conjugates. Any attempt to make international standards for these antibodies needs to take into account the different specificities of the conjugates that are used in different laboratories.

The cutoff value between negative and positive in a test that measures autoantibodies is extremely important. In subjective tests such as IIF, the technician examining the slide under the microscope has to decide what strength of immunofluorescence and what pattern should be considered positive. Different people and microscopes may give different results. The results with Ouchterlony immunodiffusion are less subjective than IIF but still depend on the sharpness of the eyes, the indirect light source, and the attention to detail of the viewer.

One of the main advantages of ELISA over many other techniques to measure autoantibodies is that it is objective. The optical density (O.D.) of the patient is compared to that of a calibrator or standard curve and given a value. The biggest challenge to anyone developing an ELISA is setting the value that divides negative or indeterminate from positive. Kits made by various in-house methods and by different manufacturers may yield opposite results on a given sample simply because the cutoffs are quite different. This dichotomy arises because different statistical methods and different control groups are used to determine the cutoff between negative and positive.

The most egregious approach occurs when normal blood donors are used as the control group and a value of two or three standard deviations above the mean is chosen as the cutoff. In this case, both the control group and the statistical analysis are inappropriate. Very rarely is the blood from a healthy person, such as the average blood donor, sent to a clinical laboratory for autoantibody tests. Usually the person is sick. Thus, the correct control group should consist of people with autoimmune diseases who are expected to be negative for the autoantibody in question and people with infectious diseases with symptoms similar to those of an autoimmune disease. Very often these latter groups have higher antibody levels, and higher binding on ELISA, than normal blood donors. The average and standard deviation are useful statistical tools only when the distribution of values in a population yields a normal, or bell-shaped, curve. In an ELISA, the distribution of values in the negative population is not bell shaped but usually resembles the right half of a bell. That is, a large percentage of the population will yield the lowest results, with smaller and smaller percentages yielding higher and higher results.

The best way to determine the correct cutoff is to perform a simple nonparametric statistical analysis of the expected negative and positive groups [61]. All the samples should be put in rank order from highest O.D. to lowest O.D. At least 60, but preferably about 200, patients who are expected to be negative for the autoantibody but have symptoms related to the disease in question should be tested. In addition, more than 20, or as many as possible, people with the disease or known to be positive for the autoantibody should also be tested. After all the patients and controls are put in rank order, one can examine the results and determine the best cutoff to yield the optimum sensitivity and specificity for that ELISA.

A recent paper showed great differences in the specificity, but only moderate changes in the sensitivity, of the anti-chromatin ELISA depending on the cutoff that was chosen. When a cutoff was used that yielded 98% specificity (i.e., 2% positive) in blood donors, the sensitivity was 86% in SLE patients, the group who were expected to be positive [62]. However, the specificity in other groups that were expected to be negative was poor. People with infectious diseases also showed 2% false-positive results, while 13% of SSc patients were positive. With this cutoff this test has a high sensitivity but poor specificity, and it may not help doctors in their diagnosis. When the value for the cutoff was raised so that no blood donors were positive, then no one with infectious diseases or SSc was positive, while the sensitivity in the SLE patients only dropped to 71% (A. Doria, personal communication). With this cutoff the test is still quite sensitive, but is now very specific and has significant clinical utility.

8.4
Comparison of Multiplexed Assays

Many hundreds of different autoantibodies have been identified in the literature, but only a small percentage of them have proven to be clinically useful. Sometimes an autoantibody profile in a person can help a doctor determine whether the person has an autoimmune disease or not, and which one they have [53]. The autoantibody profiles for people with systemic rheumatic diseases show that certain sets of autoantibodies are associated with SLE, SS, SSc, RA, and PM (Fig. 8.4). It is clearly useful to measure all autoantibodies associated with rheumatic diseases at one time, but would it be an advantage to the doctor to detect all of the clinically useful autoantibodies to all autoimmune diseases in a single test?

The majority of the clinically useful autoantibody tests have been cleared by the FDA for *in vitro* use to help diagnose autoimmune diseases. These include those to help diagnose connective tissue diseases such as RA, SLE, SS, SSc, and PM/DM; gastrointestinal diseases such as celiac disease, Crohn's disease, and ulcerative colitis; autoimmune liver diseases such as PBC and autoimmune hepatitis types I and II; autoimmune vasculitides such as Wegener's granulomatosis and Goodpasture's syndrome; autoimmune endocrine diseases such as Hashimoto's thyroiditis and Graves' disease; and autoimmune coagulation disorders such as antiphospholipid syndrome. Examples of clinically useful autoantibody tests that have not been cleared by the FDA include antibodies to help diagnose pernicious anemia, autoimmune skin-blistering diseases such as pemphigus and pemphigoid, and some autoimmune neurological diseases. Auto-

ANA Profiles

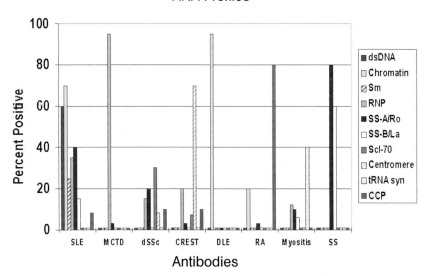

Fig. 8.4 Illustration of ANA profiles in people with rheumatic diseases. The Y-axis shows the percentage of people who are positive for a given autoantibody, while the X-axis is divided into various rheumatic diseases. For example, many people with SLE have numerous antibodies: 60% have anti-DNA, 70% have anti-chromatin, 25% have anti-Sm, etc. Some other diseases have less diversity of autoantibodies. Anti-RNP is almost the only autoantibody seen in patients with MCTD. Antibodies to SS-A/Ro and SS-B/La are found in a high percentage of patients with SS and in a smaller percentage of patients with SLE.
Abbreviations: MCTD = mixed connective tissue disease; dSSc = diffuse systemic sclerosis; CREST = calcinosis, Raynaud's phenomenon, esophageal dysmotility, sclerodactyly, and telangiectasia; DLE = drug-induced lupus; SS = Sjögren's syndrome.

antibodies may be useful prognostic markers in people with type 1 diabetes if a method is discovered for preventing diabetes in those who are most at risk.

Sometimes, the symptoms found in people with the above autoimmune diseases are actually caused by infectious diseases. Ulcers caused by infection with *Helicobacter pylori* yield the same symptoms as autoimmune gastrointestinal disease; infectious liver disease can be similar to autoimmune liver disease; people with hepatitis C virus or Lyme disease often have symptoms similar to RA. Would it be clinically useful to test for a wide variety of antibodies to infectious disease organisms at the same time one tested for autoantibodies?

Using multiplex technology, dozens, hundreds, or even thousands of parameters can be measured simultaneously on a single sample. In one way, a technique such as IIF on HEp-2 cells is a multiplexed test. There are thousands of antigens that are present in the fixed HEp-2 cell. Reactivity to many of them can be detected by immunofluorescence. A few reactivities, such as centromere, can even be identified at the molecular level by their pattern. But testing sera for reactivity on HEp-2 cells is more generally considered a screening test because most positive results cannot be clearly identified at the molecular level. Also, at this time pattern-recognition software is not advanced enough to automate evaluation of the slide. Similarly, Western blot – where proteins are separated by gel electrophoresis and transferred to a membrane, and then antibodies against them are detected – is a multiplex technology. However, a positive reaction is often ambiguous because many different proteins may migrate to the same spot on the gel.

Another system that is related to a true multiplexed assay is the large automated ELISA machine. The multiple tests are performed sequentially rather than simultaneously, but because all of the tests are finished in one day, the results are similar to a true multiplexed test. A large automated ELISA system can run tests on eight ELISA plates at one time. Each plate can have up to four different assays on it (three strips of eight wells each). Thus, a total of 24 samples and controls can be tested on 32 different assays in real time. This yields the performance of a small multiplexed assay by brute force.

There are a large number of true multiplex technologies available in research today (reviewed in [63]). Some types of multiplex technology, such as the ordered arrangement of expressed cDNA clones or any other large array of unknown proteins or peptides, are more like screening assays than multiplexed assays. These techniques can be used in research to discover new autoantibody reactivities but not in the clinical laboratory. It is not clear whether technologies such as the Nanobarcode will be appropriate for measuring autoantibodies.

Three of the multiplex technologies have progressed to the point where they are available to measure autoantibodies against known antigens today. Two are used in both research and the clinical lab, while one is still in the research phase. The first of these three is line blot, which is related to Western blot. However, in a line blot purified antigens are put on a membrane in known locations [64]. A narrow strip of membrane typically 7–10 cm long has 10–20 narrow lines of antigen sprayed on it with easily visible space between each line. If it becomes important to test more antigens simultaneously, the strip can be made longer. For applications manufactured in-house, antigens can be applied by a pipette in dots. When large numbers of line blots are manufactured, the same technology used in inkjet printers is used to transfer the lines of antigen onto the membrane. As in a Western blot and ELISA, diluted patient serum is incubated with the strip and washed away, and then conjugated detecting antibody is incubated with the strip and finally washed away. Although other detection technologies are available, bound antibodies are typically detected by a chemical reaction in which a dye becomes insoluble in the presence of the conjugated enzyme and precipitates out as a dark gray line. The readout for this test is an estimate of the intensity of any lines by eye; alternatively, the strip can be put in a scanner and the intensity of each line can be quantitated. Each line is a known antigen and can have an intensity used for the cutoff between negative and positive that is specific for that antigen. Machines have been developed to automate almost the entire process. They can perform the entire test from diluting the patient sample up to the step of stopping the development of the chemical reaction used to detect conjugated antibody. The only thing that needs to be done manually is to either read the strips by eye or manually place them in a scanner and run the scanning program. The limits to this technology are the number of strips that can be processed in a given time, the size of a strip that can be easily handled, and the number of lines that can be reliably separated by eye or a scanner. About 50 different lines or dots with a different antigen for each line could fit on a 20-cm strip. Making the strip wide enough for two columns would allow 100 different tests per strip.

Microarrays are similar to line blots in which everything has been miniaturized and compacted to the size of a microscope slide [65]. The slide can be made of glass or plastic and can be treated in various ways. Alternatively, the slide can be covered by a membrane made of nylon, nitrocellulose, or PVDF. Thousands of dots of antigen can be placed on the slide or membrane in known places using a computer-controlled robotic arm and a micropipette capable of dispensing nanoliters of liquid [66]. The micropipette technique, or the technology used in inkjet printers, can be used to put antigens on a membrane. Often the same antigen is put in several locations in the microarray, allowing for redundancy in measuring reactions, which decreases the number of false-positive and false-negative results due to assay variability.

The assay conditions for the microarray are very similar to those for IIF. Diluted patient sample is incubated with the slide and washed off, and then the slide is incubated with a detecting antibody conjugated to a fluorescent probe and finally washed. The processed slide is placed in a fluorescent microscope, and the amount of fluorescence at each dot in the microarray is recorded. Special software recognizes the pattern of known negative and positive control dots and thus identifies the location of every dot on the slide. Obviously, the antigen at each location is known. The amount of fluorescence from each dot is measured, repeat measurements of the same antigens are combined, and a quantitative or semi-quantitative result is given for each antigen. This is a very powerful technique because of the large numbers of reactions that can be measured on one sample at the same time. In research, this technology allows the investigator to ask questions and obtain answers about autoantibodies that could not be addressed previously. It is not clear how the microarray technique will be used in clinical laboratories. At this time the main drawbacks to this technique are the specialized equipment necessary to make the slides and the time it takes to read each sample and process the data from an entire slide. Results are generally not available in real time.

The third multiplex technique uses a dual laser flow cytometer from Luminex Corporation that can measure antibody reactivity on 100 different antigens simultaneously [67]. Specifically, the flow cytometer has been specially set up to measure beads that are dyed internally with various amounts of two different fluorescent dyes. These dyes are both stimulated with the same wavelength of light, but they emit their fluorescence at wavelengths that are different enough from each other that they can be separated by filters with no cross-contamina-

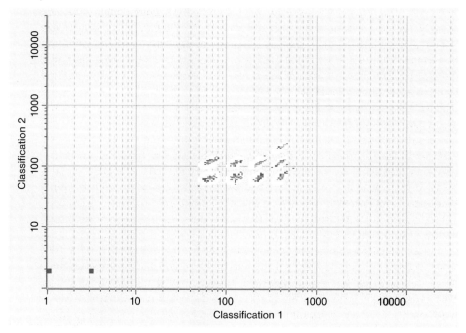

Fig. 8.5 Nine of the 100 bead regions available to the Luminex 100. The X-axis is the fluorescent intensity of classification dye #1 and the Y-axis is the fluorescent intensity of classification dye #2. The white circles designate the regions, and the dots inside each region represent beads that have the appropriate fluorescent intensities of dye #1 and dye #2. This is an example of an assay using nine different bead sets.

tion. This allows the accurate measurement of the intensity of the fluorescence from each dye in each bead to be done in real time using a single laser and appropriate filters and detectors (Fig. 8.5). Based on the amount of fluorescence of each dye, 100 different beads can be identified. To be precise, the beads are identified by "different absolute amounts of two fluorescent dyes," but usually it is said that the beads have 100 different "colors." Luminex Corporation owns the patent on using two different dyes per bead and is the only company offering this technology.

The beads are all 5.6 microns in diameter. Because of the uniform size of all the beads, aggregates of two or more can be detected based on the side scatter of each particle passing through the first laser. Data collected from aggregated beads are not used. The second laser of the flow cytometer can stimulate a fluorescent dye such as phycoerythrin, which is used on the detecting antibody.

The beads are made of the same type of carboxylated polystyrene, also called "latex," that has been used in antibody-antigen tests for over 50 years. Using standard chemistry, the carboxyl groups on the beads are activated to bind to amino groups on the antigen of interest [68]. The antigen is incubated with the beads and is covalently attached to them. Other types of chemistries can be used to cross-link hydroxyl [69] rather than amino groups to the beads. It is also possible to modify the antigen by adding amino groups to it so that it can react with the bead. It takes about two hours to perform the coupling reaction of antigen to the bead, and it is straightforward to couple enough beads to perform tens of thousands of tests. Many differently colored beads can be processed at the same time. Once antigens have been coupled to their individual bead sets, the beads are all mixed together to form the multiplex assay.

The Luminex 100 flow cytometer sips the beads from a 96-well plate. Up to 100 different bead sets can be in each well, and each bead set can be coated with a different antigen. One way to maximize the potential for multiplexing in the Luminex is to coat the 100 bead sets in the first well with one group of 100 antigens, the 100 bead sets in the second well with a group of 100 different antigens, etc. In this way, 9600 antigens could be tested in a microtiter plate.

The assay is performed similarly to those described above, except there are no wash steps. The diluted patient sample is incubated with the beads in the well of a microtiter plate. Then the phycoerythrin-conjugated detecting antibody is added. Finally, the beads are read on the Luminex 100 flow cytometer. Fifty beads from each bead set are analyzed, and the median fluorescent intensity of each set is calculated. It takes about 20 s for the beads in each well to be analyzed. Thus, the entire 96-well plate is read and all of the results are reported in about 30 min. At some point Luminex may make a three-laser flow cytometer that will be capable of measuring 1000 different bead sets.

What are the pros and cons of each of the three types of multiplex technologies? Two of the three technologies, line blot and the Luminex flow cytometer, are commercially available today and are used in many clinical laboratories to report patient results and in many research laboratories. The microarray technology at this time is restricted to research laboratories that build their own systems. The three technologies have different limits to the number of autoantibodies that they can simultaneously measure. The Luminex system is limited to 100 sets now, and possibly 1000 in the future. Thus, 100, or eventually 1000, autoantibody reactivities can be measured in a single well. If one considers the whole microtiter plate as a reaction vessel, then 9600–96,000 autoantibodies could be measured at one time. The Luminex beads use approximately 10% the amount of antigen needed for an ELISA. The line blot is limited by the number of lines that can be separated without magnification and can fit into a reasonably sized strip. This is probably in the range of 50–100 lines. It also utilizes about 10% of the antigen needed for an equivalent ELISA. The microarray has the most potential for measuring large numbers of different autoantibodies simultaneously. Currently, more than 1000 dots can be put on a slide. If the slide were made larger or the dots more dense, 5000–10,000 dots could be put on a single slide. The manufacture of the slide can be automated to a large degree. The biggest advantage of the microarray is that extremely small amounts of antigen are used in each test, perhaps 10,000–100,000 fewer than needed for ELISA. Scaling up the manufacture of the slides for microarrays requires better machines, but not large-scale production of antigens.

Both the line blot and the Luminex technologies yield reportable results in real time, i.e., within seconds or minutes after performing the test. At this time the microarray requires a large amount of scanning on a microscope and data analysis in a computer, so results are not available in real time. If enough work were put into automating the detection system, it is probable that results for the microarray could be reported in near real time.

The largest problem facing multiplex testing is validating every test in the multiplex. A certain percentage of antigens will not attach to a given substrate in an antigenic form, and a certain number of antibody-antigen systems require unique buffers or other conditions for optimal performance. As more and more antigens are put on the line blot, on the matrix for the microarray, or on different beads, there is a greater chance that certain antibody-antigen pairs will not work as expected, yielding either false-negative or false-positive results. There are a number of possible solutions.

One option is to spend all the time necessary to optimize the coating of every antigen onto the substrate and the detection of every type of autoantibody. This requires a large effort for each antigen-antibody set. Since multiplexing by definition is the measurement of many different things at the same time, it is impossible to optimize most variables for each antibody-antigen system. The patient dilution, buffers, incubation time, and detecting reagent must be the same for all autoantibody-antigen pairs. Thus, these parameters are determined, and the only remaining variable is the way that each antigen is attached to the substrate.

Each technology has limits to the flexibility of attaching antigens to the substrate. A large amount is known about ways to coat antigens onto latex beads because immunologists have been doing that for over 50 years. Standard procedures are available to coat proteins and polysaccharides via covalent linkage through amino and hydroxyl groups, respectively. Many cross-linking agents are readily available to try novel methods of covalent attachment of macromolecules to latex beads.

One way to add flexibility in attaching antigens to either the line immunoassay or the microarray is to manufacture the substrate out of more than one material. Two or more treatments of the glass or several types of membranes could be put together. Antigens that did not attach in an immunogenic way to one substrate could be bound to one of the others.

Another option is to ignore any troublesome antigens and assume that the large quantity of antigens that do work will overcome the lack of antigens that do not work. This approach is very useful in a research setting where the objective is to study a global autoimmune response or to detect novel autoantibodies. It also can be used to detect new profiles of autoantibodies because of the ease of testing such a large number of antigens at one time. However, certain autoantibodies have been proven over the years to have important clinical utility. If these key autoantibody-antigen systems do not work extremely well, the system as a whole will not have a good clinical utility.

Even with the large number of autoantibodies that can be measured on these multiplex tests at one time, it will probably not be possible to measure all clinically important autoantibodies simultaneously. For one reason, some clinically important autoantibodies are IgA, such as anti-gliadin and tTG, while others are IgM, such as RF, anti-cardiolipin, and β2-GP1. The vast majority of diagnostically important autoantibodies are IgG. Thus, in most systems an IgG-specific detecting antibody is preferred over a polyspecific detecting antibody. In fact, it is known that some IgM autoantibodies are not clinically important and can yield positive results in normal blood donors [70]. Thus, a polyspecific detecting reagent would probably yield too many false-positive results to be clinically useful. Also, IgG anti-f-actin helps to diagnose autoimmune hepatitis [6], but IgA anti-f-actin autoantibodies may be useful in diagnosing celiac disease [71]; therefore, it would be clinically useful to know the class of antibody bound to this antigen.

It is possible that a system could be devised to spectrally discriminate IgG, IgA, and IgM detecting reagents in these multiplex assays. For example, the proposed third laser in the Luminex flow cytometer could be used to detect a second conjugate instead of expanding the number of beads counted from 100 to 1000. In the microarray, class-specific detecting antibodies with different fluorescent probes on them could be mixed together, and the scanning microscope could have a series of filters that would allow the system to detect each conjugate separately. In the line immunoassay, it might be possible to make enzyme-substrate pairs that yielded differently colored precipitates. Of course the simplest solution would be to run the exact same test three times, once each with the three different detecting systems.

Besides the potential difficulty with the conjugate, another problem with an assay that tries to measure all important autoantibodies at the same time is that there are a number of known autoantibodies that cannot easily be measured in a solid-phase assay. One example is anti-fibrillarin, an autoantibody found in patients with SSc. These antibodies can be detected in immunofluorescence and immunoprecipitation assays, but not in ELISA [72]. Another reason is that the specificity of some autoantibodies, such as atypical or X-ANCA, is not known [73]. A specific test to measure this autoantibody cannot be developed until the antigen is known.

What are the advantages of multiplex testing for autoantibodies in a clinical laboratory? The new multiplex technologies will likely decrease labor costs because many different tests are run simultaneously. Another advantage is that a very high percentage of all autoantibodies of known clinical significance can be detected at one time. Perhaps some new clinically important patterns of autoantibody reactivity will be discovered because of multiplex technology. However, it will be difficult to detect all important autoantibodies in one multiplex test for the reasons mentioned above. Similarly, some autoantibodies may not be detected at the most optimal sensitivity and specificity because they are part of a multiplex and not a stand-alone assay optimized for their detection. Nonetheless, sometimes laboratories are willing to switch to new technologies as long as the results are still satisfactory to the doctor. Examples of this are changing from the Farr assay to the anti-DNA ELISA, and from IIF on HEp-2 cells to the

ANA ELISA for ANA screening. Neither of the new ELISAs is as clinically useful as the original test, but both are still good and are much easier to perform than the original test. If doctors do not complain, the labs will use the cheaper and more convenient technology even if it is slightly less clinically relevant. This approach is acceptable in diagnosing autoimmune diseases because there is usually no single laboratory test that can rule in or rule out a diagnosis. Because there are no formal standards set by the FDA for autoimmune tests, 510(k) clearance has been given to tests that have over 15% false-positive rates in the normal population [74], or less than 50% agreement for positive samples with the predicate device [75]. Thus, for autoimmune tests, both the doctor and the clinical laboratory must understand the systems that they are using. There is not much variability allowed for most tests for infectious diseases because the laboratory test is often the one and only diagnostic criterion. Only a perfect result is acceptable in many types of infectious disease assays.

What disadvantages exist in multiplex testing in a clinical laboratory? The two largest problems with performing multiplex testing in clinical laboratories concern performing tests that are not ordered by the doctor and performing tests that are not clinically relevant even if they were ordered by a doctor. In the first instance, a doctor may want to measure the titer of anti-DNA antibodies just to see whether an SLE patient has responded to therapy to decrease a flare-up in their disease [76]. Similarly, a doctor may want to measure anti-SS-A and SS-B autoantibodies in a pregnant woman just to see whether her child is at risk for being born with a form of congenital heart block [77]. Should these samples be tested on a multiplex of 10 or 100 or 1000 autoantigens? Assuming that the software can suppress the results of all tests except the ones ordered, is it legally or ethically right to do so? Some countries and U.S. states have passed laws stating that a clinical laboratory may not perform a test that was not ordered on a sample. These laws were designed to prevent fraudulent billing on chemistry panels where all tests were performed (and billed) because the machine performed all tests at once, even if only one was ordered. Even in places where it is not the law, some laboratories have internal regulations stating that they are not allowed to perform a test that was not ordered. Some countries have a law where a lab must report the results of all tests performed on a patient, even if only one test was ordered and paid for. Even though multiplex tests for autoantibodies were not envisioned when these laws and regulations were passed, the tests could well fall under the shadow of these rules.

A clinical lab could get around these problems by offering only the multiplex autoantibody profile, not individual autoantibody tests. Thus, the doctor would always order the entire autoantibody profile. Laws and regulations that were passed to stop previous abuses in clinical laboratories may make this approach difficult, too. In some countries and U.S. states, it is illegal to perform clinical tests for conditions that the patient does not have. Thus, if a patient has symptoms of rheumatic disease, it is reasonable to test them for autoantibodies found in any of the autoimmune rheumatic diseases. In this case a small multiplex test is easily justified. However, is it also reasonable to test them for autoantibodies found in people with autoimmune liver, gastrointestinal, coagulation, vasculitic, and endocrine diseases and related infectious diseases? It may be possible to get around the above restrictions by using software and billing practices that report only the tests ordered by the doctor and bill the patient only for tests that are reported. These practices would be within the spirit of most laws and regulations.

Assuming that legal and ethical questions about multiplex testing for autoantibodies are resolved, the issue then comes down to the cost of the technology to the laboratory. Clinical laboratories are not willing to increase the cost of reagents even if they can more than make up for this increased cost with the decreased cost of labor. This occurs because the lab rarely fires workers when laborsaving technology is adopted. Thus, it is extremely difficult for a lab to justify an increase in the cost of reagents, regardless of the theoretical savings in labor. This means that the price of the multiplex test must be relatively inexpensive. A way to roughly calculate the allowable price of a multiplex test is to add up the costs of all reagents and kits used for autoimmune testing in a laboratory and divide that sum by the number of patients that were tested. This yields the average cost of autoantibody tests per patient. Assuming that the perfect multiplexed test can measure all autoantibodies at one time, this sets an upper limit on the value of the test to a clinical laboratory.

As described above, some patients with symptoms of systemic rheumatic disease may be tested for up to 10 different autoantibodies. Most patients with symptoms of other autoimmune diseases such as celiac disease, autoimmune liver disease, vasculitis, and thyroiditis are tested only for the presence of two to four autoantibodies. This constraint probably limits the price of an all-encompassing autoantibody multiplex test to no more than five times the price of an individual test. If a great savings in labor were achieved, the price could be somewhat higher. If measuring large autoantibody profiles yields a powerful clinical utility, a higher cost could also be justified.

What technology might be most suited for a clinical laboratory? Currently, less than 50 different autoantibody tests are approved by the FDA for use in diagnosing autoimmune diseases. Perhaps that number will more than double to around 100 different specificities in the next decade or two. If that is the case, then any of the multiplex technologies will work because all can detect 100 different reactivities at one time. Market forces such as price, ease of use, and clinical sensitivity and specificity would determine which multiplex technology, if any, will predominate. Legal and ethical decisions also need to be made about multiplex testing in clinical laboratories. If small profiles of autoantibodies become the norm in clinical laboratories, then the two technologies currently in use, line blot and the Luminex flow cytometer, will probably continue to dominate the market for multiplex autoantibody testing. If it becomes clear that there is a clinical utility in measuring 1000 or more different antibodies at one time, then the microarray on a slide will become a staple for testing autoantibodies in clinical laboratories.

References

1 Von Mühlen CA, EM Tan. Autoantibodies in the Diagnosis of Systemic Rheumatic Diseases. *Semin Arthritis Rheum.* **1995.** 24:323–358.

2 Anderson JR, Gray KG, Beck JS, Buchanan WW, McElhinney AJ. Precipitating auto-antibodies in the connective tissue diseases. *Ann. Rheum. Dis.* **1962.** 21:360–369.

3 Carpenter AB. Antibody based methods. In: Manual of Clinical Laboratory Immunology, 6th ed. Rose NR, Hamilton RG, Detrick B, eds. ASM Press, Washington, DC. **1997.**

4 Dieterich W, Ehnis T, Bauer M, Volta U, Riecken EO, Schuppan D. Identification of tissue transglutaminase as the autoantigen of celiac disease. *Nat Med.* **1997.** 3:797–801.

5 Shellekens GA, de Jong BAW, van den Hoogen FHJ, van de Putte LBA, van Venrooij WJ. Citrulline is an essential constituent of antigenic determinants recognized by rheumatoid arthritis-specific autoantibodies. *J Clin Invest.* **1998,** 101:273–281.

6 Czaja AJ, Cassani F, Cataleta M, Valentini P, Bianchi FB. Frequency and significance of antibodies to actin in type 1 autoimmune hepatitis. *Hepatology* **1996.** 24:1068–1073.

7 Luettig B, Boeker KH, Schoessler W, Will H, Loges S, Schmidt E, Worman HJ,Gershwin ME, Manns MP. The antinuclear autoantibodies Sp100 and gp210 persist after orthotopic liver transplantation in patients with primary biliary cirrhosis. *J Hepatol.* **1998.** 28:824–828.

8 Czaja AJ, Donaldson PT, Lohse AW. Antibodies to soluble liver antigen/liver pancreas and HLA risk factors for type 1 autoimmune hepatitis. *Am J Gastroenterol.* **2002.** 97:413–419.

9 Teml A, Kratzer V, Schneider B, Lochs H, Norman GL, Gangl A, Vogelsang H, Reinisch W. Anti-Saccharomyces cerevisiae antibodies: a stable marker for Crohn's disease during steroid and 5-aminosalicylic acid treatment. *Am J Gastroenterol* **2003.** 98:2226–2231.

10 Van Venrooj WJ and Maini RN editors: Manual of Biological Markers of Disease, section B: Autoantigens **1994.** Kluwer Academic Publishing, Boston.

11 Rose NR, Hamilton RG, Detrick B editors: Manual of Clinical Laboratory Immunology, sixth edition, **2002.** ASM Press, Washington, D.C.

12 Wild D editor: The Immunoassay Handbook, second edition **2001.** Nature Publishing Group, New York.

13 Tan EM, Cohen AS, Fries JF, et al. The 1982 revised criteria for the classification of systemic lupus erythematosus. *Arthritis Rheum* **1983.** 25:1271–1277.

14 Tan EM, Feltkamp TE, Smolen JS, Butcher B, Dawkins R, Fritzler MJ, Gordon T, Hardin JA, Kalden JR, Lahita RG, Maini RN, McDougal JS, Rothfield NF, Smeenk RJ,Takasaki Y, Wiik A, Wilson MR, Koziol JA. Range of Antinuclear antibodies in "healthy" individuals. *Arthritis Rheum* **1997.** 40:1601–1611.

15 Harmon C, Deng JS, Peebles CL, Tan EM. The importance of tissue substrate in the SS-A/Ro antigen-antibody system. *Arthritis Rheum* **1984.** 27:166–173.

16 Miyachi K, Fritzler MJ, Tan EM. Autoantibody to a nuclear antigen in proliferating cells. *J Immunol.* **1978.** 121:2228–2234.

17 Moroi Y, Peebles C, Fritzler MJ, Steigerwald J, Tan EM. Autoantibody to centromere (kinetochore) in scleroderma sera. *Proc Natl Acad Sci.* **1980.** 77:1628–1631.

18 Koh WH, Dunphy J, Whyte J, Dixey J, McHugh NJ. Characterisation of anti-cytoplasmic antibodies and their clinical associations. *Ann Rheum Dis.* **1995.** 54:269–273.

19 Monce NM Jr, Cappel VL, Saqueton CB. A comparison of two fixatives on IFA HEp-2 slides for the detection of antinuclear antibodies. *J Immunoassay.* **1994.** 15:55–68.

20 Smolen JS, Butcher B, Fritzler MJ, Gordon T, Hardin J, Kalden JR, Lahita R, Maini RN, Reeves W, Reichlin M, Rothfield N, Takasaki Y, van Venrooij WJ, Tan EM. Reference sera for antinuclear anti-

bodies. II. Further definition of antibody specificities in international antinuclear antibody reference sera by immunofluorescence and western blotting. *Arthritis Rheum.* **1997.** 40:413–418.

21 Tonuttia E, Bassetti D, Piazza A, Visentini D, Poletto M, Bassetto F, Caciagli P, Villalta D, Tozzoli R, Bizzaro N. Diagnostic accuracy of ELISA methods as an alternative screening test to indirect immunofluorescence for the detection of antinuclear antibodies. Evaluation of five commercial kits. *Autoimmunity.* **2004.** 37:171–176.

22 Russell AS, Johnston C. Relative value of commercial kits for ANA testing. *Clin Exp Rheumatol.* **2003.** 21:477–480.

23 Wold RT, Young FE, Tan EM, Farr RS. Deoxyribonucleic acid antibody: a method to detect its primary interaction with deoxyribonucleic acid. *Science.* **1968.** 161:806–807.

24 Rubin RL, Joslin FG, Tan EM. An improved ELISA for anti-native DNA by elimination of interference by anti-histone antibodies. *J Immunol Methods.* **1983.** 63:359–366.

25 Aarden LA, deGroot ER, Feltkamp TEW. Immunology of DNA. III. Crithidia luciliae, a simple substrate for the determination of anti-dsDNA with the immunofluorescence technique. *Ann NY Acad Sci.* **1975.** 254:505–515.

26 Werle E, Blazek M, Fiehn W. The clinical significance of measuring different anti-dsDNA antibodies by using the Farr assay, an enzyme immunoassay and a Crithidia luciliae immunofluorescence test. *Lupus.* **1992.** 1:369–377.

27 Tipping PG, Buchanan RC, Riglar AG, Dimech WJ, Littlejohn GO, Holdsworth SR. Measurement of anti-DNA antibodies by ELISA: a comparative study with Crithidia and a Farr assay. *Pathology.* **1991.** 23:21–24.

28 Hylkema MN, van Bruggen MC, ten Hove T, de Jong J, Swaak AJ, Berden JH, Smeenk RJ. Histone-containing immune complexes are to a large extent responsible for anti-dsDNA reactivity in the Farr assay of active SLE patients. *J Autoimmun.* **2000.** 14:159–68.

29 Savige J, Davies D, Falk RJ, Jennette JC, Wiik A. Antineutrophil cytoplasmic antibodies and associated diseases: a review of the clinical and laboratory features. *Kidney Int.* **2000.** 57:846–862.

30 Franssen CF, Stegeman CA, Kallenberg CG, Gans RO, De Jong PE, Hoorntje SJ, Tervaert JW. Antiproteinase 3- and anti-myeloperoxidase associated vasculitis. *Kidney Int.* **2000.** 57:2195–2206.

31 Schonermarck U, Lamprecht P, Csernok E, Gross WL. Prevalence and spectrum of rheumatic diseases associated with proteinase 3-antineutrophil cytoplasmic antibodies (ANCA) and myeloperoxidase-ANCA. *Rheumatology* (Oxford). **2001.** 40:178–184.

32 Terjung B, Worman HJ, Herzog V, Sauerbruch T, Spengler U. Differentiation of antineutrophil nuclear antibodies in inflammatory bowel and autoimmune liver diseases from antineutrophil cytoplasmic antibodies (p-ANCA) using immunofluorescence microscopy. *Clin Exp Immunol.* **2001.** 126:37–46.

33 Van Meensel B, Hiele M, Hoffman I, Vermeire S, Rutgeerts P, Geboes K, Bossuyt X. Diagnostic accuracy of ten second-generation (human) tissue transglutaminase antibody assays in celiac disease. *Clin Chem.* **2004.** 50:2125–2135.

34 Rutz R, Ritzler E, Fierz W, Herzog D. Prevalence of asymptomatic celiac disease in adolescents of eastern Switzerland. *Swiss Med Wkly.* **2002** 132:43–47.

35 McPherson RA. Commentary: advances in the laboratory diagnosis of celiac disease. *J Clin Lab Anal.* **2001.** 15:105–107.

36 Waaler E. On the occurrence of a factor in human serum activating the specific agglutination of sheep blood corpuscles. *Acta Pathol Microbiol Scand.* **1940.** 17:172–178.

37 Tuffanelli DL, Wuepper KD, Bradford LL, Wood RM. Fluorescent treponemal-antibody adsorption tests: studies of false-positive reactions to tests for syphilis. *N Engl J Med.* **1967.** 276:258–262.

38 Hargraves MM, H Richmond and R Moreton. Presentation of two bone marrow elements: The "tart" cells and the "L.E." cell. *Mayo Clin Proc.* **1948.** 27:25–28.

39 Nielen MM, van Schaardenburg D, Reesink HW, van de Stadt RJ, van der Horst-Bruinsma IE, de Koning MH, Habibuw MR, Vandenbroucke JP, Dijkmans BA. Specific autoantibodies precede the symptoms of rheumatoid arthritis: a study of serial measurements in blood donors. *Arthritis Rheum.* **2004**. 50:380–386.

40 Wener MH: Rheumatoid Factors. Manual of Clinical Laboratory Immunology, sixth edition, **2002**. ASM Press, Washington, D.C. 961–972.

41 Schellekens GA, Visser H, de Jong BA, van den Hoogen FH, Hazes JM, Breedveld FC, van Venrooij WJ. The diagnostic properties of rheumatoid arthritis antibodies recognizing a cyclic citrullinated peptide. *Arthritis Rheum.* **2000**. 43:155–163.

42 Vallbracht I, Rieber J, Oppermann M, Forger F, Siebert U, Helmke K. Diagnostic and clinical value of anti-cyclic citrullinated peptide antibodies compared with rheumatoid factor isotypes in rheumatoid arthritis. *Ann Rheum Dis.* **2004**. 63:1079–1084.

43 Hochberg MC. Updating the American College of Rheumatology revised criteria for the classification of systemic lupus erythematosus. *Arthritis Rheum.* **1997**. 40:1725.

44 Koike T, Sueishi M, Funaki H, Tomioka H, Yoshida S. Anti-phospholipid antibodies and biological false positive serological test for syphilis in patients with systemic lupus erythematosus. *Clin Exp Immunol.* **1984**. 56:193–199.

45 McNeil HP, Simpson RJ, Chesterman CN, Krilis SA. Anti-phospholipid antibodies are directed against a complex antigen that includes a lipid-binding inhibitor of coagulation: β_2-glycoprotein I (apolipoprotein H). *Proc Natl Acad Sci USA.* **1990**. 87:4120–4124.

46 Galli M, Comfurius P, Maassen C, Hemker HC, De Baets MH, Van Breda-Vriesman PJC, Barbui T, Zwaal RFA, Bevers EM. Anticardiolipin antibodies (ACA) directed not to cardiolipin but to a plasma protein cofactor. *Lancet.* **1990**. 335:1544–1547.

47 Urbanus RT, de Laat HB, de Groot PG, Derksen RH. Prolonged bleeding time and lupus anticoagulant: a second paradox in theantiphospholipid syndrome. *Arthritis Rheum.* **2004** Nov;50(11):3605–3609.

48 Holman R and HR Deicher. The reaction of the lupus erythematosus (L.E.) cell factor with deoxyribonucleoprotein of the cell nucleus. *J Clin Invest* **1959**. 38:2059–2072.

49 Lachman PJ: An attempt to characterize the lupus erythematosus cell antigen. *Immunology.* **1961**. 4:153–163.

50 Schett G, Rubin RL, Steiner G, Hiesberger H, Muller S, Smolen J. The lupus erythematosus cell phenomenon: comparative analysis of antichromatin antibody specificity in lupus erythematosus cell-positive and -negative sera. *Arthritis Rheum.* **2000**. 43:420–428.

51 Burlingame RW. The clinical utility of antihistone antibodies. Autoantibodies reactive with chromatin in systemic lupus erythematosus and drug-induced lupus. *Clin Lab Med* **1997**; 17:367–377.

52 Burlingame RW. Recent advances in understanding the clinical utility and underlying cause of antinucleosome (antichromatin) autoantibodies. *Clin Appl Immun Rev.* **2004**. 4:351–366.

53 Tan EM. Antinuclear Antibodies: Diagnostic Markers for Autoimmune Diseases and Probes for Cell Biology. *Advances in Immunology* **1989**. 44:95–151.

54 Rosa MD, Hendrick Jr JP, Lerner MR, Steitz JA, and Reichlin M. A mammalian tRNA His-containing antigen is recognized by the polymyositis-specific antibody anti-Jo-1. *Nucleic Acids Re.* **1983**. 11:853–870.

55 Burlingame RW, Boey ML, Starkebaum G, Rubin RL. The central role of chromatin in autoimmune responses to histones and DNA in systemic lupus erythematosus. *J Clin Invest* **1994**. 94:184–192.

56 Burlingame RW and Rubin RL. Drug-induced anti-histone autoantibodies display two patterns of reactivity with substructures of chromatin. *J Clin Invest* **1991**. 88:680–690.

57 Murakami A, Kojima K, Ohya K, Imamura K, Takasaki Y. A new conformational epitope generated by the binding of recombinant 70-kdprotein and U1 RNA to anti-U1 RNP autoantibodies in sera from patients with mixed connective tissue disease. *Arthritis Rheum*. **2002**. 46:3273–3282.

58 Doire G, Lopez-Longo FJ, Lapointe S, Menard HA. Sera from patients with autoimmune disease recognize conformational determinants on the 60-kd Ro/SS-A protein. *Arthritis Rheum*. **1991**. 34:722–730.

59 Elkon K, Skelly S, Parnassa A, Moller W, Danho W, Weissbach H, Brot N. Identification and chemical synthesis of a ribosomal protein antigenic determinant in systemic lupus erythematosus. *Proc Natl Acad Sci U S A*. **1986**. 83:7419–7423.

60 Itoh Y, Reichlin M. Autoantibodies to the Ro/SSA antigen are conformation dependent. I: Anti-60 kD antibodies are mainly directed to the native protein; anti-52 kD antibodies are mainly directed to the denatured protein. *Autoimmunity*. **1992**. 14:57–65.

61 National Committee for Clinical Laboratory Standards. How to Define and Determine Reference Intervals in the Clinical Laboratory: Approved Guideline. **1995**. NCCLS Document C28-A, Vol 15, No. 4. 771 East Lancaster Avenue, Villanova, PA 19085.

62 Ghiradello A, Doria A, Zampieri S, Tarricone E, Tozzoli R, Villata D, Bizzaro N, Piccoli A, Gambari PF, Antinucleosome antibodies in SLE: a two-year follow-up study of 101 patients, *J Autoimmun* **2004**. 22:235–240.

63 Hueber W, Utz PJ, Steinman L, Robinson WH. Autoantibody profiling for the study and treatment of autoimmune disease. *Arthritis Res* **2002**. 4:290–295.

64 Pottel H, Wiik A, Locht H, Gordon T, Roberts-Thomson P, Abraham D, Goossens K, Dobbels C, De Bosschere K, Hulstaert F, Meheus L. Clinical optimization and multicenter validation of antigenspecific cut-off values on the INNO-LIA ANA update for the detection of autoantibodies in connective tissue disorders. *Clin Exp Rheumatol*. **2004**. 22:579–588.

65 Graham KL, Robinson WH, Steinman L, Utz PJ. High-throughput methods for measuring autoantibodies in systemic lupus erythematosus and other autoimmune diseases. *Autoimmunity*. **2004**. 37:269–272.

66 Robinson WH, DiGennaro C, Hueber W, Haab BB, Kamachi M, Dean EJ, Fournel S, Fong D, Genovese MC, de Vegvar HE, Skriner K, Hirschberg DL, Morris RI, Muller S, Pruijn GJ, van Venrooij WJ, Smolen JS, Brown PO, Steinman L, Utz PJ. Autoantigen microarrays for multiplex characterization of autoantibody responses. *Nat Med*. **2002**. 8:295–301.

67 Martins TB, Burlingame R, von Muhlen CA, Jaskowski TD, Litwin CM, Hill HR. Evaluation of multiplexed fluorescent microsphere immunoassay for detection of autoantibodies to nuclear antigens. *Clin Diagn Lab Immunol*. **2004**. 11:1054–1059.

68 Griffin C, Sutor J, Shull B. Microparticle Reagent Optimization. **1994**. Serydyn, Inc. Part No. 0347835. Indianapolis, Indiana.

69 Pickering JW, Martins TB, Greer RW, Schroder MC, Astill ME, Litwin CM, Hildreth SW, Hill HR. A multiplexed fluorescent microsphere immunoassay for antibodies to pneumococcal capsular polysaccharides. *Am J Clin Pathol*. **2002**. 117:589–596.

70 Comtesse N, Heckel D, Maldener E, Glass B, Meese E. Probing the human natural autoantibody repertoire using an immunoscreening approach. *Clin Exp Immunol*. **2000**. 121:430–436.

71 Granito A, Muratori P, Cassani F, Pappas G, Muratori L, Agostinelli D, Veronesi L, Bortolotti R, Petrolini N, Bianchi FB, Volta U. Anti-actin IgA antibodies in severe coeliac disease. *Clin Exp Immunol*. **2004**. 137:386–392.

72 Arnett FC, Reveille JD, Goldstein R, Pollard KM, Leaird K, Smith EA, Leroy EC, Fritzler MJ. Autoantibodies to fibrillarin in systemic sclerosis (scleroderma). An immunogenetic, serologic and clinical analysis. *Arthritis Rheum*. **1996**. 39:1151–1160.

73 Terjung B, Worman HJ, Herzog V, Sauerbruch T, Spengler U. Differentiation of antineutrophil nuclear antibodies in inflammatory bowel and autoimmune liver diseases from antineutrophil cytoplasmic antibodies (p-ANCA) using immunofluorescence microscopy. *Clin Exp Immunol.* **2001**. 126:37–46.

74 *http://www.accessdata.fda.gov/scripts/cdrh/cfdocs/cfPMN/pmn.cfm?ID=14120,* see "Decision Summary".

75 *http://www.accessdata.fda.gov/scripts/cdrh/cfdocs/cfPMN/pmn.cfm?ID=14419,* see "Decision summary".

76 El Hachmi M, Jadoul M, Lefebvre C, Depresseux G, Houssiau FA. Relapses of lupus nephritis: incidence, risk factors, serology and impact on outcome. *Lupus.* **2003**. 12:692–696.

77 Buyon JP, Ben-Chetrit E, Karp S, Roubey RA, Pompeo L, Reeves WH, Tan EM, Winchester R. Acquired congenital heart block. Pattern of maternal antibody response to biochemically defined antigens of the SS-A/Ro–SS-B/La system in neonatal lupus. *J Clin Invest.* **1989**. 84:627–634.

9

Synthetic Peptides for the Analysis of B-cell Epitopes in Autoantigens *

Jean-Paul Briand and Sylviane Muller

9.1
Introduction

While it is well known that serologic markers are only an aid to diagnosis, they are regarded with great interest for monitoring or predicting the evolution of autoimmune diseases. Validated biomarkers and surrogate markers are sorely needed for evaluating the risk of developing an autoimmune disease in predisposed patients or for identifying the onset of overlapping syndromes that often complicate long-term follow-up of patients. Such markers are also critical for research based on clinical trials [1]. Proteins recognized by circulating antibodies from patients with autoimmune diseases have been intensively studied over the two decades since cDNA-encoding autoantigens have become available. Analysis of sera from auto-immune patients with recombinant fragments of different lengths and with short overlapping peptides in immunoprecipitation assays or in solid-phase assays, such as enzyme-linked immunosorbent assays (ELISA) and Western immunoblotting, has revealed the presence of dominant B-cell epitopes, recognized by most if not all sera, and minor epitopes, recognized by only a fraction of the sera tested. Detailed studies of large series of patient's sera collected longitudinally have demonstrated that some of these epitopes are targeted by antibodies from patients with specific diseases or disease subsets, while others are not specific to a single disease but the corresponding peptides can advantageously replace the natural protein, which is often difficult to extract and purify.

Innovative technologies, such as peptide arrays and biosensors, as well as the exploitation of large peptide libraries have recently opened up new perspectives. Completely novel strategies for high-throughput screening have emerged and new reactivities have been characterized from arrays constructed with hundreds of proteins and peptides. Peptides bearing natural or non-natural modifications, as well as peptide mimics of protein or non-protein antigens (DNA, RNA, carbohydrates), have been designed and might replace native antigens in routine

---

* A list of abbreviations used is located at the end of this chapter.

Autoantibodies and Autoimmunity: Molecular Mechanisms in Health and Disease. Edited by K. Michael Pollard
Copyright © 2006 WILEY-VCH Verlag GmbH & Co. KGaA, Weinheim
ISBN: 3-527-31141-6

immunoassays. Although numerous conformational epitopes have not yet been characterized and cannot be identified by the approaches classically used in epitope-mapping studies, peptides and peptide analogues may represent valuable probes for establishing specific and sensitive early diagnostic tests. They may also lead to the design of high-affinity ligands for purifying autoantibodies and for the development of tolerogenic peptidomimetics relevant to immunointervention. These different past and recent advances will be reviewed followed by examples of epitope-mapping studies with peptides and recombinant fragments (when available) from a set of selected autoantigens.

9.2
Autoantibodies as Diagnostic Markers

Some of the antibodies produced by patients with systemic (non-organ-specific) or organ-specific autoimmune diseases are clinically useful for diagnosis, since their appearance is restricted to certain diseases or disease subtypes. These include antibodies to double-stranded (ds)DNA, Sm antigen, and ribosomal P proteins in systemic lupus erythematosus (SLE); DNA-topoisomerase I in systemic sclerosis (SSc); citrullinated-modified proteins in rheumatoid arthritis (RA); tRNA synthetase in myositis; glutamic acid decarboxylase and the protein tyrosine phosphatase–like molecule (known as IA-2) in insulin-dependent diabetes mellitus (IDDM); thyroid peroxidase and thyroglobulin in autoimmune thyroiditis; and the E2 component of pyruvate dehydrogenase (PDC-E2) in primary biliary cirrhosis (PBC) [2–8]. While many antibodies are highly specific to a particular disease, the usefulness of some of them as diagnostic markers is relatively poor due to their low prevalence. For example, this is the case for anti-Sm antibodies, which are a good marker for SLE but are found in only 5% (in Europe) to 20% (in North America) of lupus patients. On the other hand, the levels of some antibodies remain relatively constant in the serum of patients during the course of a disease, while other antibodies have fluctuating levels, depending on the phase, active or quiescent, of the disease. In the latter case, monitoring particular serum antibody subsets may be useful for prognosis. It is worth noting that the presence of particular antibody subsets in the serum of healthy individuals seems to predict the subsequent development of autoimmune diseases [6, 7]. This observation obviously complicates the setup and interpretation of assays since the serum of any "healthy" individual used to determine the threshold for positivity for each test may happen to be unexpectedly positive.

Before we describe in more detail the methodologies used to characterize serum autoantibodies with peptides and give some results that are relevant for a better definition of autoantibody specificity, it is important to highlight some basic concepts that are fundamental for a proper interpretation of data. As pointed out by Kavanaugh in his editorial [9], "improper use of (laboratory) tests may result in misdiagnosis, needless additional testing, and inappropriate therapy." As is the case with other laboratory tests, it is important to be aware of possible pitfalls of each peptide-based assay, to include the appropriate positive and negative controls, and to know the limitations of interpretation (sensitivity, intra-test variability, specificity) of each test. At the peptide level, improper synthesis or the use of peptides of low quality can dramatically affect the data and lead to false conclusions. In addition to summarizing well-established results, the object of this chapter is also to lay emphasis on the weak links of peptide-based diagnostic assays and to propose some solutions for the standardization of such tests. We will first set out two domains of peptide chemistry that have been intensively developed and have resulted in expansion of peptide-based-immuno-chemistry — namely, multiple peptide synthesis and multiple peptide presentation.

9.3
Synthetic Peptides

The phenomenal range of current applications of synthetic peptides is the consequence of the development of the chemistry of peptide synthesis over the last 50 years. It was in 1954 that Du Vigneaud and colleagues [10] accomplished the synthesis of oxytocin and in 1963 that the first chemical synthesis of human insulin was achieved by the team of Meienhoffer. These two hormones were produced by applying the classical methods of synthesis in solution, which require purification and characterization of intermediate peptides at every step. This approach generally requires many months of efforts and is the prerogative of experienced organic chemists.

The introduction in 1963 of the concept of solid-phase peptide synthesis (SPPS) by Merrifield considerably modified the existing state of the art [11]. This methodology revolutionized the synthesis of peptides and allowed the rapid production of synthetic antigens, biologically active peptides, artificial proteins, active enzymes, and peptide libraries.

In this approach, an *N-a-tert*-butyloxycarbonyl (Boc) amino acid is covalently linked to a solid support. The Boc group is removed by trifluoroacetic acid (TFA) and a second Boc amino acid is coupled to the free amino terminus of the resin-bound amino acid. Since most of the side products of reaction and degradation are dissolved in the reaction mixture, all of the intermediate steps of purification, which are necessary for synthesis in solution, are reduced to simple washings. At the final step of the procedure, the peptide is cleaved from the resin by a strong acid, usually hydrogen fluoride (HF). The advantages of SPPS are to be found in its speed, the relative ease of its implementation, and the fact that it is a method that can be completely automated. At present, the maximal amount of peptide synthesized on solid phase can vary from grams to kilograms, but quite often a few milligrams are amply sufficient to meet the needs of immunologists.

In essence, the central protocol detailed by Merrifield in his original paper has changed very little. However, the development of combinations of amino acid–protecting groups has been continuously refined to allow the selective regeneration of the α amino function in the presence of side chain–protecting groups and to achieve complete deprotection of the final peptide with clean removal from the inert support.

In particular, a very successful and extensively explored "orthogonal" SPPS approach using the base labile 9-fluorenylmethyl-oxycarbonyl (Fmoc) group has been developed since 1978 [12, 13]. This method of synthesis uses the Fmoc group for protecting the α-NH$_2$ function [14] and the *tert*-butyl group for protecting the side chain functionalities of the amino acids. This combination avoids both repeated acid treatments and the use of HF inherent in the Boc/benzyl procedure. The approach is called "orthogonal" because Fmoc is cleaved by a base (usually piperidine) and the peptide is cleaved from the resin by an acid (TFA). The use of TFA for the final cleavage of the peptide from the resin requires an ester linkage that is relatively labile to acids. This requirement has led to the introduction of handles (or linkers) between the C-terminal amino acid and the resin. Handles are generally defined as bifunctional spacers that attach the initial residue to the polymeric support in two steps. These handles are all designed so that the final release of the peptide chain from the support can be carried out without the use of strong acids or bases to provide the C-terminal residue as a free acid (-COOH), carboxamide (-CONH$_2$), peptide hydrazine, or one of a number of less common carboxyl derivatives. The handle approach is appropriate for a wide range of parent supports. Overall, such advances in the Fmoc procedure have contributed to a wide acceptance of this synthesis method throughout the international scientific community.

This part of the present review is meant not as a review of all of the possibilities that exist in the field of solid-phase peptide chemistry, but rather to provide specific information to the reader who is seeking an introduction to multiple peptide synthesis and multiple peptide presentation for immunological applications. It is also meant to warn immunologists against the pitfalls created by the use of poor-quality peptides.

9.3.1
Multiple Peptide Synthesis on Classical Resin Supports

The increasing use of peptides for immunological research and the steady discovery of new natural peptides endowed with biological activity have led over the last 20 years to the development of new methods and new devices for the preparation of individual peptides in large numbers.

9.3.1.1 Resin Supports
To be suitable for use in peptide synthesis, the solid support must meet a number of well-defined criteria. Since the synthesis of peptides takes place within swollen beads, the polymeric support must demonstrate physical and chemical stability when subjected to the various steps of synthesis and allow solvents and

reagents to diffuse readily to the peptide chain, during both synthesis itself and cleavage of the peptide from the resin.

Fmoc SPPS can be carried out as either a batch or a continuous flow process. In the former technique, the peptide resin is contained in a reaction vessel and the reagents are added and removed manually or by using a fully automated device. In the continuous flow method, the resin is contained in a column through which reagents and solvents are pumped continuously. Equipments necessary for this type of continuous flow synthesis are commercially available and have been adapted in some cases to automated multiple peptide synthesis.

Polystyrene Resin The beaded polystyrene resin introduced by Merrifield is still commonly used, and this support is well adapted to batch SPPS using either Boc or Fmoc amino acids. The first support successfully used by Merrifield [11] was a copolymer of polystyrene cross-linked with 2% divinylbenzene. In 1971, Gutte and Merrifield recommended polystyrene cross-linked with 1% divinylbenzene as the support of choice for the large majority of applications. Beads of polymer are swollen in an organic solvent and molecular events take place within the swollen resin matrix in the same manner as they do in a homogeneous solution ([15] and references therein). All of the reactive sites on the polymer network are fully and equally accessible in less than 10^{-6} s. The peptide-resin beads thus have to be kept highly swollen throughout the synthesis. Based on these characteristics, robots have been successfully developed for multiple peptide synthesis, using simple diffusion of solvents and reagents during all the steps of peptide assembly.

Polyethylene Glycol-Polystyrene Graft Supports Polyethylene glycol-polystyrene graft supports, such as Tentagel (PEG-PS/POE-PS), are another range of widely used solid supports that are suitable for both continuous flow and batch synthesis in Fmoc SPPS. Their architecture is based on a cross-linked polystyrene backbone grafted with polyethylene glycol (PEG) or polyoxyethylene (POE) [16, 17]. Due to the spacer effect of polyoxyethylene, the reactive sites located at the end of the spacers are totally separated from the cross-linked backbone and are totally solvated. In continuous flow, chemical efficiency is improved by the physical stability and compression strength of the graft supports, which allow for ultrahigh-speed continuous flow synthesis. Based on the same principle, a flow-stable polyethylene glycol dimethyl acrylamide (PEGA) support has been synthesized by Meldal [18]. PEG resins are also widely used for the synthesis of resin-bound peptide libraries.

PEG-based resins have interesting immunological applications: the peptide may be synthesized in a usual way attached to the resin via a stable amide bond. A one-step side-chain deprotection using TFA yields a polyoxyethylene-linked peptide epitope conjugate [19] that can be used as an antigen and an immunogen.

9.3.1.2 Devices

Semiautomated Simultaneous Multiple Peptide Synthesis   The first approach involving semiautomated simultaneous multiple peptide synthesis was developed by Houghten and was called the "Tea-bag method" [20]. In this system, the individual resins for simultaneous peptide synthesis are contained in separated solvent-permeable polypropylene bags enabling optimal applications of the many identical repetitive steps involved in SPPS. Peptides can be assembled using either a Boc-based process and cleavage in a multiple vessel HF apparatus [20] or a Fmoc-based process [21]. The Tea-bag method is said to allow one person to synthesize 120 different 15-residue peptides in two to four weeks in amounts of 10–1000 mg each. However, this method is designed for manual operation and involves numerous sorting steps that must be carried out with the greatest care.

Machine-based Multiple Peptide Synthesis   To eliminate any errors during synthesis, some fully automated simultaneous multi-channel synthesizers have been developed (see, e.g., [22]). Using such synthesizers, it is possible to assemble eight to 12 different peptides in parallel, which allows the chemist to prepare about 40 peptides of 15–20 residues in amounts of tens of milligrams per week, thus easily meeting the needs of a research laboratory.

A series of laboratory robots have also been adapted to Fmoc multiple peptide synthesis of a large number of peptides in milligram quantities [23–25]. The synthesis is carried out in a rack of 48 to 96 test tubes with reagents supplied by one arm of the robot, while all of the washing procedures are handled by the other arm. This method satisfies most of the criteria for successful multiple synthesis and it is automatic. However, the operation of a conventional laboratory robot is time-consuming and serial in nature. On some models, active vortex mixing ensures production of peptides at a quality comparable to that obtained with classical monosynthesizers.

Manually operated devices for parallel multiple column SPPS in continuous flow version have also been proposed [26]. A fully automatic, online-monitored, multiple-column synthesizer was later developed by the Meldal's team.

9.3.2
Multiple Peptide Synthesis on Specific Matrices

In spite of the rapidity and efficiency of classical SPPS, the amount of work required for synthesizing the hundreds and thousands of different peptide analogues needed for epitope mapping and for screening immunological and biological activities of proteins has quickly become prohibitive. For many preliminary studies, only a small amount (less than 1 mg) of each peptide is required. As a result, considerable effort has been made to develop supports and techniques for multiple peptide synthesis. Incidentally, it can be mentioned that polystyrene-grafted polyethylene film matrices [27] and cotton fabric [28] have been used in an novel manner for multiple peptide synthesis, but this section will focus on two supports that are easily available to a research laboratory and widely used by the scientific community: polyethylene supports and cellulose paper.

9.3.2.1 Polyethylene Supports for the Multi-pin Synthesis Technology

The multi-pin peptide synthesis procedure was originally developed for epitope mapping using ELISA [29]. It is referred to as PEPscan, a term widely used by immunochemists (see Section 9.4.2). Using a Boc procedure, peptide synthesis was performed on polyethylene rods, also known as "pins," that had been previously immersed in a solution of acrylic acid and γ-irradiated, producing about 50–100 nmol peptide per pin. Using this technique, it was not possible to cleave the synthesized peptides from the support. Later, the introduction of the Fmoc procedure and cleavable linkers made it possible to obtain peptides in solution. Since then, the scope of the multi-pin method has been extended by changing the pin shape to a two-piece format consisting of a support stem and a detachable crown. In addition, higher levels of polymer grafted to the crowns have been achieved. Grafting of 2-hydroxy-ethyl-methacrylate (HEMA) to polyethylene crowns proved to be the most reproducible procedure and yielded surfaces well suited to peptide synthesis. Radiation grafting of HEMA to the polyethylene crowns generated a hydroxylated polymer, and it was therefore possible to attach suitably protected amino acids or handles, as in the case of classical solid supports. Loading in the range of 1–2 μmol per crown was then achieved [30]. Larger pin formats and new graft polymers have since allowed further improvements of this technology, which is now an alternative to beaded cross-linked resins and allows handling large numbers of peptides in multiple parallel synthesis ([31] and references therein).

9.3.2.2 Cellulose Paper for SPOT Synthesis

Simultaneous syntheses at distinct positions on a membrane support were introduced by Frank in the late 1980s [32]. This allowed a PEPscan-like approach to be designed with parallel synthesis of large numbers (thousands) of peptides on distinct areas of one sheet of paper. Cellulose paper has excellent resistance to most organic solvents, and Fmoc SPPS is perfectly compatible with the cellulose support. The concept of SPOT synthesis is suitable for both manual and automated operations using robots. The SPOT method provides simple, economical, and rapid access to large numbers of short peptide sequences at the nanomolar scale for biological screening purposes. The scale of synthesis can be easily increased to the range of μmol/spot using a thicker paper such as Whatman 3MM. As in the case of classical resins, the paper sheet needs to be chemically derivatized to introduce suitable anchors for the synthesis of immobilized or dissolved peptides. Overlapping peptides spanning an entire protein sequence can be synthesized to localize epitopes (SPOTscan method). Each peptide can be further analyzed to determine the contribution of each individual amino acid residue (see Section 9.4.3).

Alternatively, as many as 100 discs can be tightly stacked in column reactors or sealed in "Tea-bags" and then allowed to react simultaneously with the same amino acid derivative in each column or "Tea-bag" [33, 34]. For example, using 146 "Tea-bags," Van't Hof and coworkers synthesized 146×100 peptides on paper discs and were able to test 100 antisera with 146 different peptides in a reasonable time [35].

At the same time, Laursen and coworkers [36] developed a method for the simultaneous synthesis of peptides as spots on a derivatized polypropylene membrane. This method presents some similarities with the multi-spot method of Frank but uses a membrane that is not commercially available.

SPOT synthesis is simple, easily accessible, and, unlike polypropylene pin methods, very economical in terms of solvents and reagents. However, the quality control of the synthesized peptides is not easy to manage and the size of the peptides is limited.

9.3.3
The Quality of Peptides

It has long been assumed that immunologists/immunochemists need only crude or partially purified peptides. As crude or improperly purified peptides generally rapidly degrade, even if they are kept freeze-dried at 2–6 °C, this belief has certainly caused the publication of many results that could not be reproduced in the same laboratory or by other research teams. Moreover, there have been several examples of unexpected immune responses to contaminants and altered peptides formed during a synthesis ([37] and references therein). In fact, despite all the refinements brought to peptide chemistry, side reactions still occur during synthesis and cleavage of the peptides, and these have to be taken into account.

For example, problems associated with incomplete couplings and deprotection have not been totally solved. Problem-causing, or "difficult," sequences are characterized by reproducible stretches or repetitive incomplete aminoacylations and/or incomplete deprotection. They are caused by the tendency of the peptide chain to form hydrogen-bonded aggregates either with other peptide chains or with the polymeric support [15]. Few authors have proposed approaches for predicting difficult sequences ([38] and references therein), and they all point to intermolecular aggregation caused by β-sheet hydrogen bonding as the major source of difficulties in peptide coupling. This effect of aggregation is easily visible in batch synthesis, where resin swelling is reduced, and in continuous flow synthesis, where a broadening of the deprotection peak is observed. The net result of incomplete peptide-bond formation is that the peptide chains formed are closely related to the target peptide but are missing one or more amino acid residues.

These difficult sequences generally occur at 5–15 residues from the resin. There is a general relationship between the side chain structure of a peptide and its tendency for aggregation: Ala, Val, Ile, unprotected Asn, and Gln are effective in promoting association, while trityl (Trt) protection of Gln and small hydrophilic groups, such as acetamido methyl (Acm), reverse the aggregation effect. Amino acid residues such as Pro and Ser are virtually never found within difficult sequences, presumably because these residues impose a turn in the peptide chain. The loading of the resin also has a significant effect. High loading can exaggerate the phenomenon, but the nature of the solid support apparently has no major effect on aggregation.

With the Boc procedure, the problem of difficult sequences does not seem to be related to incomplete removal of the Boc group, but rather to incomplete acylation. With the Fmoc procedure, a slow acylation is generally linked to an incomplete or slow Fmoc deprotection of the preceding amino acid. On sophisticated machines with feedback control, the problem is in part solved by using repeated deprotection and increased time in the following acylation step. Several sophisticated approaches have been used for breaking the peptide conformation on the solid support and promoting a coupling reaction. They include the use of dimethyl sulfoxide/N-methylpyrrolidinone (NMP) mixtures, NMP/dimethyl formamide mixtures containing 1% Triton, chaotropic salts in organic solvents, and higher temperatures. However, the most novel solution used to solve the aggregation problem has been reported by Sheppard and coworkers [39]. These authors have proposed introducing reversibly N-substituted amino acids into the peptide chain for preventing the formation of intermolecular hydrogen bonds. Only occasional residues need to be substituted in order to inhibit interchain association during an entire synthesis. The pseudoproline-protected dipeptide building blocks developed by Mutter and coworkers [40] act similarly by preventing inter- and intramolecular hydrogen bonding, a limitation of this approach being that serine or threonine must be present in the sequence.

Besides problems related to difficult sequences, other undesired reactions and racemization of amino acids may occur during peptide assembly. For example, in the Boc procedure, the formation of aspartimide and its opening via addition of bases has long been observed [41]. In the Fmoc procedure, unexpectedly high aspartimide and piperidide formation has been detected in crude products when, in the peptide sequence, Asp (OtBu) is followed by Asn, Gln (trityl-protected or not), Gly, Arg (2,2,5,7,8-pentamethylchroman-6-sulfonyl, Pmc), Cys (Acm), Cys (Trt), Ser, and Thr [42].

It is important to realize that each peptide behaves individually, not only during peptide assembly but also during the purification process. Mainly hydrophilicity, but also the size and conformation that characterize each peptide, governs its solubility in a given solvent and its retention time measured by high-performance liquid chromatography (HPLC). This makes it almost impossible to automate purification processes. As a consequence, purification and analysis (mass spectrometry and/or amino acid analysis) constitute the main bottlenecks of the multiple synthesis approach.

Last but not least, since at the end of the purification procedure peptides are present as salts (e.g., trifluoroacetates when the last purification step has been performed in solvents containing 0.1% TFA), lyophilized peptides inevitably contain counterions and residual water. Therefore, even if a peptide is said to be 95% pure, the net amount of peptide (the so-called net peptide content), which depends on its amino acid composition, may only account for 50–85% of the powder. Companies proposing peptides generally advertise whether they are selling peptides by net peptide weight. Obviously, this parameter is of the highest importance for quantitatively evaluating the reactivities of antibodies with a particular peptide.

In conclusion, immunologists/immunochemists have to be aware that each peptide must be considered as a unique reagent that should be handled with great care.

9.3.4
Branched Peptides or Peptide Dendrimers

Synthetic branched polypeptides were introduced by Hudecz and coworkers (see [43] for a review) in the early 1980s. They have emerged as a new class of artificial proteins with potential biomedical application, particularly in vaccine design and serodiagnosis. They were based on a poly[Lys-(DL-Ala3)] backbone. Since then, several variations of branched peptides have been developed, which differ only in the design of the core matrix (Fig. 9.1). Some can be produced by classical solid-phase synthesis methods, such as the multiple antigen peptide (MAP) system, whose core contains two or three levels of geometrically branched lysine residues [44]; the template-assembled synthetic protein (TASP), whose core template is made of linear or cyclic peptides with lysine side chains for peptide anchoring [45]; and, more recently, a sequential oligopeptide carrier (SOCn) formed by the repetitive [Lys-Aib-Gly] moiety [46]. Such branched peptides are also known as peptide dendrimers [47].

9.3.4.1 The MAP System
The MAP system (Fig. 9.1) is certainly the most popular type of peptide dendrimer and has been demonstrated to be a very efficient immunogen as well as a useful antigen for ELISA. The core matrix of lysine residues can be designed for anchoring multiple copies of the same peptide (monoepitope MAPs) or two different peptides (diepitope MAPs). In the case of monoepitope MAPs, the core matrix is built using Boc Lys (Boc) derivative in the Boc procedure or Fmoc Lys (Fmoc) derivative in the Fmoc procedure to reach the desired branched level. The diepitope core matrix is synthesized using the same strategy, but a Boc Lys (Fmoc) derivative is introduced at the last branching level, allowing the synthesis of two different peptide antigens on separate branches. One peptide sequence is synthesized using a Boc procedure and the other by a Fmoc procedure. Alternatively, introduction of Fmoc Lys (Dde) derivatives makes possible the synthesis of diepitope MAPs using a Fmoc procedure exclusively ([48] and references therein).

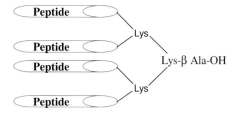

MAP system

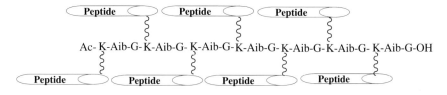

SOCn

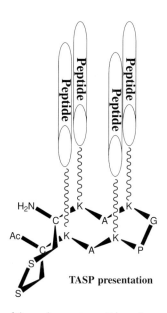

TASP presentation

Fig. 9.1 Schematic illustration of three oligomeric peptide systems.

9.3.4.2 The TASP Construct

Originally, the TASP construct (Fig. 9.1) was designed to enhance intramolecular folding of amphiphilic helices covalently attached to a template, but this type of construct has also been used to raise peptide antibodies that cross-react with the native protein. Molecular dynamics calculations suggest that the template folds as an anti-parallel β-sheet connected by a type II β-turn and cyclized via a disulfide bridge ([49] and references therein). The four attachment sites of the peptides (amino groups of Lys residues) are oriented on the same side of the template plane.

9.3.4.3 The SOCn Construct

Like the TASP construct, the SOCn (Fig. 9.1) has been designed with a predetermined three-dimensional structure that defines the spatial arrangement of the attached antigenic peptides. Nuclear magnetic resonance experiments and molecular dynamics suggest that the average structure of the template is a distorted 3_{10} helix. A detailed conformational study of SOCn conjugates indicated that antigenic peptides covalently linked to the template do not interact with each other or with the carrier [46], which is certainly not the case in the MAP system. On the other hand, it seems that antigenic peptides presented as SOCn conjugates retain the initial conformation of the free peptide, thus preserving their topological characteristics.

9.3.4.4 Synthesis of Dendrimers

As mentioned above, MAPs, TASPs, and SOCn can all be made by classical solid-phase synthesis by using appropriate Lys derivatives. However, these are high-molecular-weight macromolecules, often exceeding 15 kDa, which makes their synthesis by stepwise solid-phase methods and subsequent purification to high homogeneity challenging, even though impressive pieces of work have been published. To overcome this problem, a convenient modular strategy has been proposed by several authors [47, 49, 50] who developed chemoselective strategies for the preparation of branched peptides by ligating unprotected purified peptide segments to a purified core matrix. In this approach, maximal advantage is taken of the ability to synthesize, purify, and characterize separately the different compounds (template and peptides of interest). Then, the target dendrimer is produced directly in the final unprotected form.

9.4
Peptide-based Methods for Detection and Quantification of Autoantibodies

After problems associated with synthesis and purification of peptides have been discussed in the first part of this chapter, the next step is to find an appropriate assay to determine whether these synthetic peptides are recognized by autoantibodies present in the patient's sera. Solid-phase immunoassays such as ELISAs remain the most widely used technique for detection and quantification of autoantibodies using synthetic peptides. However, a new generation of tests providing for simultaneous screening of several hundred or even thousands of peptides using autoimmune sera has been recently introduced. These emerging methods allow investigators to considerably improve epitope-mapping studies by using, for example, overlapping peptides covering the total sequence of large proteins as well as peptides bearing post-translational modifications. The number and potential diversity of the peptides tested also provide for identification of valuable peptide mimics of non-protein autoantigens, such as carbohydrates or dsDNA. Identifying peptide mimotopes should not only improve detection of autoantibodies recognizing non-protein autoantigens but also allow characterization of conformational epitopes that, generally, cannot be identified by classical tests using a limited number of peptides corresponding to linear sequences in the cognate protein.

9.4.1
ELISA Using Synthetic Peptides

Several ELISA formats can be used with peptides to delineate linear and conformational epitopes of a protein [51–53]. In a classical approach, the capacity of a candidate peptide tested in the liquid-phase to inhibit the interaction between a protein adsorbed on the plastic surface of a microtiter plate and antibodies contained in the patient's serum is measured. Bound antibodies are subsequently revealed by adding a second antibody against human IgG and/or IgM conjugated to an enzyme, generally horseradish peroxidase, alkaline phosphatase, or -galactosidase. Finally, the absorbance of colored product is measured. It is important to understand that this type of immunoassay will select autoantibodies reacting with the solid-phase immobilized parent protein only, to the exclusion of any other antibody subsets, which may be important for diagnosis. Also, it is important to bear in mind that this approach reveals only the epitopes presented by the immobilized protein and mimicked by the peptide in solution.

Alternatively, an indirect assay can be set up, wherein peptides are directly adsorbed to the wells of a microtiter plate, serial dilutions of patients' sera are incubated in the peptide-coated wells, and bound antibodies are revealed by a second antibody against human Ig linked to a selected enzyme. For B-cell epitope mapping, a complete set of overlapping peptides covering the whole length of the protein is used. This strategy has been applied, for example, to histones [54–56]; 52-kD SSA/Ro protein (Ro52, [57]); D1 protein of Sm antigen (SmD1, [58–60]); A, C, and 70K proteins of the U1 small nuclear ribonucleoprotein (snRNP) antigen (U1A, U1C, U1-70K; [61–63]); hnRNP A2/B1 protein [64]; and human thyroprotein receptor [65]. This ELISA format presents numerous advantages insofar as it is simple, fast, and easily automatable, but it also has a number of conceptual limitations directly related to peptide adsorption to plastic. Direct adsorption of a peptide can affect its conformation and mask a portion of its surface. Furthermore, the efficacy of adsorption of a peptide can vary widely according to its length, charge, and solubility; the pH and composition of coating buffer; and the type of plastic of the microtiter plates (polyvinyl, polystyrene with or without plastic activation) (Fig. 9.2; Dali and Muller, unpublished). Based on our experience, peptides that comprise at least 15 residues are

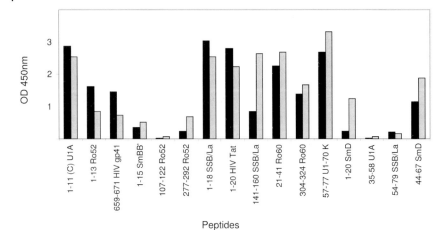

Fig. 9.2 Relative coating efficacy of various synthetic peptides on polystyrene microtiter plates. Biotinylated peptides of different lengths and charges were allowed to adsorb onto polystyrene microtiter plates (MaxiSorp, Nunc, Roskilde, Denmark) overnight at 37 °C. For coating the plates, peptides were suspended in 0.1 M carbonate buffer pH 9.6 at a concentration of 0.5 μM (black) and 2 μM (gray). Adsorption of biotinylated peptides was evaluated by incubating peptide-coated plates with streptavidin conjugated with peroxidase. The final reaction was visualized by adding 3,3',5,5' tetramethylbenzidine in the presence of H_2O_2. The peptides are arranged by length in the figure (the shortest are on the left and the longest are on the right) (Dali and Muller, unpublished data).

in general efficiently adsorbed to plastic after incubating the peptide solution in the wells overnight, at room temperature or 4 °C. However, even for experts, it remains difficult to predict whether a peptide will be a "good" or a "moderate" plastic binder, and when a careful internal calibration of the tests has not been performed, it is often impossible to compare quantitatively the various absorbance values measured with a panel of peptides.

To overcome such drawbacks, some authors (see, e.g., [66]) recommended the use of peptides conjugated to a carrier protein (bovine serum albumin, ovalbumin) to increase the coating efficiency and diminish the amount of peptide used per assay. Others proposed the use of multi-presentation systems such as MAPs, TASPs, and SOCn (see Sections 9.3.4 and 9.5) to avoid coupling the peptides with a carrier. When unconjugated peptides are used, their effective binding to the plate must be checked, e.g., by using anti-peptide antibodies or by incubating with enzyme-conjugated streptavidin when biotinylated peptides are used (Fig. 9.2). Likewise, when peptide conjugates are used as antigens, the yield of effective peptide coupling must be controlled and the stability of conjugates checked over time [67, 68]. Moreover, the choice of a conjugation procedure is crucial since the antigenic activity of a peptide can be dramatically affected by different coupling procedures [68, 69]. Consequently, the chemical agent used to conjugate the peptide with an appropriate carrier must be carefully chosen according to each specific sequence.

To ensure reliability of peptide-based ELISAs used to monitor autoimmune sera, several important points must be routinely checked:

- Unrelated peptides or, preferably, scrambled peptides containing the same amino acid residues in a different order compared to the parent sequence should always be tested in parallel as controls; because patients' sera can contain a diversity of autoantibodies whose range of specificities is not known with certainty, control peptides need to be selected with care.

- When conjugated peptides are used, it is necessary to verify the absence of reaction with the carrier or, preferably, with the carrier presenting the control peptide; false reactions have been found with patient's antibodies cross-reacting, for instance, with bovine serum albumin or ovalbumin.

- The absence of a reaction of enzyme-labeled second antibodies with peptides in the absence of antibodies must be verified.

- A large number of sera from normal donors must be tested in the same ELISA conditions to define the cutoff value for positivity for each peptide. It is known that certain classes of autoantibodies are surprisingly common in the normal population; for example, low levels of anti-SSA/Ro antibodies are present in 5–15% of the normal population [70].

- In isotyping studies, particular attention should be paid to the specificity of secondary enzyme-labeled antibodies with regard to their ability to reveal equally well all IgG subclasses, as certain minor subclasses can be increased in autoimmune situations, e.g., peptide-reacting antibodies of the IgG3 subclass in lupus mice [71], and are poorly detected with most commercial enzyme–labeled anti-IgG antibodies [72].

- Finally, it should be stressed that several factors can generate high ELISA background. False positivity may be due to aggregates present in sera from collections that have been stored for a long time, even in good conditions. Many laboratories routinely heat sera to 56 °C, which can cause major problems in nonspecific binding in ELISAs due to the presence of aggregates in sera. False positivity can also result from cross-reaction of antibodies with nonfat bovine milk or normal serum used as blocking agents to prevent nonspecific adsorption of proteins to wells. These added reagents can contain self-antigens such as DNA and histones [73]. Bovine IgG can contaminate bovine serum albumin [51]. Patients' sera can also contain circulating self-antigens. For example, the presence of nucleosomes and proteinase-3 (a neutrophil primary granule that is recognized by cytoplasmic anti-neutrophil cytoplasmic antibodies, cANCA) in the serum of normal and/or autoimmune patients has been demonstrated. Rheumatoid factors also can cause a high level of false positives. Finally, anti-albumin autoantibodies have been detected in the serum of autoimmune and infected patients [74, 75]. Many of these recommendations are also useful when other types of solid-phase immunoassays are utilized.

9.4.2
The PEPscan Technique

To perform a fast concurrent synthesis of peptides for epitope-mapping studies, Geysen et al. [29] introduced a method of linear peptide epitope scanning that can be used for the synthesis of hundreds of peptides on polyethylene pins and direct testing of their antigenic activity without removing them from the support (see Section 9.3.2.1). The initial method used radiation-grafted polyethylene pins arranged in an 8×12 matrix with the format and the spacing of a microtiter plate, which allowed the pin-attached peptides to be directly tested by ELISA [76]. Complete sets of overlapping peptides have been used to map various antigens with autoantibodies. For example, the complete sequence of Ro60 protein [77]; SSB/La protein [78]; SmD1 and BB′ proteins [79–82]; U1A, U1C, and U1-70K proteins [83–85]; proteinase-3 [86]; heat shock protein (Hsp) 60 in children with IDDM [87]; and human sperm protein Sp17 [88] were assayed in this manner.

In the period between 1984 and 1995, the method was greatly improved [89, 90]. Peptides were made on a similar solid support but were biotinylated and cleaved before recapture and testing. This additional cleavage step made it possible to analyze the purity and identity of the peptides, which could not be done with the earlier test format. Moreover, a spacer was introduced between the crown and the antigenic sequence to minimize steric interference between the simultaneous binding of the peptide to the capture molecule (avidin or streptavidin) and to the antibody. This method is also attractive because only small serum aliquots are required for each test. Replicates are possible, compatible with statistical analysis. Biotinylated peptides can also be used in modes other than direct binding, e.g., as competitors in a solution-phase antigen-antibody reaction or on tissue slices.

9.4.3
The SPOTscan Technique

Another method for systematically screening autoepitopes with short overlapping peptides is based on the SPOTsynthesis introduced by Frank (see Section 9.3.2.2). Detection of antibodies bound to peptides immobilized on paper can be achieved by conventional solid-phase ELISA or Western immunoblotting procedures. In general, highly sensitive chemiluminescent reagents are used. Membrane-bound peptides are reusable many times (>50) if the peptides are not irreversibly modified by the assay procedure and if bound antibodies have been completely removed [91]. Signal patterns can be documented and quantitatively evaluated utilizing the most recent image analysis tools. This method has been widely used for the mapping of autoantigens such as U1C [62]; SSB/La [92]; SmD1 [60]; the ribosomal phospho (P) proteins P0, P1, and P2 [93]; the Goodpasture antigen contained in human α3 chain of collagen IV [94]; proteinase-3 [95]; centromere-associated protein A (CENP-A) [96, 97]; the so-called PM/Scl-

100 antigen recognized by antibodies from patients with polymyositis-scleroderma overlap syndrome [98]; and early endosome antigen 1 (EEA1) [99]. We have shown in our laboratory that the results obtained with overlapping peptides covering U1C protein prepared using either the SPOTsynthesis method or conventional techniques leading to free peptides tested by indirect ELISA largely agreed [62].

9.4.4
Biosensors

Optical biosensors have been used for a large range of immunological applications. They can be used for quick measurements of biomolecular interactions in real time without requiring label reactants. Many review articles have analyzed the scope and limitations of optical biosensors [100, 101]. In the domain of autoepitope mapping with peptides, however, very few reports have been published. They concern, for example, the characterization of major epitopes recognized by cANCA in the proteinase-3 using the surface plasmon resonance BIAcore biosensor [102] and the test of monoclonal autoantibodies generated from lupus mice using nucleosomes, dsDNA, and peptide 83–100 of histone H3 [103]. Screening for epitope-specific autoantibodies using biotinylated peptides immobilized on streptavidin chips in the BIAcore system has also been used to detect autoantibodies against the β1-adrenergic receptor in sera of patients with idiopathic dilated cardiomyopathy [104] and the angiotensin II receptor 1 in patients with preeclampsia [105]. While positive responses were obtained in both cases, the low level of specific antibodies present in IgG fractions did not permit kinetic analysis. Thus, surface plasmon resonance had no obvious advantages for screening autoantibodies over more simple techniques such as ELISA. In the case of sera from patients with Chagas' disease, analysis for anti-receptor autoantibodies was made difficult by the presence of antibodies directed against polyanionic epitopes, resulting in a high background on the carboxylated dextran matrices used in the BIAcore system [106]. However, autoantibodies from the same patients were successfully used after purification by affinity chromatography to quantify the affinities of the various antibodies for epitopes on *T. cruzi* ribosomal proteins compared to those on human ribosomal proteins [107].

9.4.5
Autoantigen Microarray Technologies

In the past few years, miniaturized autoantigen-array technology has been developed to perform large-scale antibody screenings [108–115]. In this method, thousands of autoantigens (proteins and peptides) can be distributed onto 10-cm^2 microscope slides coated with poly-L-lysine. These "chips" maintain reactivity for months. The protein- and peptide-coated slides are incubated with diluted patients' sera and subsequently revealed with an anti-human Ig secondary antibody labeled with a fluorescent marker. For one slide presenting several hundred (up to ≈ 1000) different antigens, 0.2–2 μL of undiluted serum sample is required. It has been shown that results obtained with this method fit well with those obtained with ELISA, in particular when the sera from autoimmune patients were tested with peptides [116]. A large-scale array analysis including synthetic peptides has been applied to sera from mice with experimental autoimmune encephalomyelitis (EAE), a model of multiple sclerosis (MS) [117]. Similar strategies are currently used to screen sera from animal models and patients with SLE, IDDM, RA, and PBC [115].

There are a number of obvious advantages of miniaturized multiplexing methodology. First, many autoantigens and candidate autoantigens can be studied simultaneously, using small amounts of biological fluids such as serum, cerebrospinal fluid, synovial fluid, or antibodies eluted from diseased tissue such as kidney or brain plaques. Second, isotyping of autoantibodies that bind to individual antigens becomes possible, allowing an even finer analysis of the immune response. Third, deposition of antigens on slides allows one to study essentially any biomolecule, including lipids, carbohydrates, nucleic acids, protein complexes, polypeptides, truncation mutants, peptides, and post-translationally modified proteins and peptides. Finally, the sensitivity of such tests has been found to exceed that obtained by standard ELISAs, and with the introduction of newly developed detection methods (new fluorophores in particular), even higher sensitivities should be reached.

The major limitation of planar array-based autoantibody profiling is that many antigens do not adhere to the poly-L-lysine surface (particularly negatively charged proteins and peptides) and many proteins denature when the slides dry within minutes of spotting. Several technologies are being developed to overcome these limitations, including identification of novel surfaces for planar arrays and creation of liquid-phase assays (reviewed in [113, 114]).

9.4.6
Emerging Technologies for Biomarker Identification with Peptides

Novel nanomaterials have been developed, such as carbon nanotubes that can be functionalized with a large variety of components, including synthetic peptides [118, 119]. New specific biosensors based on this technology should soon be available for screening autoantibodies with peptides. Feasibility has been recently demonstrated with monoclonal antibodies and whole U1A snRNP autoantigen [120]. Furthermore, novel methods for detection are undergoing rapid development, including, for example, addressable laser bead assays based on microspheres embedded with laser reactive dyes coupled to peptides. Such an assay is commercially available for the testing of autoantibodies to ribosomal proteins P0, P1, and P2 present in the serum of patients with SLE [121]. In this test, beads are coated with a peptide called C22 located at the conserved C-terminus of the three proteins [122, 123] and routinely used in various homemade and other commercial immunoassays [93, 121, 124].

9.5
Multiple Peptide Presentation

The multi-presentation of a reactive peptide (e.g., as a MAP or SOCn; see Section 9.3.4) is often used to increase the sensitivity of tests. Multi-presentation of antigenic motifs on a scaffold considerably enhances the avidity of the interaction and improves the level of detection of autoantibodies. It may also be seen as a valuable alternative to assays using peptides that adsorb poorly onto plastic supports, such as the C22 peptide of ribosomal P proteins [125]. For example, MAPs have been used successfully with SmD1 C-terminal peptide [59], the ribosomal C22 peptide [121, 124, 126], and a peptide of the mitochondrial PDC-E2 antigen associated to lipoic acid [127]. Examples of constructions with SOCn include peptides of the La/SSB antigen, the motif PPGMRPP present in several RNP proteins, and peptides of the α-subunit of the Torpedo nicotinic acetylcholine receptor (AchR), a target of autoantibodies from patients with myasthenia gravis [46, 128–130].

Multi-presentation of autoantigenic peptides as MAPs and SOCn may thus have important applications in diagnostic assays. Actually, it is possible that, in the case of autoantigens, such constructions mimic the structure of self-antigens better than single peptide copies do. It has been observed that epitopes of self-antigens are often made of repeated sequences, either as a single molecule (typical examples include DNA or RNA, CENP-A, and histone H1 [131, 132]) or within macromolecular complexes. For example, autoantibodies react frequently with the well-studied PPPGMRPP motif present in several snRNPs (SmB/B', U1A, and U1C), with RG-rich regions present in SmD proteins, hnRNPA1, fibrillarin, and nucleolin, and with the RNA-binding motif called RNP1 present in U1-70K, U1A, hnRNPA2/B1, SSB/La, and SSA/Ro proteins [133–135]. This multi-presentation considerably enhances the avidity of the interaction and may be important pathologically, e.g., for the spreading of the autoimmune response during the course of the disease [136].

While some peptides seem to be highly antigenic when presented as MAPs or at the surface of pins or phages, in certain cases the respective monomeric sequences do not exhibit the same properties. As pointed out above, such findings may be linked to the sensitivity of assays based on multimeric constructions. They may also result from the fact that the conformation of peptides free in solution is quite different from that of the same sequence in the MAP construct or synthesized at the surface of pins or phages. In the case of a peptide anchored to SOCn, however, it has been demonstrated that the original structure of the free peptide seems to be preserved [46]. Furthermore, a multivalent binding of antibodies is possible with MAPs, pins, or phages. Thus, there are some limitations to keep in mind when multimeric presentations are used. These can include higher background in ELISA, possible false-positive reactions, and a lower solubility of constructions compared to monomeric peptides [137].

9.6
Peptides Containing Natural Modifications and Structural Motifs

It is well recognized today that synthetic peptides are valuable antigenic probes because they are chemically controlled and can be produced in large numbers and amounts at a moderate cost compared to peptides generated from purified or recombinant proteins. In addition, peptides offer the possibility of introducing during synthesis modified residues and cofactors that are normally present in natural molecules or added at specific stages of the cell cycle. This strategy is particularly attractive since several antigens targeted by autoantibodies contain such modified residues and cofactors, the presence of which is necessary for the antigen to be recognized by patients' antibodies. This is the case, for example, for PDC-E2 antigen (which contains lipoyl cofactors and is recognized by autoantibodies from patients with PBC); glycosylated p68 autoantigen, glycosylated collagen, and deiminated fibrin (which are closely associated with RA); phosphorylated components of RNA polymerase I and II and phosphorylated proteins of the serine/arginine family (which are associated with SLE); and SmD1/D3 proteins (associated with SLE) and myelin basic protein (MBP; associated with MS), which both contain symmetrical dimethyl arginine [138–146]. Studies describing the reactivity of patients' antibodies have been reported with ubiquitinated peptides [147], with peptides containing a lipoyl acid moiety [127, 148] or symmetrical dimethyl arginine [146], and with a cyclic peptide called CCP containing deiminated arginine (citrulline) residues. CCP-based kits are commercially available for detecting antibodies in RA [149–151]. Some of these modifications play a spectacular "all-or-nothing" role. For example, the synthetic C-terminal peptide 95–119 of SmD1 containing symmetrical dimethyl arginine was recognized by most of the anti-Sm patients' sera and by the monoclonal antibody Y12, whereas homologous peptides with asymmetrical dimethyl arginine residues or non-modified arginine residues were not recognized [146].

Detailed studies of several autoantigens have shown that in patients' sera, antibodies react specifically with zinc finger motifs. This intriguing feature has been described for Ro60, which contains a zinc finger motif in residues 305–323 [152], and poly(ADP ribose) polymerase (PARP), which contains two zinc fingers, called F1 and F2, involved in DNA strand-break repair [153–155]. In the latter case, antibodies from patients with SLE and mixed connective tissue disease (MCTD) showed much weaker reactivity with peptides mutated at the cysteine residues involved in zinc coordination.

Natural modifications of peptides have been shown in certain instances to be necessary to maintain their recognition by autoantibodies. It is unclear whether this means that, *in vivo*, such post-translational modifications do occur in the cognate proteins and are directly involved in the breakdown of tolerance and initiation of the autoimmune response. However, this possibility and its many potential implications in the etiology of autoimmune diseases are actively being explored [156–158].

9.7
Peptides Containing Non-natural Modifications

N-acetylation, carboxamidation, and introduction of peptide bond surrogates are supposed to reduce the susceptibility of peptides to proteases and/or generate structures that are more stable in solution and therefore more reactive with antibodies. In some cases, it is enough to introduce an acetyl group at the N-terminus end and/or a carboxamide group at the C-terminus of the peptide to increase its reactivity with patients' antibodies. For example, it has been observed that peptide 304–324 of Ro60 is much more reactive with sera from patients with SLE and SS when it is blocked at both ends [159]. However, this result is difficult to predict because, as discussed by Saitta et al. [160], depending on the position of the epitopes recognized by autoantibodies, blocking the free amino group at the N-terminus of the peptide may also alter its antigenicity [161, 162]. This observation requires attention since in several mapping methods (e.g., PEPscan, SPOTscan), peptides are immobilized via their C-terminus and are generally acetylated at their N-terminus.

Peptide analogues containing modified peptide bonds have also been tested with autoimmune sera. Thus, the activity of retro-inverso peptide analogues of the sequences 130–135 of histone H3, 304–324 of Ro60 protein, and 277–291 of Ro52 protein has been evaluated with the sera from lupus mice and patients with SLE and SS [159]. In these analogues, also referred to as retro-all-D peptides, the amino acid side chains are oriented in the same way as in the original sequence, while the direction of the CO-NH bond in the backbone is reversed [163, 164]. Depending on the sequences, the retro-inverso analogues were recognized by autoantibodies as well or even better than their natural counterpart [159]. Since autoimmune sera generally contain elevated levels of proteases due to peripheral inflammation in autoimmune individuals, such stable analogues might represent valuable probes for immunodiagnostic assays. Their stability in the serum of autoimmune mice or in the presence of protease cocktails has been shown to be increased by a factor of 10 to 700 [164–166]. Other backbone modifications might lead to heteroclitic peptide analogues of interest. Notable examples are peptides containing reduced peptide bond CH_2-NH or β3-amino acid residues giving rise to analogues with NH_2-CH(R)-CH_2-COOH bonds [167–169].

9.8
Mimotopes

In recent years, several formats of chemical peptide libraries and phage-display libraries have yielded numerous sequences considered to be good binders for autoantibodies. To reveal high affinity for autoantibodies and to identify specific binders, these libraries have often been used with monoclonal autoantibodies of interest. However, they have also been used with human sera that contain subpopulations of antibodies directed against known or unknown antigens. These sequences of linear or conformational epitopes have been identified as sequences of so-called "mimotopes." According to the definition introduced by Geysen's group, mimotopes are not peptide structures with one or two natural amino acid exchanges only (which are simple peptide analogues), but "molecules able to bind to the antigen combining site of an antibody molecule, not necessarily identical with the epitope inducing the antibody, but an acceptable mimic of the essential features of the epitope" [170]. Therefore, mimotopes can be peptides capable of mimicking epitopes of carbohydrates, lipids, lipopeptides, or nucleic acids. It is beyond the scope of this chapter to describe the technical aspects of the strategy used to identify such mimotopes. Numerous review articles are available that describe this approach in full methodological detail (see, e.g., [171–175]) and discuss their potential [176–178]. We will mention only a few examples of mimotopes specifically recognized by autoantibodies, such as mimotopes recognized by serum antibodies from patients with polymyositis-scleroderma overlapping syndrome [179], Cogan's syndrome [180], or MS [181] and mimotopes recognized by synovial fluid antibodies from patients with RA [182]. In the former case, for example, the sequence of the mimotope, a 16-amino-acid peptide, was identified in the PM/Scl-100 antigen [179]. However, the sequence of peptides identified using phage-display or chemical libraries generally cannot be identified in any proteins present in available databases [183]. Carbohydrate-mimicking peptides have also been identified by using chemical libraries [184]. Because it is much easier to synthesize and manipulate peptides than complex sugars, identifying mimics of carbohydrate surrogates may yield valuable probes for selecting autoantibodies and for further therapeutic use.

The same strategy was used to identify DNA mimotopes recognized by antibodies from lupus patients (reviewed in [185]). A series of DNA mimotopes was identified using monoclonal or polyclonal antibodies from lupus individuals and mice, corresponding, for example, to the sequences D/EWD/EEYS/G [186–189], RLTSSLRYNP [190], or XXXDCTXNT$\Phi\Phi$CQL/Y/DXE (where Φ is an aromatic residue [F, Y, or W] and X is any residue) [191]. A 44-amino-acid fragment recognized by pathogenic anti-DNA antibody 3E10 has also been identified [192]. Contrary to the findings of other studies, this monomeric peptide was found to correspond to a sequence of HP8, a protein of the osteonectin/SPARC family of extracellular matrix proteins. Several experiments including mutagenesis have demonstrated that binding of both dsDNA and HP8 protein occurs through overlapping portions of the antibody-binding site.

Identifying carbohydrate, DNA, or nucleosome peptide mimics can have huge applications for both diagnosis and therapy. Therefore, this line of research is being actively pursued by several teams, but numerous limitations hamper the development of this strategy. It has been shown in particular that mimotopes identified using phage-display libraries are poorly reactive in their monomeric form [193, 194]. It seems that their multi-presentation either as MAPs or as carrier protein conjugates, for example, is required for their recognition by the antibodies used for their selection. Furthermore, in contrast to multimeric peptide constructs, immunization of animals with the monomeric peptide form does not generate cross-reacting and pathogenic antibodies. These findings may be related to some of the limitations exposed above [69]. Affinity measurements as well as thermodynamic and structural studies should help us to understand the mechanisms involved in the recognition of these DNA mimics.

9.9
Cross-reactivity of Autoantibodies with Synthetic Peptides and the Cognate Protein

Numerous studies of autoimmune sera and monoclonal autoantibodies using synthetic peptides to identify epitopes of a protein have failed to locate autoepitopes in the sequence of the cognate protein. This finding was expected since it is well known that short peptides rarely mimic the conformational epitopes that constitute the large majority of antigenic sites of a protein or a complex. Such results, although always disappointing, are generally well accepted. However, systematic studies of several autoantigens have revealed the presence, in sera from patients or from lupus-prone mice, of antibodies reacting with peptides but not with the whole protein itself. These antibody subsets coexist with other antibody subpopulations reacting with both the peptides and the full-length parent protein or with the whole protein only. The presence of the former antibody population often has been ignored because, in general, investigators first select sera that react with a particular protein, examining the reactivity of positive sera with peptides only later to delineate the epitopes recognized in the parent protein. In fact, these antibody subsets might be more important than initially recognized. In longitudinal studies, antibodies cross-reacting with peptides are often detected significantly before antibodies reacting with the cognate protein. This phenomenon has been described in the case of histones [54, 103, 195], several ribonucleoproteins such as SmBB′/N [128, 196], SmD1 protein [58–60, 64, 134], U1-70K protein [63], U1A protein [197], hnRNP A2/B1 protein [64], Ro52 protein [57], and PARP [153, 154].

It is difficult to know whether truly distinct antibody populations are effectively produced in autoimmune patients and animals. It could be argued that the fact that the reaction observed with peptides is stronger than with the parent protein simply reflects a difference in the inherent sensitivity of the respective assays. Visualization of cross-reactions is better when peptides bearing a major epitope, rather than whole purified or recombinant proteins, are tested in optimal conditions. We should also bear in mind that most antigens (including antigens in apoptotic bodies) are complexed *in vivo* with other proteins and/or nucleic acids, which may lead to exposure of epitopes that might not be readily accessible when the isolated protein is used in ELISA or Western immunoblotting. On the other hand, we cannot exclude the possibility that, besides antibodies reacting with native proteins and nucleoprotein complexes, antibodies reacting with denatured proteins are also produced. Such antibodies might be better revealed by using short peptides, rather than the whole protein from which they are issued. A hypothesis has been proposed in which such "non-native" proteins (denatured/defolded or damaged self-proteins) might participate in the initiation or propagation of the autoimmune response [86, 198–200]. Finally, another explanation rests on the fact that cleavage of autoantigens during apoptosis is responsible for generating autoantibodies that preferentially recognize fragments rather than full-length proteins [201–207]. Thus, this subpopulation of autoantibodies should not be ignored in our investigations or interpreted as an insignificant antibody subset, as they might reflect important features of the autoimmune response.

9.10
Selected Examples of Epitope Mapping with Synthetic Peptides

Systematic studies using the same antibodies under different conditions have revealed that epitope mapping is largely affected by the type of assay used (ELISA, Western immunoblotting, precipitation) and the nature of the antigen (short or long peptides, recombinant fragments, monomeric vs. multimeric presentation). For example, in some cases the free peptide used in solution as inhibitor is most active, while in others antibodies react preferentially with immobilized peptides adsorbed to a solid phase or conjugated to a carrier [208, 209]. As illustrated above, the level of conformational mimicry between peptide and protein can be increased by presenting the peptide in a particular way, for example, after coupling to a carrier protein [152] or as a MAP or a SOCn construct [193]. Conversely, such types of multi-presentation can be deleterious and induce an unsuitable conformation in the peptide. All these considerations, added to the fact that very different antibody probes (patients' sera and monoclonal antibodies) are used in different laboratories, may explain some of the discrepancies noted in the literature regarding the identification of B-cell autoepitopes. Several recent articles provide a comprehensive review of autoepitope mapping illustrated by specific examples [68, 210–215]. Although notable discrepancies were found between independent studies, these reviews also mention a number of important similarities in the results, allowing one to identify emerging dominant epitopes or antigenic regions of patho-physiological importance that may serve as valuable probes for diagnosis or for developing therapeutic strategies.

This chapter was not intended to provide the reader with a compilation of autoepitopes described so far in the current literature, but rather to describe the advantages and limitations of different approaches used in this field and to highlight the potential interest in using synthetic peptides for diagnostic purposes. Below we have selected a few model antigens that belong to very different classes of proteins and whose epitopes have been studied in different laboratories with a variety of approaches (Fig. 9.3). For other examples, see [213], in which a similar representation of epitopes in the histones H1, H2A, H2B, H3, and H4 and of RNP protein U1-70K, U1A, U1C, SmD1, SmBB', hnRNPA2, Ro60, Ro52, and SSB/La can be found. See also [214] for additional information

(A) Proteinase-3 (29-32 kDa)

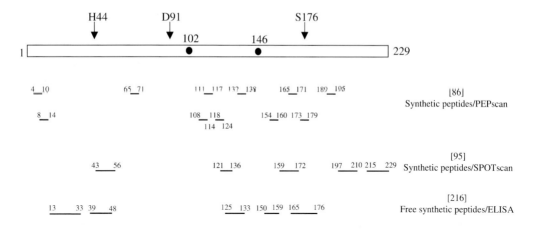

(B) Calreticulin (46 kDa)

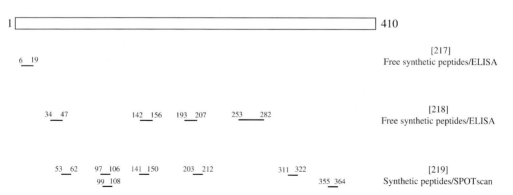

Fig. 9.3 Schematic representation of linear epitopes recognized by autoantibodies from patients and mice with systemic autoimmune diseases. Adapted from the original references indicated on the right. The data generated from studies using experimental animals immunized with autoantigens are not reported. In proteinase-3 (A), residues H^{44}, D^{91}, and S^{176} form the catalytic triad; there are two glycosylation sites in residues N^{102} and N^{146} (●) and four disulfide bridges. In calreticulin (B), distinct sequences were recognized by IgA antibodies from patients with PBC, autoimmune hepatitis, or celiac disease [219]. They are not individualized in the figure. In DNA topoisomerase I (C), the globular core and the COOH-terminal domain (C-t) are responsible for the catalytic activity of the protein. The Y^{723} residue in the human sequence is critical for topoisomerase I activity. The antigen named Scl-70 (70 kDa) is a degradation product of the 100-kDa protein. In the figure, the reactivity of IgG, IgA, and IgM from patients with SSc or from subsets of patients with SSc is shown. Recombinant fragments were tested by Western immunoblotting and in some cases also by ELISA and immunoprecipitation assays [226, 227].

(C) DNA Topoisomerase I (100–110 kDa)

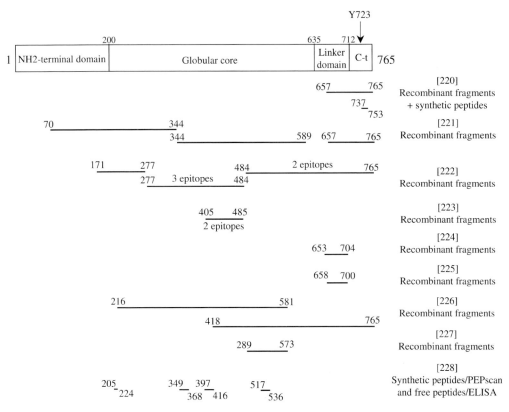

Fig. 9.3 (continued)

on calreticulin, Ku70, and Ku80 antigens, 60S ribosomal protein P2, filaggrin, histidyl-tRNA synthetase, and PM/Scl 100 antigen. The examples we have selected are (1) proteinase-3, a 29–32-kDa serine proteinase recognized by antibodies from patients with Wegener's granulomatosis (for a review on proteinase-3 epitopes, see [215]); (2) calreticulin, a 46-kDa calcium-binding protein with multiple regulatory functions that is targeted by autoantibodies in various diseases, including SLE, subacute and neonatal lupus, SS, RA, MCTD, hepatic and celiac disease, and hepatocellular carcinoma, as well as some parasitic diseases; and (3) DNA topoisomerase I, a 100–110-kDa nuclear protein that relaxes supercoiled DNA for cellular functions such as replication, recombination, transcription, and DNA repair. Anti–DNA topoisomerase I antibodies are disease-specific diagnostic marker antibodies for SSc. Figure 9.3 presents the results obtained in humans by using synthetic peptides in different test formats and recombinant fragments when available.

9.11
Concluding Remarks

It is unrealistic to believe that the complete map of epitopes of a protein can be established, as there are several levels of complexity. First, an epitope is defined as a structural element recognized by the paratope of the antibody tested. This means that, by definition, each antibody, which is unique, will define a unique epitope. Second, with the method used routinely, only linear epitopes are identified. It is well known that conformational epitopes represent the large majority of epitopes of a protein or a macromolecular complex. In the case of autoimmune diseases, since the antigen that gave rise to antibodies is generally far from known, identifying the "true" epitopes recognized by serum circulating antibodies is virtually impossible. Third, perception of what constitutes an epitope is largely operational. It is beyond the scope of this review to debate on the concept of epitopes and paratopes and their thermodynamic interaction. From a practical point of view, however, as discussed by several authors, discrepancies found in the literature result mostly from the fact that investigators have used different techniques (and therefore have visualized different types of interaction), different antigenic probes, and different serum samples. Fourth, with regard to the latter aspect, an important drawback comes from the inherent nature of the immune response, which changes and matures with time. This phenomenon, called "epitope spreading", has been studied by several teams of investigators in animals immunized with peptides or in autoimmune patients and animals, and it has been observed at both the B-cell and T-cell level in systemic and organ-specific autoimmune diseases (e.g., SLE, MS, and IDDM) as well as in individuals infected by different pathogens. Epitope spreading complicates the design of sensitive diagnostic tests developed to identify a maximum of patients suffering from the same disease subset. A possible solution would be to use a cocktail of peptides to cover a majority of individuals and improve the sensitivity of assays. Several peptides, e.g., in SmD1, Ro60, Ro52 and ribosomal P proteins, have already shown great potential for distinguishing SLE patients from patients with other rheumatic or inflammatory diseases [59, 60, 81, 152, 230–232]. CCP is an important marker for patients with RA [233], and a lipoylated peptide of the E2 antigen has proved to be specifically recognized by patients with PBC and not by non-PBC patients with anti-mitochondrial M2 antibodies [148]. As advocated by Leslie et al. [234], screening the general population to identify individuals at high risk for some autoimmune diseases or particular forms of these debilitating diseases could have an important impact. This requires simple, rapid, inexpensive, and discriminative assays. Newly introduced methods, based on peptides or peptidomimetics, might represent powerful approaches to predict, quantify, and follow the progression of the disease, allowing some patients to receive early an adapted treatment that can prevent progression to clinical disease and limit the impact of the disease. It is anticipated that emerging multiplexed assays, as well as new peptide probes containing post-translational modifications to better mimic the natural antigens or mimotopes identified from random libraries, should give rise in the near future to highly specific and valuable peptide-based diagnostic assays for autoimmune diseases.

Abbreviations

AchR	acetylcholine receptor
Boc	*N-a-tert*-butyloxycarbonyl
cANCA	cytoplasmic anti-neutrophil cytoplasmic antibodies
CCP	cyclic citrullinated peptide
CENP-A	centromere-associated protein A
Dde	1-(4,4-dimethyl-2,6-dioxo-cyclohexylidene)ethyl
ds	double-stranded
EAE	experimental autoimmune encephalomyelitis
ELISA	enzyme-linked immunosorbent assay
Fmoc	9-fluorenylmethyl-oxycarbonyl
HIV	human immunodeficiency virus
hnRNP	heterogeneous nuclear ribonucleoprotein
HPLC	high-performance liquid chromatography
HSP	heat shock protein
IDDM	insulin-dependent diabetes mellitus
MAP	multiple antigen peptide system
MBP	myelin basic protein
MCTD	mixed connective tissue disease
MS	multiple sclerosis
PARP	poly(ADP ribose) polymerase
PBC	primary biliary cirrhosis
PDC-E2	E2 component of pyruvate dehydrogenase
PEG	polyethylene glycol
RA	rheumatoid arthritis
Ro52, Ro60	52- and 60-kDa SSA/Ro protein
SLE	systemic lupus erythematosus
SmD1	protein D1 of Sm antigen
snRNP	small nuclear ribonucleoprotein
SOCn	sequential oligopeptide carrier
SPPS	solid-phase peptide synthesis
SS	Sjögren's syndrome
SSc	systemic sclerosis
TASP	template assembled synthetic protein
TFA	trifluoroacetic acid
Trt	trityl
U1A, U1C, U1-70K	proteins A, C, and 70K of the U1 snRNP antigen

References

1 G. G. Illei, E. Tackey, L. Lapteva and P. E. Lipsky, Arthritis Rheum. **2004**, *50*, 1709–1720.

2 W. J. Van Venrooij and R. N. Maini, in *Manual of biological markers of disease*, Kluwer Acad. Publ., Dordrecht **1994**.

3 C. A. von Mühlen and E. M. Tan, *Semin. Arthritis Rheum.* **1995**, *24*, 323–358.

4 J. B. Peter and Y. Shoenfeld, in *Autoantibodies*, Elsevier, Amsterdam **1996**, pp 880.

5 E. M. Tan, *The immunologist* **1999**, *7/8*, 85–92.

6 D. Leslie, P. Lipsky and A. L. Notkins, *J. Clin. Invest.* **2001**, *108*, 1417–1422.

7 A. Lernmark, *J. Clin. Invest.* **2001**, *108*, 1091–1096.

8 M. A. van Boekel, E. R Vossenaar, F. H. van den Hoogen and W. J. van Venrooij, *Arthritis Res.* **2002**, *4*, 87–93.

9 A. Kavanaugh, *Arthritis Rheum.* **2001**, *44*, 2221–2223.

10 V. Du Vigneaud, C. Ressler, J. M. Swann, C. W. Roberts and P. G. Katsoyannis, *J. Am. Chem. Soc.* **1954**, *76*, 3115–3121.

11 R. B. Merrifield, *J. Am. Chem. Soc.* **1963**, *85*, 2149–2154.

12 E. Atherton, H. Fox, D. Harkiss, C. J. Logan, R. C. Sheppard and B. J. Williams, *J. Chem. Soc. Chem. Commun.* **1978**, 537–539.

13 C. D. Chang and J. Meienhofer, *Int. J. Peptide Protein Res.* **1978**, *11*, 246–249.

14 L. A. Carpino and G. Y. Han, *J. Am. Chem. Soc.* **1970**, *92*, 5748–5749.

15 S. B. H. Kent, *Ann. Rev. Biochem.* **1988**, *57*, 957–989.

16 E. Bayer, *Angew. Chem., Int. Ed. Engl.* **1991**, *30*, 113–129.

17 S. Zalipsky, J. L. Chang, F. Albericio and G. Barany, *React. Polym.* **1994**, *22*, 243–258.

18 M. Meldal, *Tetrahedron lett.* **1992**, *33*, 3077–3080.

19 M. Zeppezauer, R. Hoffmann, A. Schönberger, S. Rawer, W. Rapp and E. Bayer, *Z. Naturforsch.* **1993**, *48b*, 1801–1806.

20 R. A. Houghten, *Proc. Natl. Acad. Sci.* **1985**, *82*, 5131–5135.

21 A. G. Beck-Sickinger, H. Dürr and G. Jung, *Peptide Res.* **1991**, *4*, 88–94.

22 J. Neimark and J.-P. Briand, *Peptide Res.* **1993**, *6*, 219–228.

23 G. Schnorrenberg and H. Gerhardt, *Tetrahedron* **1989**, *45*, 7759–7764.

24 R. N. Zuckermann, J. M. Kerr, M. A. Siani and S. C. Banville, *Int. J. Peptide Protein Res.* **1992**, *40*, 498–507.

25 H. Gausepohl, C. Boulin, M. Kraft and R. W. Frank, *Peptide Res.* **1992**, *5*, 315–320.

26 M. Meldal, C. B. Holm, G. Bojesen, M. A. Jakobsen and A. Holm, *Int. J. Peptide Protein Res.* **1993**, *41*, 250–260.

27 R. H. Berg, K. Almdal, W. B. Pedersen, A. Holm, J. P. Tam and R. B. Merrifield, *J. Am. Chem. Soc.* **1989**, *111*, 8024–8026.

28 J. Eichler, M. Bienert, A. Stierandova and M. Lebl, *Peptide Res.* **1991**, *4*, 296–307.

29 H. M. Geysen, S. J. Barteling and R. H. Meloen, *Proc. Natl. Acad. Sci. USA* **1985**, *82*, 178–182.

30 R. M. Valerio, A. M. Bray, R. A. Campbell, A. DiPasquale, C. Margellis, S. J. Rodda, H. M. Geysen and N. J. Maeji, *Int. J. Peptide Protein Res.* **1993**, *42*, 1–9.

31 N. J. Ede, *J. Immunol. Methods* **2002**, *267*, 3–11.

32 R. Frank, *Tetrahedron* **1992**, *48*, 9217–9232.

33 R. Frank and R. Döring, *Tetrahedron* **1988**, *44*, 6031–6040.

34 V. Krchnak, J. Vagner, J. Novak, A. Suchankova and J. Roubal, *Anal. Biochem.* **1990**, *189*, 80–83.

35 W. Van't Hof, M. Van den Berg and R. C. Aalberse, *J. Immunol. Methods* **1993**, *161*, 177–186.

36 Z. Wang and R. Laursen, *Peptide Res.* **1992**, *5*, 275–280.

37 A. W. Purcell, W. Chen, N. J. Ede, J. J. Gorman, J. Fecondo, D. C. Jackson, Y. Zhao and J. McCluskey, *J. Immunol.* **1998**, *160*, 1085–1090.

38 J. Bedford, C. Hyde, T. Johnson, W. Jun, D. Owen, M. Quibell and R. C. Sheppard, *Int. J. Peptide Protein Res.* **1992**, *40*, 300–307.

39 T. Johnson, M. Quibell and R. C. Sheppard, *J. Pept. Sci.* **1995**, *1*, 11–25.

40 T. Woehr, F. Wahl, A. Nefzi, B. Rohwedder, T. Sato, X. Sun and M. Mutter, *J. Am. Chem. Soc.* **1996**, *118*, 9218–9227.

41 M. Bodanszky and J. Z. Kwei, *Int. J. Peptide Protein Res.* **1978**, *12*, 69–74.

42 R. Dölling, M. Beyermann, J. Haenel, F. Kernchen, E. Krause, P. Franke, M. Brudel and M. Bienert, *J. Chem. Soc. Chem. Commun.* **1994**, 853–858.

43 G. Mezö, J. Kajtar, I. Nagy, M. Szekerke and F. Hudecz, *Biopolymers* **1997**, *42*, 719–730.

44 J. P. Tam, *Proc. Natl. Acad. Sci. USA* **1988**, *85*, 5409–5413.

45 M. Mutter and G. Tuchscherer, *Macomol. Chem. Rapid Commun.* **1988**, *9*, 437–443.

46 M. Sakarellos-Daitsiotis, V. Tsikaris, C. Sakarellos, P. G. Vlachoyiannopoulos, A. G. Tzioufas and H. M. Moutsopoulos, *Vaccine* **1999**, *18*, 302–310.

47 J. P. Tam and J. C. Spetzler, *Biomedical Peptides, Proteins and Nucleid Acids* **1995**, *1*, 123–132.

48 N. Ahlborg, *J. Immunol. Methods* **1999**, *179*, 269–275.

49 G. Tuchscherer and M. Mutter, *J. Pept. Sci.* **1995**, *1*, 3–10.

50 P. E. Dawson and S. B. H. Kent, *J. Am. Chem. Soc.* **1993**, *115*, 7263–7266.

51 J. R. Crowther, in *ELISA, theory and practice*, Methods in Molecular Biology, Humana Press, Totowa, New Jersey, **1995**, Vol 42, pp 223.

52 G. E. Morris, in *Epitope mapping protocols*, Methods in Molecular Biology, Humana Press, Totowa, New Jersey, **1996**, Vol 66, pp 416.

53 M. H. V. Van Regenmortel and S. Muller, in *Synthetic peptides as antigens*, Laboratory Techniques in Biochemistry and Molecular Biology, Elsevier, Amsterdam, **1999**, Vol 28, pp 381.

54 C. Stemmer, J.-P. Briand and S. Muller, *Mol. Immunol.* **1994**, *31*, 1037–1046.

55 M. Monestier, P. Decker, J.-P. Briand, J. L. Gabriel and S. Muller, *J. Biol. Chem.* **2000**, *275*, 13558–13563.

56 S. Fournel, S. Neichel, H. Dali, B. Maillère, J.-P. Briand and S. Muller, *J. Immunol.* **2003**, *171*, 636–644.

57 V. Ricchiuti, J.-P. Briand, O. Meyer, D. A. Isenberg, G. Pruijn and S. Muller, *Clin. Exp. Immunol.* **1994**, *95*, 397–407.

58 S. Barakat, J.-P. Briand, J.-C. Weber, M. H. V. Van Regenmortel and S. Muller, *Clin. Exp. Immunol.* **1990**, *81*, 256–262.

59 A. Sabbatini, M. P. Dolcher, B. Marchini, S. Bombardieri and P. Migliorini, *J. Rheumatol.* **1993**, *20*, 1679–1683.

60 G. Riemekasten, J. Marell, G. Trebeljahr, R. Klein, G. Hausdorf, T. Haupl, J. Schneider-Mergener, G. R. Burmester and F. Hiepe, *J. Clin. Invest.* **1998**, *102*, 754–763.

61 S. Barakat, J.-P. Briand, N. Abuaf, M. H. V. Van Regenmortel and S. Muller, *Clin. Exp. Immunol.* **1991**, 86, 71–78.

62 H. Halimi, H. Dumortier, J.-P. Briand and S. Muller, *J. Immunol. Methods* **1996**, *199*, 77–85.

63 F. Monneaux, J.-P. Briand and S. Muller, *Eur. J. Immunol.* **2000**, *30*, 2191–2200.

64 H. Dumortier, F. Monneaux, B. Jahn-Schmid, J.-P. Briand, K. Skriner, P. L. Cohen, J. S. Smolen, G. Steiner and S. Muller, *J. Immunol.* **2000**, *165*, 2297–2305.

65 J. C. Morris, J. L. Gibson, E. J. Haas, E. R. Bergert, J. S. Dallas and B. S. Prabhakar, *Autoimmunity* **1994**, *17*, 287–299.

66 K. B. Elkon, *Mol. Biol. Rep.* **1992**, *16*, 207–212.

67 J.-P. Briand, S. Muller, M. H. V. Van Regenmortel, *J. Immunol. Methods* **1985**, *78*, 59–69.

68 S. Muller, in *Synthetic peptides as antigens* (eds. M. H. V. Van Regenmortel and S. Muller) Elsevier, Amsterdam **1999**, pp. 247–280.

69 J.-P. Briand, C. Barin, M. H. V. Van Regenmortel and S. Muller, *J. Immunol. Methods* **1992**, *156*, 255–265.

70 K. K. Gaither, O. F. Fox, H. Yamagata, M. J. Mamula, M. Reichlin and J. B. Harley, *J. Clin. Invest.* **1987**, *79*, 841–846.

71 C. Mézière, F. Stöckl, S. Batsford, A. Vogt and S. Muller, *Clin. Exp. Immunol.* **1994**, *98*, 287–294.

72 N. Benkirane, M. Friede, G. Guichard, J.-P. Briand, M. H. V. Van Regenmortel and S. Muller, *J. Biol. Chem.* **1993**, *268*, 26279–26285.

73 S. Waga, E. M. Tan and R. L. Rubin, *Biochem. J.* **1987**, *244*, 675–682.

74 D.E. Sansonno, P. DeTomaso, M.A. Papanice, O.G. Manghisi, *J. Immunol. Methods* **1986**, *90*, 131–136.

75 P.J. Kilshaw, F.J. McEwan, K.C. Baker and A.J. Cant, *Clin. Exp. Immunol.* **1986**, *66*, 481–489.

76 S.J. Rodda, H.M. Geysen, T.J. Mason and P.G Schoofs, *Mol. Immunol.* **1986**, *23*, 603–610.

77 R.H. Scofield and J.B. Harley, *Proc. Natl. Acad. Sci. USA* **1991**, *88*, 3343–3347.

78 A.G. Tzioufas, E. Yiannaki, M. Sakarellos-Daitsiotis, J.G. Routsias, C. Sakarellos and H.M. Moutsopoulos, *Clin. Exp. Immunol.* **1997**, *108*, 191–198.

79 D.G. Williams, N.G. Sharpe, G. Wallace and D.S. Latchman, *J. Autoimmun.* **1990**, *3*, 715–725.

80 J.A. James and J.B. Harley, *J. Immunol.* **1992**, *148*, 2074–2079.

81 J.A. James, M.J. Mamula and J.B. Harley, *Clin. Exp. Immunol.* **1994**, *98*, 419–426.

82 M.T. McClain, P.A. Ramsland, K.M. Kaufman and J.A. James *J. Immunol.* **2002**, *168*, 2054–2062.

83 J.A. James and J.B. Harley, *Clin. Exp. Rheumatol.* **1995**, *13*, 299–305.

84 J.A. James and J.B. Harley, *J. Immunol.* **1996**, *156*, 4018–4026.

85 J.A. James, R.H. Scofield and J.B. Harley, *Scand. J. Immunol.* **1994**, *39*, 557–566.

86 R.C. Williams Jr, R. Staud, C.C. Malone, J. Payabyab, L. Byres and D. Underwood, *J. Immunol.* **1994**, *152*, 4722–4737.

87 L. Horvath, L. Cervenak, M. Oroszlan, Z. Prohaszka, K. Uray, F. Hudecz, E. Baranyi, L. Madacsy, M. Singh, L. Romics, G. Fust and P. Panczel, *Immunol. Lett.* **2002**, *80*, 155–162.

88 I.A. Lea, P. Adoyo and M.G. O'Rand, *Fertility Sterility* **1997**, *67*, 355–361.

89 S.J. Rodda and G. Tribbick, *Methods* **1996**, *9*, 473–481.

90 G. Tribbick, *J. Immunol. Methods* **2002**, *267*, 27–35.

91 R. Frank, *J. Immunol. Methods* **2002**, *267*, 13–26.

92 L.R. Haaheim, A.K. Halse, R. Kvakestad, B. Stern, O. Normann and R. Jonsson, *Scand. J. Immunol.* **1996**, *43*, 115–121.

93 M. Mahler, K. Kessenbrock, J. Raats, R. Williams, M.J. Fritzler and M. Blüthner, *J. Mol. Med.* **2003**, *81*, 194–204.

94 J.B. Levy, J.A. Coulthart and C.D. Pusey, *J. Am. Soc. Nephrol.* **1997**, *8*, 1698–1705.

95 M.E. Griffith, A. Coulthart, S. Pemberton, A.J. George and C.D. Pusey, *Clin. Exp. Immunol.* **2001**, *123*, 170–177.

96 M. Mahler, R. Mierau and M. Blüthner, *J. Mol. Med.* **2000**, *78*, 460–467.

97 Y. Muro, N. Azuma, H. Onouchi, M. Kunimatsu, Y. Tomita, M. Sasaki and K. Sugimoto, *Clin. Exp. Immunol.* **2000**, *120*, 218–223.

98 M. Blüthner, M. Mahler, D.B. Müller, H. Dünzl and F.A. Bautz, *J. Mol. Med.* **2000**, *78*, 47–54.

99 S. Selak, M. Mahler, K. Miyachi, M.L. Fritzler and M.J. Fritzler, *Clin. Immunol.* **2003**, *109*, 154–164.

100 S.S. Pathak and H.F.J. Savelkoul, *Immunol. Today* **1997**, *18*, 464–467.

101 R.L. Rich and D.G. Myszka, *J. Mol. Recognit.* **2002**, *15*, 352–376.

102 A.A. Rarok, Y.M. van der Geld, C.A. Stegeman, P.C. Limburg and C.G. Kallenberg, *J. Clin. Immunol.* **2003**, *23*, 460–468.

103 C. Stemmer, P. Richalet-Secordel, M. van Bruggen, K. Kramers, J. Berden and S. Muller, *J. Biol. Chem.* **1996**, *271*, 21257–21261.

104 R. Mobini, A. Staub, S.B. Felix, G. Baumann, G. Wallukat, J. Deinum, H. Svensson, A. Hjalmarson and M. Fu, *J. Autoimmunity* **2003**, *20*, 345–350.

105 D. Dragun, D.N. Muller, J.H. Bräsen, L. Fritsche, M. Nieminen-Kelhä, R. Dechend, U. Kintescher, B. Rudolph, J. Hoebeke, D. Eckert, I. Mazak, R. Plehm, C. Schönemann, T. Unger, K. Budde, H.-H.Neumayer, F.C. Luft and G. Wallukat, *N. Engl. J. Med.* **2005**, *352*, 558–569.

106 R. Elies, I. Ferrari, G. Wallukat, D. Lebesgue, P. Chiale, M. Elizari, M. Rosenbaum, J. Hoebeke and M.J. Levin, *J. Immunol.* **1996**, *157*, 4203–4211.

107 D. Kaplan, I. Ferrari, P.L. Bergami, E. Mahler, G. Levitus, P. Chiale, J. Hoebeke, M.H.V. Van Regenmortel and M.J. Levin, *Proc. Natl. Acad. Sci. USA* **1997**, *94*, 10301–10306.

108 T.O. Joos, M. Schrenk, P. Hopfl, K. Kroger, U. Chowdhury, D. Stoll, D. Schorner, M. Durr, K. Herick, S. Rupp,

K. Sohn and H. Hammerle, *Electrophoresis* **2000**, *21*, 2641–2650.

109 D. Stoll, M. F. Templin, M. Schrenk, P. C. Traub, C. F. Vohringer and T. O. Joos, *Front Biosci.* **2002**, *7*, c13–32.

110 M. F. Templin, D. Stoll, M. Schrenk, P. C. Traub, C. F. Vohringer and T. O. Joos, *Trends Biotechnol.* **2002**, *20*, 160–166.

111 U. Reimer, U. Reineke and J. Schneider-Mergener, *Curr. Opin. Biotechnol.* **2002**, *13*, 315–320.

112 W. H. Robinson, L. Steinman and P. J. Utz , *Arthritis Rheum.* **2002**, *46*, 885–893.

113 W. Hueber, P. J. Utz, L. Steinman and W. H. Robinson, *Arthritis Res.* **2002**, *4*, 290–295.

114 W. H. Robinson, L. Steinman and P. J. Utz, *Proteomics* **2003**, *3*, 2077–2084.

115 P. J. Utz, *Lupus* **2004**, *13*, 304–311.

116 W. H. Robinson, C. DiGennaro, W. Hueber, B. B. Haab, M. Kamachi, E. J. Dean, S. Fournel, D. Fong, M. C. Genovese, H. E. de Vegvar, K. Skriner, D. L. Hirschberg, R. I. Morris, S. Muller, G. J. Pruijn, W. J. van Venrooij, J. S. Smolen, P. O. Brown, L. Steinman and P. J. Utz, *Naure Med.* **2002**, *8*, 295–301.

117 W. H. Robinson, P. Fontoura, B. J. Lee, H. E. Neuman de Vegvar, J. Tom, R. Pedotti, C. D DiGennaro, D. J Mitchell, D. Fong, P. P. K Ho, P. J. Ruiz, E. Maverakis, D. B. Stevens, C. C. A. Bernard, R. Martin, V. K. Kuchroo, J. M. van Noort, C. P. Genain, S. Amor, T. Olsson, P. J. Utz, H. Garren and L. Steinman, *Nature Biotech.* **2003**, *21*, 1033–1039.

118 D. Pantarotto, C. D. Partidos, J. Hoebeke, F. Brown, E. Kramer, J.-P. Briand, S. Muller, M. Prato and A. Bianco, *Chem Biol.* **2003**, *10*, 961–966.

119 D. Pantarotto, J.-P. Briand, M. Prato and A. Bianco, *Chem. Commun.* **2004**, 16–17.

120 R. J. Chen, S. Bangsaruntip, K. A. Drouvalakis, N. Wong Shi Kaam, M. Shim, Y. Li, W. Kim, P. J. Utz and H. Dai, *Proc. Natl. Acad. Sci. USA* **2003**, *100*, 4984–4989.

121 M. Mahler, K. Kessenbrock, J. Raats and M. J. Fritzler, *J. Clin. Lab. Analysis* **2004**, *18*, 215–223.

122 K. Elkon, S. Skelly, A. Parnassa, W. Moller, W. Danho, H. Weissbach and N. Brot, *Proc. Natl. Acad. Sci. USA* **1986**, *83*, 7419–7423.

123 D. A. Isenberg, M. Garton, M. W. Reichlin and M. Reichlin, *Br. J. Rheumatol.* **1997**, *36*, 229–233.

124 A. Ghirardello, L. Caponi, F. Franceschini, S. Zampieri, M. Quinzanini, R. Bendo, S. Bombardieri, P. F. Gambari and A. Doria, *J. Autoimmunity* **2002**, *19*, 71–77.

125 S. Hirohata, K. Isshi and S. Toyoshima, *Arthritis Rheum.* **1998**, *41*, 1137–1140.

126 L. Caponi, S. Pegoraro, V. Di Bartolo, P. Rovero, R. Revoltella and S. Bombardieri, *J. Immunol. Methods* **1995**, *179*, 193–202.

127 J.-P. Briand, C. André, N. Tuaillon, L. Hervé, J. Neimark and S. Muller, *Hepatology* **1992**, *16*, 1395–1403.

128 C. J. Petrovas, P. G. Vlachoyiannopoulos, A. G. Tzioufas, C. Alexopoulos, V. Tsikaris, M. Sakarellos-Daitsiotis, C. Sakarellos and H. M. Moutsopoulos, *J. Immunol. Methods* **1998**, *220*, 59–68.

129 E. E. Yiannaki, A. G. Tzioufas, M. Bachmann, J. Hantoumi, V. Tsikaris, M. Sakarellos-Daitsiotis, C. Sakarellos and H. M. Moutsopoulos, *Clin. Exp. Immunol.* **1998**, *112*, 152–158.

130 V. Tsikaris, C. Sakarellos, M. Sakarellos-Daitsiotis, P. Orlewski, M. Marraud, M. T. Cung, E. Vatzaki and S. Tzartos, *Int. J. Biol. Macromol.* **1996**, *19*, 195–205.

131 M. Mahler, R. Mierau, W. Schlumberger and M. Blüthner, *J. Mol. Med.* **2001**, *79*, 722–731.

132 C. Stemmer, J.-P. Briand and S. Muller, *Mol. Immunol.* **1994**, *31*, 1037–1046.

133 J. A. James, T. Gross, R. H. Scofield and J. B. Harley, *J. Exp. Med.* **1995**, *181*, 453–461.

134 F. Monneaux and S. Muller, *Scand. J. Immunol.* **2001**, *54*, 45–54.

135 F. Monneaux and S. Muller, *Arthritis Rheum.* **2002**, *46*, 1430–1438.

136 G. W. Zieve and P. R. Khusial, *Autoimmunity Rev.* **2003**, *2*, 235–240.

137 J.-P. Briand, C. Barin, M. H. V. Van Regenmortel and S. Muller, *J. Immunol. Methods* **1992**, *156*, 255–265.

138 D. A. Stetler and S. T. Jacob, *J. Biol. Chem.* **1984**, *259*, 13629–13632.

139 S. P. Fussey, S. T. Ali, J. R. Guest, O. F. James, M. F. Bassendine and S. J. Yeaman, *Proc. Natl. Acad. Sci. USA* **1990**, *87*, 3987–3991.

140 M. Satoh, A. K. Ajmani, T. Ogasawara, J. J. Langdon, M. Hirakata, J. Wang and W. H. Reeves, *J. Clin. Invest.* **1994**, *94*, 1981–1989.

141 G. Shen, in *Autoantibodies* (eds. J. B. Peter, Y. Shoenfeld), Elsevier, Amsterdam, **1996**, pp. 185–194.

142 P. J. Utz, M. Hottelet, P. H. Schur and P. Anderson, *J. Exp. Med.* **1997**, *185*, 843–854.

143 S. Bläss, C. Meier, H. W. Vohr, M. Schwochau, C. Specker and G. R. Burmester, *Ann. Rheum. Dis.* **1998**, *57*, 220–225.

144 K. M. Neugebauer, J. T. Merrill, M. H. Wener, R. G. Lahita and M. B. Roth, *Arthritis Rheum.* **2000**, *43*, 1768–1778.

145 C. Masson-Bessière, M. Sebbag, E. Girbal-Neuhauser, L. Nogueira, C. Vincent, T. Senshu and G. Serre, *J. Immunol.* **2001**, *166*, 4177–4184.

146 H. Brahms, J. Raymackers, A. Union, F. de Keyser, L. Meheus and R. Lührmann, *J. Biol. Chem.* **2000**, *275*, 17122–17129.

147 S. Plaué, S. Muller and M. H. V. Van Regenmortel, *J. Exp. Med.* **1989**, *169*, 1607–1617.

148 N. Tuaillon, C. André, J.-P. Briand, E. Penner and S. Muller, *J. Immunol.* **1992**, *148*, 445–450.

149 G. A. Schellekens, B. A. W. de Jong, F. H. J. van den Hoogen, L. B. A. van de Putte and W. J. van Venrooij, *J. Clin. Invest.* **1998**, *101*, 273–281.

150 E.-J. A. Kroot, B. A. W. de Jong, M. A van Leeuwen, H. Swinkels, F. H. J. van den Hoogen, M. van't Hof, L. B. A. van de Putte, M. H. van Rijswijk, W. J. van Venrooij and P. L. C. M. van Riel, *Arthritis Rheum.* **2000**, *43*, 1831–1835.

151 S. Dubucquoi, E. Solau-Gervais, D. Lefranc, L. Marguerie, J. Sibilia, J. Goetz, V. Dutoit, A.-L. Fauchais, E. Hachulla,

R.-M. Flipo and L. Prin, *Ann. Rheum. Dis.* **2004**, *63*, 415–419.

152 S. Barakat, O. Meyer, F. Torterotot, P. Youinou, J.-P. Briand, M.-F. Kahn and S. Muller, *Clin. Exp. Immunol.* **1992**, *89*, 38–45.

153 S. Muller, J.-P. Briand, S. Barakat, J. Lagueux, G. G. Poirier, G. de Murcia and D. A. Isenberg, *Clin. Immunol. Immunopathol.* **1994**, *73*, 187–196.

154 P. Decker, J.-P. Briand, G. de Murcia, R. W. Pero, D. A. Isenberg and S. Muller, *Arthritis Rheum.* **1998**, *41*, 918–926.

155 P. Decker, D. Isenberg and S. Muller, *J. Biol. Chem.* **2000**, *275*, 9043–9046.

156 P. J. Utz, T. J. Gensler and P. Anderson, *Arthritis Res.* **2000**, *2*, 101–114.

157 R. J. T. Rodenburg, J. M. H. Raats, G. J. M. Pruijn and W. J. van Venrooij, *BioEssays* **2000**, *22*, 627–636.

158 P. A. C. Cloos and S. Christgau, *Biogerontology* **2004**, *5*, 139–158

159 J.-P. Briand, G. Guichard, H. Dumortier and S. Muller, *J. Biol. Chem.* **1995**, *270*, 20686–20691.

160 M. R. Saitta, F. C. Arnett and J. D. Keene, *J. Immunol.* **1994**, *152*, 4192–4202.

161 L. A. Rokeach, M. Jannatipour and S. O. Hoch, *J. Immunol.* **1990**, *144*, 1015–1022.

162 Y. Ou, D. Sun, G. C. Sharp and S. O. Hoch, *Clin. Immunol. Immunopathol.* **1997**, *83*, 310–317.

163 M. Chorev and M. Goodman, *Acc. Chem. Res.* **1993**, *26*, 266–273.

164 G. Guichard, N. Benkirane, G. Zeder-Lutz, M. H. V. Van Regenmortel, J.-P. Briand and S. Muller, *Proc. Natl. Acad. Sci. USA* **1994**, *91*, 9765–9769.

165 J.-P. Briand, N. Benkirane, G. Guichard, J. F. E. Newman, M. H. V. Van Regenmortel, F. Brown and S. Muller, *Proc. Natl. Acad. Sci. USA* **1997**, *94*, 12545–12550.

166 T. Ben-Yedidia, A.-S. Beignon, C. D. Partidos, S. Muller and R. Arnon, *Mol. Immunol.* **2002**, *39*, 323–331.

167 N. Benkirane, G. Guichard, M. H. V. Van Regenmortel, J.-P. Briand and S. Muller, *J. Biol. Chem.* **1996**, *271*, 33218–33224.

168 J. M. Lozano, F. Espejo, D. Diaz, L. M. Salazar, J. Rodriguez, C. Pinzon, J. C.

Calvo, F. Guzman and M. E. Pararroyo, *J. Peptide Res.* **1998**, *52*, 457–469.

169 A. Phan Chan Du, D. Limal, V. Semetey, H. Dali, M. Jolivet, C. Desgranges, M. T. Cung, J.-P. Briand, M.-C. Petit and S. Muller, *J. Mol. Biol.* **2002**, *323*, 503–521.

170 H. M. Geysen, S. J. Rodda and T. J. Mason, *Mol. Immunol.* **1986**, *23*, 709–715.

171 C. Pinilla, J. Appel, S. Blondelle, C. Dooley, B. Dörner, J. Eichler, J. Ostresh and R. A. Houghten, *Biopolymers* **1995**, *37*, 221–240.

172 S. Cabilly, In *Combinatorial peptide library protocols*, Methods in Molecular Biology, Humana Press, Totowa, New Jersey, **1998**, vol 87, pp 313.

173 R. H. Meloen, W. C. Puijk and J. W. Slootstra, *J. Mol. Recognit.* **2000**, *13*, 352–359.

174 U. Reineke, C. Ivascu, M. Schlief, C. Landgraf, S. Gericke, G. Zahn, H. Herzel, R. Volkmer-Engert and J. Schneider-Mergener, *J. Immunol. Methods* **2002**, *267*, 37–51.

175 C. Pinilla, J. R. Appel, E. Borras and R. A. Houghten, *Nat. Med.* **2003**, *9*, 118–122.

176 M. Sioud, Ø. Førre and A. Dybwad, *Clin. Immunol. Immunopathol.* **1996**, *79*, 105–114.

177 C. D. Partidos, *Curr. Opin. Mol. Ther.* **2000**, *2*, 74–79.

178 G. Tribbick, *J. Immunol. Methods* **2002**, *267*, 27–35.

179 M. Blüthner, E. K. F. Bautz and F. A. Bautz, *J. Immunol. Methods* **1996**, *198*, 187–198.

180 C. Lunardi, C. Bason, M. Leandri, R. Navone, M. Lestani, E. Millo, U. Benatti, M. Cilli, R. Beri, R. Corrocher and A. Puccetti, *Lancet* **2002**, *360*, 915–921.

181. C. Jolivet-Reynaud, H. Perron, F. Ferrante, L. Bequart, P. Dalbon and B. Mandrand, *Clin. Immunol.* **1999**, *93*, 283–293.

182 A. Dybwad, Ø. Førre, J. B. Natvig and M. Sioud, *Clin. Immunol. Immunopathol.* **1995**, *75*, 45–50.

183 D. Barchan, M. Balass, M. C. Souroujon, E. Katchalski-Katzir and S. Fuchs, *J. Immunol.* **1995**, *155*, 4264–4269.

184 C. Pinilla, J. R. Appel, G. D. Campbell, J. Buencamino, N. Benkirane, S. Muller and N. S. Greenspan, *J. Mol. Biol.* **1998**, *283*, 1013–1025.

185 S. Fournel and S. Muller, *Cell. Mol. Life Sci.* **2002**, *59*, 1280–1284.

186 B. Gaynor, C. Putterman, P. Valadon, L. Spatz, M. D. Scharff and B. Diamond, *Proc. Natl. Acad. Sci. USA* **1997**, *94*, 1955–1960.

187 C. Putterman and B. Diamond, *J. Exp. Med.* **1998**, *188*, 29–38.

188 C. Putterman, B. Deocharan and B. Diamond, *J. Immunol.* **2000**, *164*, 2542–2549.

189 E. Beger, B. Deocharan, M. Edelman, B. Erblich, Y. Gu and C. Putterman, *J. Immunol.* **2002**, *168*, 3617–3626.

190 Y. Sun, K. Y. Fong, M. C. Chung and Z. J. Yao, *Int. Immunol.* **2001**, *13*, 223–232.

191 P. Sibille, T. Ternynck, F. Nato, G. Buttin, D. Strosberg and A. Avrameas, *Eur. J. Immunol.* **1997**, *27*, 1221–1228.

192 D. J. Zack, K. Yamamoto, A. L. Wong, M. Stempniak, C. French and C. R. H. Weisbart, *J. Immunol.* **1995**, *154*, 1987–1994.

193 A. Sharma, D. Isenberg and B. Diamond, *Rheumatology* **2003**, *42*, 453–460.

194 G. Cunto-Amesty, P. Luo, B. Monzavi-Karbassi, A. Lees, T. Kieber-Emmons, *Vaccine* **2001**, *19*, 2361–2368.

195 N. Tuaillon, S. Muller, J.-L. Pasquali, P. Bordigoni, P. Youinou and M. H. V. Van Regenmortel, *Int. Arch. Allergy Appl. Immunol.* **1990**, *91*, 297–305.

196 J. J. Hines, W. Danho and K. B. Elkon, *Arthritis Rheum.* **1991**, *34*, 572–579.

197 H. Dumortier, M. Abbal, M. Fort, J.-P. Briand, A. Cantagrel and S. Muller, *Int. Immunol.* **1999**, *11*, 249–257.

198 C. Atanassov, J.-P. Briand, D. Bonnier, M. H. V. Van Regenmortel. and S. Muller, *Clin. Exp. Immunol.*, **1991**, *86*, 124–133.

199 Y. Itoh, K. Itoh, M. B. Frank and M. Reichlin, *Autoimmunity* **1992**, *14*, 89–95.

200 M. J. Rico, N. J. Korman, J. R. Stanley, T. Tanaka and R. P. Hall, *J. Immunol.* **1990**, *145*, 3728–3733.

201 L. A. Casciola-Rosen, G. J. Anhalt and A. Rosen, *J. Exp. Med.* **1995**, *182*, 1625–1634.

202 C. A. Casiano, S. J. Martin, D. R. Green and E. M. Tan, *J. Exp. Med.* **1996**, *184*, 765–770.

203 L. A. Casciola-Rosen, F. Andrade, D. Ulanet, W. B. Wong and A. Rosen, *J. Exp. Med.* **1999**, *190*, 815–825.

204 P. J. Utz, T. Gensler and P. Anderson, *Arthritis Res.* **2000**, *2*, 101–114.

205 K. M. Pollard, *Arthritis Rheum.* **2002**, *46*, 1699–1702.

206 L. Schachna, F. M. Wigley, S. Morris, A. C. Gelber, A. Rosen and L. A. Casciola-Rosen, *Arthritis Rheum.* **2002**, *46*, 1873–1884.

207 E. L. Greidinger, M. F. Foeckling, J. Magee, L. Wilson, S. Ranatunga, R. A. Ortmann and R. W. Hoffman, *J. Immunol.* **2004**, *172*, 709–716.

208 S. Muller, S. Plaué, M. Couppez and M. H. V. Van Regenmortel, *Mol. Immunol.* **1986**, *23*, 593–601.

209 V. Ricchiuti, G. J. Pruijn, J. P. Thijssen, W. J. van Venrooij and S. Muller, *J. Autoimmun.* **1997**, *10*, 181–191.

210 M. Wahren-Herlenius, S. Muller and D. Isenberg, *Immunol. Today* **1999**, *20*, 234–240.

211 N. M. Moutsopoulos, J. G. Routsias, P. G. Vlachoyiannopoulos, A. G. Tzioufas and H. M. Moutsopoulos, *Mol. Medicine* **2000**, *6*, 141–151.

212 M. Mahler, M. Blüthner and K. M. Pollard, *Clin. Immunol.* **2003**, *107*, 65–79.

213 S. Fournel and S. Muller, *Current Protein & Peptide Science* **2003**, *4*, 261–276.

214 J. G. Routsias, A. G. Tzioufas and H. M. Moutsopoulos, *Clin. Chim. Acta* **2004**, *340*, 1–25.

215 Y. M. Van der Geld, C. A. Stegeman and C. G. M. Kallenberg, *Clin. Exp. Immunol.* **2004**, *137*, 451–459.

216 Y. M. Van der Geld, A. Simpelaar, R. van der Zee, J. W. C. Tervaert, C. A. Stegeman, P. C. Limburg and C. G. M. Kallenberg, *Kidney International* **2001**, *59*, 147–159.

217 T.-S. Lieu, M. M. Newkirk, F. C. Arnett, L. A. Lee, J.-S. Deng, J. D. Capra and R. D. Sontheimer, *J. Autoimmunity* **1989**, *2*, 367–374.

218 P. Eggleton, F. J. Ward, S. Johnson, M. A. Khamashta, G. R. V. Hughes, V. A. Hajela, M. Michalak, E. F. Corbett, N. A. Staines and K. B. M. Reid, *Clin. Exp. Immunol.* **2000**, *120*, 384–391.

219 D. Sánchez, L. Tucková, T. Mothes, W. Kreisel, Z. Benes, H. Tlaskalová-Hogenová, *J. Autoimmunity* **2003**, *21*, 383–392.

220 G. G. Maul, S. A. Jimenez, E. Riggs and D. Ziemnicka-Kotula, *Proc. Natl. Acad. Sci. USA* **1989**, *86*, 8492–8496.

221 R. Verheijen, F. van den Hoogen, R. Beijer, A. Richter, E. Penner, W. J. Habets and W. J. van Venrooij, *Clin. Exp. Immunol.* **1990**, *80*, 38–43.

222 P. d'Arpa, H. White-Cooper, D. W. Cleveland, N. F. Rothfield and W. C. Earnshaw, *Arthritis Rheum.* **1990**, *33*, 1501–1511.

223 G. Piccinini, E. Cardellini, G. Reimer, F. C. Arnett and E. Durban, *Molecular Immunol.* **1991**, *28*, 333–339.

224 T. M. Meesters, M. Hoet, F. H. J. van den Hoogen, R. Verheijen, W. J. Habets and W. J. van Venrooij, *Mol. Biol. Reports* **1992**, *16*, 117–123.

225 M. Kuwana, J. Kaburaki, T. Mimori, T. Tojo and M. Homma, *Arthritis Rheum.* **1993**, *36*, 1406–1413.

226 H. P. Seelig, H. Schröter, H. Ehrfeld and M. Renz, *J. Immunol. Meth.* **1993**, *165*, 241–252.

227 M. Kuwana, J. Kaburaki, T. A. Medsger, Jr. and T. M. Wright, *Arthritis Rheum.* **1999**, *42*, 1179–1188.

228 C. Rizou, J. P. A. Ioannidis, E. Panou-Pomonis, M. Sakarellos-Daitsiotis, C. Sakarellos, H. M. Moutsopoulos and P. G. Vlachoyiannopoulos, *Am. J. Respir. Cell. Mol. Biol.* **2000**, *22*, 344–351.

229 P. A. Henry, S. P. Atamas, V. V. Yurovsky, I. Luzina, F. M. Wigley and B. White, *Arthritis Rheum.* **2000**, *43*, 2733–2742.

230 B. Bozic, G. J. Pruijn, B. Rozman and W. J. van Venrooij, *Clin. Exp. Immunol.* **1993**, *94*, 227–235.

231 J.G. Routsias, A.G. Tzioufas, M. Sakar-ellos-Daitsiotis, C. Sakarellos and H.M. Moutsopoulos, *Eur. J. Clin. Invest.* **1996**, *26*, 514–521.

232 M. Reichlin, T.F. Broyles, O. Hubscher, J. James, T.A. Lehman, R. Palermo, H.A. Stafford, E. Taylor-Albert and M. Wolfson-Reichlin, *Arthritis Rheum.* **1999**, *42*, 69–75.

233 F.A. van Gaalan, S.P. Linn-Rasker, W.J. van Venrooij, B.A. de Jong, F.C. Breedveld, C.L. Verweij, R.E.M. Toes and T.W.J. Huizinga, *Arthritis Rheum.* **2004**, *50*, 709–715.

234 D. Leslie, P. Lipsky and A.L. Notkins, *J. Clin. Invest.* **2001**, *108*, 1417–1422.

10
Autoantibodies and Systemic Autoimmune Diseases

Karsten Conrad and Michael Bachmann

10.1
Characteristics and Classification of Systemic Autoimmune Diseases

Diseases can be characterized as autoimmune by direct, indirect, and circumstantial evidence [1]. Direct evidence is given by the presence of disease-specific autoantibodies (AABs) and/or autoreactive T cells that cause organ dysfunction and/or chronic inflammation. Animal models with spontaneously developed or induced diseases that resemble autoimmune diseases (AIDs) in humans may provide indirect evidence. Circumstantial evidence includes the association with other AIDs, the presence of AABs (regardless of their pathogenic role), the association with major histocompatibility complex (MHC) haplotypes, the infiltration of lymphocytes into target organ(s), germinal centers in the lesions, infiltrating lymphocytes with restricted V-gene usage, and favorable response to immunosuppression. The etiologies and pathological mechanisms involved in the development of AIDs are incompletely understood. There is no doubt that genetic as well as environmental factors are responsible for the induction, development, and progression of AIDs. According to clinical manifestations and autoimmune responses, AIDs may be considered organ-specific or non-organ-specific (systemic).

Systemic autoimmune diseases represent a very heterogeneous group of AIDs with manifestations on multiple tissues or organs and include rheumatoid arthritis (RA, see Chapter 12), connective tissue diseases (CTDs), anti-phospholipid syndrome, and systemic vasculitides. The CTDs can be classified as systemic lupus erythematosus (SLE; see Chapter 11), systemic sclerosis (SSc, scleroderma), Sjögren's syndrome (SjS), idiopathic inflammatory myopathies (autoimmune myositides, including polymyositis [PM] and dermatomyositis [DM]), as well as various overlap syndromes (mixed connective tissue disease [MCTD] and PM-SSc overlap syndrome) and undifferentiated (unclassifiable) CTDs. Even within a defined disease entity (e.g., SLE according to the criteria of the American College of Rheumatology), there is large heterogeneity, and hence added complexity, regarding clinical manifestations, genetic background, and autoantibody profiles.

Autoantibodies and Autoimmunity: Molecular Mechanisms in Health and Disease. Edited by K. Michael Pollard
Copyright © 2006 WILEY-VCH Verlag GmbH & Co. KGaA, Weinheim
ISBN: 3-527-31141-6

Table 10.1 Nature and examples of disease-specific autoantibodies.

Disease group	Autoantibodies directed against	Examples of autoantibody reactivities
Non-organ-specific (systemic) AIDs	Widely distributed autoantigens:	
• Rheumatoid arthritis	Citrullinated proteins/peptides	Citrullinated filaggrin
• Connective tissue diseases	Non-organ-specific, highly conserved nuclear or cytoplasmic antigens	Double-stranded DNA DNA topoisomerase I tRNA synthetases
• Antiphospholipid syndrome	Phospholipids (PL) and PL-associated proteins	Cardiolipin β2-glycoprotein I
• Systemic vasculitides	Enzymes of neutrophil granulocytes and monocytes	Myeloperoxidase Proteinase 3
Organ-specific AID	Tissue/organ-specific antigen(s)	Acetylcholine receptor Intrinsic factor Thyroperoxidase
Multiple organ-specific AID	Tissue/organ-specific antigens of different organs	

Furthermore, there is strong and accumulating support for familial clustering of specific manifestations of multiple systemic autoimmune diseases caused by genetic but perhaps also shared environmental factors [2].

Circulating disease–specific AABs are hallmarks of AIDs regardless of their pathogenic role. Whereas AABs in organ-specific AIDs are directed against antigens that are expressed in the targeted organ(s), AABs in systemic AIDs respond to widely distributed antigens. In autoimmune polyglandular endocrine syndromes that do not represent systemic but multiple organ-specific diseases, different organ-specific AABs are present (Table 10.1).

10.2
Distinguishing Features of Systemic Autoimmune Disease-specific Autoantibodies

There are striking differences in most features between naturally occurring AABs and disease-related AABs that are induced during the pathogenesis of organ-specific and systemic AIDs. Here we will focus on the main aspects of the humoral autoimmune response associated with systemic AIDs.

10.2.1
Heterogeneity of the Autoimmune Response

Although the autoimmune response in a defined AID is characterized by major molecular recognition patterns to the main autoantigen(s), this response is not uniform among patients with the same disease but may be heterogeneous with regard to the AAB's isotype, affinity/avidity, and epitope specificity as well as with regard to the intra- and intermolecular epitope spreading. Those variations may be in part responsible for differences in the results obtained by different AAB detection assays (see Section 10.2.4) and in variations in AAB profiles, in the pathogenicity of AABs, and in the clinical course of the disease. For example, proteinase 3 (PR3) antibodies of different patients with Wegener's granulomatosis (WG) recognize a limited number of epitopes of overlapping regions on PR3, but with interindividual differences in epitope specificity at the time of diagnosis and with intraindividual changes of epitope specificity during the course of disease [3]. Further investigation is required to determine whether the epitope specificity is responsible for the pathogenicity of PR3 autoantibodies. Anti-dsDNA antibodies in sera of patients with SLE are heterogeneous in relation to cross-reactivity with some proteins [4, 5]. The cross-reactivity of human SLE anti-dsDNA antibodies with a-actinin may contribute to the pathogenesis of lupus nephritis [5]. Heterogeneity may also occur regarding the recognition of distinctly modified forms of the respective autoantigen(s). An association between recognition of either apoptotically or oxidatively modified forms of the U1-70-kDa autoantigen with different clinical disease manifestations has been described [6].

10.2.2
Racial/Ethnic Variations in Frequency, Epitope Recognition, and Clinical Relevance of Disease-related Autoantibodies

Many studies have shown differences in the clinical as well as autoimmunologic presentation of systemic autoimmune diseases by race or ethnicity. This could be explained in part by different distributions of major histocompatibility complex (MHC) class II alleles as well as polymorphisms of genes coding for immunoglobulins, immune mediators, and regulators or genes coding for the appropriate autoantigen(s) itself. The distribution of many of the SLE-, SSc-, and myositis-related AABs differs among patients of various ethnic backgrounds. For example, Caucasian SSc patients have the highest frequency of anti-centromere antibodies (ACA), whereas American blacks have a higher frequency of anti-topoisomerase, anti-fibrillarin, and anti-fibrillin 1 antibodies [7, 8]. Anti-Sm antibodies were significantly more frequently seen in American black, Afro-Caribbean, and black South African SLE patients than in Caucasians [9, 10]. Besides such different AAB frequencies, striking ethnic differences in epitope recognition have been reported for some disease-specific AABs. For example, the frequency of reactivity of anti-topoisomerase antibodies to the region adjacent to the amino terminus of DNA topoisomerase I was lower in Caucasian and American black than in Japanese and Choctaw Native American SSc patients. Conversely, the frequency of reactivity to the region adjacent to the carboxyl terminus was lower in Japanese patients compared to patients from other ethnic groups [11]. Using three recombinant peptides of human fibrillin 1, spanning the N-terminal end, the proline-rich C region, and the epidermal growth factor-like calcium-binding repeats, significant differences in epitope recognition among Caucasian, African American, Choctaw Native American, and Japanese SSc patients were found [8]. Furthermore, ethnic variations in clinical presentations may occur even in immunologically similar groups. All anti-fibrillarin antibody-positive Afro-Caribbean patients had diffuse cutaneous SSc (dcSSc) compared to only 47% of the Caucasian patients. Therefore, the anti-fibrillarin antibody-positive limited cutaneous SSc (lcSSc) subset seems to be almost of Caucasian origin [12]. Anti-Ku antibodies in Japanese patients are strongly associated with scleroderma-polymyositis and SLE-scleroderma-polymyositis overlap syndromes, whereas in African American patients these AABs are associated with SLE [10]. Anti-PR3 antibody is a highly specific marker for Wegener's granulomatosis in Caucasians, whereas a marked variability in the spectrum of diseases associated with this AAB was described in the Chinese population [13]. In summary, the prevalence, epitope specificity, and clinical associations of disease-related AAB vary considerably among different racial/ethnic groups. This should be considered if the relevance of a defined AAB will be evaluated in retrospective and/or prospective studies. The racial/ethnic differences may reflect genetic, social, or environmental factors that have to be discovered. Because ethnic differences are seen for MHC [14] and also non-MHC genes [7], those genetic factors may be in part accountable for the described impact of ethnicity on the immunological and clinical presentation of systemic AIDs.

10.2.3
Autoantibodies as Predictors (Early Markers) of Disease

Most AIDs are characterized by a subclinical prodrome, during which the only evidence of the developing disorder may be the manifestation of disease-specific autoimmunity. Indeed, AABs that are typically produced in defined disease manifestations are detectable months to years before appearance of the respective clinical symptoms [15–26]. This has been shown for SLE-, RA-, SSc-, SjS-, and PM-typical AABs by retrospective (use of stored sera) and prospective (follow-up) studies (Table 10.2). Therefore, certain AABs might predict disease development in risk groups or even in the general population. The prediction of AIDs becomes more and more important as effective novel immune intervention therapies become available. Recently, the most important clinical utility of AAB testing has been diagnosis of the respective AIDs as early as possible or diagnosis of limited or non-typical forms of the disease (for examples, see Section 10.3.4.1).

Table 10.2 Autoantibodies as early indicators of the development
of systemic autoimmune diseases.

Autoantibodies directed against	Diseases	Retrospective (R) or prospective (P) studies	Ref.
Cyclic-citrullinated peptides (CCP)	Rheumatoid arthritis (RA)	**R:** analysis of stored sera from blood donors who developed RA showed that anti-CCP antibodies predate RA by several years (mean 4.5 years; range 0.1–13.8 years)	19, 20
Double-stranded DNA (dsDNA)	Systemic lupus erythematosus (SLE)	**R:** testing of stored sera from US Armed Services Serum Repository from former military personal who developed SLE showed that anti-dsDNA antibodies may appear up to 9 years (mean: 2.2 years) before onset of SLE	15
Sm	SLE	**R** (see dsDNA): anti-Sm antibodies may appear up to 8 years (mean: 1.5 years) before onset of SLE	15
Ro/SS-A	SLE, Sjögren's syndrome (SjS)	**R** (see dsDNA): anti-Ro/SS-A antibodies appeared as early as 10 years before the first onset of disease (mean 3.6 years) **P:** a 5–10-year follow-up of anti-Ro/SS-A–positive asymptomatic women who gave birth to babies with neonatal lupus showed that approximately half of these persons developed SLE, SjS, or undifferentiated syndromes	15–17
La/SS-B	SLE, SjS	**R** (see dsDNA): anti-La/SS-B antibodies may appear up to 8 years (mean: 3.6 years) before onset of SLE	15
Centromere proteins (CENP-B, ACA)	Systemic sclerosis (SSc)	**P:** patients with Raynaud's phenomenon (RP) initially positive for ACA or ATA had a 63-fold increased risk for developing signs of CTD/SSc compared to the remaining patients with RP **P:** more than one-third of asymptomatic ACA-positive uranium miners developed SSc manifestations or definite SSc	22–24, 26
DNA topoisomerase I (scl-70, ATA)	Systemic sclerosis	**P:** see ACA **P:** nearly one-third of asymptomatic ATA-positive uranium miners developed SSc manifestations or definite SSc	23, 24–26

10.2.4
Problems of Standardization of AAB Testing

Recent methods of AAB determination used in clinical laboratories lack universal standards. In most cases the "golden standard" for the evaluation of AAB detection assays is the typical clinical expression of the respective disease. The methods currently used include indirect immunofluorescence (IIF), immunodiffusion (Ouchterlony technique), Western blotting, dot/line blotting, and FARR- and enzyme-linked immunosorbent assays (ELISA). The results of these different assays are usually hard to compare. Furthermore, the diagnostic value of an autoantibody specificity varies according to the type of detection method used. Higher assay sensitivity usually results in higher diagnostic sensitivity, but often results in a lower specificity of a given autoantibody for the corresponding disease. For example, the autoantibodies to various "extractable nuclear antigens," which are used in double radial immunodiffusion (Ouchterlony technique), are highly specific for connective tissue diseases, though their sensitivity is limited. The use of highly sensitive ELISA increases the diagnostic sensitivity, but usually does so at the expense of diagnostic specificity. The optimal sensitivity:specificity ratio of a new assay should therefore be carefully determined before the assay is introduced for routine diagnostics. In general, it is hardly possible to use only one assay for optimal diagnostics because of the heterogeneity of the autoimmune response (see Section 10.2.1).

As a consequence of the above-mentioned points, one has to realize that effective and high-grade successful diagnostics cannot be exercised without tight collaboration among patients, clinicians, the diagnostic industry, and laboratory immunologists [27].

10.3
Autoantibodies as Diagnostic and/or Prognostic Markers in Systemic Autoimmune Diseases

A large variety of AABs with more or less disease specificity are detectable in systemic AIDs. With regard to the relevance, AABs may be classified as (1) AABs that are more frequently found in an AID than in controls but do not have any significant pathological or clinical relevance; (2) AABs that serve as disease markers regardless of their role in etiopathogenesis; and (3) AABs that are involved in pathological processes of disease progression or organ manifestations. Categories 2 and 3 are not mutually exclusive, as is shown for dsDNA antibodies (1: ACR criteria for the classification of SLE; 2: involved in kidney manifestation).

10.3.1
Autoantibodies in Rheumatoid Arthritis

Several AABs with more or less disease specificity have been described in RA patients. Although not specific for RA, rheumatoid factors belong to the classification criteria. Recently, it was shown that AABs with high specificity for RA are directed against proteins or peptides that are citrullinated in a sequence-specific manner (see Chapter 12).

10.3.2
Autoantibodies in Systemic Lupus Erythematosus

In sera of SLE patients more than 100 AAB specificities have been described so far [28]. The clinically relevant AABs are described in Chapter 11.

10.3.3
Autoantibodies in Sjögren's Syndrome

SjS is a chronic inflammatory autoimmune disease of unknown origin characterized by lymphocytic infiltration into exocrine glands. Its primary symptoms are keratoconjunctivitis sicca and xerostomia, but several extraglandular manifestations may occur. There are two types of SjS: primary SjS and secondary SjS, which is associated with another underlying autoimmune disease. Ro/SS-A and La/SS-B antibodies are included in the classification criteria for SjS [29] and are detectable in 60–75% and 30–50% of patients, respectively. Anti-La/SS-B antibodies are mostly found in SjS and SLE patients. Therefore, La/SS-B antibodies in the absence of SLE-specific AABs are highly specific for SjS. If negative for Ro/La AAB, α-fodrin antibodies may be determined. The sensitivity and specificity of these AABs for SjS are lower than described earlier, however [30]. Some rarely detectable AABs (Coilin-p80, NuMA, Golgi apparatus antibodies) have no relevance for the diagnosis of SjS. AABs reacting with the M3 muscarinic acetylcholine receptor (M3R) are described as highly sensitive and highly specific SjS. Those AABs are probably involved in the pathogenesis of SjS [31, 32].

10.3.4
Autoantibodies in Systemic Sclerosis (Scleroderma)

10.3.4.1 Characteristics, Heterogeneity, and Subsets of Systemic Sclerosis
Systemic sclerosis (SSc), also called scleroderma, is a generalized autoimmune disorder characterized by vascular damage and fibrosis within the skin and visceral organs, notably the gut, lung, heart, kidney, joints, and muscles. With regard to the extent of skin and internal organ involvement, the pace of disease progression and, consequently, the prognosis, patients with SSc present a high degree of variability. According to the preliminary ACR criteria for the classification of SSc, the presence of either the major criterion (symmetric skin sclerosis proximal to the MCP and/or MTP joints) or two or more of the minor criteria (sclerodactyly, digital pitting scars, bibasilar lung fibrosis) classify a condition as SSc with 97% sensitivity and 98% specificity [33]. If used for the diagnosis in the single patient, these criteria may be quite misleading, because they do not allow the diagnosis of early SSc or "sclerosis sine scleroderma," a disorder with primary organ involvement in the absence of or prior to skin fibrosis. In the presence of SSc-specific autoantibodies (Table 10.3), patients with Raynaud's phenomenon (RP) or other symptoms of a peripheral vascular disease or pa-

Table 10.3 Diagnostic relevant autoantibodies in patients with systemic sclerosis overlap syndromes with scleroderma.

Autoantibody	Disease association	Prognosis and organ manifestations
Anti-centromere (ACA)	SSc (lcSSc) CREST syndrome	Gastrointestinal complications and increased risk of pulmonary hypertension; otherwise lower frequency of internal organ manifestation Lower mortality than SSc patients with anti-scl-70 or anti-nucleolar antibodies
Anti-scl-70 (ATA)	SSc (dcSSc)	Increased frequency of pulmonary fibrosis Relation with cancer? Worse prognosis
Anti-U3-RNP/ fibrillarin (AFA)	SSc (dcSSc)	Myositis, pulmonary hypertension, renal disease
Anti-Th/To	SSc (lcSSc)	Milder skin and systemic involvement Worse prognosis because of more severe pulmonary involvement
Anti-RNAP	SSc (dcSSc)	High frequency of systemic involvement (heart, lung, kidney) Increased mortality
Anti-PM/Scl	PM/Scl-overlap, but also in SSc and myositis alone Juvenile sclero-myositis	Benign course with better response to steroids
Anti-U1-RNP	MCTD, but also in SSc alone	More benign course
Anti-Ku	Overlap syndrome with scleroderma features	

tients with RP plus internal organ involvement (hypomotility of the distal esophagus and/or small bowel, interstitial lung disease, pulmonary hypertension, SSc-typical renal or cardiac manifestations) may suffer from SSc without satisfying ACR criteria, especially if other CTDs can be excluded [34, 35].

Because of the extreme variability of SSc, various disease subsets have been defined with the aim of prognosticating different disease courses, such as pace of disease progression and development of internal organ involvement [36, 37]. Patients with diffuse cutaneous (dc) SSc are characterized by diffuse involvement of the skin and early occurrence of internal organ involvement, whereas limited cutaneous (lc) SSc remains confined to the face and to regions distal to the elbow or knee joints. Patients with lcSSc develop less organ involvement than those with dcSSc. The so-called CREST syndrome characterized by calcinosis cutis, RP, esophageal dysfunction, sclerodactyly, and telangiectasia belongs to the limited SSc subset. Furthermore, a distinct intermediate cutaneous (ic) SSc subset, which differs from both lcSSc and dcSSc in terms of evolution and prognosis, should be differentiated [38, 39].

Scleroderma-specific autoantibodies associate strongly with distinct clinical phenotypes, making serologic testing of great diagnostic aid. Out of the several autoantibody specificities detected in the sera of SSc patients (Table 10.3) anti-centromere antibodies (ACAs), anti-scl-70 antibodies, and anti–RNA polymerase III antibodies are useful for defining subgroups in the clinical setting. For example, ACAs are confined to patients with lcSSc and are associated with calcinosis, telangiectasia, and a longer survival. Anti-scl-70 antibodies are more prevalent in, but not specific of, dcSSc (and icSSc) and are associated with interstitial lung fibrosis [40]. Anti-RNA polymerase III antibodies are associated with heart and kidney involvement in patients with dcSSc [41]. Therefore, clinical and serological subsets can be useful in diagnostic approaches, disease monitoring, and treatment decisions. For example, anti-scl-70-positive dcSSc patients should be carefully searched for alveolitis early on.

10.3.4.2 Anti-centromere Antibodies

ACAs that are relevant for scleroderma diagnosis are directed against the centromere-associated proteins (CENP) CENP-A (17 kDa), CENP-B (80 kDa), and CENP-C (140 kDa). CENP-B is the antigen most commonly targeted by ACAs. Autoantibodies directed against other centromeric proteins (e.g., proteins only transiently associated with the centromere) are not included in the "diagnostic-category" ACAs. The method of choice for detecting ACAs is indirect immunofluorescence (IIF) using monolayers of tumor cells (usually HEp-2). The number of spots corresponds to the number of chromosomes in interphase nuclei and in the equatorial plane of mitotic cells. If the typical ACA pattern is masked by other autoantibodies, an enzyme immunoassay using recombinant CENP-B protein should be used. ACAs are diagnostic markers for systemic sclerosis with a specificity of >95% (SSc versus other CTD) to nearly 100% (SSc versus normal controls) and a sensitivity of 20–30% in general (reviewed in [42]). The frequency varies in different ethnic and clinical groups. ACAs are most often seen in CREST syndrome and similar variants, with a relatively mild clinical course and lower mortality compared to SSc patients with anti-scl-70 or antinucleolar antibodies. The prevalence of interstitial pulmonary fibrosis and renal involvement in ACA-positive scleroderma patients is very low. However, ACA-positive patients do have an increased risk of pulmonary hypertension and ischemic digital loss. The occurrence of ACAs in high-risk patients or patients with Raynaud's phenomenon is an important indicator of the potential for SSc development [22–24, 26]. ACAs can be detected years before the occurrence of specific symptoms of scleroderma. ACAs are also detectable in patients with primary biliary cirrhosis (PBC). Roughly half of these patients have concomitant scleroderma or signs of the development of scleroderma (e.g., Raynaud's phenomenon). ACAs are infrequently detectable in circumscribed forms of scleroderma as well as in SLE, polymyositis/dermatomyositis, primary pulmonary hypertension, and chronic active hepatitis. Positive ACA test results can also indicate the potential for the development of scleroderma in these patients.

10.3.4.3 Anti-topoisomerase I Antibodies

The so-called anti-topoisomerase I (anti-scl-70) antibodies target DNA topoisomerase I, which is found in the nucleoplasm and nucleolus and catalyzes the cleavage and rebinding of single-stranded DNA during the relaxation phase of supercoiled DNA. Although the name "Scl-70 antibody" is still used, the scientifically more correct name is "anti-topoisomerase I antibody" (ATA). IIF using HEp-2 cells usually reveals fine granular to homogeneous staining of the nucleoplasm with or without (depending on the substance used for fixation) staining of the nucleoli and chromatin of mitotic cells. Immunodiffusion, enzyme immunoassay, and Western blot are used in routine diagnostic testing. ATAs are marker antibodies with a diagnostic specificity of >99%. The sensitivity for diagnosis of SSc is 15–43% (reviewed in [42]). ATAs are associated with diffuse skin involvement and internal manifestations (lung, heart, kidney). ATA-positive scleroderma patients generally have a more severe clinical course and a poorer prognosis than their ACA-positive counterparts. The co-occurrence of ATA with other SSc marker antibodies is extremely rare. ATA detection in high-risk patients (e.g., miners with a history of silica exposure) or patients with Raynaud's phenomenon is an important warning of the possible development of SSc [23, 24, 26].

10.3.4.4 Anti-nucleolar and Anti-RNA Polymerase Antibodies

The term "anti-nucleolar antibodies" describes all autoantibodies that show a nucleolar pattern by IIF on Hep-2 cells. The autoantigenic targets that are relevant for SSc are fibrillarin, PM-Scl, RNA polymerase I, and To/Th antigen. High-titer anti-nucleolar antibodies are diagnostic markers for SSc, but may also be detected in patients with tumors (especially hepatocellular carcinoma) and other diseases, depending on the target specificity.

Anti-fibrillarin antibodies (AFAs) are directed against fibrillarin, the main protein component of the nucleolar U3-RNP complex, which is involved in pre-rRNA processing. Fibrillarin is also a component of other small nucleolar ribonucleoprotein (snoRNP) complexes. By IIF on Hep-2 cells, AFAs reveal a granular (clumpy) nucleolar immunofluorescence pattern. Chromosomal staining in metaphase may also be observed. Specific, highly sensitive methods for detection of fibrillarin antibodies are not yet available for routine use. AFAs are detectable in fewer than 10% of patients with SSc (associated with dcSSc) but have also been described in patients with SLE and localized scleroderma (reviewed in [42]). Fibrillarin antibody production was induced using mercury salts in a mouse model [43]. This suggests that exogenous factors may play a role in pathogenesis.

Anti-Th/To antibodies target components of the ribonuclease MRP and the ribonuclease P complexes. IIF using HEp-2 cells reveals a homogeneous nucleolar staining pattern. They are detectable in 2–5% of patients with SSc and are associated with milder skin and organ involvement, with one exception: pulmonary arterial hypertension (reviewed in [42]).

Anti-RNA polymerase antibodies target RNA polymerases (RNAPs) of the RNAP multiprotein complexes consisting of 8–14 proteins weighing 10–220 kDa. There are three classes of RNAPs (RNAPs I, II, III). Whereas only RNAP-I is localized in the nucleolus, RNAPs II and III are localized in the nucleoplasm. Since the different types of RNAP antibodies often occur in combination, it is hardly possible to make a differential assessment of the clinical relevance of the individual specificities. RNAP-I antibodies are observed in 4–11% of patients with systemic sclerosis (scleroderma) but are rarely detected in other autoimmune diseases. They are associated with severe, diffuse forms of scleroderma. These patients have a poor prognosis because they tend to have a higher frequency of cardiac, hepatic, and renal involvement. RNAP-III antibodies are detected in 12–23% of patients with systemic sclerosis and are frequently associated with RNAP-I and RNAP-II antibodies. RNAP-III antibodies seem to be specific for scleroderma since they have not yet been found in any other disease. They are associated with diffuse or extensive skin manifestations and with heart and kidney involvement [41]. RNAP-III antibodies have also been detected during a renal crisis in the absence of skin manifestations, i.e., sclerosis without scleroderma [44].

10.3.5
Autoantibodies in Idiopathic Inflammatory Myopathies

The idiopathic inflammatory myopathies (IIMs, autoimmune myositides) comprise a heterogeneous group of rare diseases characterized by skeletal muscle inflammation and a variety of systemic symptoms. The two most common types are dermatomyositis (DM) and polymyositis (PM). The typical features are muscle soreness and increasing muscle weakness that ultimately progresses to muscular atrophy. PM and DM have different pathogenetic bases and histomorphological features: DM is characterized by complement-dependent membranolysis of the intramuscular capillaries, whereas PM is associated with cytotoxic T lymphocytes. In patients with IIM, a variety of myositis-specific autoantibodies (MSAs) and myositis-associated autoantibodies (MAAs) have been described (Table 10.4). MAAs are found also in connective tissue diseases without the presence of myositis, whereas MSAs are highly specific for IIM. Despite this high specificity, MSAs are (up to now) not included in the widely used classification criteria for the diagnosis of DM and PM [45]. Furthermore, some MSAs are specific markers for different subtypes of IIMs that differ in clinical manifestation, disease severity, response to immunosuppressive therapy, prognosis, and pathogenesis (for review, see [46]). Most of the known MSAs are directed against cytoplasmic ribonucleoproteins involved in the process of protein syn-

Table 10.4 Autoantibodies in patients with idiopathic inflammatory myopathies.

Myositis-specific autoantibodies (MSA)	Disease association	Prognosis and organ manifestations
Anti-Mi-2	Classic DM	Good prognosis; however, association with malignancies
Anti-aminoacyl-tRNA synthetases Anti-Jo-1 (His-tRNA synthetase) Anti-PL-7 (Thr-tRNA synthetase) Anti-PL-12 (Ala-tRNA synthetase) Anti-EJ (Glu-tRNA synthetase) Anti-OJ (Ile-tRNA synthetase) Anti-KS (Asp-tRNA synthetase)	PM (anti-synthetase syndrome)	Fibrosing alveolitis, polysynovitis More severe clinical course, frequent active episodes, and a poor prognosis
Anti-SRP	PM (anti-SRP syndrome)	Relatively rapid progression to severe muscle weakness Cardiac involvement? Poor prognosis

thesis. The currently used diagnostic markers are directed to several tRNA-synthetases (anti-Jo-1 antibodies among others), to components of the signal recognition particle (anti-SRP antibodies), and to components of a nucleosome-remodeling complex (anti-Mi-2 antibodies).

Anti-aminoacyl-tRNA synthetase antibodies (anti-synthetase antibodies) are directed against cytoplasmic enzymes that catalyze the binding of a specific amino acid to the corresponding transfer RNA (tRNA) molecule. The most frequently detectable anti-synthetase antibody is the anti-Jo-1 antibody, which binds the histidyl-tRNA synthetase. Aminoacyl-tRNA synthetase antibodies are specific markers for IIM, especially PM. The diseases associated with these autoantibodies usually have similar symptoms and are therefore referred to as anti-Jo-1 or anti-synthetase syndrome [46, 47]. This subset of IIM is characterized by the additional occurrence of fibrosing alveolitis and polysynovitis. Except for Jo-1 antibodies, the individual aminoacyl-tRNA synthetase antibodies are very rarely found in IIM (<1–3%). The sensitivity and specificity of Jo-1 antibodies for IIM in adults is approximately 30% and >99%, respectively. In juvenile myositis, Jo-1 antibodies are seldom found. Myositis patients positive for Jo-1 antibodies tend to have a more severe clinical course, frequent active episodes, and a poor prognosis.

Anti-SRP antibodies are directed against proteins of the cytoplasmatic signal recognition particles (SRPs). SRPs are ribonucleoprotein complexes consisting of one 7SL RNA and six different proteins (SRP9, SRP14, SRP19, SRP54, SRP68, and SRP74). SRP antibodies mainly react with protein SRP54, and some also react with SRP68 and SRP72. They are diagnostic markers for IIM with a diagnostic specificity of virtually 100% and a sensitivity of roughly 4%. SRP antibodies may define a relatively homogeneous group of patients with similar clinical symptoms [46, 48]. In contrast to myositis patients with aminoacyl-tRNA synthetase antibodies, patients with SRP antibodies do not exhibit involvement of the joints, lungs, or skin. Many of the patients do not respond well to immunosuppressants. They have the poorest prognosis of all patients with myositis!

Anti-Mi-2 antibodies are diagnostic markers for IIM with a diagnostic sensitivity of 5–12%. They can be found more frequently in DM than in PM. Roughly 95% of patients who test positive for anti-Mi-2 antibodies have DM, and around 3% have PM. Compared to the myositis patients who test positive for aminoacyl-tRNA synthetase or SRP antibodies, those positive for Mi-2 antibodies generally have a relatively mild clinical course; rarely exhibit synovitis, lung manifestations, or Raynaud's phenomenon; and respond well to glucocorticosteroids. However, the clinical association may differ depending on the detection method used (Ouchterlony versus ELISA; see also Sections 10.2.1 and 10.2.4) or the ethnic background of the studied patients [49, 50].

10.3.6
Autoantibodies in Mixed Connective Tissue Disease

Mixed connective tissue disease (MCTD) or Sharp syndrome combines features of SLE, SSc, and IIM [51]. The sera of these patients contain high titers of antinuclear antibodies (granular fluorescence pattern) directed against U1-RNP. Whether or not the corresponding clinical picture first described by Gordon Sharp in 1971 is really a separate nosological entity remains a subject of debate.

Anti-U1-RNP autoantibodies are directed against the U1-snRNP-specific proteins A (34 kDa), C (22 kDa), and 68 kDa (70 kDa). Indirect immunofluorescence using cell monolayers (HEp-2) reveals moderately granular staining (these granules mark the foci of spliceosomal components) superimposed on diffuse nucleoplasmic fluorescence. The nucleoli are negative. Ouchterlony, ELISA, and dot-blot/line assays are used in routine diagnostics. In the absence of Sm and dsDNA antibodies, U1-RNP antibodies are diagnostic markers of MCTD that belong to the classification criteria [51]. According to these criteria, the absence of U1-RNP antibodies essentially rules out the Sharp syndrome. U1-RNP antibodies are also found in 13–32% of patients with SLE. The data on the association of the antibodies to different manifestations of SLE are very inconsistent, but the positive association between U1-RNP antibodies and vasculitic skin and mucosal manifestations (discoid lesions, oral ulcers) and Raynaud's phenomenon is relatively well confirmed. In SSc, U1-RNP antibodies are found in up to 10% of the affected patients and are associated with pulmonary fibrosis and joint involvement.

10.3.7
Autoantibodies in Polymyositis-Scleroderma Overlap Syndrome (Scleromyositis)

Overlap syndromes with features of both PM and SSc are associated with PM-Scl and Ku antibodies. However, negative tests for these AABs do not exclude the possibility of PM-scleroderma overlap syndrome.

PM-Scl antibodies are directed against components of the exosome, a complex consisting of 11–16 proteins (20–110 kDa) located in the granular part of the nucleoli and in the nucleoplasm. The main targets of PM-Scl antibodies are proteins of 100 kDa (PM-Scl-100) and of 75 kDa (PM-Scl-75). PM-Scl antibodies are highly characteristic of, although not specific for, PM-scleroderma overlap syndrome [52]. They are detectable in approximately 24% of patients with PM-scleroderma overlap syndrome, in 8–12% with IIM, and in 1–16% with SSc. Apart from myositis, arthritis and Raynaud's phenomenon are the most common manifestations observed in PM-Scl antibody-positive patients. Cardiac and renal involvement is very rare. The prognosis for these patients is therefore relatively good. In childhood, the PM-Scl antibody-positive scleromyositis appears to be the most common scleroderma-like disease [53]. The clinical course is relatively benign compared to that of juvenile dermatomyositis or scleroderma.

Ku antibodies are directed against DNA-binding, non-histone proteins (p70/p80 heterodimers) and the catalytic subunit (p350) of DNA-dependent protein kinase (DNA-PK). Ku antibodies are detectable in patients with myositis-scleroderma overlap syndrome but can also be found in patients with primary pulmonary hypertension, SLE, and other connective tissue diseases (reviewed in [42]).

10.3.8
The Antiphospholipid Syndrome

The Antiphospholipid Syndrome (APS), also called Hughes syndrome, is a multi-system thrombophilic disorder associated with circulating AABs directed against negatively charged phospholipids (PL) and PL-binding proteins [54, 55]. APS may occur as an isolated disease entity (primary APS) or in combination with another autoimmune disease, especially systemic lupus erythematosus (secondary APS). The clinical features of APS are caused by venous and/or arterial thrombosis and/or pregnancy morbidity. According to the localization and severity of thrombosis, the clinical picture is extremely variable, and the complications arising from the disease may be minimal to life-threatening. International clinical and laboratory criteria have provided consensus on the typical features of the syndrome [54]. Several manifestations are relatively common in APS patients (deep vein occlusions affecting the lower limbs, stroke, large vessel occlusions, fetal loss, thrombocytopenia, livedo reticularis). However, many other clinical manifestations with lower prevalence have been described – such as chorea, acute encephalopathy, or avascular necrosis of the bone – showing that the full expression of this syndrome is more heterogeneous [56]. In clinical practice, the lupus anticoagulant (LA) detected by clotting assays as well as the anticardiolipin (aCL) and anti-β2-glycoprotein I antibodies detected by ELISA are the most widely used tests for the serological diagnosis of APS. However, according to the heterogeneous entity of this syndrome, other AABs against phospholipids (phosphatidylserine, phosphatidylinositol, phosphatidyl-ethanolamine, phosphatidylcholine) or PL-binding proteins (prothrombin, annexin V, protein C, protein S) are or may be involved in APS patients.

The laboratory criteria for the classification of APS include antiphospholipid antibodies (aPLs) determined by the standardized β2-dependent anticardiolipin (IgG and/or IgM) and the lupus anticoagulant assay. These assays must be positive on two or more occasions at least six weeks apart [54]. A definite APS can be diagnosed if at least one of the clinical criteria (manifestation of vascular thrombosis and pregnancy morbidity) and one of the laboratory criteria is present. Anti-CL antibodies are also frequently detectable in patients with other systemic AIDs (especially SLE) and are associated with the presence or development of thrombotic manifestations (secondary APS). However, aCLs predict the development of thrombosis only at a low frequency in those patients. An anticoagulant therapy is not recommended in aCL-positive patients in the absence of a thrombotic event. Because the morbidity following thrombosis is significant, it is necessary to look for risk factors with a high predictive value to prevent serious thrombotic events by early anticoagulant therapy. For example, a high-titer aPL and the presence of more than one aPL increase the association with clinical symptoms of APS [57, 58]. Prospective studies should be done to evaluate the predictive value of different aPL antibody profiles. Such profiles should also include novel aPL assays such as the aPS/PT assay for the determination of AABs against phosphatidylserine-prothrombin complexes [59].

10.3.9
ANCA-associated Vasculitides

ANCA-associated vasculitides, which include Wegener's granulomatosis (WG), microscopic polyangiitis (MPA), and Churg-Strauss syndrome (CSS), are characterized by interactions between anti-neutrophil cytoplasm autoantibodies (AN-CAs) and neutrophils initiating endothelial and vascular injury. Focal necrotizing lesions are the common vascular pathology of the ANCA-associated disorders. According to the localization and severity of those lesions, a variety of symptoms and signs can be seen. In contrast to anti-glomerular basement membrane disease, IgA nephropathy, or lupus nephritis, the immunohistology shows little deposition of immune reactants. Myeloperoxidase (MPO) was identified as the target antigen of MPA-associated ANCAs, and proteinase 3 (PR3) as that of WG-associated ANCAs [60, 61]. ANCAs are determined by IIF using ethanol-fixed human neutrophils and by ELISA using MPO or PR3 as target antigen. Most PR3 antibodies produce a granular cytoplasmic (cANCA) pattern, whereas most MPO antibodies produce a perinuclear (pANCA) immunofluorescence pattern.

10.3.9.1 Anti-proteinase 3 Antibodies (PR3-ANCAs)

Proteinase 3 (PR3) is a multifunctional protein found in the azurophil (primary) granules of neutrophils, in the granules of monocytes, and in the cytoplasm of endothelial cells. Antibodies against PR3 are highly specific for WG. The diagnostic sensitivity of these AABs is dependent on the stage and activity of disease: roughly 50% in the inactive initial stage, roughly 60% in active mono- or oligosymptomatic forms (kidney or lung involvement), and virtually 100% in the active generalized phase. A positive PR3-ANCA result is highly specific and permits the definitive diagnosis of early and abortive forms of WG as well as a number of limited forms of WG, e.g., in patients with scleritis, episcleritis, subglottic stenosis, Tolosa-Hunt syndrome, facial paresis, cranial polyneuritis, peripheral neuropathy, secondary polychondritis, pulmonary hemorrhage, idiopathic progressive necrotizing nephritis, and hemodialysis patients with renal failure of unclear origin (reviewed in [62]). PR3-ANCAs are also found at low frequencies in other vasculitic diseases associated with WG (e.g., microscopic polyangiitis, Churg-Strauss syndrome, classical panarteritis nodosa). In WG, PR3-ANCA titers correlate with disease activity, i.e., they decrease in remission (response to therapy) and increase when exacerbation is imminent. PR3-ANCA monitoring can therefore be used to ensure optimal patient management.

10.3.9.2 Anti-myeloperoxidase Antibodies (MPO-ANCAs)

Myeloperoxidase (MPO), an enzyme found in the azurophil (primary) granules of neutrophils, is a homodimer with a molecular weight of approximately 140 kDa. MPO-ANCA is the diagnostic marker for MPA in general (sensitivity 60–80%) as well as a diagnostic marker for immunohistologically negative ("pauci-immune") focal necrotizing glomerulonephritis, which – when inadequately managed – can transform into extracapillary proliferative, rapidly progressive glomerulonephritis (RPNG). Pauci-immune glomerulonephritis can occur as a component of systemic vasculitis (especially MPA) or as an "idiopathic" type (without signs of extrarenal vasculitis). MPO-ANCAs are detectable in roughly 65% of patients with this type of glomerulonephritis. Exogenous factors such as medications (mainly hydralazine and propylthiouracil, but also penicillamine, methimazole, allopurinol, and sulfasalazine) or silica exposure are currently being discussed as potential triggers in some of these cases. MPO-ANCAs are also found in 30–40% of patients with renopulmonary syndrome ("anti-GBM disease"). The patients tend to be older and respond to immunosuppressant therapy better than patients with GBM antibodies alone. Low frequencies of MPO-ANCAs have been found in WG, CSS, and classical panarteritis nodosa. The MPO-ANCA titer is frequently associated with the disease activity of ANCA-associated vasculitis. MPO-ANCAs have also been described in non-ANCA-associated diseases such as vasculitic lesions in patients treated with thyreostatic drugs, connective tissue diseases (up to 10%), hydralazine-induced lupus erythematosus (10–100%), and chronic inflammatory bowel disease (reviewed in [62]). The prevalence of drug-induced MPO-ANCA-associated vasculitis may be higher than was previously assumed [63].

To ensure a timely and effective initiation of treatment, MPO-ANCA antibodies should be determined at even the slightest suspicion of renal vasculitis. Without adequate treatment, the development of terminal renal failure is often inevitable.

10.4
Summary and Perspectives

Disease-specific and even disease-associated AABs are important biomarkers not only to confirm the diagnosis of the respective systemic AID but also to diagnose the disease at very early stages (mono- or oligosymptomatic manifestations) or to diagnose the respective disease without the typical clinical manifestations (atypical forms). A confirmation of the diagnosis in early stages is required if patients are to benefit from early therapeutic intervention. For example, it has been shown that treatment with disease-modifying anti-rheumatic drugs initiated within only three months of symptom onset of RA (very early RA) is beneficial when compared to even a short delay of such therapy [64]. Because the clinical picture of early systemic AIDs is not always characteristic and the classification criteria are frequently not fulfilled at early disease stages, AAB tests with high diagnostic specificity and high predictive values are necessary. Such assays may also replace more invasive and costly diagnostic techniques. Furthermore, some AAB specificities are predictors of certain organ manifestations and can help in the early recognition of fatal complications of systemic diseases such as pulmonary hypertension (PHT) or renal crisis. For example, anti-U3-RNP antibody is strongly associated with PHT in SSc patients [65]. As a novel and successful medication of PHT with endothelin receptor blocker became recently available, AABs together with other risk factors are very helpful in early therapy decisions. Early therapy may possibly prevent, delay, or attenuate this severe complication [65].

Another valuable use of AABs is that they facilitate an understanding of the complex pathogenesis of systemic AIDs. AABs may amplify autoimmune responses by alterations of antigen presentation (leading to intra- and intermolecular epitope spreading of the immune response) or by direct pathogenicity [66]. Direct pathogenicity of diagnostically relevant AABs has been shown only for Ro/SS-A antibodies (congenital heart block), ANCAs (vasculitides), and perhaps aPLs (thrombosis). However, there is increasing evidence that other disease-specific AABs may play a direct role in disease pathogenesis. For example, it was demonstrated recently that anti-topoisomerase I antibodies bind specifically to determinants of the fibroblast surface [67]. The molecular identity of these determinants and the possible role of an anti-fibroblast activity are being studied. Furthermore, novel AABs with a probable pathogenic role in general (e.g., matrix metalloproteinase-inhibiting AABs in SSc) or in special manifestations (e.g., anti-carbonic anhydrase II antibodies in pulmonary involvement of SSc) have been described [68, 69]. Although many clinically useful novel AAB specificities are not yet available in routine practice, the rapid development of new technologies that permit detection of multiple AABs in a single platform (e.g., addressable laser bead assays or microchip arrays) may bring these into widespread use.

References

1 Rose NR: Foreword – The uses of autoantibodies. In: Autoantibodies (Eds: Shoenfeld Y and Peter JB), Amsterdam: Elsevier, Amsterdam 1996, p. xxvii–xxixv.

2 Criswell LA: Familial clustering of disease features: Implications for the etiology and investigation of systemic autoimmune diseases. Arthritis Rheum 2004; 50:1707–1708.

3 Rarok AA, van der Geld Y, Stegeman CA, Limburg PC, Kallenberg CGM: Diversity of PR3-ANCA epitope specificity in Wegener's granulomatosis. Analysis using biosensor technology. J Clin Immunol 2003; 23:460–468.

4 Takeda I, Rayno K, Wolfson-Reichlin M, Reichlin M: Heterogeneity of anti-dsDNA antibodies in their cross-reaction with ribosomal P proteins. J Autoimmun 1999; 13:423–428.

5 Zhao Z, Weinstein E, Tuzova M, Davidson A, Mundel P, Marambio P, Putterman C: Cross-reactivity of human lupus anti-DNA antibodies with α-actinin and nephritogenic potential. Arthritis Rheum 2005; 52:522–530.

6 Greidinger EL, Casciola-Rosen L, Morris SM, Hoffman RW, Rosen A: Autoantibody recognition of distinctly modified forms of the U1-70-kd antigen is associated with different clinical disease manifestations. Arthritis Rheum 2000; 43:881–888.

7 Reveille JD: Ethnicity and race and systemic sclerosis: how it affects susceptibility, severity, antibody genetics, and clinical manifestations. Curr Rheumatol Rep 2003; 5:160–167.

8 Tan FK, Arnett FC, Reveille JD, Ahn C, Antohi S, Sasaki T, Nishioka K, Bona CA: Autoantibodies to fibrillin 1 in systemic sclerosis. Ethnic differences in antigen recognition and lack of correlation with specific clinical features or

HLA alleles. Arthritis Rheum 2000; 43:2464–2471.

9 Cooper GS, Parks CG, Treadwell EL, StClair EW, Gilkeson GS, Cohen PL, Roubey RAS, Dooley MA: Differences by race, sex and age in the clinical and immunologic features of recently diagnosed systemic lupus erythematosus patients in the southeastern United States. Lupus 2002; 11:161–167.

10 Wang J, Satoh M, Kabir F, Shaw M, Domingo MA, Mansoor R, Behney KM, Dong X, Lahita RG, Richards HB, Reeves WH: Increased prevalence of autoantibodies to Ku antigen in African American versus white patients with systemic lupus erythematosus. Arthritis Rheum 2001; 44:2367–2370.

11 Kuwana M, Kaburaki J, Arnett FC, Howard RF, Medsger TA, Wright TM: Influence of ethnic background on clinical and serologic features in patients with systemic sclerosis and anti-DNA topoisomerase I antibody. Arthritis Rheum 1999; 42:365–474.

12 Tormey VJ, Bunn CC, Denton CP, Black CM: Anti-fibrillarin antibodies in systemic sclerosis. Rheumatology 2001; 40:1157–1162.

13 Lee SS, Lawton JWM: Heterogeneity of anti-PR3 associated disease in Hong Kong. Postgrad Med J 2000; 76:287–288.

14 Takeuchi F, Nabeta H, Füssel M, Conrad K, Frank KH: Association of the TNFα13 microsatellite with systemic sclerosis in Japanese patients. Ann Rheum Dis 2000; 59:293–296.

15 Airbuckle MR, McClain MT, Rubertone MV, Scofield H, Dennis GJ, James JA, Harley JB: Development of autoantibodies before the clinical onset of systemic lupus erythematosus. N Engl J Med 2003; 349:1526–1533.

16 Waltuck J, Buyon JP: Autoantibody-associated congenital heart block: outcome in mothers and children. Ann Intern Med 1994; 120:544–551.

17 Julkunen H, Eronen M: Long-term outcome of mothers of children with isolated heart block in Finland. Arthritis Rheum 2001; 44:647–652.

18 Del Puente A, Knowler WC, Pettitt DJ, Bennett PH: The incidence of rheumatoid arthritis is predicted by rheumatoid factor titer in a longitudinal population study. Arthritis Rheum 1988; 31:1239–1244.

19 Nielen MMJ, van Schaardenburg D, Reesink HW, van de Stadt RJ, van der Horst-Bruinsma IE, de Koning MHMT, Habibuw MR, Vandenbroucke JP, Dijkmans BAC: Specific autoantibodies precede the symptoms of rheumatoid arthritis: a study of serial measurements in blood donors. Arthritis Rheum 2004; 50:380–386.

20 Rantapää-Dahlqvist S, de Jong BAW, Berglin E, Hallmans G, Wadell G, Stenlund H, Sundin U, van Venrooij WJ: Antibodies against cyclic citrullinated peptide and IgA rheumatoid factor predict the development of rheumatoid arthritis. Arthritis Rheum 2003; 48:2741–2749.

21 Iijima T, Tada H, Hidaka Y, Yagoro A, Mitsuda N, Kanzaki T, Murata Y, Amino N: Prediction of postpartum onset of rheumatoid arthritis. Ann Rheum Dis 1998; 57:460–463.

22 Tramposch HD, Smith CD, Senécal JL, Rothfield NF: A long-term longitudinal study of anticentromere antibodies. Arthritis Rheum 1984; 27:121–124.

23 Weiner ES, Hildebrandt S, Senécal JL, Daniels L, Noell S, Joyal F, Roussin A, Earnshaw W, Rothfield NF: Prognostic significance of anticentromere antibodies and anti-topoisomerase I antibodies in Raynaud's disease. Arthritis Rheum 1991; 34:68–77.

24 Conrad K, Mehlhorn J: Diagnostic and prognostic relevance of autoantibodies in uranium miners. Int Arch Allergy Immunol 2000; 123:77–91.

25 Satoh M, Miyazaki K, Mimori T, Akizuki M, Ichikawa Y, Homma M, Ajimani AK, Reves WH: Changing autoantibody profiles with variable clinical manifestations in a patient with relapsing systemic lupus erythematosus and polymyositis. Br J Rheumatol 1995; 34:915–919.

26 Kallenberg CG, Wouda AA, Hoet MH, van Venrooij WJ: Development of connective tissue disease in patients presenting with Raynaud's phenomenon: a six year follow up with emphasis on the predictive value of antinuclear antibodies as detected by immunoblotting. Ann Rheum Dis 1988; 47:634–641.

27 Wiik AS, Gordon TP, Kavanaugh AF, Lahita RG, Reeves W, van Venrooij WJ, Wilson MR, Fritzler M, and the IUIS/WHO/AF/CDC Committee for the Standardization of Autoantibodies in Rheumatic and Related Diseases: Cutting Edge Diagnostics in Rheumatology: The Role of Patients, Clinicians, and Laboratory Scientists in Optimizing the Use of Autoimmune Serology. Arthritis Rheum 2004; 51:291–298.

28 Sherer Y, Gorstein A, Fritzler MJ, Shoenfeld Y: Autoantibody explosion in systemic lupus erythematosus: more than 100 different antibodies found in SLE patients. Semin Arthritis Rheum 2004; 34:501–537.

29 Vitali C, Bombardieri S, Jonsson R, Moutsopoulos HM, Alexander HL, Carsons SE, Daniels TE, Fox PC, Fox RI, Kassan SS, Pillemer SR, Talal N, Weisman HM: Classification criteria for Sjögren's syndrome: a revised version of the European criteria proposed by the American-European Consensus Group. Ann Rheum Dis 2002; 61:554–558.

30 Zandbelt MM, Vogelzangs J, van de Putte LBA, van Venrooij WJ, van den Hoogen FHJ: Anti-fodrin antibodies do not add much to the diagnosis of Sjögren's syndrome. Arthritis Res Ther 2004; 6:R33–R38.

31 Bacman S, Sterin-Borda L, Camusso JJ, Arana R, Hubscher O, Borda E: Circulating antibodies against rat parotid gland M3 muscarinic receptors in primary Sjögren's syndrome. Clin Exp Immunol 1996; 104:454–459.

32 Naito Y, Matsumoto I, Wakamatsu E, Goto D, Sugiyama T, Matsumura R, Ito S, Tsutsumi A, Sumida T: Muscarinic

acetylcholine receptor autoantibodies in patients with Sjögren's syndrome. Ann Rheum Dis 2005; 64:510–511.

33 Masi AT, Rodnan GP, Medsger TA, et al. (Subcommittee for scleroderma criteria of the American Rheumatism Association Diagnostic and Therapeutic Criteria Committee): Preliminary criteria for the classification of systemic sclerosis (scleroderma). Arthritis Rheum 1980; 23:581–590.

34 LeRoy EC, Medsger TA Jr: Criteria for the classification of early systemic sclerosis. J Rheumatol 2001; 28:1573–1576.

35 Poormoghim H, Lucas M, Fertig N, Medsger TA Jr: Systemic sclerosis sine scleroderma: demographic, clinical, and serologic features and survival in forty-eight patients. Arthritis Rheum 2000; 43:444–451.

36 LeRoy EC, Black C, Fleichmajer R, Jablonska S, Krieg T, Medsger TA Jr, Rowell N, Wollheim F: Scleroderma (systemic sclerosis). Classification, subset and pathogenesis. J Rheumatol 1988; 15:202–205.

37 Giordano M, Valentini G, Migliaresi S, Picillo U, Vatti M: Different antibody patterns and different prognoses in patients with scleroderma with various extent of skin sclerosis. J Rheumatol 1986; 13:911–916.

38 Ferri C, Valentini G, Cozzi F, Sebastiani M, Michelassi C, La Montagna G, Bullo A, Cazzato M, Tirri E, Storino F, Giuggioli D, Cuomo G, Rosada M, Bombardieri S, Todesco S, Tirri G: Systemic sclerosis. Demographic, clinical and serologic features and survival in 1,012 Italian patients. Medicine 2002; 81:139–153.

39 Scussel-Lonzetti L, Joyal F, Raynauld J-P, Roussin A, Rich E, Goulet JR, Raymond Y, Senecal JL: Predicting mortality in systemic sclerosis. Analysis of a cohort of 309 French Canadian patients with emphasis on features at diagnosis as predictive factors for survival. Medicine 2002; 81:154–167.

40 Weiner ES, Earnshaw WC, Senecal JL, Bordwell B, Johnson P, Rothfield NF: Clinical association of anticentromere antibodies and antibodies to topoisomerase I. A study of 355 patients. Arthritis Rheum 1988; 31:378–385.

41 Harvey GR, Butts S, Rands AL, Patel Y, McHugh NJ: Clinical and serological associations with anti-RNA polymerase antibodies in systemic sclerosis. Clin Exp Immunol 1999; 117:395–402.

42 Cepeda EJ, Reveille JD: Autoantibodies in systemic sclerosis and fibrosing syndromes: clinical indications and releance. Curr Opin Rheumatol 2004; 16:723–732.

43 Pollard KM, Lee DK, Casiano CA, Blüthner M, Johnston MM, Tan EM: The autoimmunity-inducing xenobiotic mercury interacts with the autoantigen fibrillarin and modifies its molecular and antigenic properties. J Immunol 1997; 158:3521–3528.

44 Phan TG, Cass A, Gillin A, Trew P, Fertig N, Sturgess A: Anti-RNA polymerase III antibodies in the diagnosis of scleroderma renal crisis sine scleroderma. J Rheumatol 1999; 26:2489–2492.

45 Bohan A, Peter JB: Polymyositis and dermatomyositis (first of two parts). N Engl J Med 1975; 292:344–347.

46 Hengstman GJD, van Engelen BGM, van Venrooij WJ: Myositis specific autoantibodies: changing insights in pathophysiology and clinical associations. Curr Opin Rheumatol 2004; 16:692–699.

47 Imbert-Masseau A, Hamidou M, Agard C, Grolleau J-Y, Chérin P: Antisynthetase Syndrome. Joint Bone Spine 2003; 70:161–168.

48 Miller T, Al-Lozi MT, Lopate G, Pestronk A: Myopathy with autoantibodies to the signal recognition particle: clinical and pathological features. J Neurol Neurosurg Psychiatry 2002; 73:420–428.

49 Love LA, Leff RL, Fraser DD, Targoff IN, Dalakas M, Plotz PH, Miller FW: A new approach to the classification of idiopathic inflammatory myopathy: myositis-specific autoantibodies define useful homogeneous patient groups. Medicine 1991; 70:360–374.

50 Hengstman GJD, Brouwer R, Vree Egberts WTM, Seelig HP, Jongen PJH, van Venroiij WJ, van Engelen BGM: Clinical and serological characteristics of 125 Dutch myositis patients. Myositis specific autoantibodies aids in the differential diagnosis of the idiopathic inflammatory myopathies. J Neurol 2002; 249:69–75.

51 Sharp GC, Irvin WS, Tan EM, Gould RG, Holman HR: Mixed connective tissue disease – an apparently distinct rheumatic disease syndrome associated with a specific antibody to an extractable nuclear antigen (ENA). Am J Med 1972; 52:148–159.

52 Reichlin M, Maddison PJ, Targoff I, Bunch T, Arnett F, Sharp G, Treadwell F, Tan EM: Antibodies to a nuclear/nucleolar antigen in patients with polymyositis overlap syndromes. J Clin Immunol 1984; 4:40–44.

53 Blaszczyk M, Jablonska S, Szymanska-Jagiello W, Jarzabek-Chorzelska M, Chorzelski T, Mohamed AH: Childhood scleromyositis: an overlap syndrome associated with PM-Scl antibody. Pediatric Dermatol 1991; 8:1–8.

54 Wilson WA, Gharavi AE, Koike T, Lockshin MD, Branch DW, Piette JC, Brey R, Derksen R, Harris EN, Hughes GRV, Triplett DA, Khamashta MA: International consensus statement on preliminary classification for definite antiphospholipid syndrome. Arthritis Rheum 1999; 42:1309–1311.

55 Hughes GRV, Harris EN, Gharavi AE: The antiphospholipid syndrome. J Rheumatol 1986; 13:486–489.

56 Asherson RA, Cervera R: The antiphospholipid syndrome: multiple faces beyond the classical presentation. Autoimmunity Rev 2003; 2:140–151.

57 Obermoser G, Bitterlich W, Kunz F, Sepp NT: Clinical significance of anticardiolipin and anti-β2-glycoprotein I antibodies. Int Arch Allergy Immunol 2004; 135:148–153.

58 Sairam S, Baethge BA, McNearney T: Analysis of risk factors and comorbid diseases in the development of thrombosis in patients with anticardiolipin antibodies. Clin Rheumatol 2003; 22:24–29.

59 Atsumi T, Koike T: Clinical relevance of prothrombin antibodies. Autoimmun Rev 2002; 1:49–53.

60 Falk RJ, Jennette JC: Anti-neutrophil cytoplasmic autoantibodies with specificity for myeloperoxidase in patients with systemic vasculitis and idiopathic necrotizing and crescentic glomerulonephritis. N Engl J Med. 1988; 318:1651–1657.

61 Jenne DE, Tschopp J, Lüdemann J, Utecht B, Gross WL: Wegener's autoantigen decoded. Nature 1990; 346:520.

62 Conrad K, Schößler W, Hiepe F: Autoantibodies in Systemic Autoimmune Diseases. A Diagnostic Reference. Pabst Science Publishers, Lengerich 2002.

63 Choi HK, Merkel PA, Walker AM, Niles JL: Drug-associated antineutrophil cytoplasmic antibody-positive vasculitis: prevalence among patients with high titers of antimyeloperoxidase antibodies. Arthritis Rheum 2000; 43:405–413.

64 Nell VP, Machold KP, Eberl G, Stamm TA, Uffmann M, Smolen JS: Benefit of very early referral and very early therapy with disease-modifying anti-rheumatic drugs in patients with early rheumatoid arthritis. Rheumatology 2004; 43:906–914.

65 Steen V, Medsger TA Jr: Predictors of isolated pulmonary hypertension in patients with systemic sclerosis and limited cutaneous involvement. Arthritis Rheum 2003; 48:516–522.

66 Harris ML, Rosen A: Autoimmunity in scleroderma: the origin, pathogenetic role, and clinical significance of autoantibodies. Curr Opin Rheumatol 2003; 15:778–784.

67 Hénault J, Tremblay M, Clément I, Raymond Y, Senécal JL: Direct binding of anti-DNA topoisomerase I autoantibodies to the cell surface of fibroblasts in patients with systemic sclerosis. Arthritis Rheum 2004; 50:3265–3274.

68 Nishijima C, Hayakawa I, Matsushita T, Komura K, Hasegawa M, Takehara K, Sato S: Autoantibody against matrix metalloproteinase-3 in patients with systemic sclerosis. Clin Exp Immunol 2004; 138:357–363.

69 Alessandri C, Bombardieri M, Scrivo R, Viganego F, Conti F: Anti-carbonic anhydrase II antibodies in systemic sclerosis: association with lung involvement. Autoimmunity 2003; 36:85–89.

11
Autoantibodies in Systemic Lupus Erythematosus

Falk Hiepe

11.1
Introduction and Historical Perspective

Systemic lupus erythematosus (SLE) is a multi-systemic autoimmune disease that can involve almost any organ of the human body. The diverse clinical manifestations of SLE are accompanied by a huge number of autoantibodies. The number of antibodies associated with SLE was recently reported to be 116 [1]. No other autoimmune disease is similar to SLE with regard to the vast number of autoantibodies linked with it. SLE autoantibodies can react with nuclear, cytoplasmic, and surface cellular antigens as well as with complement components and coagulation system factors.

In 1948, Malcom Hargraves, Helen Richmond, and Robert Morton from the hematology laboratory of the Mayo Clinic in Rochester noted the presence of previously unknown cells in the bone marrow of a patient with acute SLE. These cells, which they called LE cells, were described as mature neutrophilic polymorphonuclear leukocytes that phagocytose Feulgen-stained nuclear material [2]. This historic finding ultimately led to the discovery of a broad variety of autoantibodies directed against nuclear antigens, which are now known as antinuclear antibodies (ANAs). In 1949, Haserick and Bortz made the important observation that, when incubated with normal bone marrow, serum from SLE patients was able to induce the formation of LE cells [3]. The inducing factor, called LE factor, was found to be associated with the gamma-globulin fraction of SLE serum [4], which was suspected to be an antibody. For the next 10 years, the detection of LE cells in the peripheral blood remained the most popular laboratory test for the diagnosis of SLE. In 1953, Peter Miescher observed that the sera from rabbits immunized with cell nuclei were able to induce LE cell formation using normal human leukocytes. One year later, Miescher demonstrated that absorption of SLE serum by cell nuclei isolated from calf thymus cells made the serum incapable of inducing LE cell formation. Based on these experiments, the LE factor was confirmed to be an ANA [5]. These pivotal findings resulted in the simultaneous reporting of antibodies to DNA in the sera of SLE patients by at least four different groups in 1957 [5–9].

Autoantibodies and Autoimmunity: Molecular Mechanisms in Health and Disease. Edited by K. Michael Pollard
Copyright © 2006 WILEY-VCH Verlag GmbH & Co. KGaA, Weinheim
ISBN: 3-527-31141-6

Because the spectrum of autoantibodies associated with SLE is so broad, this article will focus on autoantibodies of high diagnostic relevance. Table 11.1 summarizes the characteristics of important autoantigen–autoantibody systems in SLE.

A recent publication has shown that autoantibodies are typically present many years before the diagnosis of SLE. Furthermore, the appearance of autoantibodies tends to follow a predictable course, with a progressive accumulation of specific autoantibodies before the onset of SLE, while patients are still asymptomatic [10].

11.2
Antinuclear Antibodies

Since ANAs are present in almost all patients with SLE, the ANA test is the most sensitive test for lupus. In a recent study, ANAs were found in 280 out of 291 (96.2%) SLE patients [11]. However, ANAs are not specific for SLE because they occur in a variety of autoimmune, rheumatic, and infectious diseases. Moreover, ANAs are sometimes detected in healthy individuals, especially in the elderly. In any case, the absence of ANAs makes the diagnosis of SLE much less likely, although still possible. Indirect immunofluorescence with tissue or cell culture substrates is the most widely used method for detection of ANAs. Because of their large nucleus and prominent nuclear constituents, human esophageal tumor cells (HEp-2) are most commonly used for this purpose. HEp-2 cells have virtually replaced mouse kidney or liver tissue sections because they are much more sensitive for ANAs. The rare anti-Ro/SSA precipitin-positive lupus patient continues to be ANA negative because of the paucity of the Ro/SSA antigen and the loss of its antigenicity after cell fixation.

The ANA test is interpreted both by titer and by pattern. Higher titers loosely correlate with pathologic significance. Since the ANA test is dependent upon immunologic reagents and laboratory conditions, there is substantial interlaboratory variation [12]. The different antigenic targets bound by the autoantibody lead to different ANA immunofluorescence patterns, depending on their location within the cell and on the specific changes caused by fixation (Fig. 11.1, see page 253).

Counterimmunoelectrophoresis and immunodiffusion techniques were previously used to detect specific ANAs, but more sensitive techniques have now been developed, for instance, enzyme-linked immunosorbent assays (ELISA) and line immunoassays (LIA) using whole cell nuclei, affinity-purified antigens, recombinant proteins, or synthetic peptides. Immunoblotting [13, 14] and immunoprecipitation [15, 16] are valuable tools for characterizing many autoantibodies that react with nuclear and cytoplasmic antigens. New developments for miniaturization and simultaneous determination of different ANAs and other autoantibodies include novel autoantigen microarrays [17–19] and a laser-based flow technology (Luminex) [20, 21].

Table 11.1 Characterization of autoantigen–autoantibody systems in SLE (modified according to [1, 12, 180, 181]).

Autoantibody to	Characterization of antigen	Biological function	Prevalence	Disease specificity	Correlation with disease activity	Clinical associations and comments
ANA	Multiple nuclear antigens (see below)		95–100%	No	No	One of the revised ACR criteria of SLE; indirect immunofluorescence assay for ANAs is a useful screening test
dsDNA	Double-stranded, native DNA	Genetic code	40–80%	High	Yes	Included in the revised ACR criteria of SLE, important marker for the diagnosis of SLE; nephritis, CNS involvement
Histones	H1, H2A, H2B, H3, H4, H5, [H2A-H2B]-DNA dimer	Organization of nucleosomes		No	Controversial	Nephritis? Frequently positive in drug-induced lupus
Nucleosome	140 base pairs of DNA wrapped around 4 pairs of core histones	Organization of nuclear DNA	50–90%	High	Yes	Nephritis, psychosis
Sm	Core proteins B (28), B' (29), D (16), E (13), F and G of U1, U2, U4, U5, and U6 snRNPs	Splicing of pre-mRNA	5–70%	High	Yes	Included in the revised ACR criteria of SLE; more frequent in Asians and Afro-Americans; CNS involvement, milder form of nephritis, lung fibrosis, pericarditis, oral ulcer, thrombopenia, leukopenia, lower prevalence of sicca symptoms; usually found with anti-U1RNP
U1-nRNP	Proteins 70 kDa, A (33) and C (22) of U1-sn RNP	Splicing of pre-mRNA	23–40%	No	Controversial	Raynaud's phenomenon, myositis, arthritis, lower chance for nephritis

Table 11.1 (continued)

Autoantibody to	Characterization of antigen	Biological function	Prevalence	Disease specificity	Correlation with disease activity	Clinical associations and comments
RA33	Protein A1 (34 kDa) of hnRNP	Splicing of pre-mRNA	9–40%	No	No	Erosive arthritis
Ro/SS-A	52-kDa and 60-kDa ribonucleo-protein containing small uridine-rich nucleic acids (hY1, hY3, hY4, hY5)	DNA binding protein (52 kDa Ro); quality control for 5S rRNA production/ involvement in translation of ribosomal protein mRNA (60 kDa Ro)	24–60%	No	Controversial	Secondary Sjögren's syndrome, subacute-cutaneous lupus, photo-sensitivity; neonatal lupus, inter-stitial lung disease, lympho-penia, nephritis and anti-DNA in patients without anti-La/SSB
La/SS-B	Phosphoprotein (48 kDa) asso-ciated with a variety of small RNAs (precursors of cellular 5S RNA and tRNA, 7S RNA, viral RNAs, Ro/SS-A cytoplasmic hY RNAs)	Probably tran-scription termi-nation factor of RNA polymer-ase III	6–35%	No	No	Secondary Sjögren's syndrome, neonatal lupus, subacute cuta-neous lupus, cytopenia, pneumo-nitis, leukocytoclastic vasculitis, C2 and C4 deficiency; lower prevalence of nephritis and anti-dsDNA in patients with anti-Ro/SSA and anti-La/SSB
PCNA	Cyclin (36 kDa)	Auxiliary protein of DNA-poly-merase	2–7%	High	Not known	Young age of onset, proliferative nephritis

Table 11.1 (continued)

Autoantibody to	Characterization of antigen	Biological function	Prevalence	Disease specificity	Correlation with disease activity	Clinical associations and comments
Ku	Heterodimer consisting of 70-kDa and 80–86-kDa protein subunits, DNA binding component of a 350-kDa catalytic subunit with DNA-dependent kinase activity	Repairs dsDNA breaks, V(D)J recombination	10–40%	No	No	Mild disease by a low incidence of renal and CNS involvement, Raynaud's phenomenon, arthritis, pulmonary hypertension, esophageal reflux
Ribosomal RNP	Phosphoproteins P0 (15 kDa), P1 (16 kDa), and P2 (38 kDa)	Active in elongation step of protein synthesis	8–42%	High	Yes	Frequencies differ in different ethnic groups; more prevalent in juvenile-onset and Asians; psychosis, hepatitis
Proteasome	Cytoplasmic and nuclear-localized proteinase complex (20S), arranged in a cylindrical structure of 4 stacked rings, each composed of 7 subunits (α-type subunits form the outer rings, β-type subunits form the inner rings carrying the proteolytic sites	Involved in the ubiquitin-dependent selective degradation of short-lived and abnormal proteins; processing of antigens presented by MHC class I molecules	58%	No	Not known	SLE, Sjögren's syndrome, myositis
C1q	Collagen-like region of C1q	Complement protein that initiates classic pathway of complement cascade	30–50%	No	Yes	Nephritis, hypocomplementemia, urticarial vasculitis, predicts relapses of lupus nephritis, correlates with anti-dsDNA

Table 11.1 (continued)

Autoantibody to	Characterization of antigen	Biological function	Prevalence	Disease specificity	Correlation with disease activity	Clinical associations and comments
Phospholipids, Lupus anticoagulant (LAC)	Negatively charged phospholipids (e.g., cardiolipin, phosphatidylserine), phospholipid-binding proteins (β2 glycoprotein 1)	Role in coagulation	20–60%	No	aCL yes LAC no	Included in the revised ACR criteria of SLE; secondary antiphospholipid syndrome in SLE: thrombosis recurrent fetal loss, thrombocytopenia, hemolytic anemia, CNS involvement
Red blood cells	Protein and glycoprotein antigens on RBC membrane		10–50%	No	No	Hemolytic anemia, often positive without anemia, warm antibodies usually detected
Platelets	Major platelet surface glycoproteins (GPIb: 143- and 22-kDa subunits; GPIIb: 132- and 23-kDa subunits; IIIa: 114 kDa; IX: 17–22 kDa)		10–62%	No	Yes	Thrombocytopenia
	CD36	Signal transduction, scavenger receptor, and adhesion molecule	nd	nd	No	Thrombopenia, recurrent early fetal loss
Endothelial cells	Numerous intracellular and membrane antigens		7–86%	No	Yes	Nephritis, CNS involvement, pulmonary hypertension, digital vasculitis, Raynaud's phenomenon, serositis, aCL

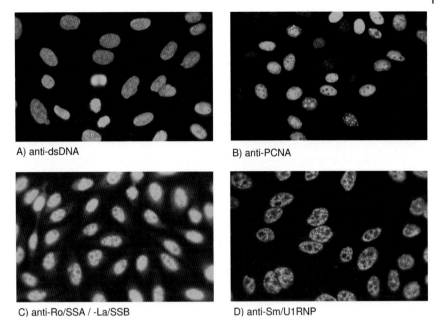

A) anti-dsDNA

B) anti-PCNA

C) anti-Ro/SSA / -La/SSB

D) anti-Sm/U1RNP

Fig. 11.1 Immunofluorescence patterns on HEp-2 cells seen in SLE.

11.2.1
Antibodies Directed Against the Nucleosome Family

11.2.1.1 Anti-DNA Antibodies
Antibodies to DNA were first described in 1957 [6–9]. They constitute a subgroup of ANAs that bind single-stranded and/or double-stranded DNA. They may be IgM antibodies or any IgG antibody subclass. In general, tests for IgG complement-fixing antibodies to DNA, especially those that bind double-stranded DNA, have the greatest diagnostic value in patients in whom SLE is suspected. Therefore, anti-dsDNA antibodies were included in the American College of Rheumatology classification criteria [22, 23]. In addition to serving as a laboratory marker for SLE, these antibodies may contribute to the development of associated diseases, such as nephritis. The underlying stimulus for anti-DNA antibody production in SLE patients remains unknown [24].

Antibodies that bind exclusively to single-stranded DNA can bind its component bases, nucleosides, nucleotides, oligonucleotides, or ribose-phosphate backbone, all of which are exposed in single-stranded DNA. In contrast, anti-double-stranded DNA antibodies bind to the ribose-phosphate backbone, base pairs, or specific conformations of the double helix. Double-stranded DNA exists primarily in a right-handed helical form called B DNA. There is also a left-handed helical form called Z DNA. Most widely available tests for measuring anti-DNA antibodies are based on reactivity with B DNA. Most anti-dsDNA antibodies bind both double-stranded and single-stranded DNA [24].

There is a high potency of anti-DNA antibodies to cross-react with non-DNA antigens such as laminin, heparan sulfate, type IV collagen, and α-actinin, which are located in the kidney. The cross-reactivity with renal antigens may contribute to the pathogenesis of lupus nephritis in which anti-DNA antibodies clearly play a central role [24, 25]. Recently, it was demonstrated that the penta-peptide Asp/Glu-Trp-Asp/Glu-Tyr-Ser/Gly is a molecular mimic of dsDNA. The sequence that is also present in the extracellular ligand-binding domain of murine and human N-methyl-D-aspartate (NMDA) receptor subunits NR2a and NR2b is recognized by a subset of both murine and human anti-DNA antibodies. These antibodies can signal neuronal death and can be detected in the cerebrospinal fluid of SLE patients [26]. Very recently, an association between neuropsychiatric disturbances in SLE and antibodies against a decapeptide containing this sequence motif present in the extracellular NMDA receptor was shown [27].

Enzyme-linked immunosorbent assays (ELISA) and indirect immunofluorescence using the substrate *Crithidia luciliae* are currently the most widely used techniques for the detection of anti-DNA antibodies. Radioimmunoassays such as the Farr assay are still available, but their use has decreased sharply. There are important differences between these techniques. The Farr assay measures the precipitation of radiolabeled dsDNA using anti-dsDNA antibodies under stringent conditions (high saline concentrations) to ensure that only high-affinity antibodies are detected. However, this assay may also detect other proteins capable of precipitating dsDNA; furthermore, it may occasionally be contaminated by ssDNA in the test preparation, and the test does not distinguish between isotypes. The *Crithidia* test detects binding of anti-dsDNA to the kinetoplast of the organism, which contains circular dsDNA unrelated to histone proteins. This test can be used to measure IgG, IgM, or all isotypes of anti-dsDNA [28]. In ELISA, the wells of a test plate are coated with dsDNA, the test serum is added as a source of anti-dsDNA, and the target anti-DNA antibody is detected by a second antibody. Although the ELISA can be used to detect various antibody isotypes, IgG anti-dsDNA detection normally suffices for clinical purposes. The ELISA detects both low- and high-affinity antibodies, which could make it less specific than other assays [29]. Therefore, when interpreting the results of anti-DNA antibody tests, the clinician should consider the technique used, the type of laboratory in which the test was performed, and the laboratory's ranges for that test.

After a review of all relevant available literature, guidelines for anti-DNA antibody testing were recently published with the conclusions that a positive anti-dsDNA test offers strong evidence for the diagnosis of SLE but that a negative test does not exclude the diagnosis. Anti-DNA testing should be reserved for patients who tested ANA positive. Anti-DNA antibodies correlate with overall disease activity in SLE. However, as the correlations are modest at best, test results must be interpreted in the overall clinical context. Similarly, anti-DNA antibodies correlate with the activity of renal disease in SLE, but to a limited extent. Higher titers of anti-DNA antibodies have a stronger correlation with disease activity. Concerning longitudinal assessment, a positive anti-DNA test does not predict a flare-up of disease. Increasing titers of anti-DNA may precede or accompany flare-ups of disease activity. However, the number of high-quality studies addressing this issue is limited, and a number of important questions concerning the optimal use of anti-DNA testing longitudinally remain to be answered [30].

11.2.1.2 Antibodies to Nucleosomes (Chromatin)

Antibodies to nucleosomes have had a "comeback" in the last few years. This has to do with both the clinical utility of these antibodies in the diagnosis of SLE and drug-induced lupus (DIL) and new evidence suggesting that nucleosomes may be major candidate autoimmunogens in lupus. Since it is generally accepted that anti-nucleosome antibodies cause the LE cell phenomenon, they were actually among the first autoantibodies discovered. Of note, autoantibodies against individual components of nucleosomes, i.e., DNA or histone, cannot induce LE cell formation. For decades, the LE cell test introduced in 1948 was one of the most common immunological tests performed in clinical laboratories to diagnose SLE. Different names for anti-nucleosome antibodies have caused some confusion. They have been referred to as anti-DNP or anti-sNP antibodies in older publications and as anti-nucleosome, anti-chromatin, and anti-(H2A-H2B)-DNA antibodies in more recent articles [31–33].

The nucleosome is the fundamental unit of chromatin. It consists of a core particle composed of an octamer with two copies each of histones H2A, H2B, H3, and H4, around which is wrapped helical DNA with approximately 146 base pairs (bp) [34, 35]. Chromatin, the native complex of histones and DNA found in the cell nucleus of eukaryotes, is comprised of approximately 40% DNA, 40% histones, and 20% non-histone proteins, RNA, and other macromolecules. The periodic arrangement of histones along the DNA gives chromatin a "beads-on-a string" appearance in electron micrographs. The "beads" can be isolated by digesting the linker DNA between them with micrococcal nuclease, yielding nucleosomes. Thus, polynucleosomes and chromatin are identical [33].

Anti-nucleosome/chromatin antibodies are defined as antibodies that react with the portion of histones exposed in chromatin/nucleosome, the structure of DNA found in chromatin/nucleosome, or an epitope comprised of the native histone–DNA complex. Specifically excluded are antibodies that react with non-histone proteins, with epitopes on histones buried in chromatin, and with histone–DNA structures, such as A, C, and Z forms not present in chromatin. Thus, some but not all DNA-reactive antibodies have anti-nucleosome reactivity [31–33].

The new strategy in lupus research is to define a broad anti-nucleosome antibody family, including nucleosome-specific antibodies (anti-nucleosome antibodies without anti-dsDNA and anti-histone reactivities), anti-nucleosome antibodies with anti-dsDNA reactivity (bona fide anti-dsDNA antibodies), and anti-nucleosome antibodies with anti-histone reactivity (bona fide anti-histone antibodies) [31].

Anti-nucleosome antibodies are clinically important for several reasons. The nucleosome is emerging as one of the major nuclear autoantigen targets, and 70–80% of SLE patients are anti-nucleosome antibody positive [36–41]. Independent studies have shown that the contribution of anti-dsDNA and anti-histone antibodies to serum reactivity against nucleosomes in SLE patients is only 25–30% at most [36, 37]. One-third of SLE sera studied have high anti-nucleosome activity and little if any anti-dsDNA or anti-histone reactivity [36, 37, 41]. The level of the anti-nucleosome antibody titer correlates with the level of disease activity [39, 42–46]. This finding was also observed in SLE patients negative for anti-dsDNA antibodies [43, 44]. Anti-nucleosome antibodies are also associated with lupus nephritis [36, 39, 42–45], which is not surprising considering the bulk of evidence suggesting that they contribute to the pathogenesis of lupus nephritis [47–50]. An increase in IgG3 anti-nucleosome titers was observed during SLE flare-ups, and this increase was found to be closely associated with active nephritis. IgG1 anti-nucleosome antibody titers tended to correlate inversely with SLE disease activity [45]. One group found an association between anti-nucleosome antibodies and lupus psychosis [42].

A very recent study showed that measurement of anti-nucleosome antibodies can help to predict the development of SLE in patients with primary antiphospholipid syndrome (PAPS). The authors followed 18 PAPS patients (15 female, three male) for a mean 11 years to evaluate the potential for SLE development. When PAPS was diagnosed, nine patients were positive for anti-nucleosome antibodies, and six of them developed clinical manifestations of SLE. In contrast, none of the patients who were anti-nucleosome–negative developed SLE [51].

Almost all patients with procainamide-induced lupus, half of those with quinidine-induced lupus, and some with hydralazine-induced lupus were positive for anti-nucleosome antibodies [52]. Most procainamide patients without drug-induced lupus were negative for anti-nucleosome antibodies. A few other drugs infrequently cause drug-induced lupus, and these patients often demonstrate anti-nucleosome activity [53].

In some studies, a high percentage of patients with systemic sclerosis were positive for anti-nucleosome antibodies [32, 41]. This was surprising because scleroderma patients do not exhibit a typical ANA immunofluorescence pattern when tested using HEp-2 cells. Methodological reasons for anti-nucleosomes reacting with scleroderma sera include the use of DNA reconstituted with the denatured antigens H2A and H2B, use of whole chromatin containing residual topoisomerase I protein as the antigen, and use of an inappropriate cutoff. When H1-stripped chromatin or nucleosome core particles are used as the antigen with a cutoff that properly distinguishes between positive and negative, virtually no patients with systemic sclerosis should test positive for anti-nucleosome antibodies [53–55]. In one study, 50% of 36 patients with autoimmune hepatitis type I were anti-chromatin positive, while 5–13% of patients with other liver diseases were positive [56].

11.2.2
Anti-Sm and Anti-U1RNP Antibodies

Both anti-Sm and anti-U1RNP are specificities of various components of the spliceosome, which splices pre-messenger RNA. These antibodies consist of RNA–protein complex particles, known as snRNPs (small nuclear ribonuclear proteins): U1–U6 RNA complexes with members of a set of different protein subunits [57]. Sm is associated with U2, U4, and U6 RNA and with the B, B', D1, D2, D3, E, F, and G polypeptides. U1 snRNP is associated with anti-U1RNP, which is composed of U1 RNA and A, C, or 70-kDa polypeptides.

Anti-Sm antibodies, which were first described by Tan and Kunkel [58], are detected in about 10–25% of Caucasian American lupus patients and in a substantially higher percentage of African American patients [59]. In fact, a recent study of 114 lupus patients (68% African American, 19% Hispanic American, and 13% Caucasian) reported the finding of anti-Sm antibodies in 40% of patients [60]. The presence of anti-Sm antibodies is virtually pathognomonic for lupus. Therefore, they are included in the ACR classification criteria for SLE [22, 23]. There are no particularly strong clinical associations for anti-Sm, but these antibodies have been associated with CNS involvement, nephritis, serositis, oral ulcers, thrombopenia, leukopenia, and pulmonary fibrosis as well as with a lower prevalence of sicca symptoms [61–64]. These associations could not be confirmed in a recent study using a line immunoassay (LIA) for detection of anti-Sm [11]. There is a correlation between SLE disease activity and the anti-Sm level [65].

Anti-U1RNP was first described by Mattioli and Reichlin [66]; it is present in more than 20% of Caucasian Americans with SLE compared to about 40% of African Americans with SLE. Lupus patients with anti-U1RNP autoantibodies tend to have myositis, Raynaud's phenomenon, and arthritis but are less likely to develop lupus nephritis [11, 62, 63, 67]. Since anti-U1RNP antibodies are found in a variety of autoimmune diseases, they are not specific for SLE [68]. High titers of anti-U1RNP are characteristic for mixed connective tissue disease (MCTD); this association was first described by Sharp et al. in 1971 [69].

Nearly all patients with high anti-Sm titers will eventually develop anti-U1RNP antibodies [70]; hence, there is a correlation between the two specificities. The basis for the association is thought to be their coexistence on the same U1 snRNP.

The first epitope in the anti-Sm B/B' system is defined by the peptide PPPGMRPP [71, 72]. No exceptions have yet been identified. This autoimmune response later expands to involve the multiple epitopes on the Sm B/B' antigen in a process referred to as epitope spreading. Immunization with PPPGMRPP results in anti-PPPGMRPP antibody production; the antibodies subsequently bind to different epitopes of the B/B' subunit. Epitope spreading then carries the humoral immune response to the rest of the spliceosome, including A, C, and 70 kDa polypeptides. Some immunized animals also develop anti-dsDNA, thrombocytopenia, seizures, or proteinuria [73, 74].

PPPGMRPP closely resembles PPPGRRP from Epstein-Barr nuclear antigen-1 (EBNA-1); anti-Sm antibodies cross-react with both peptides. This molecular mimicry may partially explain the strong association of Epstein-Barr virus infection with lupus [75–77]. A recent study reported that Epstein-Barr virus in lupus patients was approximately 40 times higher than in controls and that this increase was unrelated to disease activity and immunosuppressant use [78].

Since anti-U1RNP sera can also react, to a variable extent, with B and B' proteins [79], D proteins appear to be the most important Sm antigens. A C-terminal SmD1 peptide was identified as an important conformational autoantigenic epitope with an extraordinarily high sensitivity and specificity for SLE. Seventy percent of Caucasian SLE sera reacted with this SmD1 peptide in ELISA [65]. The sensitivity and specificity of this anti-SmD1 (83–119) ELISA was confirmed in other lupus cohorts [80, 81]. Casein added to the blocking buffer in ELISA seems to be an important cofactor in autoantibody reactivity directed against the C-terminal SmD1 (83–119) peptide; it probably functions by changing the conformation of the peptide's critical epitope [82]. This C-terminal SmD1 peptide contains a supercharged GR repeat and shows homology to EBNA-1 [83, 84]. Of note, the anti-SmD1 (83–119) reactivity was significantly higher in anti-dsDNA-positive sera [65]. Immunization of NZB/W F_1 mice with this C-terminal SmD1 peptide led to an acceleration of nephritis and stimulated anti-dsDNA production [85]; the peptide was found to generate T-cell help for autoantibodies, including anti-dsDNA [86]. Very recently, our group showed that high-dose tolerance to SmD1 delays the production of autoantibodies, postpones the onset of lupus nephritis (confirmed by histology), and prolongs survival [87]. Tolerance to SmD1 83–119 was adoptively transferred by CD90$^+$ T cells, which reduce T-cell help for autoreactive B cells *in vitro*. One week after SmD1 83–119 tolerance induction in pre-nephritic mice, we detected cytokine changes in cultures of CD90$^+$ T and B220$^+$ B cells with decreased expression of IFN-gamma and IL-4 and an increase in TGF-beta. Increased frequencies of regulatory IFN-gamma$^+$ and IL10$^+$ CD4$^+$ T cells were later detected. Such regulatory IL-10$^+$/IFN-gamma$^+$ type 1 regulatory T cells prevented autoantibody generation and anti-CD3-induced proliferation of naive T cells. These results indicate that SmD1 83–119 peptide may play a dominant role in the activation of helper and regulatory T cells that influence autoantibody generation and murine lupus [88].

Post-translational modifications of the C-terminal SmD1 and SmD3 peptides by dimethylation may play an essential role in the formation of major autoepitopes [89–91].

11.2.3
Anti-Ro/SSA and Anti-La/SSB

Autoantibodies to the Ro/SSA and La/SSB antigens were first reported in 1961 in sera from patients with Sjögren's syndrome and in 1969 in SLE patients [92, 93]. Two precipitin reactions in SLE sera were designated Ro and La based on the names of the patients in whom they were first identified [93]. The anti-Ro and anti-La precipitins were shown later to be identical to the anti-SSA and anti-SSB precipitins, respectively, reported in sera from patients suffering from Sjögren's syndrome [94]. Both antibody types are more common in Sjögren's syndrome.

The Ro/SSA–La/SSB complex consists of three different proteins (52-kDa Ro/SSA, 60-kDa Ro/SSA, and 48-kDa La/SSB) and four small RNAs [95].

Nearly all anti-Ro/SSA-positive sera bind the Ro/SSA 60-kDa protein, which is complexed with small RNA molecules known as Y RNA. Humans have four types of Y RNA: hY1, hY3, hY4, and hY5. A specific subset of Y RNA is present in some cells. For example, erythrocytes contain hY1 and hY4 [96], and platelets contain hY3 and hY4 [97]. Sera from some anti-Ro/SSA 60-kDa antibody–positive patients also bind the Ro/SSA 52-kDa autoantigen. The 52-kDa Ro/SSA protein associated with this complex was later described [98]. It is antigenically and structurally distinct from 60-kDa Ro/SSA and La/SSB and contains zinc finger and leucine finger motifs [99, 100]. However, the question of whether the Ro/SSA-60 kDa and the Ro/SSA-52 kDa are physically related continues to be controversial. It was shown that antibodies binding the leucine zipper, a major linear epitope in the Ro/SSA 52-kDa autoantigen, also bind native Ro/SSA-60 kDa; this would provide a basis for the cross-reaction [101]. Anti-Ro/SSA and anti-La/SSB are similar in that high titers of anti-La/SSB are almost never present in the absence of anti-Ro/SSA. The La/SSB particle is a 48-kDa protein believed to function as a termination factor for RNA polymerase III [102]. It is also associated with small RNA molecules, most of which terminate with polyuridine. The association of anti-La/SSB with anti-Ro/SSA has been attributed to the physical association between Ro/SSA and La/SSB RNA proteins, at least at times.

The function of the Ro/SSA particle is not well understood. Recent evidence suggests that the Ro/SSA particle might be involved in quality control of misfolded small RNAs and in preventing cellular damage induced by ultraviolet light [103, 104]. It is remarkable in this context that a murine knockout for 60-kDa Ro/SSA is susceptible to UV damage [105]. There is evidence that Ro/SSA plays a role in telomerase function [106]. Other data suggest that Ro/SSA modulates the immune response to other proteins, for example, calreticulin, thereby influencing autoimmunity [87]. Mice lacking the 60-kDa Ro/SSA protein develop signs of autoimmunity resembling human SLE. They exhibit anti-ribosome and anti-chromatin antibodies, photosensitivity, and glomerulonephritis [105].

The presence of anti-Ro/SSA and anti-La/SSB autoantibodies is associated with subacute cutaneous lupus erythematosus [107], photosensitivity, secondary Sjögren's syndrome, and neonatal lupus [108]. Neonatal lupus provides perhaps the strongest clinical evidence for a pathogenic role of these autoantibodies. This syndrome, related to the presence of anti-Ro/SSA and anti-La/SSB antibodies in the mother, is characterized by skin rash, cytopenia, cholestasis, and/or congenital heart block (CHB) [108]. In recent prospective studies of women with anti-Ro/SSA antibodies, the risk of complete CHB was found to be 1–2% [109, 110] and of transient cutaneous neonatal lupus about 5% [110]. Of note, no effect on pregnancy outcome was observed [111]. The risk of occurrence of CHB in a subsequent child is estimated to be 10–16% [112–114]. The congenital heart block is especially associated with high levels of antibodies binding 52-kDa Ro/SSA [108, 115], whereas the best single test to identify high-risk mothers was detection of these antibodies by immunoblot [114]. Fine epitope mapping revealed a striking difference in which the response in mothers with affected children was dominated by antibodies to amino acids 200–239 of the 52-kDa Ro/SSA protein, whereas the primary activity in control mothers was against amino acids 176–196. Furthermore, eight of nine mothers of children with CHB had antibody reactivity against amino acids 1–135 of the 52-kDa Ro/SSA protein, containing two putative zinc fingers reconstituted under reducing conditions [116]. The analysis of CHB cohorts suggests a higher frequency in female infants [113, 114, 117].

11.2.4
Anti-PCNA/Cyclin Antibodies

PCNA/cyclin is a highly conserved auxiliary protein of DNA polymerase-delta, which is essential for leading strand DNA replication [118, 119]. Autoantibodies against it give a polymorphic nuclear pattern in indirect immunofluorescence on HEp-2 cells, corresponding to different phases of the cell cycle, because it associates with different sites of the cell nucleus where DNA is being replicated [120, 121]. Depending on the level of PCNA/cyclin expression, there may be strong and variable staining in the S phase and weak or negative staining in the G0 or G1 phases [121, 122]. The antibodies first described in 1978 are considered specific for SLE [121]. However, the frequency of these autoantibodies is rather low: they are detected in 2–7% of SLE patients [123–125]. Because of their low frequency, little is known about their clinical associations. Positive subjects show a higher incidence of diffuse proliferative glomerulonephritis and hematological disorders than the general SLE population [124]. Another study describes an association with arthritis in five of five anti-PCNA-positive SLE patients, with diffuse proliferative glomerulonephritis in four of five patients and with hypocomplementemia in four of five patients [126].

11.3
Antibodies to Cytoplasmic Antigens

11.3.1
Anti-ribosomal P Antibodies

Autoantibodies to the ribosomal phosphoproteins first described in 1985 are a serological feature of patients with SLE [127, 128]. Rib-P autoantigens consist of three protein components of the 60S ribosomal subunit designated P0 (38 kDa), P1 (19 kDa), and P2 (17 kDa). A pentameric complex composed of one copy of

P0 and two copies each of P1 and P2 interacts with the 28S rRNA molecule to form a GTPase domain, which is active during the elongation step of protein translation. The major immunoreactive epitope of these ribosomal antigens has been localized to the carboxy-terminal domain, which is highly conserved in all three proteins; moreover, it contains two phosphorylated serine residues (e.g., Ser^{102} and Ser^{105} of human P2) [129–131]. Several studies have shown that both the acidic and hydrophobic clusters are critical for autoantibody binding and that P protein phosphorylation is not [130, 132]. Furthermore, epitope mapping studies have shown that the major epitope domain is located within the last six C-terminal amino acids (GFGLFD) [132].

This amino acid motif is also present in several microorganisms, which raises the possibility of a molecular mimicry mechanism in the development of anti-P antibody in lupus. Some anti-ribosomal P antibodies cross-react with other autoantigens, particularly the Sm D and Sm B/B′ spliceosomal subunits [133], nucleosomal molecules, and DNA [134]. As in the case of anti-dsDNA, anti-ribosomal P antibodies also are capable of penetrating living cells and of profoundly suppressing protein synthesis [135].

The reported prevalence of anti-ribosomal P antibodies in SLE ranges from 10–40%; prevalence is higher in Asian patients than in black and Caucasian patients [136]. A correlation between anti-ribosomal P and lupus psychosis was reported soon after the discovery of this antibody [127]. Several subsequent studies confirmed this association and also reported an association with depression [137, 138], although other researchers disagree [139]. Anti-ribosomal P antibody correlates with the activity of lupus [140], particularly lupus nephritis [141, 142]. Furthermore, the coexistence of anti-dsDNA and anti-ribosomal P antibodies is more closely associated with lupus nephritis than is the presence of either of them alone [143]. Anti-ribosomal P antibody is also associated with lupus hepatitis [144]. Indeed, the association between anti-ribosomal P and lupus hepatitis does not apply to patients with autoimmune hepatitis except when lupus is present; this again emphasizes the high specificity of anti-ribosomal P with lupus [145].

Although anti-ribosomal P protein autoantibodies were discovered approximately 20 years ago, they have not achieved the same attention and clinical impact as anti-Sm or anti-dsDNA antibodies. This may be due to the limited reliability of ANA screening by indirect immunofluorescence for the detection of anti-ribosomal P antibodies or to the absence of an international reference serum. It is noteworthy that a reference standard human Rib-P antibody has recently become available (Centers for Disease Control, Atlanta, GA: Catalogue #2706). This should be an important step in standardizing assays from different sources.

Because of the high specificity of anti-ribosomal P for SLE, some researchers have put forward the proposal that, like anti-Sm and anti-dsDNA antibodies, Rib-P antibodies should be considered for inclusion as a criterion for the classification of SLE [136].

11.4
Antiphospholipid Antibodies

Antiphospholipid antibodies are a wide and heterogeneous group of mainly IgG and/or IgM antibodies and, less frequently, IgA antibodies directed against phospholipid–protein complexes or phospholipid-binding proteins, such as β2-glycoprotein I, prothrombin, protein C, protein S, thrombomodulin, annexin V, and kininogen. The term "antiphospholipid antibody" is therefore incorrect, because the antibody is actually directed against a phospholipid–protein complex, but the name has been retained for historical reasons. Although the negatively charged phospholipid cardiolipin plays the most important role, phosphatidylserine, phosphatidylethanolamine, and phosphatidylcholine may also form part of the complex. The target epitope is still not fully explained [146, 147].

Lupus anticoagulants and anticardiolipin antibodies were the first such antibodies to be described. The "Sapporo" laboratory criteria for definite antiphospholipid syndrome require both assays to be present on two or more occasions at least six weeks apart [148]. Lupus anticoagulant must be diagnosed according to the criteria proposed by the Subcommittee of Standardization of Lupus Anticoagulants/Phospholipid-dependent Antibodies [149]. Anticardiolipin antibodies must be measured using a standardized ELISA for β2-glycoprotein I–dependent antibodies; medium or high titers of IgG and/or IgM antibodies are required for a positive result. According to the Sapporo criteria, the diagnosis of definite antiphospholipid syndrome (APS) occurring as a secondary disease in SLE is established when at least one clinical criterion and one laboratory criterion are met. The clinical criteria include thrombotic events and recurrent pregnancy loss [148].

The prevalence of antiphospholipid antibodies in SLE varies widely; figures between 22% and 69% have been reported. This variation may be due to differences in methods or patient selection. Antiphospholipid antibodies are found less frequently in African American SLE patients. Generally, antiphospholipid antibodies appear to be more easily suppressed by treatments for active SLE [150]. In SLE, disease activity was accompanied by significantly increased IgG-aCL, whereas no elevation was found in other diseases with detectable aCL antibodies [151].

Antiphospholipid syndrome is characterized by a wide spectrum of clinical manifestations that, pathophysiologically, are mainly caused by venous or arterial thrombosis, which is also associated with SLE. Dermatologic manifestations are extremely frequent in APS. The most common is livedo reticularis. Cardiac manifestations, especially valve disease, are frequently observed. Thrombocytopenia and Coombs-positive hemolytic anemia are also often found in APS [147, 150].

A recent single-center study of 600 SLE patients showed that the prevalence of antiphospholipid antibodies was 24%; 15% had IgG aCL, 9% IgM aCL, and 15% lupus anticoagulant [67]. A cluster of clinical events, characterized by neurologic involvement, thrombocytopenia, and IgG aCL, was observed in this study. The association of neurologic involvement with clinical or laboratory features found in APS (e.g., livedo reticularis or thrombocytopenia) was also described in previous SLE studies [152, 153]. High titers of IgG aCL were strongly associated with CNS involvement [152]. A multivariate analysis showed that aPLs are independently associated with cerebrovascular disease, headache, and seizures in SLE. The presence of lupus anticoagulant (LAC) was independently associated with white matter hyperintensity lesions on MRI [154].

Catastrophic APS is an uncommon but potentially life-threatening condition that requires high clinical awareness. Thirty percent of patients with this condition have definitive SLE. The majority of patients with this condition clearly manifest microangiopathy, i.e., occlusive vascular disease that mainly affects small vessels of different organs, particularly the kidneys, lungs, brain, heart, and liver; the minority of patients experience only the typical large vessel–type occlusions seen in simple APS. The occurrence of sudden and essential aPL-induced coagulation or fibrinolysis disorders is highly probable in this group of patients, but precipitating factors remain unknown in most cases [155].

11.5
Anti-C1q Antibodies

C1q (460 kDa), a highly conserved protein, is part of the first component of the complement system. The biological function of C1q is to bind immune complexes via its six globular domains and of a variety of other "non-immune" activators of the complement system, including CRP, DNA, fibronectin, fibrinogen, and lipopolysaccharides, by its collagen-like region (CLR). In immune complexes, C1q is normally bound to Fc regions of IgG in order to fulfill the activation function of C1q within the classical pathway [156]. For many years, C1q was therefore used in radioimmunoassays and ELISAs to detect circulating immune complexes (CIC) in numerous diseases, including SLE [157–159]. In SLE, the CIC titers determined by C1q assays correlated well with disease activity and renal involvement. However, an alternative means of binding C1q has also been described for use in cases where high-affinity autoantibodies directly recognize the CLR of C1q through the antibody F(ab) antigen-combining sites rather than via the Fc domain. Since they were first described [160–162], anti-C1q autoantibodies have been commonly identified in patients with autoimmune diseases such as SLE, rheumatoid vasculitis, MCTD, Felty's syndrome, ankylosing spondylitis, polyarteritis, mixed cryoglobulinemia, membranoproliferative glomerulonephritis, glomerulosclerosis, anti-glomerular basement membrane nephritis, and hypocomplementemic urticarial vasculitis syndrome [163–165].

Anti-C1q autoantibodies are thought to be closely associated with nephritis in SLE. IgG anti-C1q autoantibodies correlate with nephritis, hypocomplementemia, and anti-dsDNA autoantibodies [166–168]. Because significant increases in serum anti-C1q autoantibody titers precede clinical manifestation of nephritis, they have a predictive value [169]. Recently, anti-C1q autoantibodies were identified postmortem in the glomeruli of four of five patients with proliferative glomerulonephritis. The concentrations of these autoantibodies in the glomerular tissue was at least 50 times higher than the serum concentration; this is the first evidence suggesting that anti-C1q autoantibodies collect and concentrate in the renal glomeruli of patients with SLE. Therefore, anti-C1q autoantibodies may contribute to the pathogenesis of lupus glomerulonephritis [170, 171]. Conversely, lupus nephritis does not develop in the absence of anti-C1q autoantibodies, [172, 173]. Anti-C1q autoantibodies also occur in murine models of SLE [174, 175]. A recent study showed that anti-C1q antibodies cause renal pathologies in combination with glomerular C1q-containing immune complexes [176].

11.6
Autoantibody Assessment in Clinical Routine

Patients exhibiting symptoms of suspected SLE should be screened for ANAs using indirect immunofluorescence on HEp-2 cells. Because ANAs are detectable in more than 95% of SLE patients, a negative result largely excludes this diagnosis. In extremely rare cases with clinical continuity of suspicion of SLE, a wide variety of autoantibody tests should be performed. The subsequent analysis of autoantibodies and their profile characteristic in SLE helps to consolidate the diagnosis and to predict lupus subsets with typical organ manifestations (Fig. 11.2).

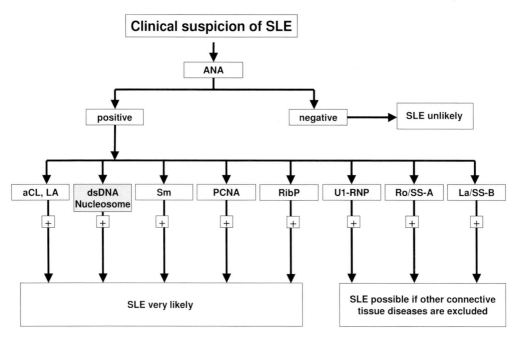

Fig. 11.2 Decision tree of autoantibody testing in patients with clinical suspicion of SLE.

Some of them are included in the revised criteria of the American College of Rheumatology for the classification of SLE [22, 23]. A person is said to have SLE if four or more of the 11 criteria are present, either serially or simultaneously, during any interval or observation.

1. Malar rash
2. Discoid rash
3. Photosensitivity
4 Oral ulcers
5. Arthritis
6. Serositis
   a) Pleuritis or
   b) Pericarditis
7. Renal disorder
   a) Persistent proteinuria (>0.5 g/24 h or 3+) or
   b) Cellular casts
8. Neurologic disorder
   a) Seizures or
   b) Psychosis (having excluded other causes, e.g., drugs)
9. Hematologic disorder
   a) Hemolytic anemia or
   b) Leukopenia (<4/nl) or
   c) Lymphopenia (<1.5/nl) or
   d) Thrombocytopenia (<100/nl)
10. Immunological disorders
    a) Raised anti-dsDNA antibody binding or
    b) Anti-Sm antibody or
    c) Positive finding of antiphospholipid antibodies based on:
       i. IgG/M anticardiolipin antibodies
       ii. Lupus anticoagulant
       iii. False positive serological test for syphilis, present for at least 6 months
11. Antinuclear antibody in raised titer

The majority of autoantibodies do not correlate with disease activity. Therefore, it seems to be sufficient to control these antibodies in annual periods. Only antibodies to dsDNA, which may fluctuate with lupus activity in many patients but not in all, belong together with measurement of complement levels to the routine tools in monitoring disease activity.

It remains to be seen whether one or more other antibody tests such as antinucleosome, anti-ribosomal P, and anti-C1q will be accepted in routine parameters. Assumedly, future therapeutic options more selectively targeting the (auto)-immune system will require new biomarkers that include an extended palette of autoantibody tests [177–179].

References

1 Sherer Y, Gorstein A, Fritzler MJ, Shoenfeld Y. Autoantibody explosion in systemic lupus erythematosus: More than 100 different antibodies found in SLE patients. Semin Arthritis Rheum. 2004, 34:501–537.

2 Hargraves MM, Richmond H, Morton RJ. Presentation of two bone marrow elements: the "tart" cell and the "LE" cell. Proc Mayo Clin. 1948, 23:2558.

3 Haserick JR, Bortz DW. Normal bone marrow inclusion phenomena induced by lupus erythematosus plasma. J Invest Dermatol. 1949, 13:47–49.

4 Haserick JR, Lewis LA, Bortz DW. Blood factor in acute disseminated lupus erythematosus. I. Determination of γ-globulin as specific plasma fraction. Am J Med Sci. 1950, 219:660–663.

5 Miescher P, Fouconnet M. L'absorption du facteur "LE" par des noyaux cellulaires isolés. Experimentia. 1954, 10:252–254.

6 Ceppellini R, Polli E, Celada FA. DNA-reacting factor in serum of a patient with lupus erythematosus diffuses. Proc Soc Exp Biol. 1957, 96:572–574.

7 Holman HR, Kunkel HG. Affinity between the LE factor and cell nucleic acid nucleoprotein. Science. 1957, 126:162–163.

8 Seligmann M. Mise en evidence dans le serum de malades atteints de lupus erythemateux dissemine diune substance determinant une reaction de precipitation avec liacide desoxyribonucleique. CR Acad Sci (Paris). 1957, 245: 243–245.

9 Miescher P, Straessle R. New serological methods for the detection of the LE factor. Vox Sang. 1957, 2:283–287.

10 Arbuckle MR, McClain MT, Rubertone MV, Scofield RH, Dennis GJ, James JA, Harley JB. Development of autoantibodies before the clinical onset of systemic lupus erythematosus. N Engl J Med. 2003, 349:1526–1533.

11 Hoffman IE, Peene I, Meheus L, Huizinga TW, Cebecauer L, Isenberg D, De Bosschere K, Hulstaert F, Veys EM, De Keyser F. Specific antinuclear antibodies are associated with clinical features in systemic lupus erythematosus. Ann Rheum Dis. 2004, 63:1155–1158.

12 Sawalha AH, Harley JB. Antinuclear autoantibodies in systemic lupus erythematosus. Curr Opin Rheumatol. 2004, 16:534–540.

13 Chan EKL, Pollard KM. Autoantibodies to ribonucleoprotein particles by immunoblotting. In: Rose NR, de Macario EC, Fahey JL, Friedman H, Penn GM, eds. Manual of clinical laboratory immunology. Washington,D.C.: American Society for Microbiology, 1992:755–761.

14 Verheijen R, Salden M, van Venrooij WJ. Protein blotting. In: van Venrooij WJ, Maini RN, eds. Manual of Biological Markers of Disease. Kluwer Academic Publishers, 1993:A4-1–A4/25.

15 Lerner MR, Steitz JA. Antibodies to small nuclear RNAs complexed with proteins are produced by patients with systemic lupus erythematosus. Proc Natl Acad Sci USA. 1979, 76:5495–5499.

16 Pettersson I, Hinterberger M, Mimori T, Gottlieb E, Steitz JA. The structure of mammalian small nuclear ribonucleoproteins. Identification of multiple protein components reactive with anti-(U1)ribonucleoprotein and anti-Sm autoantibodies. J Biol Chem. 1984, 259:5907–5914.

17 Hentschel Ch, Schoessler W, Schulte-Pelkum J, Kreutzberger J, Hiepe F. Development of a sensitive and reliable biochip for detection of autoantibodies in rheumatic diseases. In: Conrad K, Sack U, eds. Autoantigens, Autoantibodies, Autoimmunity. 4. Pabst, 2004: 484–489.

18 Robinson WH, DiGennaro C, Hueber W, Haab BB, Kamachi M, Dean EJ, Fournel S, Fong D, Genovese MC, de Vegvar HE, Skriner K, Hirschberg DL, Morris RI, Muller S, Pruijn GJ, van Venrooij WJ, Smolen JS, Brown PO, Steinman L, Utz PJ. Autoantigen microarrays for multiplex characterization of autoantibody responses. Nat Med. 2002, 8:295–301.

19 Joos TO, Schrenk M, Hopfl P, Kroger K, Chowdhury U, Stoll D, Schorner D, Durr M, Herick K, Rupp S, Sohn K, Hammerle H. A microarray enzyme-

linked immunosorbent assay for autoimmune diagnostics. Electrophoresis. 2000, 21:2641–2650.

20 Rouquette AM, Desgruelles C, Laroche P. Evaluation of the new multiplexed immunoassay, FIDIS, for simultaneous quantitative determination of antinuclear antibodies and comparison with conventional methods. Am J Clin Pathol. 2003, 120:676–681.

21 Buliard A, Fortenfant F, Ghillani-Dalbin P, Musset L, Oksman F, Olsson NO. Analysis of nine autoantibodies associated with systemic autoimmune diseases using the Luminex technology. Results of a multicenter study. Ann Biol Clin (Paris). 2005, 63:51–58.

22 Hochberg MC. Updating the American College of Rheumatology revised criteria for the classification of systemic lupus erythematosus. Arthritis Rheum. 1997, 40:1725.

23 Tan EM, Cohen AS, Fries JF, Masi AT, McShane DJ, Rothfield NF, Schaller JG, Talal N, Winchester RJ. The 1982 revised criteria for the classification of systemic lupus erythematosus. Arthritis Rheum. 1982, 25:1271–1277.

24 Hahn BH. Antibodies to DNA. N Engl J Med. 1998, 338:1359–1368.

25 Pisetsky DS. Anti-DNA and autoantibodies. Curr Opin Rheumatol. 2000, 12:364–368.

26 DeGiorgio LA, Konstantinov KN, Lee SC, Hardin JA, Volpe BT, Diamond B. A subset of lupus anti-DNA antibodies crossreacts with the NR2 glutamate receptor in systemic lupus erythematosus. Nat Med. 2001, 7:1189–1193.

27 Omdal R, Brokstad K, Waterloo K, Koldingsnes W, Jonsson R, Mellgren SI. Neuropsychiatric disturbances in SLE are associated with antibodies against NMDA receptors. Eur J Neurol. 2005, 12:392–398.

28 Aarden LA, de Groot ER, Feltkamp TE. Immunology of DNA. III. Crithidia luciliae, a simple substrate for the determination of anti-dsDNA with the immunofluorescence technique. Ann NY Acad Sci. 1975, 254:505–515.

29 Tan EM, Smolen JS, McDougal JS, Butcher BT, Conn D, Dawkins R, Fritzler MJ, Gordon T, Hardin JA, Kalden JR, Lahita RG, Maini RN, Rothfield NF, Smeenk R, Takasaki Y, van Venrooij WJ, Wiik A, Wilson M, Koziol JA. A critical evaluation of enzyme immunoassays for detection of antinuclear autoantibodies of defined specificities. I. Precision, sensitivity, and specificity. Arthritis Rheum. 1999, 42:455–464.

30 Kavanaugh AF, Solomon DH. Guidelines for immunologic laboratory testing in the rheumatic diseases: anti-DNA antibody tests. Arthritis Rheum. 2002, 47:546–555.

31 Amoura Z, Piette JC, Bach JF, Koutouzov S. The key role of nucleosomes in lupus. Arthritis Rheum. 1999, 42:833–843.

32 Amoura Z, Koutouzov S, Piette JC. The role of nucleosomes in lupus. Curr Opin Rheumatol. 2000, 12:369–373.

33 Burlingame RW, Cervera R. Anti-chromatin (anti-nucleosome) autoantibodies. Autoimmun Rev. 2002, 1:321–328.

34 Bavykin SG, Usachenko SI, Zalensky AO, Mirzabekov AD. Structure of nucleosomes and organization of internucleosomal DNA in chromatin. J Mol Biol. 1990, 212:495–511.

35 Luger K, Mader AW, Richmond RK, Sargent DF, Richmond TJ. Crystal structure of the nucleosome core particle at 2.8 A resolution. Nature. 1997, 389:251–260.

36 Burlingame RW, Boey ML, Starkebaum G, Rubin RL. The central role of chromatin in autoimmune responses to histones and DNA in systemic lupus erythematosus. J Clin Invest. 1994, 94:184–192.

37 Chabre H, Amoura Z, Piette JC, Godeau P, Bach JF, Koutouzov S. Presence of nucleosome-restricted antibodies in patients with systemic lupus erythematosus. Arthritis Rheum. 1995, 38:1485–1491.

38 Ghillani-Dalbin P, Amoura Z, Cacoub P, Charuel JL, Diemert MC, Piette JC, Musset L. Testing for anti-nucleosome antibodies in daily practice: a monocentric evaluation in 1696 patients. Lupus. 2003, 12:833–837.

39 Cervera R, Vinas O, Ramos-Casals M, Font J, Garcia-Carrasco M, Siso A, Ramirez F, Machuca Y, Vives J, Ingelmo

M, Burlingame RW. Anti-chromatin antibodies in systemic lupus erythematosus: a useful marker for lupus nephropathy. Ann Rheum Dis. 2003, 62:431–434.

40 Lefkowith JB, Kiehl M, Rubenstein J, DiValerio R, Bernstein K, Kahl L, Rubin RL, Gourley M. Heterogeneity and clinical significance of glomerular-binding antibodies in systemic lupus erythematosus. J Clin Invest. 1996, 98:1373–1380.

41 Wallace DJ, Lin HC, Shen GQ, Peter JB. Antibodies to histone (H2A-H2B)-DNA complexes in the absence of antibodies to double-stranded DNA or to (H2A-H2B) complexes are more sensitive and specific for scleroderma-related disorders than for lupus. Arthritis Rheum. 1994, 37:1795–1797.

42 Bruns A, Bläss S, Hausdorf G, Burmester GR, Hiepe F. Nucleosomes are major T and B cell autoantigens in systemic lupus erythematosus. Arthritis Rheum. 2000, 43:2307–2315.

43 Simon JA, Cabiedes J, Ortiz E, Alcocer-Varela J, Sanchez-Guerrero J. Anti-nucleosome antibodies in patients with systemic lupus erythematosus of recent onset. Potential utility as a diagnostic tool and disease activity marker. Rheumatology (Oxford). 2004, 43:220–224.

44 Min DJ, Kim SJ, Park SH, Seo YI, Kang HJ, Kim WU, Cho CS, Kim HY. Anti-nucleosome antibody: significance in lupus patients lacking anti-double-stranded DNA antibody. Clin Exp Rheumatol. 2002, 20:13–18.

45 Amoura Z, Koutouzov S, Chabre H, Cacoub P, Amoura I, Musset L, Bach JF, Piette JC. Presence of antinucleosome autoantibodies in a restricted set of connective tissue diseases: antinucleosome antibodies of the IgG3 subclass are markers of renal pathogenicity in systemic lupus erythematosus. Arthritis Rheum. 2000, 43:76–84.

46 Benucci M, Gobbi FL, Del Rosso A, Cesaretti S, Niccoli L, Cantini F. Disease activity and antinucleosome antibodies in systemic lupus erythematosus. Scand J Rheumatol. 2003, 32:42–45.

47 Berden JH, Licht R, van Bruggen MC, Tax WJ. Role of nucleosomes for induction and glomerular binding of autoantibodies in lupus nephritis. Curr Opin Nephrol Hypertens. 1999, 8:299–306.

48 Berden JH, van Bruggen MC. Nucleosomes and the pathogenesis of lupus nephritis. Kidney Blood Press Res. 1997, 20:198–200.

49 van Bruggen MC, Kramers C, Walgreen B, Elema JD, Kallenberg CG, van den BJ, Smeenk RJ, Assmann KJ, Muller S, Monestier M, Berden JH. Nucleosomes and histones are present in glomerular deposits in human lupus nephritis. Nephrol Dial Transplant. 1997, 12:57–66.

50 Koutouzov S, Jeronimo AL, Campos H, Amoura Z. Nucleosomes in the pathogenesis of systemic lupus erythematosus. Rheum Dis Clin North Am. 2004, 30:529–558.

51 Abraham SJ, Rojas-Serrano J, Cabiedes J, Alcocer-Varela J. Antinucleosome antibodies may help predict development of systemic lupus erythematosus in patients with primary antiphospholipid syndrome. Lupus. 2004, 13:177–181.

52 Burlingame RW, Rubin RL. Drug-induced anti-histone autoantibodies display two patterns of reactivity with substructures of chromatin. J Clin Invest. 1991, 88:680–690.

53 Burlingame RW. The clinical utility of antihistone antibodies. Autoantibodies reactive with chromatin in systemic lupus erythematosus and drug-induced lupus. Clin Lab Med. 1997, 17:367–378.

54 Hmida Y, Schmit P, Gilson G, Humbel RL. Failure to detect antinucleosome antibodies in scleroderma: comment on the article by Amoura et al. Arthritis Rheum. 2002, 46:280–282.

55 Suer W, Dahnrich C, Schlumberger W, Stocker W. Autoantibodies in SLE but not in scleroderma react with protein-stripped nucleosomes. J Autoimmun. 2004, 22:325–334.

56 Li L, Chen M, Huang DY, Nishioka M. Frequency and significance of antibodies to chromatin in autoimmune hepatitis type I. J Gastroenterol Hepatol. 2000, 15:1176–1182.

57 Zieve GW, Khusial PR. The anti-Sm immune response in autoimmunity and cell biology. Autoimmun Rev. 2003, 2:235–240.

58 Tan EM, Kunkel HG. Characteristics of a soluble nuclear antigen precipitating with sera of patients with systemic lupus erythematosus. J Immunol. 1966, 96:464–471.

59 Arnett FC, Hamilton RG, Roebber MG, Harley JB, Reichlin M. Increased frequencies of Sm and nRNP autoantibodies in American blacks compared to whites with systemic lupus erythematosus. J Rheumatol. 1988, 15:1773–1776.

60 Ignat GP, Rat AC, Sychra JJ, Vo J, Varga J, Teodorescu M. Information on diagnosis and management of systemic lupus erythematosus derived from the routine measurement of 8 nuclear autoantibodies. J Rheumatol. 2003, 30:1761–1769.

61 Yasuma M, Takasaki Y, Matsumoto K, Kodama A, Hashimoto H, Hirose S. Clinical significance of IgG anti-Sm antibodies in patients with systemic lupus erythematosus. J Rheumatol. 1990, 17:469–475.

62 Cervera R, Khamashta MA, Font J, Sebastiani GD, Gil A, Lavilla P, Domenech I, Aydintug AO, Jedryka-Goral A, de Ramon E. Systemic lupus erythematosus: clinical and immunologic patterns of disease expression in a cohort of 1000 patients. The European Working Party on Systemic Lupus Erythematosus. Medicine (Baltimore). 1993, 72:113–124.

63 ter Borg EJ, Groen H, Horst G, Limburg PC, Wouda AA, Kallenberg CG. Clinical associations of antiribonucleoprotein antibodies in patients with systemic lupus erythematosus. Semin Arthritis Rheum. 1990, 20:164–173.

64 Vlachoyiannopoulos PG, Karassa FB, Karakostas KX, Drosos AA, Moutsopoulos HM. Systemic lupus erythematosus in Greece. Clinical features, evolution and outcome: a descriptive analysis of 292 patients. Lupus. 1993, 2:303–312.

65 Riemekasten G, Marell J, Trebeljahr G, Klein R, Hausdorf G, Haupl T, Schneider-Mergener J, Burmester GR, Hiepe F. A novel epitope on the C-terminus of SmD1 is recognized by the majority of sera from patients with systemic lupus erythematosus. J Clin Invest. 1998, 102:754–763.

66 Mattioli M, Reichlin M. Physical association of two nuclear antigens and mutual occurrence of their antibodies: the relationship of the SM and RNAprotein (MO) systems in SLE sera. J Immunol. 1973, 110:1318–1324.

67 Font J, Cervera R, Ramos-Casals M, Garcia-Carrasco M, Sents J, Herrero C, del Olmo JA, Darnell A, Ingelmo M. Clusters of clinical and immunologic features in systemic lupus erythematosus: analysis of 600 patients from a single center. Semin Arthritis Rheum. 2004, 33:217–230.

68 von Muhlen CA, Tan EM. Autoantibodies in the diagnosis of systemic rheumatic diseases. Semin Arthritis Rheum. 1995, 24:323–358.

69 Sharp GC, Irvin WS, LaRoque RL, Velez C, Daly V, Kaiser AD, Holman HR. Association of autoantibodies to different nuclear antigens with clinical patterns of rheumatic disease and responsiveness to therapy. J Clin Invest. 1971, 50:350–359.

70 Fisher DE, Reeves WH, Wisniewolski R, Lahita RG, Chiorazzi N. Temporal shifts from Sm to ribonucleoprotein reactivity in systemic lupus erythematosus. Arthritis Rheum. 1985, 28:1348–1355.

71 Arbuckle MR, Reichlin M, Harley JB, James JA. Shared early autoantibody recognition events in the development of anti-Sm B/B' in human lupus. Scand J Immunol. 1999, 50:447–455.

72 James JA, Harley JB. Linear epitope mapping of an Sm B/B' polypeptide. J Immunol. 1992, 148:2074–2079.

73 James JA, Gross T, Scofield RH, Harley JB. Immunoglobulin epitope spreading and autoimmune disease after peptide immunization: Sm B/B'-derived PPPGMRPP and PPPGIRGP induce spliceosome autoimmunity. J Exp Med. 1995, 181:453–461.

74 James JA, Harley JB. A model of peptide-induced lupus autoimmune B cell epitope spreading is strain specific and is not H-2 restricted in mice. J Immunol. 1998, 160:502–508.

75 Harley JB, James JA. Epstein-Barr virus infection may be an environmental risk factor for systemic lupus erythematosus in children and teenagers. Arthritis Rheum. 1999, 42:1782–1783.

76 James JA, Kaufman KM, Farris AD, Taylor-Albert E, Lehman TJ, Harley JB. An increased prevalence of Epstein-Barr

virus infection in young patients suggests a possible etiology for systemic lupus erythematosus. J Clin Invest. 1997, 100:3019–3026.

77 James JA, Neas BR, Moser KL, Hall T, Bruner GR, Sestak AL, Harley JB. Systemic lupus erythematosus in adults is associated with previous Epstein-Barr virus exposure. Arthritis Rheum. 2001, 44:1122–1126.

78 Kang I, Quan T, Nolasco H, Park SH, Hong MS, Crouch J, Pamer EG, Howe JG, Craft J. Defective control of latent Epstein-Barr virus infection in systemic lupus erythematosus. J Immunol. 2004, 172:1287–1294.

79 Habets WJ, de Rooij DJ, Hoet MH, van de Putte LB, van Venrooij WJ. Quantitation of anti-RNP and anti-Sm antibodies in MCTD and SLE patients by immunoblotting. Clin Exp Immunol. 1985, 59:457–466.

80 Jaekel HP, Klopsch T, Benkenstein B, Grobe N, Baldauf A, Schoessler W, Werle E. Reactivities to the Sm autoantigenic complex and the synthetic SmD1-aa83-119 peptide in systemic lupus erythematosus and other autoimmune diseases. J Autoimmun. 2001, 17:347–354.

81 Tsao BP, Grossman JM, Riemekasten G, Strong N, Kalsi J, Wallace DJ, Chen CJ, Lau CS, Ginzler EM, Goldstein R, Kalunian KC, Harley JB, Arnett FC, Hahn BH, Cantor RM. Familiality and co-occurrence of clinical features of systemic lupus erythematosus. Arthritis Rheum. 2002, 46:2678–2685.

82 Riemekasten G, Marell J, Hentschel C, Klein R, Burmester GR, Schoessler W, Hiepe F. Casein is an essential cofactor in autoantibody reactivity directed against the C-terminal SmD1 peptide AA 83-119 in systemic lupus erythematosus. Immunobiology. 2002, 206:537–545.

83 Rokeach LA, Haselby JA, Hoch SO. Molecular cloning of a cDNA encoding the human Sm-D autoantigen. Proc Natl Acad Sci USA. 1988, 85:4832–4836.

84 Rokeach LA, Jannatipour M, Haselby JA, Hoch SO. Mapping of the immunoreactive domains of a small nuclear ribonucleoprotein-associated Sm-D autoantigen.

Clin Immunol Immunopathol. 1992, 65:315–324.

85 Riemekasten G, Kawald A, Weiss C, Meine A, Marell J, Klein R, Hocher B, Meisel C, Hausdorf G, Manz R, Kamradt T, Burmester GR, Hiepe F. Strong acceleration of murine lupus by injection of the SmD1 (83-119) peptide. Arthritis Rheum. 2001, 44:2435–2445.

86 Riemekasten G, Langnickel D, Ebling FM, Karpouzas G, Kalsi J, Herberth G, Tsao BP, Henklein P, Langer S, Burmester GR, Radbruch A, Hiepe F, Hahn BH. Identification and characterization of SmD 183-119-reactive T cells that provide T cell help for pathogenic anti-double-stranded DNA antibodies. Arthritis Rheum 2003, 48:475–485.

87 Staikou EV, Routsias JG, Makri AA, Terzoglou A, Sakarellos-Daitsiotis M, Sakarellos C, Panayotou G, Moutsopoulos HM, Tzioufas AG. Calreticulin binds preferentially with B cell linear epitopes of Ro60 kD autoantigen, enhancing recognition by anti-Ro60 kD autoantibodies. Clin Exp Immunol. 2003, 134:143–150.

88 Riemekasten G, Langnickel D, Enghard P, Undeutsch R, Humrich J, Ebling FM, Hocher B, Humaljoki T, Neumayer H, Burmester GR, Hahn BH, Radbruch A, Hiepe F. Intravenous injection of a D1 protein of the Smith proteins postpones murine lupus and induces type 1 regulatory T cells. J Immunol. 2004, 173:5835–5842.

89 Brahms H, Raymackers J, Union A, De Keyser F, Meheus L, Luhrmann R. The C-terminal RG dipeptide repeats of the spliceosomal Sm proteins D1 and D3 contain symmetrical dimethylarginines, which form a major B-cell epitope for anti-Sm autoantibodies. J Biol Chem. 2000, 275:17122–17129.

90 Mahler M, Stinton LM, Fritzler MJ. Improved serological differentiation between systemic lupus erythematosus and mixed connective tissue disease by use of an SmD3 peptide-based immunoassay. Clin Diagn Lab Immunol. 2005, 12:107–113.

91 Mahler M, Fritzler MJ, Bluthner M. Identification of a SmD3 epitope with a

single symmetrical dimethylation of an arginine residue as a specific target of a subpopulation of anti-Sm antibodies. Arthritis Res Ther. 2005, 7:R19–R29.

92 Anderson JR, Gray KG, Beck JS, Kinnear WF. Precipitating autoantibodies in Sjögren's disease. Lancet. 1961, 2:456–460.

93 Clark G, Reichlin M, Tomasi TB, Jr. Characterization of a soluble cytoplasmic antigen reactive with sera from patients with systemic lupus erythematosus. J Immunol. 1969, 102:117–122.

94 Alspaugh MA, Tan EM. Antibodies to cellular antigens in Sjogren's syndrome. J Clin Invest. 1975, 55:1067–1073.

95 Franceschini F, Cavazzana I. Anti-Ro/SSA and La/SSB antibodies. Autoimmunity. 2005, 38:55–63.

96 O'Brien CA, Harley JB. A subset of hY RNAs is associated with erythrocyte Ro ribonucleoproteins. EMBO J. 1990, 9:3683–3689.

97 Itoh Y, Reichlin M. Ro/SS-A antigen in human platelets. Different distributions of the isoforms of Ro/SS-A protein and the Ro/SS-A-binding RNA. Arthritis Rheum. 1991, 34:888–893.

98 Ben Chetrit E, Chan EK, Sullivan KF, Tan EM. A 52-kD protein is a novel component of the SS-A/Ro antigenic particle. J Exp Med. 1988, 167:1560–1571.

99 Chan EK, Hamel JC, Buyon JP, Tan EM. Molecular definition and sequence motifs of the 52-kD component of human SS-A/Ro autoantigen. J Clin Invest. 1991, 87:68–76.

100 Itoh K, Itoh Y, Frank MB. Protein heterogeneity in the human Ro/SSA ribonucleoproteins. The 52- and 60-kD Ro/SSA autoantigens are encoded by separate genes. J Clin Invest. 1991, 87: 177–186.

101 Kurien BT, Chambers TL, Thomas PY, Frank MB, Scofield RH. Autoantibody to the leucine zipper region of 52 kDa Ro/SSA binds native 60 kDa Ro/SSA: identification of a tertiary epitope with components from 60 kDa Ro/SSA and 52 kDa Ro/SSA. Scand J Immunol. 2001, 53:268–276.

102 Stefano JE. Purified lupus antigen La recognizes an oligouridylate stretch common to the 3' termini of RNA polymerase III transcripts. Cell. 1984, 36:145–154.

103 Chen X, Quinn AM, Wolin SL. Ro ribonucleoproteins contribute to the resistance of Deinococcus radiodurans to ultraviolet irradiation. Genes Dev. 2000, 14:777–782.

104 Chen X, Smith JD, Shi H, Yang DD, Flavell RA, Wolin SL. The Ro autoantigen binds misfolded U2 small nuclear RNAs and assists mammalian cell survival after UV irradiation. Curr Biol. 2003, 13:2206–2211.

105 Xue D, Shi H, Smith JD, Chen X, Noe DA, Cedervall T, Yang DD, Eynon E, Brash DE, Kashgarian M, Flavell RA, Wolin SL. A lupus-like syndrome develops in mice lacking the Ro 60-kDa protein, a major lupus autoantigen. Proc Natl Acad Sci USA. 2003, 100:7503–7508.

106 Ramakrishnan S, Sharma HW, Farris AD, Kaufman KM, Harley JB, Collins K, Pruijn GJ, van Venrooij WJ, Martin ML, Narayanan R. Characterization of human telomerase complex. Proc Natl Acad Sci USA. 1997, 94:10075–10079.

107 Sontheimer RD, Maddison PJ, Reichlin M, Jordon RE, Stastny P, Gilliam JN. Serologic and HLA associations in subacute cutaneous lupus erythematosus, a clinical subset of lupus erythematosus. Ann Intern Med. 1982, 97:664–671.

108 Dörner T, Feist E, Pruss A, Chaoui R, Göldner B, Hiepe F. Significance of autoantibodies in neonatal lupus erythematosus. Int Arch Allergy Immunol. 2000, 123:58–66.

109 Brucato A, Frassi M, Franceschini F, Cimaz R, Faden D, Pisoni MP, Muscara M, Vignati G, Stramba-Badiale M, Catelli L, Lojacono A, Cavazzana I, Ghirardello A, Vescovi F, Gambari PF, Doria A, Meroni PL, Tincani A. Risk of congenital complete heart block in newborns of mothers with anti-Ro/SSA antibodies detected by counterimmunoelectrophoresis: a prospective study

of 100 women. Arthritis Rheum. 2001, 44:1832–1835.

110 Costedoat-Chalumeau N, Amoura Z, Lupoglazoff JM, Thi Huong dL, Denjoy I, Vauthier D, Sebbouh D, Fain O, Georgin-Lavialle S, Ghillani P, Musset L, Wechsler B, Duhaut P, Piette JC. Outcome of pregnancies in patients with anti-SSA/Ro antibodies: a study of 165 pregnancies, with special focus on electrocardiographic variations in the children and comparison with a control group. Arthritis Rheum. 2004, 50: 3187–3194.

111 Brucato A, Doria A, Frassi M, Castellino G, Franceschini F, Faden D, Pisoni MP, Solerte L, Muscara M, Lojacono A, Motta M, Cavazzana I, Ghirardello A, Vescovi F, Tombini V, Cimaz R, Gambari PF, Meroni PL, Canesi B, Tincani A. Pregnancy outcome in 100 women with autoimmune diseases and anti-Ro/SSA antibodies: a prospective controlled study. Lupus. 2002, 11:716–721.

112 Buyon JP, Hiebert R, Copel J, Craft J, Friedman D, Katholi M, Lee LA, Provost TT, Reichlin M, Rider L, Rupel A, Saleeb S, Weston WL, Skovron ML. Autoimmune-associated congenital heart block: demographics, mortality, morbidity and recurrence rates obtained from a national neonatal lupus registry. J Am Coll Cardiol. 1998, 31:1658–1666.

113 Eronen M, Siren MK, Ekblad H, Tikanoja T, Julkunen H, Paavilainen T. Short- and long-term outcome of children with congenital complete heart block diagnosed in utero or as a newborn. Pediatrics. 2000, 106:86–91.

114 Julkunen H, Kaaja R, Siren MK, Mack C, McCready S, Holthofer H, Kurki P, Maddison P. Immune-mediated congenital heart block (CHB): identifying and counseling patients at risk for having children with CHB. Semin Arthritis Rheum. 1998, 28:97–106.

115 Buyon JP, Winchester RJ, Slade SG, Arnett F, Copel J, Friedman D, Lockshin MD. Identification of mothers at risk for congenital heart block and other neonatal lupus syndromes in their children. Comparison of enzyme-linked immunosorbent assay and immunoblot for measurement of anti-SS-A/Ro and anti-SS-B/La antibodies. Arthritis Rheum. 1993, 36:1263–1273.

116 Salomonsson S, Dorner T, Theander E, Bremme K, Larsson P, Wahren-Herlenius M. A serologic marker for fetal risk of congenital heart block. Arthritis Rheum. 2002, 46:1233–1241.

117 Dörner T, Feist E, Chaoui R, Hiepe F. Enhanced frequency of autoimmune congenital heart block in female offspring. Rheumatology (Oxford). 1999, 38:380–382.

118 Bravo R, Frank R, Blundell PA, Macdonald-Bravo H. Cyclin/PCNA is the auxiliary protein of DNA polymerase-delta. Nature. 1987, 326:515–517.

119 Prelich G, Tan CK, Kostura M, Mathews MB, So AG, Downey KM, Stillman B. Functional identity of proliferating cell nuclear antigen and a DNA polymerase-delta auxiliary protein. Nature. 1987, 326:517–520.

120 Chou CH, Satoh M, Wang J, Reeves WH. B-cell epitopes of autoantigenic DNA-binding proteins. Mol Biol Rep. 1992, 16:191–198.

121 Miyachi K, Fritzler MJ, Tan EM. Autoantibody to a nuclear antigen in proliferating cells. J Immunol. 1978, 121:2228–2234.

122 Takasaki Y, Fishwild D, Tan EM. Characterization of proliferating cell nuclear antigen recognized by autoantibodies in lupus sera. J Exp Med. 1984, 159:981–992.

123 Tan EM. Antinuclear antibodies: diagnostic markers for autoimmune diseases and probes for cell biology. Adv Immunol. 1989, 44:93–151.

124 Asero R, Origgi L, Crespi S, Bertetti E, D'Agostino P, Riboldi P. Autoantibody to proliferating cell nuclear antigen (PCNA) in SLE: a clinical and serological study. Clin Exp Rheumatol. 1987, 5:241–246.

125 Grimaudo SA, Guilleron CMJA. Immunoblotting for detectionof anti-self reactivities in collagen diseases: autoantibody profiles and clinical significance in patients with SLE. Lupus. 2005, 4:160.

126 Grimaudo SA, Guilleron CMJA. Immunoblotting for detection of anti-self reactivities in collagen diseases: autoantibody profiles and clinical significance in patients with SLE. Lupus. 1995, 4:160.

127 Bonfa E, Golombek SJ, Kaufman LD, Skelly S, Weissbach H, Brot N, Elkon KB. Association between lupus psychosis and anti-ribosomal P protein antibodies. N Engl J Med. 1987, 317:265–271.

128 Elkon KB, Parnassa AP, Foster CL. Lupus autoantibodies target ribosomal P proteins. J Exp Med. 1985, 162:459–471.

129 Elkon K, Bonfa E, Llovet R, Danho W, Weissbach H, Brot N. Properties of the ribosomal P2 protein autoantigen are similar to those of foreign protein antigens. Proc Natl Acad Sci USA. 1988, 85:5186–189.

130 Hasler P, Brot N, Weissbach H, Parnassa AP, Elkon KB. Ribosomal proteins P0, P1, and P2 are phosphorylated by casein kinase II at their conserved carboxyl termini. J Biol Chem. 1991, 266:13815–13820.

131 Hasler P, Brot N, Weissbach H, Danho W, Blount Y, Zhou JL, Elkon KB. The effect of phosphorylation and site-specific mutations in the immunodominant epitope of the human ribosomal P proteins. Clin Immunol Immunopathol. 1994, 72:273–279.

132 Mahler M, Kessenbrock K, Raats J, Williams R, Fritzler MJ, Bluthner M. Characterization of the human autoimmune response to the major C-terminal epitope of the ribosomal P proteins. J Mol Med. 2003, 81:194–204.

133 Caponi L, Bombardieri S, Migliorini P. Anti-ribosomal antibodies bind the Sm proteins D and B/B′. Clin Exp Immunol. 1998, 112:139–143.

134 Caponi L, Chimenti D, Pratesi F, Migliorini P. Anti-ribosomal antibodies from lupus patients bind DNA. Clin Exp Immunol. 2002, 130:541–547.

135 Reichlin M. Cellular dysfunction induced by penetration of autoantibodies into living cells: cellular damage and dysfunction mediated by antibodies to dsDNA and ribosomal P proteins. J Autoimmun. 1998, 11:557–561.

136 Mahler M, Kessenbrock K, Reeves W, Takasaki Y, Garcia-De La Torre I, Shoenfeld Y, Hiepe F, Shun-le C, von Mühlen C, Wiik A, Höpfl P, Szmyrka M, Fritzler MJ. Multi-centre evaluation of a new assay to detect autoantibodies to ribosomal P proteins. Arthritis Res Ther (in press).

137 Nojima Y, Minota S, Yamada A, Takaku F, Aotsuka S, Yokohari R. Correlation of antibodies to ribosomal P protein with psychosis in patients with systemic lupus erythematosus. Ann Rheum Dis. 1992, 51:1053–1055.

138 Schneebaum AB, Singleton JD, West SG, Blodgett JK, Allen LG, Cheronis JC, Kotzin BL. Association of psychiatric manifestations with antibodies to ribosomal P proteins in systemic lupus erythematosus. Am J Med. 1991, 90:54–62.

139 Gerli R, Caponi L, Tincani A, Scorza R, Sabbadini MG, Danieli MG, De AV, Cesarotti M, Piccirilli M, Quartesan R, Moretti P, Cantoni C, Franceschini F, Cavazzana I, Origgi L, Vanoli M, Bozzolo E, Ferrario L, Padovani A, Gambini O, Vanzulli L, Croce D, Bombardieri S. Clinical and serological associations of ribosomal P autoantibodies in systemic lupus erythematosus: prospective evaluation in a large cohort of Italian patients. Rheumatology (Oxford). 2002, 41:1357–1366.

140 Sato T, Uchiumi T, Ozawa T, Kikuchi M, Nakano M, Kominami R, Arakawa M. Autoantibodies against ribosomal proteins found with high frequency in patients with systemic lupus erythematosus with active disease. J Rheumatol. 1991, 18:1681–1684.

141 Chindalore V, Neas B, Reichlin M. The association between anti-ribosomal P antibodies and active nephritis in systemic lupus erythematosus. Clin Immunol Immunopathol. 1998, 87:292–296.

142 Reichlin M, Wolfson-Reichlin M. Evidence for the participation of anti-ribosomal P antibodies in lupus nephritis. Arthritis Rheum. 1999, 42:2728–2729.

143 Reichlin M, Wolfson-Reichlin M. Correlations of anti-dsDNA and anti-ribosomal P autoantibodies with lupus nephritis. Clin Immunol. 2003, 108: 69–72.

144 Hulsey M, Goldstein R, Scully L, Surbeck W, Reichlin M. Anti-ribosomal P antibodies in systemic lupus erythematosus: a case-control study correlating hepatic and renal disease. Clin Immunol Immunopathol. 1995, 74:252–256.

145 Ohira H, Takiguchi J, Rai T, Abe K, Yokokawa J, Sato Y, Takeda I, Kanno T. High frequency of anti-ribosomal P antibody in patients with systemic lupus erythematosus-associated hepatitis. Hepatol Res. 2004, 28:137–139.

146 Galli M. Antiphospholipid syndrome: association between laboratory tests and clinical practice. Pathophysiol Haemost Thromb. 2003, 33:249–255.

147 Gromnica-Ihle E, Schossler W. Antiphospholipid syndrome. Int Arch Allergy Immunol. 2000, 123:67–76.

148 Wilson WA, Gharavi AE, Koike T, Lockshin MD, Branch DW, Piette JC, Brey R, Derksen R, Harris EN, Hughes GR, Triplett DA, Khamashta MA. International consensus statement on preliminary classification criteria for definite antiphospholipid syndrome: report of an international workshop. Arthritis Rheum. 1999, 42:1309–1311.

149 Brandt JT, Triplett DA, Alving B, Scharrer I. Criteria for the diagnosis of lupus anticoagulants: an update. On behalf of the Subcommittee on Lupus Anticoagulant/Antiphospholipid Antibody of the Scientific and Standardisation Committee of the ISTH. Thromb Haemost. 1995, 74:1185–1190.

150 Petri M. Diagnosis of antiphospholipid antibodies. Rheum Dis Clin North Am. 1994, 20:443–469.

151 Buttgereit F, Grunewald T, Schuler-Maue W, Burmester GR, Hiepe F. Value of anticardiolipin antibodies for monitoring disease activity in systemic lupus erythematosus and other rheumatic diseases. Clin Rheumatol. 1997, 16:562–569.

152 Karassa FB, Ioannidis JP, Touloumi G, Boki KA, Moutsopoulos HM. Risk factors for central nervous system involvement in systemic lupus erythematosus. Q JM. 2000, 93:169–174.

153 West SG, Emlen W, Wener MH, Kotzin BL. Neuropsychiatric lupus erythematosus: a 10-year prospective study on the value of diagnostic tests. Am J Med. 1995, 99:153–163.

154 Sanna G, Bertolaccini ML, Cuadrado MJ, Laing H, Khamashta MA, Mathieu A, Hughes GR. Neuropsychiatric manifestations in systemic lupus erythematosus: prevalence and association with antiphospholipid antibodies. J Rheumatol. 2003, 30:985–992.

155 Asherson RA, Cervera R, Piette JC, Font J, Lie JT, Burcoglu A, Lim K, Munoz-Rodriguez FJ, Levy RA, Boue F, Rossert J, Ingelmo M. Catastrophic antiphospholipid syndrome. Clinical and laboratory features of 50 patients. Medicine (Baltimore). 1998, 77:195–207.

156 Hiepe F, Pfüller B, Wolbart K, Bruns A, Leinenbach H-P, Hepper M, Schössler W, Otto V. C1q – a multifunctional ligand for a new immunoadsorption treatment. Ther Apher. 1999, 3:246–251.

157 Nydegger UE, Lambert PH, Gerber H, Miescher PA. Circulating immune complexes in the serum in systemic lupus erythematosus and in carriers of hepatitis B antigen. Quantitation by binding to radiolabeled C1q. J Clin Invest. 1974, 54:297–309.

158 Hay FC, Nineham LJ, Roitt IM. Routine assay for the detection of immune complexes of known immunoglobulin class using solid phase C1q. Clin Exp Immunol. 1976, 24:396–400.

159 Schössler W, Hiepe F, Montag T, Schmidt HE. The use of glass as solid phase in enzyme immunoassay as exemplified by the detection of circulating immune complexes. Biomed Biochim Acta. 1985, 44:1247–1253.

160 Uwatoko S, Aotsuka S, Okawa M, Egusa Y, Yokohari R, Aizawa C, Suzuki K. C1q solid-phase radioimmunoassay: evidence for detection of antibody directed against the collagen-like region of C1q in sera from patients with sys-

temic lupus erythematosus. Clin Exp Immunol. 1987, 69:98–106.

161 Uwatoko S, Mannik M. Low-molecular weight C1q-binding immunoglobulin G in patients with systemic lupus erythematosus consists of autoantibodies to the collagen-like region of C1q. J Clin Invest. 1988, 82:816–824.

162 Wisnieski JJ, Naff GB. Serum IgG antibodies to C1q in hypocomplementemic urticarial vasculitis syndrome. Arthritis Rheum. 1989, 32:1119–1127.

163 Wener MH, Uwatoko S, Mannik M. Antibodies to the collagen-like region of C1q in sera of patients with autoimmune rheumatic diseases. Arthritis Rheum. 1989, 32:544–551.

164 Siegert CE, Daha MR, van der Voort EA, Breedveld FC. IgG and IgA antibodies to the collagen-like region of C1q in rheumatoid vasculitis. Arthritis Rheum. 1990, 33:1646–1654.

165 Seelen MA, Trouw LA, van der Hoorn JW, Fallaux-van den Houten FC, Huizinga TW, Daha MR, Roos A. Autoantibodies against mannose-binding lectin in systemic lupus erythematosus. Clin Exp Immunol. 2003, 134:335–343.

166 Siegert C, Daha M, Westedt ML, van dV, Breedveld F. IgG autoantibodies against C1q are correlated with nephritis, hypocomplementemia, and dsDNA antibodies in systemic lupus erythematosus. J Rheumatol. 1991, 18:230–234.

167 Moroni G, Trendelenburg M, Del Papa N, Quaglini S, Raschi E, Panzeri P, Testoni C, Tincani A, Banfi G, Balestrieri G, Schifferli JA, Meroni PL, Ponticelli C. Anti-C1q antibodies may help in diagnosing a renal flare in lupus nephritis. Am J Kidney Dis. 2001, 37:490–498.

168 Marto N, Bertolaccini ML, Calabuig E, Hughes GR, Khamashta MA. Anti-C1q antibodies in nephritis: correlation between titres and renal disease activity and positive predictive value in systemic lupus erythematosus. Ann Rheum Dis. 2005, 64:444–448.

169 Siegert CE, Daha MR, Tseng CM, Coremans IE, van EL, Breedveld FC. Predic-

tive value of IgG autoantibodies against C1q for nephritis in systemic lupus erythematosus. Ann Rheum Dis. 1993, 52:851–856.

170 Mannik M, Wener MH. Deposition of antibodies to the collagen-like region of C1q in renal glomeruli of patients with proliferative lupus glomerulonephritis. Arthritis Rheum. 1997, 40:1504–1511.

171 Mannik M, Merrill CE, Stamps LD, Wener MH. Multiple autoantibodies form the glomerular immune deposits in patients with systemic lupus erythematosus. J Rheumatol. 2003, 30:1495–1504.

172 Fremeaux-Bacchi V, Noel LH, Schifferli JA. No lupus nephritis in the absence of antiC1q autoantibodies? Nephrol Dial Transplant. 2002, 17:2041–2043.

173 Trendelenburg M, Marfurt J, Gerber I, Tyndall A, Schifferli JA. Lack of occurrence of severe lupus nephritis among anti-C1q autoantibody-negative patients. Arthritis Rheum. 1999, 42:187–188.

174 Hogarth MB, Norsworthy PJ, Allen PJ, Trinder PK, Loos M, Morley BJ, Walport MJ, Davies KA. Autoantibodies to the collagenous region of C1q occur in three strains of lupus-prone mice. Clin Exp Immunol. 1996, 104:241–246.

175 Trinder PK, Maeurer MJ, Schorlemmer HU, Loos M. Autoreactivity to mouse C1q in a murine model of SLE. Rheumatol Int. 1995, 15:117–120.

176 Trouw LA, Groeneveld TW, Seelen MA, Duijs JM, Bajema IM, Prins FA, Kishore U, Salant DJ, Verbeek JS, Van Kooten C, Daha MR. Anti-C1q autoantibodies deposit in glomeruli but are only pathogenic in combination with glomerular C1q-containing immune complexes. J Clin Invest. 2004, 114:679–688.

177 Illei GG, Tackey E, Lapteva L, Lipsky PE. Biomarkers in systemic lupus erythematosus: II. Markers of disease activity. Arthritis Rheum. 2004, 50:2048–2065.

178 Illei GG, Tackey E, Lapteva L, Lipsky PE. Biomarkers in systemic lupus erythematosus. I. General overview

of biomarkers and their applicability. Arthritis Rheum. 2004, 50:1709–1720.

179 Schiffenbauer J, Hahn B, Weisman MH, Simon LS. Biomarkers, surrogate markers, and design of clinical trials of new therapies for systemic lupus erythematosus. Arthritis Rheum. 2004, 50:2415–2422.

180 Hiepe F, Dorner T, Burmester G. Antinuclear antibody- and extractable nuclear antigen-related diseases. Int Arch Allergy Immunol. 2000, 123:5–9.

181 von Mühlen CA, Tan EM. Autoantibodies in the diagnosis of systemic rheumatic diseases. Semin Arthritis Rheum. 1995, 24:323–358.

12

Autoantibodies in Rheumatoid Arthritis

Tsuneyo Mimori

12.1
Introduction

Rheumatoid arthritis (RA) is a systemic inflammatory disease that is characterized by chronic and erosive polyarthritis or by abnormal growth of synovial tissue (pannus) and causes irreversible joint disability. Recent studies show that joint injury in RA patients progresses within two years from onset, and aggressive treatments from the early stage can prevent the progression of the disease. Hence, the necessities of early diagnosis and early treatment have been emphasized. However, RA patients do not always show typical symptoms at the early stages and are often difficult to diagnose since they may not fulfill the classification criteria for RA.

RA is also categorized among systemic autoimmune diseases because of the presence of rheumatoid factor (RF), autoantibodies against the Fc portion of IgG, and other autoantibodies. RF has been clinically utilized as the only serologic marker of RA so far. However, the sensitivity of RF is 60–80% in RA, and the specificity is rather low since RF is also detected widely and frequently in many other conditions, including various connective tissue diseases, chronic liver diseases, and infectious diseases, and even in a few percentages of healthy people. Therefore, although RF is adopted into the criteria for classification of RA, its diagnostic value is unsatisfactory especially in the early stages of the disease.

In recent years, a number of novel autoantibodies have been described in RA, and their clinical significance and possible pathogenic roles have been discussed. In particular, new autoantibodies to citrullinated filaggrin and its circular form (cyclic citrullinated peptide, CCP) are the most remarkable because of their reasonable sensitivity and high specificity in RA patients, which may be able to serve as an early diagnostic marker and a prognostic factor of joint destruction. This chapter reviews and discusses the target autoantigens as well as the clinical and possible etiopathogenic significance of recently found autoantibodies in RA.

Autoantibodies and Autoimmunity: Molecular Mechanisms in Health and Disease. Edited by K. Michael Pollard
Copyright © 2006 WILEY-VCH Verlag GmbH & Co. KGaA, Weinheim
ISBN: 3-527-31141-6

12.2
Anti-citrullinated Protein Antibodies

12.2.1
Identification of Citrullinated Proteins as RA-specific Autoantigens

In the 1960s, an autoantibody called anti-perinuclear factor (APF) was first described as an RA-specific autoantibody that reacted with keratohyaline granules scattered around the perinuclear region of human buccal epithelial cells in indirect immunofluorescence [1]. In the 1970s, so-called "anti-keratin" antibodies (AKA) were reported as another RA-specific autoantibody recognized by indirect immunofluorescent study using rat esophagus cryostat sections [2]. Although termed as AKA since keratin-like structures in the cornified layer of esophageal epithelia were specifically stained, the true target antigen had not been clarified. These two antibodies appeared to be highly specific for RA patients, and it was suspected that they were the same autoantibodies because they tended to be detected simultaneously. However, these autoantibodies had not been in routine clinical use as target antigens had not been identified and there were some practical difficulties in detecting techniques.

In 1993, Simon et al. found that 75% of RA patient sera recognized a 40-kDa protein isolated from human skin tissue [3]. They finally demonstrated, by absorption study, that this protein was the target antigen of AKA and, by peptide mapping, that it was a molecule called filaggrin, which was involved in the aggregation of intracellular cytokeratin filaments. They further recognized that AKA and APF had almost the same specificity because the target molecule of APF was profilaggrin, the precursor molecule of filaggrin [4].

Filaggrin is first produced as a profilaggrin of ~400 kDa in the late stage of skin differentiation and is stored in the keratohyaline granules of keratinocytes. Profilaggrin is a phosphorylated protein with 10–12 repeated motifs of 324 amino acid sequences (filaggrin unit) that is dephosphorylated and cleaved during keratinization and turns into filaggrin molecules. Furthermore, arginine residues of filaggrin molecules are converted to citrullines by the enzyme peptidylarginine deiminase (PADI). These citrulline residues on the filaggrin are important for epitopes recognized by RA autoantibodies [5].

Cyclic citrullinated peptide (CCP) is an artificial molecule in which two serine residues in a major epitope peptide from filaggrin are converted to cysteine and the circular form is made by an S-S bond. It has been reported that the sensitivity in RA patients increased and the specificity was unchanged by using CCP as the antigen for ELISA [6]. However, the results of anti-filaggrin and anti-CCP antibodies are not always identical, which suggests the diversity of autoantigenic epitopes of citrullinated peptides recognized by the heterogeneous population of autoantibodies [5].

We suspect why a filaggrin molecule distributed in skin and other keratinized epithelia becomes the target of autoimmune response in the joint-affected disease. However, as discussed later, a possibility has been postulated that citrullination of proteins in the joint, rather than the filaggrin molecule itself, may be involved in autoantibody production and etiopathogenesis of RA.

12.2.2
Clinical Significance of Anti-citrullinated Protein Antibodies in the Diagnosis of RA

So far, a number of reports have demonstrated the clinical significance of auto-antibodies to citrullinated filaggrin and CCP in the diagnosis of RA, as summarized in Table 12.1 [3, 5–10]. Although the specificity of anti-filaggrin/CCP antibodies in RA is more than 90% in almost all reports, the prevalence (sensitivity) of the same antibodies ranges from 33–87.2%. Such discrepancy in sensitivity might reflect racial and genetic backgrounds as well as the differences of antigens and detection techniques used among reports. In earlier studies, natural filaggrins were used; more recently, citrullinated recombinant filaggrins and CCP have been utilized. Generally, anti-CCP appears to be more sensitive than anti-filaggrin. Furthermore, there is a first and second generation of anti-CCP kits, and the second-generation kits using peptides selected from a random peptide library have higher specificity and sensitivity than the first-generation kits.

Anti-citrullinated protein antibodies can be detected in RA patient sera from an early stage of the disease. Schellekens et al. described that anti-CCP anti-

Table 12.1 Clinical significance of anti-filaggrin/CCP antibodies in RA.

Author (year)	Subjects	Antigens (methods) [a]	Sensitivity	Specificity	Ref.
Simon (1993)	RA 48/control 56	Human skin FA (IB)	75%	89%	3
Schellekens (1998)	RA 134/control 154	CCP (ELISA)	76%	96%	5
Schellekens (2000)	RA 134/control 154	CCP (ELISA)	68%	98%	6
	Early arthritis 486	CCP (ELISA)	48%	96%	
Goldbach-Mansky (2000)	Arthritis <1 year 238 (RA 106/others 122)	Human skin FA (ELISA)	33%	93%	7
		CCP (ELISA)	41%	91%	
Bizzaro (2001)	RA 98/control 232	CCP (ELISA)	41%	97.8%	8
Vincent (2002)	RA 240/control 471	Rat r-cFA (ELISA)	67%	98.5%	9
		Human r-cFA (IB)	48%		
		CCP (ELISA)	58%		
Suzuki (2003)	RA 549/control 208	CCP (ELISA)	87.6%	88.9%	10
		Human r-cFA (ELISA)	68.7%	94.7%	
Rantapää-Dahlqvist (2003)	RA 83 from blood donors before onset	CCP (ELISA)	33.7%	98.2%	12

a) FA = filaggrin; r-cFA = recombinant citrullinated filaggrin;
    IB = immunoblotting; ELISA = enzyme-linked immunosorbant assay.

bodies were detected in 68% of RA patients. Although the sensitivity was decreased to 48% in early RA cases, the high specificity was maintained at 96% [6]. In particular, the combination of anti-CCP and IgM-RF revealed a high positive predictive value for RA. In the report of van Gaalen et al., from 318 patients with undifferentiated arthritis at the first visit, RA had later developed in 93% with positive anti-CCP and in only 25% with negative anti-CCP antibodies (OR = 37.8) [11]. Rantapää-Dahlqvist et al. reported that when preserved sera from 83 cases who had been registered as blood donors and later developed RA were studied, anti-CCP antibodies were detected in 33.7% from the disease-free period [12]. A similar result was described in the study of serial measurement in blood donors by Nielen et al., in which 49% of RA patients were positive for IgM-RF and/or anti-CCP before the development of RA symptoms (median of 4.5 years before onset, range 0.1–13.8 years) [13].

Anti-citrullinated protein antibodies may be more useful than RF as a serologic marker for RA because of their high specificity and high sensitivity in RA, and they may also serve as an early diagnostic marker.

12.2.3
Correlation Between Anti-citrullinated Protein Antibodies and Disease Severity

There have been several reports that anti-citrullinated protein antibodies might be a predictive marker for the progression of joint destruction, as summarized in Table 12.2. Schellekens et al. described that both anti-CCP and IgM-RF at the first visit predicted erosive change at two years' follow-up in RA patients and showed 91% of positive predictive value [6]. Kroot et al. reported that anti-CCP was positive in 70% of 273 RA patients who had had disease symptoms for less than one year at study entry, and patients with anti-CCP had developed significantly more severe radiological damage after six years' follow-up [14]. In multiple regression analysis, radiological damage after six years' follow-up was significantly predicted by IgM-RF, radiological score at entry, and anti-CCP status. Forslind et al. measured anti-filaggrin antibodies and AKA in 112 patients with early RA and showed that positive anti-filaggrin or AKA patients at baseline had significantly higher Larsen scores five years later than did the patients without these antibodies [15]. Later, they also reported the role of anti-CCP in the radiological outcome in 379 cases with early RA, concluding that anti-CCP as well as the baseline Larsen score and the erythrocyte sedimentation rate (ESR) were independent predictors of radiological damage and progression in multiple regression analysis [16]. In Meyer's report in which 191 RA patients within one year of onset were followed up, the likelihood of a total Sharp score increase after five years was significantly higher among patients with anti-CCP or APF but not RF and AKA [17]. Visser et al. showed that anti-CCP had a high discriminating power between persistent and self-limiting arthritis and between erosive and non-erosive arthritis in his clinical prediction model of arthritis outcome [18].

Table 12.2 Reports of anti-citrullinated antibodies as a predictive factor for prognosis of RA.

Author (year)	Subjects	Antibodies (methods)[a]	Predictability	Other prognostic factors	Ref.
Schellekens (2000)	RA 144	αCCP (ELISA)	+	IgM-RF	6
Kroot (2000)	Early RA 273	αCCP (ELISA)	+	Baseline X-ray, RF	14
Bas (2000)	RA 119	AFA (ELISA)	–	RF	19
Forslind (2001)	Early RA 112	AFA (IB)	+		15
		AKA (IF)	+		
Paimera (2001)	Early RA 78	AFA (ELISA)	–		20
Meyer (2003)	Early RA 191	αCCP (ELISA)	+		17
		APF (IF)	+		
		AKA (IF)	–		
Rantapää-Dahlqvist (2003)	RA 83 (blood donors)	αCCP (ELISA)	+	IgA-RF	12
Forslind (2004)	Early RA 378	αCCP (ELISA)	+	Baseline Larsen score, ESR	16

a) AFA = anti-filaggrin antibodies; AKA = anti-keratin antibodies;
   APF = anti-perinuclear factor; ELISA = enzyme-linked immunosorbant assay;
   IB = immunoblotting; IF = immunofluorescence.

While these reports showed anti-CCP as a good prognostic marker of radio-logical progression in RA patients, there are also several reports that anti-filaggrin antibodies are not associated with disease severity. Bas et al. measured anti-filaggrin in 199 RA patients, and the severity of erosion for a given disease duration was correlated with RF but not with anti-filaggrin [19]. In the report of Paimela et al. in which the human skin filaggrin was used as an antigen for ELISA, raised anti-filaggrin levels at entry were associated with an active and treatment-resistant disease but did not predict radiological progression [20].

As reviewed here, all reports of anti-CCP indicate a positive correlation with radiological progression, whereas anti-filaggrin and AKA tend to be independent of disease severity (Table 12.2). This discrepancy may reflect a heterogeneity of autoantigenic epitopes on citrullinated molecules and suggests a possibility that clinical significance may vary among different epitopes and different tech-niques.

12.2.4
Protein Citrullination and Etiopathogenesis of RA

Citrullinated proteins are observed in synovial tissue of RA joints but not in normal joints. Citrulline is expressed intracellularly mainly in the lining and sublining layers or is found in interstitial amorphous deposits of RA synovium [21, 22]. These citrullinated proteins are not filaggrin but were identified as ci-trullinated forms of the α- and β-chain of fibrin [22]. These results strongly suggest a possibility that citrullinated fibrins deposited in the RA synovium are the major target of anti-filaggrin and other anti-citrullinated protein antibodies. In addition, B cells from the synovial fluid, but not peripheral blood B cells, of anti-CCP-positive RA patients spontaneously produce anti-CCP antibodies [23]. This fact suggests that an antigen-driven activation of B cells specific for citrullinated proteins occurs at the site of inflammation in RA.

Recently, an interesting report concerning the correlation between the gene polymorphism of the citrullinating enzyme, PADI, and RA susceptibility has been published [24]. Japanese researchers conducted a genome-wide screening by SNPs analysis to identify disease-susceptibility genes for Japanese patients with RA. In this study, the PADI type 4 (PADI4) gene, one of the genes of four types of PADI that are located in chromosome 1p36, was identified as the locus of the RA-susceptibility gene. Haplotype 2 of PADI4 was found more frequently in RA patients (32%) than in normal controls (25%) (OR=1.97) and was thought to be the RA-susceptible haplotype. The PADI4 was mainly expressed in bone marrow cells and peripheral leukocytes and monocytes, as well as in RA synovium. Moreover, it was demonstrated that mRNA expressed from the RA-susceptible form of PADI4 had a longer half-life than mRNA from the RA-non-susceptible PADI4, and RA patients who had the homozygous RA-susceptible haplotype developed more frequent anti-filaggrin antibodies. These data suggest that proteins may be easily citrullinated in RA patients, and over-citrullinated proteins such as citrullinated fibrin might break self-tolerance and promote abnormal immune response.

However, there is also another report that contradicts this hypothesis. Shortly after the above study was published, Barton et al. reported that no correlation was found between RA patients in the UK and the PADI4 polymorphism [25]. Although genetic and racial backgrounds may be the cause of this discrepancy, further studies will be needed to clarify the role of protein citrullination in the etiopathogenesis of RA.

12.3
Anti-Sa Antibodies

Anti-Sa antibodies have been reported as RA-specific autoantibodies that recognized an unknown 50-kDa doublet protein in human spleen and placenta extracts. Anti-Sa antibodies are detected by immunoblotting in 31–43% of RA patients with very high specificity (>98%) [26–28]. The target Sa antigen was later identified as a citrullinated vimentin [29]. Therefore, anti-Sa antibodies are reactive with citrullinated proteins as well as APF, AKA, anti-filaggrin, and anti-CCP antibodies.

12.4
Anti-RA33 Antibodies

Anti-RA33 antibodies recognize a 33-kDa protein that is identified as the A2 protein complexed with heterogeneous nuclear RNA (intranuclear precursor messenger RNA), a component of spliceosome. While autoantibodies to the spliceosome complex are known as anti-U1RNP and anti-Sm (U1, U2, U4/U6, and U5-RNP) antibodies, RA33 (A2 protein) is another target of autoantibodies against spliceosome. Hassfeld et al. first described the presence of autoantibodies to RA33 in 36% of RA patients [30]. Although anti-RA33 was also detected in fairly large percentages of MCTD and SLE patients, these patient sera usually contained anti-U1RNP and/or anti-Sm antibodies [31]. Therefore, anti-RA33 seems to be specific for RA if it is detected without other autoantibodies to spliceosomes. It has also been shown that the antigenic epitope on RA33/A2 recognized by autoantibodies of RA and/or SLE was different from those of MCTD patients [32].

12.5
Anti-calpastatin Antibodies

Calpastatin is an endogenous inhibitor protein of the calcium-dependent cysteine proteinase, calpain. Canadian investigators and authors described independently the presence of autoantibodies to calpastatin in patients with RA and other systemic rheumatic diseases [33, 34].

There have been a number of reports suggesting that calpain may be involved in activating inflammatory processes and pathogenic mechanisms of rheumatic diseases. These studies propose that (1) calpain is increased in synovial cells and is secreted into synovial fluid of rheumatic patients [35], (2) calpain degrades cartilage proteoglycan [36], (3) calpain promotes exocytosis of granules and superoxide production in neutrophils [37], (4) calpain activates and secretes IL-1α through processing its precursor molecules [38], (5) autodigestion of calpain generates an oligopeptide that acts as a chemotactic factor [39], and (6) calpain irreversibly activates protein kinase C, a key enzyme of signal transduction [40]. IgG from patient sera containing anti-calpastatin specifically inhibits the biological function of calpastatin and therefore increases the proteolytic activity of calpain [33, 41]. This finding supports the hypothesis that autoantibodies to calpastatin may play a role in tissue injury and activation of inflammation through increasing calpain activity in tissues [42].

Anti-calpastatin antibodies were detected in 45–57% of patients with RA in both reports by immunoblot using recombinant human calpastatin [33, 34]. However, Despres et al. reported that the antibodies were found exclusively in RA patients [34], whereas authors found that the antibodies were also detected in 20–30% of other systemic rheumatic diseases [33]. Several reports published later described that anti-calpastatin antibodies were less frequent in RA than previously reported and that the prevalence was not significantly different between RA and other rheumatic diseases [43–46]. However, on the other hand, a recent report shows that anti-calpastatin reveals the high prevalence (82% sensitivity) and is exclusively detected (95% specificity) in RA patients [47]. Such discrepancy in the results might reflect the different assay systems, since in the former reports the synthetic C-terminal peptide containing 27 amino acids or recombinant domain I peptide was used for ELISA, whereas human erythrocyte calpastatin was utilized in the latter study. Other reports suggest that anti-calpastatin antibodies are associated with inflammatory-active scleroderma [48], lupus vasculitis [44], and deep vein thrombosis [49]. However, the true disease specificity and clinical significance of anti-calpastatin antibodies remain to be determined.

12.6
Anti-FRP Antibodies

Follistatin-related protein (FRP) is a 55-kDa molecule with unknown function that contains a domain structure similar to follistatin, an inhibitor of activin. FRP was formerly isolated as one of the proteins that were expressed from mouse osteoblasts by TGF-β1 stimulation and also were called TSC-36 [50]. The FRP molecule has FS domains that are similar to follistatin and EC domains that contain EF hands, and consists of a protein family with several other proteins that have a common FS and EC domain structure.

Tanaka et al. reported that autoantibodies to FRP were detected in 30% of RA patients (30% sensitivity and 93% specificity), and the presence of anti-FRP was correlated with the disease activity [51]. Although the physiological function of FRP is still unknown, it was demonstrated that FRP inhibited the production of inflammatory mediators such as matrix metalloproteinase (MMP)-1, MMP-3, and prostaglandin-E2 from RA synovial cells *in vitro* [52] and also suppressed the development of mouse model arthritis *in vivo* [53]. Thus, FRP appears to be one of the biological molecules with anti-inflammatory and joint-protecting effects. Anti-FRP antibodies inhibit the biological function of FRP and promote the production of inflammatory mediators [52], suggesting that they may be involved in pathogenesis of RA.

12.7
Anti-gp130-RAPS Antibodies

gp130 is a signal transduction molecule expressed on the cell membrane that acts by forming a complex with IL-6 and IL-6 receptor. A splicing variant of the gp130 molecule, termed gp130-RAPS, was identified as a novel antigen recognized by autoantibodies in RA patient sera [54]. It is known that gp130 consists of the membrane-bound molecule (110 kDa) and the short molecule (50 kDa) produced from the membrane-bound form by shedding. Another novel variant molecule, gp130-RAPS, lacks the membrane and intracellular domains and contains a novel C-terminal amino acid sequence (NIASF) by flame shift due to deletion of an 83-bp sequence. Since autoantibodies in RA patients recognize an epitope containing the C-terminal amino acid sequence, this molecule was named gp130-RAPS (gp130 of rheumatoid arthritis antigenic peptide-bearing soluble form).

Autoantibodies to the synthetic C-terminal peptide of gp130-RAPS were detected in 73% of RA but in less than 10% of other systemic rheumatic diseases [54]. Antibody titer was correlated with the ESR and with C-reactive protein and serum IL-6 levels, reflecting the disease activity of RA. gp130-RAPS inhibits the signal transduction of IL-6 by interacting with IL-6 receptor. Therefore, gp130-RAPS appears to suppress the activity of IL-6, and anti-gp130-RAPS increases the IL-6 activity by neutralizing the inhibitory function of gp130-RAPS.

12.8
Anti-GPI Antibodies

The mouse strain K/B×N, which was generated by crossing the KNR/C57BL/6 TCR transgenic mouse with the NOD mouse, develops arthritis resembling human RA [55]. This mouse strain produces arthritogenic immunoglobulins, and injection of sera from sick K/B×N mice into healthy recipients provokes arthritis within several days. The target antigen recognized by the arthritis-inducible autoantibody was identified as glucose-6-phosphate isomerase (GPI), a glycolytic enzyme [56]. GPI is demonstrated on the surface of joint cartilages in K/B×N mice, and deposition of IgG and complements is also found in the arthritis-developed mice [57]. This finding indicates that GPI-anti-GPI immune complex may deposit in the joint and provoke inflammation by activating the complement pathway.

From the observations in the mouse study, research into autoantibodies to GPI in human diseases has been performed. Schaller et al. first reported that anti-GPI was detected in 64% of RA patients with high specificity using rabbit GPI as an antigen [58]. On the other hand, in the later report by Matsumoto et al., who used recombinant human GPI for ELISA antigen and screened larger numbers of patient sera from several cohorts, anti-GPI antibodies were not as high and not as specific as in the former report [59]. Anti-GPI antibodies were positive in 15% of RA patients, while they were also detected in 12–25% of cases of psoriatic arthritis, unclassified arthritis, and ankylosing spondylitis, and even in Crohn's disease and sarcoidosis with lower prevalence. Although the pathogenicity of anti-GPI was demonstrated in the mouse model, it is still unknown whether these autoantibodies in human diseases may induce arthritis.

Table 12.3 Summary of clinical significance of autoantibodies described in RA.

Target antigens	Sensitivity in RA	Specificity in RA	Ref.
Perinuclear granule[a]	52–87%	90–95%	1, 17
So-called "keratin"[a]	37–59%	88–95%	2, 15, 17
Filaggrin[a]/CCP[a]	33–88%	89–98%	3, 5–20
Sa[a] (citrullinated vimentin)	22–43%	85–98%	26–28
RA33 (hnRNP-A2 protein)	36%	80–88%	30, 31
Calpastatin	11–82%	71–96%	33, 34, 43–49
Follistatin-related protein (FRP)	35%	93%	51
gp130-RAPS (variant soluble gp130)	73%	97%	54
Glucose-6-phosphate isomerase (GPI)	15–64%	84–95%	58, 59
Rheumatoid factor (IgG-Fc)	70–80%	~80%	
Type II collagen	27–93%	Not specific for RA	60–65
Hat-1	24% (IgM type)	100%	66
IL-1α	17%	Not defined	67
Cytokeratin-18	40% (IgA type)	90% (control=OA) Also in psoriatic arthritis	68, 69
HSP90	43%	85%	70
BiP/p68	64%	97%	71, 72
Agalactosyl IgG	78%	82%	73, 74

a) Citrullinated proteins.

12.9
Other RA-related Autoantibodies

Besides the above-reviewed autoantibodies, many other autoantibodies related to RA have been described so far. However, most of these autoantibodies appear to be neither specific nor sensitive in RA, and in most cases reproducible studies have not been described after the first reports. These autoantibodies are summarized in Table 12.3 with references.

12.10
Conclusions

In recent studies, it has been demonstrated that RA patients produce not only RF but also a variety of other autoantibodies. The possible pathogenic nature of these autoantibodies in RA is still unclear. However, several autoantibodies may play a role in pathogenesis, since certain autoantibodies inhibit the biological function of target autoantigens such as calpastatin, FRP, and soluble gp130 that may have anti-inflammatory roles and joint-protecting effects. Otherwise, some autoantibodies may be pathogenic via the formation of immune complexes with target autoantigens such as GPI and the activation of inflammatory pathway in the joints.

Although most autoantibodies are not always specific for RA, autoantibodies to citrullinated proteins (APF, AKA, anti-filaggrin, anti-CCP, and anti-Sa) appear to be exclusively detected in RA. Anti-CCP antibodies are especially noteworthy because of their high sensitivity and high specificity. These antibodies may serve as a powerful serologic marker for early diagnosis and prognostic prediction of RA. New criteria for the early diagnosis or classification of RA should be considered if routine testing for these RA-specific autoantibodies is to be utilized. Anti-citrullinated protein antibodies are locally produced in RA joints, and citrullinated proteins identified as citrullinated fibrins are localized in RA synovial tissue. This finding strongly suggests a possibility that local citrullination of intra-articular proteins might be the initial event leading to autoantibody production in RA. Genetic factors such as HLA and a gene polymorphism of the citrullinating enzyme PADI (which might express more stable mRNA and cause over-citrullination of proteins) might be associated with the breakage of self-tolerance and induction of autoimmunity against citrullinated proteins. However, further research will be necessary to elucidate the fine mechanism and significance of protein citrullination in etiopathogenesis of RA.

References

1 Nienhuis, R. L. F., Mandema, E. A. *Ann. Rheum. Dis.* **1964**, *23*, 302–305.

2 Young B. J., Mallya R. K., Leslie R. D., Clark C. J., Hamblin T. J. Anti-keratin antibodies in rheumatoid arthritis. *Br. Med. J.* **1979**, *2*, 97–99.

3 Simon, M., Girbal, E., Sebbag, M., Gomes-Daudrix, V., Vincent, C., Salama, G., Serre, G. *J. Clin. Invest.* **1993**, *92*, 1387–1393.

4 Sebbag, M., Simon, M., Vincent, C., Masson-Bessiere, C., Girbal, E., Durieux, J. J., Serre, G. *J. Clin. Invest.* **1995**, *95*, 2672–2679.

5 Schellekens, G. A., de Jong, B. A., van den Hoogen, F. H., van de Putte, L. B., van Venrooij, W. J. *J. Clin. Invest.* **1998**, *101*, 273–281.

6 Schellekens, G. A., Visser, H., de Jong, B. A., van den Hoogen, F. H., Hazes, J. M., Breedveld, F. C., van Venrooij, W. J. *Arthritis Rheum.* **2000**, *43*, 155–163.

7 Goldbach-Mansky, R., Lee, J., McCoy, A., Hoxworth, J., Yarboro, C., Smolen, J. S., Steiner, G., Rosen, A., Zhang, C., Menard, H. A., Zhou, Z. J., Palosuo, T., van Venrooij, W. J., Wilder, R. L., Klippel, J. H., Schumacher, H. R. Jr., El-Gabalawy, H. S. *Arthritis Res.* **2000**, *2*, 236–243.

8 Bizzaro, N., Mazzanti, G., Tonutti, E., Villalta, D., Tozzoli, R. *Clin. Chem.* **2001**, *47*, 1089–1093.

9 Vincent, C., Nogueira, L., Sebbag, M., Chapuy-Regaud, S., Arnaud, M., Letourneur, O., Rolland, D., Fournie, B., Cantagrel, A., Jolivet, M., Serre, G. *Arthritis Rheum.* **2002**, *46*, 2051–2058.

10 Suzuki, K., Sawada, T., Murakami, A., Matsui, T., Tohma, S., Nakazono, K., Takemura, M., Takasaki, Y., Mimori, T., Yamamoto, K. *Scand. J. Rheumatol.* **2003**, *32*, 197–204.

11 van Gaalen, F. A., Linn-Rasker, S. P., van Venrooij, W. J., de Jong, B. A., Breedveld,

F.C., Verweij, C.L., Toes, R.E., Huizinga, T.W. *Arthritis Rheum.* **2004**, *50*, 709–715.

12 Rantapää-Dahlqvist, S., de Jong, B.A., Berglin, E., Hallmans, G., Wadell, G., Stenlund, H., Sundin, U., van Venrooij, W.J. *Arthritis Rheum.* **2003**, *48*, 2741–2749.

13 Nielen, M.M., van Schaardenburg, D., Reesink, H.W., van de Stadt, R.J., van der Horst-Bruinsma, I.E., de Koning, M.H., Habibuw, M.R., Vandenbroucke, J.P., Dijkmans, B.A. *Arthritis Rheum.* **2004**, *50*, 380–386.

14 Kroot, E.J., de Jong, B.A., van Leeuwen, M.A., Swinkels, H., van den Hoogen, F.H., van't Hof, M., van de Putte, L.B., van Rijswijk, M.H., van Venrooij, W.J., van Riel, P.L. *Arthritis Rheum.* **2000**, *43*, 1831–1835.

15 Forslind, K., Vincent, C., Serre, G., Svensson, B. *Scand. J. Rheumatol.* **2001**, *30*, 221–224.

16 Forslind, K., Ahlmen, M., Eberhardt, K., Hafstrom, I., Svensson, B., BARFOT Study Group. *Ann. Rheum. Dis.* **2004**, *63*, 1090–1095.

17 Meyer, O., Labarre, C., Dougados, M., Goupille, P., Cantagrel, A., Dubois, A., Nicaise-Roland, P., Sibilia, J., Combe, B. *Ann. Rheum. Dis.* **2003**, *62*, 120–126.

18 Visser, H., Le Cessie, S., Vos, K., Breedveld, F.C., Hazes, J.M. *Arthritis Rheum.* **2002**, *46*, 357–365.

19 Bas, S., Perneger, T.V., Mikhnevitch, E., Seitz, M., Tiercy, J.M., Roux-Lombard, P., Guerne, P.A. *Rheumatology (Oxford)* **2000**, *39*, 1082–1088.

20 Paimela, L., Palosuo, T., Aho, K., Lukka, M., Kurki, P., Leirisalo-Repo, M., von Essen, R. *Ann. Rheum. Dis.* **2001**, *60*, 32–35.

21 Baeten, D., Peene, I., Union, A., Meheus, L., Sebbag, M., Serre, G., Veys, E.M., De Keyser, F. *Arthritis Rheum.* **2001**, *44*, 2255–2262.

22 Masson-Bessiere, C., Sebbag, M., Girbal-Neuhauser, E., Nogueira, L., Vincent, C., Senshu, T., Serre, G. *J. Immunol.* **2001**, *166*, 4177–4184.

23 Reparon-Schuijt, C.C., van Esch, W.J., van Kooten, C., Schellekens, G.A., de Jong, B.A., van Venrooij, W.J., Breed-

veld, F.C., Verweij, C.L. *Arthritis Rheum.* **2001**, *44*, 41–47.

24 Suzuki, A., Yamada, R., Chang, X., Tokuhiro, S., Sawada, T., Suzuki, M., Nagasaki, M., Nakayama-Hamada, M., Kawaida, R., Ono, M., Ohtsuki, M., Furukawa, H., Yoshino, S., Yukioka, M., Tohma, S., Matsubara, T., Wakitani, S., Teshima, R., Nishioka, Y., Sekine, A., Iida, A., Takahashi, A., Tsunoda, T., Nakamura, Y., Yamamoto, K. *Nat. Genet.* **2003**, *34*, 395–402.

25 Barton, A., Bowes, J., Eyre, S., Spreckley, K., Hinks, A., John, S., Worthington, J. *Arthritis Rheum.* **2004**, *50*, 1117–1121.

26 Despres, N., Boire, G., Lopez-Longo, F.J., Menard, H.A. *J. Rheumatol.* **1994**, *21*, 1027–1033.

27 Hueber, W., Hassfeld, W., Smolen, J.S., Steiner, G. *Rheumatology (Oxford)* **1999**, *38*, 155–159.

28 Hayem, G., Chazerain, P., Combe, B., Elias, A., Haim, T., Nicaise, P., Benali, K., Eliaou, J.F., Kahn, M.F., Sany, J., Meyer, O. *J. Rheumatol.* **1999**, *26*, 7–13. Erratum in: *J. Rheumatol.* **1999**, *26*, 2069.

29 Vossenaar, E.R., Despres, N., Lapointe, E., van Der Heijden, A., Lora, M., Senshu, T., van Venrooij, W.J., Menard, H.A. *Arthritis Res. Ther.* **2004**, *6*, R142-150.

30 Hassfeld, W., Steiner, G., Hartmuth, K., Kolarz, G., Scherak, O., Graninger, W., Thumb, N., Smolen, J.S. *Arthritis Rheum.* **1989**, *32*, 1515–1520.

31 Steiner, G., Skriner, K., Hassfeld, W., Smolen, J.S. *Mol. Biol. Rep.* **1996**, *23*, 167–171.

32 Skriner, K., Sommergruber, W.H., Tremmel, V., Fischer, I., Barta, A., Smolen, J.S., Steiner, G. *J. Clin. Invest.* **1997**, *100*, 127–135.

33 Mimori, T., Suganuma, K., Tanami, Y., Nojima, T., Matsumura, M., Fujii, T., Yoshizawa, T., Suzuki, K., Akizuki, M. *Proc. Natl. Acad. Sci. USA* **1995**, *92*, 7267–7271.

34 Despres, N., Talbot, G., Plouffe, B., Boire, G., Menard, H.A. *J. Clin. Invest.* **1995**, *95*, 1891–1896.

35 Yamamoto, S., Shimizu, K., Shimizu, K., Suzuki, K., Nakagawa, Y., Yamamuro, T. *Arthritis Rheum.* **1992**, *35*, 1309–1317.

36 Suzuki, K., Shimizu, K., Hamamoto, T., Nakagawa, Y., Murachi, T., Yamamuro, T. *Biochem. J.* **1992**, *285*:857–862.

37 Pontremoli, S., Melloni, E, Damiani, G., Salamino, F., Sparatore, B., Michetti, M., Horecker, B. L. *J. Biol. Chem.* **1988**, *263*, 1915–1919.

38 Kobayashi, Y., Yamamoto, K., Saido, T., Kawasaki, H., Oppenheim, J. J., Matsu shima, K. *Proc. Natl. Acad. Sci. USA* **1990**, *87*, 5548–5552.

39 Kunimatsu, M., Higashiyama, S., Sato, K., Ohkubo, I., Sasaki, M. *Biochem. Biophys. Res. Comm.* **1989**, *164*, 875–882.

40 Kishimoto, A., Mikawa, K., Hashimoto, K., Yasuda, I., Tanaka, S., Tominaga, M., Kuroda, T., Nishizuka, Y. *J. Biol. Chem.* **1989**, *264*, 4088–4092.

41 Matsumoto, M., Takada, R., Yoshida, M., Hoshiyama, K., Nojima, T., Matsumura, M., Ohosone, Y., Mimori, T. *Arthritis Rheum.* **1997**, 40, S277 (abstract).

42 Menard, H. A., El-Amine, M. *Immunol. Today* **1996**, 17, 545–547.

43 Vittecoq, O., Salle, V., Jouen-Beades, F., Krzanowska, K., Menard, J. F., Gayet, A., Fardellone, P., Tauveron, P., Le Loet, X., Tron, F. *Rheumatology (Oxford)* **2001**, *40*, 1126–1134.

44 Saulot, V., Vittecoq, O., Salle, V., Drouot, L., Legoedec, J., Le Loet, X., Godin, M., Ducroix, J. P., Menard, J. F., Tron, F., Gilbert, D. *J. Autoimmun.* **2002**, *19*, 55–61.

45 Vittecoq, O., Pouplin, S., Krzanowska, K., Jouen-Beades, F., Menard, J. F., Gayet, A., Daragon, A., Tron, F., Le Loet, X. *Rheumatology (Oxford)* **2003**, *42*, 939–946.

46 Lackner, K. J., Schlosser, U., Lang, B., Schmitz, G. *Br. J. Rheumatol.* **1998**, *37*, 1164–1171.

47 Iwaki-Egawa, S., Matsuno, H., Yudoh, K., Nakazawa, F., Miyazaki, K., Ochiai, A., Hirohata, S., Shimizu, M., Watanabe, Y. *J. Rheumatol.* **2004**, *31*, 17–22.

48 Sato, S., Hasegawa, M., Nagaoka, T., Takamatsu, Y., Yazawa, N., Ihn, H., Kikuchi, K., Takehara, K. *J. Rheumatol.* **1998**, *25*, 2135–2139.

49 Schlosser, U., Lackner, K. J., Scheckenhofer, C., Spannagl, M., Spengel, F. A., Hahn, G., Lang, B., Schmitz, G. *Thromb. Haemost.* **1997**, *77*, 11–13.

50 Shibanuma, M., Mashimo, J., Mita, A., Kuroki, T., Nose, K. *Eur. J. Biochem.* **1993**, *217*, 13–19.

51 Tanaka, M., Ozaki, S., Osakada, F., Mori, K., Okubo, M., Nakao, K. *Int. Immunol.* **1998**, *10*, 1305–1314.

52 Tanaka, M., Ozaki, S., Kawabata, D., Kishimura, M., Osakada, F., Okubo, M., Murakami, M., Nakao, K., Mimori, T. *Int. Immunol.* **2003**, *15*, 71–77.

53 Kawabata, D., Tanaka, M., Fujii, T., Umehara, H., Fujita, Y., Yoshifuji, H., Mimori, T., Ozaki, S. *Arthritis Rheum.* **2004**, *50*, 660–668.

54 Tanaka, M., Kishimura, M., Ozaki, S., Osakada, F., Hashimoto, H., Okubo, M., Murakami, M., Nakao, K. *J. Clin. Invest.* **2000**, *106*, 137–144.

55 Kouskoff, V., Korganow, A. S., Duchatelle, V., Degott, C., Benoist, C., Mathis, D. *Cell* **1996**, 87, 811–822.

56 Matsumoto, I., Staub, A., Benoist, C., Mathis, D. *Science* **1999**, *286*, 1732–1735.

57 Matsumoto, I., Maccioni, M., Lee, D. M., Maurice, M., Simmons, B., Brenner, M., Mathis, D., Benoist, C. *Nat. Immunol.* **2002**, *3*, 360–365.

58 Schaller, M., Burton, D. R., Ditzel, H. J. *Nat. Immunol.* **2001**, *2*, 746–753.

59 Matsumoto, I., Lee, D. M., Goldbach-Mansky, R., Sumida, T., Hitchon, C. A., Schur, P. H., Anderson, R. J., Coblyn, J. S., Weinblatt, M. E., Brenner, M., Duclos, B., Pasquali, J. L., El-Gabalawy, H., Mathis. D., Benoist, C. *Arthritis Rheum.* **2003**, *48*, 944–954.

60 Andriopoulos, N. A., Mestecky, J., Miller, E. J., Bradley, E. L. *Arthritis Rheum.* **1976**, 19, 613–617.

61 Clague, R. B., Shaw, M. J., Holt, P. J. *Ann. Rheum. Dis.* **1980**, *39*, 201–206.

62 Trentham, D. E., Kammer, G. M., McCune, W. J., David, J. R. *Arthritis Rheum.* **1981**, *24*, 1363–1369.

63 Stuart, J. M., Huffstutter, E. H., Townes, A. S., Kang, A. H. *Arthritis Rheum.* **1983**, *26*, 832–840.

64 Morgan, K., Clague, R. B., Collins, I., Ayad, S., Phinn, S. D., Holt, P. J. *Ann. Rheum. Dis.* **1987**, *46*, 902–907.

65 Clague, R.B. *Br. J. Rheumatol.* **1989**, *28*, 1–5.

66 Abe, Y., Inada, S., Torikai, K. *Arthritis Rheum.* **1988**, *31*, 135–139.

67 Suzuki, H., Akama, T., Okane, M., Kono, I., Matsui, Y., Yamane, K., Kashiwagi, H. *Arthritis Rheum.* **1989**, *32*, 1528–1538.

68 Borg, A.A., Dawes, P.T., Mattey, D.L. *Arthritis Rheum.* **1993**, *36*, 229–233.

69 Borg, A.A., Nixon, N.B., Dawes, P.T., Mattey, D.L. *Ann. Rheum. Dis.* **1994**, *53*, 391–395.

70 Hayem, G., De Bandt, M., Palazzo, E., Roux, S., Combe, B., Eliaou, J.F., Sany, J., Kahn, M.F., Meyer, O. *Ann. Rheum. Dis.* **1999**, *58*, 291–296.

71 Bläß, S., Specker, C., Lakomek, H.J., Schneider, E.M., Schwochau, M. *Ann. Rheum. Dis.* **1995**, *54*, 355–360.

72 Bläß, S., Union, A., Raymackers, J., Schumann, F., Ungethum, U., Muller-Steinbach, S., De Keyser, F., Engel, J.M., Burmester, G.R. *Arthritis Rheum.* **2001**, *44*, 761–771.

73 Das, H., Atsumi, T., Fukushima, Y., Shibuya, H., Ito, K., Yamada, Y., Amasaki, Y., Ichikawa, K., Amengual, O., Koike, T. *Clin. Rheumatol.* **2004**, *23*, 218–222.

74 Maeno, N., Takei, S., Fujikawa, S., Yamada, Y., Imanaka, H., Hokonohara, M., Kawano, Y., Oda, H. *J. Rheumatol.* **2004**, *31*, 1211–1217.

13
Autoantibodies and Organ-specific Autoimmunity

H. Bantel, J. Kneser, and M.P. Manns

13.1
Role of Autoantibodies in Tissue-specific Organ Damage

Autoimmune diseases affect 3–5% of the population, but they attract medical attention only when they become sustained and cause lasting tissue damage [1]. Depending on the affected organ, the clinical presentation of autoimmune diseases can be very heterogeneous and specific, or unspecific features can predominate. A common characteristic of autoimmune diseases is the presence of autoantibodies that are produced by autoreactive lymphocytes and that may be the direct cause of some of these disorders. For instance, in Graves' disease, autoantibodies bind to and stimulate the receptor for thyrotropin, resulting in unrestrained thyrocyte growth, excessive thyroid hormone production, and diffuse hyperplasia of the thyroid gland [2, 3]. In Hashimoto's thyroiditis, antibodies against thyroglobulin, thyroid peroxidase, and the thyrotropin receptor have been suggested to play a role in the progressive destruction of thyroid follicular cells [4, 5]. In pemphigus vulgaris, autoantibodies against the epidermal adhesion molecule desmoglein 3 disrupt the epidermis [6].

Although the pathogenic role played by autoantibodies is well characterized in these diseases, the cellular and molecular mechanisms underlying the initiation and the propagation of the autoimmune response remain unknown. Moreover, organ-specific damage by autoantibodies might not be sufficient to explain the progression or chronicity of an autoimmune disease. For instance, autoimmune gastritis is characterized by the production of parietal cell autoantibodies that are reactive with the alpha- and beta-subunits of the gastric H/K ATPase. However, experimental data of a murine (neonatal thymectomy) autoimmune gastritis model indicated that this autoimmune disease is mediated by $CD4^+$ T cells and not by organ-specific autoantibodies [7, 8]. Furthermore, in a variety of autoimmune diseases, such as lupus erythematosus, autoantibodies are not directed against organ-specific structures but react with widely distributed intracellular antigens.

Autoantibodies against intracellular antigens have been implicated as usually not pathogenic and instead have been viewed largely as secondary consequences

Autoantibodies and Autoimmunity: Molecular Mechanisms in Health and Disease. Edited by K. Michael Pollard
Copyright © 2006 WILEY-VCH Verlag GmbH & Co. KGaA, Weinheim
ISBN: 3-527-31141-6

of the autoimmune process. This view has also been restricted recently: in a murine model of autoimmune arthritis, the transfer of IgG from diseased animals induced arthritis in healthy recipients [9]. These pathogenic autoantibodies bind to glucose-6-phosphate isomerase, a ubiquitous intracellular antigen [10].

In summary, autoimmunity is mediated by both direct (autoantibody-associated) and indirect (cytokine-associated) immune response mechanisms. Depending on the respective autoimmune disease, one of those mechanisms may predominate. Thus, often the specificity of the autoantibodies does not correlate with clinical profiles, as exemplified by the autoimmune liver diseases. This chapter therefore deals with the relevance of autoantibodies for the diagnosis and natural history of autoimmune liver diseases including autoimmune hepatitis, primary biliary cirrhosis, and overlap syndrome.

13.2
Autoantibodies and Autoantigens in Autoimmune Hepatitis

Autoimmune hepatitis (AIH) represents a chronic, mainly periportal hepatitis upon histology, which is characterized by a female predominance, hypergammaglobulinemia, circulating autoantibodies, and a benefit from immunosuppressive treatment. The diagnosis of AIH is based on clinical, serological, and immunological features as well as on the exclusion of other hepatobiliary diseases with and without autoimmune phenomena. These include disease entities such as chronic hepatitis C, primary biliary cirrhosis, primary sclerosing cholangitis, and the so-called overlap or outlier syndromes. The revised AIH diagnostic score contributes to the establishment of the diagnosis in difficult cases by calculating a probability expressed as a numeric score [11].

Since the first description of AIH in 1950 by Waldenström [12], serological findings have attracted considerable attention not only for the diagnosis of this chronic liver disease but also as a means to study and eventually to understand its pathophysiology. Furthermore, serological detection of autoantibodies is a distinguishing feature that has been exploited for the subclassification of autoimmune hepatitis into three groups: AIH type 1, AIH type 2 and AIH type 3.

13.3
Autoantibodies Frequently Associated with Autoimmune Hepatitis Type 1

AIH type 1 represents the most common form of AIH (80% of all cases), mainly occurring between the ages of 16 and 30 years. The clinical course is usually not fulminant and an acute onset is very rare. It is characterized by the presence of antinuclear antibodies (ANAs) and/or anti–smooth muscle antibodies (SMAs). The target autoantigen(s) of type 1 autoimmune hepatitis are largely unknown but consist of multiple nuclear proteins including centromeres, ribonucleoproteins, and cyclin A as well as smooth muscle actin [13–17]. However, the molecular characterization of target antigen specificity does not supply important additional information to increase the diagnostic precision of AIH type 1. Although organ-specific autoantibodies are usually not observed, an association of AIH type 1 with other autoimmune syndromes is observed in 48% of cases, with autoimmune thyroid disease, synovitis, and ulcerative colitis as leading associations [18, 19].

13.3.1
Antinuclear Antibodies

Screening determinations of ANAs are routinely performed by indirect immunofluorescence on cryostat sections of rat liver, kidney, and stomach as well as on HEp2 cell slides. Most commonly, a homogeneous or speckled immunofluorescence pattern is detectable in all three tissues. The most precise definition of an ANA pattern is obtained using HEp2 cells, a cell line derived from laryngeal carcinoma with prominent nuclei. ANAs represent the most common autoantibodies in AIH and occur in high titers, usually exceeding 1:160. However, the titer does not correlate with disease course, disease activity, prognosis, progression, requirement of transplantation, or disease reoccurrence after transplantation. Furthermore, ANAs are not specific for autoimmune hepatitis and can also be detected in other autoimmune disorders such as systemic lupus erythematosus. In the future, more refined techniques using recombinant nuclear antigens and immunoassay formats may enable the identification of reactants and assessment of their specificity for diagnosis of and possible roles in pathogenesis.

13.3.2
Anti–Smooth Muscle Antibodies

Anti–smooth muscle antibodies (anti-SMAs) are directed against cytoskeletal proteins such as actin, troponin, and tropomyosin [20, 21]. They frequently occur in high titers in association with ANAs. However, they are not highly specific for AIH and have been shown to occur in advanced liver diseases of other etiologies as well as in infectious diseases and rheumatic disorders. In the latter cases, titers are often lower than 1:80. In pediatric patients, SMA autoantibodies may be the only marker of AIH type 1. When present in very young patients with AIH type 1, the titers may be as low as 1:40. SMAs have been found to be generally associated with HLA A1-B8-DR3 haplotype, and, possibly as a reflection of this HLA status, the affected patients are younger and have a poorer prognosis [22]. Moreover, antibodies to actin identify a subgroup of patients with SMAs who have disease at an earlier age and a poorer response to corticosteroid therapy [17].

SMA autoantibodies are also determined by indirect immunofluorescence on cryostat sections of rat stomach and kidney [23]. The examination of the kidney is of importance since this allows for visualization of the V (vessels), G (glomeruli), and T (tubuli) patterns. The V pattern is also present in non-autoimmune inflammatory liver disease, as well as in autoimmune diseases not affecting the liver and in viral infections, but VG and VGT patterns are more reliably associated with AIH, although they are not per se entirely specific for the diagnosis of AIH type I.

13.3.3
Perinuclear Anti-neutrophil Cytoplasmic Antibodies (pANCAs) and Antibodies to Asialoglycoprotein Receptor (anti-ASGPRs)

Perinuclear anti-neutrophil cytoplasmic antibodies occur in 65–96% of patients with AIH type 1 but are usually absent in patients with AIH type 2 [24, 25]. They are mainly of the IgG1 isotype, which distinguishes them from the pANCAs in primary sclerosing cholangitis [24]. Typically, these antibodies are present in high titers in AIH type 1. Actin has been proposed as target antigen; however, recent studies suggested reactivity against granulocyte-specific antigens in the nuclear lamina [26, 27]. These antibodies are of diagnostic value for those patients with AIH type 1 who have tested negative for ANA/SMA.

Anti-ASGPR is present in all forms of disease [28–30]. Seropositivity is associated with laboratory and histological indices of disease activity, and anti-ASGPRs identify patients who commonly will have a relapse after corticosteroid withdrawal [31, 32]. However, anti-ASGPRs are also found in other liver diseases including alcoholic liver disease, chronic hepatitis B and C, and primary biliary cirrhosis. The development of a commercial assay for application of anti-ASGPRs has been difficult, and their potential as diagnostic and prognostic markers has not yet been realized.

13.4
Autoantibodies and Autoantigens Associated with Autoimmune Hepatitis Type 2

AIH type 2 is a rare disorder that affects up to 20% of AIH patients in Europe but only 4% in the United States [33, 34]. The average age of onset is around 10 years, but AIH type 2 can also occur in adults, especially in Europe. In AIH type 2, patients are not only younger but also more frequently display an acute onset of hepatitis with a more severe course and rapid progression than do patients with AIH types 1 or 3.

Characteristic antibodies of AIH type 2 are liver/kidney microsomal antibodies (LKM-1) directed against cytochrome P450 (CYP)2D6 and, with lower frequency, against UDP-glucuronosyltransferases (UGT) [35]. In 10% of cases, LKM-3 autoantibodies against UGTs are also present [36, 37]. In contrast to AIH type 1, additional organ-specific autoantibodies are frequently present, such as anti-thyroid, anti–parietal cell, and anti–Langerhans' cell autoantibodies. The number of extrahepatic autoimmune syndromes such as diabetes, vitiligo, and autoimmune thyroid disease is also more prevalent compared to AIH type1 [34].

13.4.1
Liver Kidney Microsomal Antibodies

Indirect immunofluorescence first led to the description of autoantibodies reactive with the proximal renal tubule and the hepatocellular cytoplasm in 1973 [38]. These autoantibodies, termed LKM-1, were associated with a second form of ANA-negative AIH. Between 1988 and 1991, the 50-kDa antigen of LKM-1 autoantibodies was identified as CYP2D6, which belongs to the CYP superfamily of drug-metabolizing proteins located in the endoplasmic reticulum (ER) [39–42]. LKM-1 autoantibodies recognize a major linear epitope between amino acids 263 and 270 of the CYP2D6 protein [43]. These autoantibodies inhibit CYP2D6 activity *in vitro* and are capable of activating liver-infiltrating T lymphocytes, indicating the combination of B- and T-cell activity in the autoimmune process involved [44, 45]. In addition to linear epitopes, LKM-1 autoantibodies have also been shown to recognize conformation-dependent epitopes [46]. However, the recognition of epitopes located between amino acids 257 and 269 appears to be a specific autoimmune reaction of AIH and is discriminatory against LKM-1 autoantibodies associated with chronic hepatitis C virus infection [47, 48]. CYP2D6 is expressed on hepatocytes and its expression might be regulated by cytokines, giving rise to several amplification loops in the autoimmune-mediated inflammatory response [49–51].

LKM-3 autoantibodies are directed against UDP-glucuronosyltransferases (UGT1A), which are also a superfamily of drug-metabolizing proteins located in the ER. LKM-3 autoantibodies have been identified in 6–10% of patients with chronic HDV infection and in up to 10% of patients with AIH type 2 [52–54]. These autoantibodies can also occur in LKM-1-negative and ANA-negative patients and thus may become the only serological marker of AIH.

The identification of the molecular targets of autoantibodies led to the increasing use of immunoassays based on recombinant/purified antigens such as radioimmunoassays or enzyme-linked immunosorbent assays to detect the respective autoantibodies.

13.4.2
Anti-cytosol Autoantibodies Type 1 (anti-LC-1)

Anti-LC-1 are viewed as a second marker of AIH type 2, in which they have been detected in up to 50% of LKM-positive sera [55]. Other studies indicate their occurrence in combination with ANA and SMA autoantibodies and in chronic HCV [56]. In contrast to LKM autoantibodies, LC-1 autoantibodies seem to correlate with disease activity. The molecular antigen target has been identified to be formiminotransferase cyclodeaminase and commercial kits have become available [57]. However, the specificity and clinical significance of these antibodies remain unclear.

13.5
Autoantibodies and Autoantigens Associated with Autoimmune Hepatitis Type 3

AIH type 3 has a lower prevalence than AIH type 2 and has a maximum age of manifestation between 20 and 40 years. This subclass of AIH resembles AIH type 1 with respect to clinical characteristics, immunogenetic markers, and treatment response.

AIH type 3 is characterized by autoantibodies against soluble liver and pancreas antigen (SLA/LP), which are directed towards UGA-suppressor transfer RNA (tRNA)-associated protein [58–61]. Recent studies have shown that anti-SLA and the independently described anti-LP are identical [50, 62]. The exact function of this protein and its role in autoimmunity remain unclear. Anti-SLA/LP were initially detected in a patient with ANA-negative AIH. However, 74% of patients with SLA/LP autoantibodies also have other serological markers of autoimmunity, including SMAs and AMAs [58, 61, 63]. In ANA-positive patients, SLA autoantibodies appear in 11% of cases.

13.6
Autoantibodies Associated with Primary Biliary Cirrhosis

Primary biliary cirrhosis (PBC) is the inflammatory, primarily T cell–mediated, chronic destruction of intrahepatic microscopic bile ducts of unknown etiology. In 90% of cases it affects women who exhibit elevated immunoglobulin M, anti-mitochondrial antibodies (AMAs) directed against the E2 subunit of pyruvate dehydrogenase (PDH-E2), and a cholestatic liver enzyme profile leading to cirrhosis over the course of years or decades. A prominent feature is the presence of extrahepatic immune-mediated disease associations, including autoimmune thyroid disease, Sjögren's syndrome, rheumatoid arthritis, inflammatory bowel disease, and, less frequently, celiac disease and CREST syndrome. Extrahepatic syndromes frequently precede hepatic disease manifestation [64–66].

Anti-mitochondrial antibodies are found in approximately 95% of patients with PBC and are considered a serological hallmark of this disease. The targets of AMAs in PBC sera are members of an enzyme family, the 2-oxo acid dehydrogenase complexes (2-OADC), which are located on the inner membrane of the mitochondria and catalyze the oxidative decarboxylation of various alpha-keto acid substrates. Components of 2-OADC include the E2 subunit of PDC (PDC-E2), the E2 subunit of the 2-oxoglutarate dehydrogenase complex (OGDC-E2), the E2 subunit of the branched-chain 2-oxo acid dehydrogenase complex (BCOADC-E2), and the dihydrolipoamide dehydrogenase–binding protein (E3BP). The most predominant reactivity of AMAs in sera from PBC patients is directed against PDC-E2. Reactivity against OGDC-E2 and BCOADC-E2 is lower, around 50–70%. Antibodies to PDC-E1-alpha are present in lower titers. Approximately 10% of patients react only to OGDC-E2 or BCOADC-E2, or to both [67–69].

Antinuclear antibodies (ANAs) have been identified in more than 50% of patients with PBC. These include antibodies against the nuclear pore protein, gp120, which are found in 25% of patients with AMA-positive PBC and in up to 50% of patients with AMA-negative PBC. The disease specificity for the detection of such antibodies by immunoblotting is more than 90% [70]. Other autoantigens include the nuclear pore protein p62, which is recognized by PBC sera in 32% of cases [71]. In about 20–30% of PBC patients, autoantibodies are directed against the nucleoprotein Sp100, which appears to have a high specificity for PBC [72]. Less than 1% of PBC patients present antibodies to the lamin B receptor (LBR), an inner nuclear membrane protein that also has a high disease specificity for PBC [73]. In summary, the presence of PBC-associated ANAs in AMA-negative patients may be the only seroimmunological clue for establishing the diagnosis of PBC.

13.7
Autoantibodies in Overlap Syndrome Between Autoimmune Hepatitis and Primary Biliary Cirrhosis

This overlap syndrome is characterized by the coexistence of clinical, biochemical, or serological features of autoimmune hepatitis (AIH) and primary biliary cirrhosis (PBC). In about 5% of patients with a primary diagnosis of AIH, laboratory signs and clinical symptoms of PBC exist. On the other hand, 19% of patients with a primary diagnosis of PBC also have signs of AIH. The overlap of PBC and AIH is characterized by the presence of ANAs in 67% and antibodies against SMAs in 67%. Because patients with an overlap of PBC and AIH respond to corticosteroid treatment equally well as patients with primary AIH, the identification of this variant group by autoantibody characterization is required and contributes to the establishment of an efficacious therapeutic strategy [74, 75].

13.8
Discussion and Conclusions

A common feature of all autoimmune diseases is the presence of autoantibodies. Some autoantibodies are specific for the site of the disease process, as exemplified by thyroid diseases, pemphigus vulgaris, or autoimmune gastritis. However, even in instances in which the autoantibodies are not believed to be the causative agents, they always make an important contribution to the diagnosis of autoimmune diseases. Subdifferentiation of the pattern of autoantibodies allows us to distinguish not only different autoimmune types but also different subsets of autoimmune diseases. For instance, antinuclear antibodies are the most commonly detected autoantibodies in AIH type 1, but they are also frequently (50%) detected in PBC. Subclassification of ANAs shows that in PBC these autoantibodies are directed against specific nuclear antigens (gp 120, p62, Sp100) that are not detected in AIH type 1. The presence of PBC-associated ANAs in AMA-negative patients may therefore be the only diagnostic serum marker of PBC. Another example is the recognition of different epitopes by LKM-1 autoantibodies, which in the case of localizing between amino acids 257 and 269 appears to be specific for AIH and is discriminatory against LKM-1 autoantibodies associated with chronic hepatitis C virus infection.

In a number of autoimmune diseases, it is still unknown whether the autoantibodies highlight the responsible pathogenic process, thereby directly contributing to organ-specific autoimmunity and injury, or whether this is indirectly mediated by infiltrating inflammatory cells and proinflammatory cytokine production. Almost all autoimmune diseases depend on the presence of CD4$^+$ T cells that recognize self-antigens. Whether these T cells are stimulated by an autologous antigen or by an exogenous molecular mimic, they are responsible for the production of classes of autoantibodies with pathogenic capabilities or T cells that can attack and damage tissue. Production of proinflammatory cytokines including ligands of death receptors may amplify the autoimmune-mediated tissue injury. As a response to cytokines, exposed T cells become activated and differentiate into Th1 or Th2 cells. Furthermore, proinflammatory cytokines may lead to upregulation of death ligands on infiltrating/attacking T lymphocytes as well as of death receptors on parenchymal target cells, thereby contributing to apoptotic tissue injury. Proinflammatory cytokines are therefore believed to play an important role in the initiation and propagation of the autoimmune response. In addition, autoantibodies by themselves have been implicated as playing a role in the activation of T lymphocytes. In this respect, it has been demonstrated that LKM-1 autoantibodies inhibit CYP2D6 activity *in vitro* and are capable of activating liver-infiltrating T lymphocytes, indicating the combination of B- and T-cell activity in the autoimmune process involved. Liver histology from patients with autoimmune hepatitis shows a periportal infiltrate of lymphocytes and plasma cells as well as piecemeal necrosis, indicating that in this autoimmune disease an inflammatory immune response may predominately contribute to liver injury.

Although the presence of autoantibodies generally does not correlate with disease activity, disease progression, or treatment outcome, in some cases they may be of prognostic value. In the case of AIH type 1, antibodies against actin identify a subgroup of SMA-positive patients with an earlier onset of disease and a more frequent steroid treatment failure. The presence of anti-ASGPR autoantibodies is associated with laboratory and histological disease activity and more frequent relapses after corticosteroid withdrawal in patients with AIH type 1. In the case of AIH type 2, LC-1 autoantibodies seem to correlate with disease activity, whereas LKM autoantibodies do not.

The development of commercial assays for application of autoantibodies with prognostic value is needed and will give further insights into whether these antibodies are useful for monitoring the disease activity and the therapeutic response of the respective autoimmune disease.

References

1 Wanstrat A, Wakeland E (2001) The genetics of complex autoimmune diseases: Non-MHC susceptibility genes. *Nat. Immunol.* **2**, 802–809.

2 Costagliola S, Many MC, Denef JF, Pohlenz J, Refetoff S, Vassart G (2000) Genetic immunization of outbred mice with thyrotropin receptor cDNA provides a model of Graves' disease. *J. Clin. Invest.* **105**, 803–811.

3 Todaro M, Zeuner A, Stassi G (2004) Role of apoptosis in autoimmunity. *J. of Clinical Immunol.* **24**, 1–11.

4 Chiovato L, Bassi P, Santini F, Mammoli C, Lapi P, Carayon P, Pinchera A (1993) Antibodies producine complement-mediated thyroid cytotoxicity in patients with atrophic or goitrous autoimmune thyroiditis. *J. Clin. Endocrinol. Metab.* **77**, 1700–1705.

5 Bogner U, Schleuser H, Wall JR (1984) Antibody-dependent cell mediated cytotoxicity against human thyroid cells in Hashimoto's thyroiditis but not Graves' disease. *J. Clin. Endocrinol. Metab.* **59**, 734–738.

6 Amagai M, Koch PJ, Nishikawa T, Stanley JR (1996) Pemphigus vulgaris antigen (desmoglein 3) is localized in the lower epidermis, the site of blister formation in patients. *J. Invest. Dermatol.* **106**, 351–355.

7 Jones CM, Callaghan JM, Gleeson PA, Mori Y, Masuda T, Toh BH (1991) The parietal cell autoantibodies recognised in neonatal thymectomy-induced murine gastritis are the alpha and beta subunits of the gastric proton pump. *Gastroenterol.* **101**, 287–294.

8 Toh BH, Driel JR, Gleeson PA (1997) Pernicious anaemia. *N. Engl. J. Med.* **337**, 1441–1448.

9 Korganow AS, Ji H, Mangialaio S, Duchatelle V, Pelanda R, Martin T, Degott C, Kikutani H, Rajewsky K, Pasquali JL, Benoist L, Mathis D (1999) From systemic T cell self-reactivity to organ-specific autoimmune disease via immunoglobulins. *Immunity* **10**, 451–461.

10 Matsumoto I, Staub A, Benoist C, Mathis D (1999) Arthritis provoked by linked T and B cell recognition of a glycolytic enzyme. *Science* **286**, 1732–1735.

11 International Autoimmune Hepatitis Group report: review of criteria for diagnosis of autoimmune hepatitis (1999) *J. Hepatol.* **31**, 929–938.

12 Waldenström J (1950) Leber, Blutproteine und Nahrungseiweiße. *Dtsch. Gesellsch. Verd. Stoffw.* **15**, 113–119.

13 Strassburg CP, Manns MP (1999) Antinuclear antibody (ANA) patterns in hepatic and extrahepatic autoimmune disease. *J Hepatol* **31**, 751.

14 Strassburg CP, Alex B, Zindy F, Gerken G, Luttig B, Meyer zum Büschenfelde KH, Brechot C, Manns MP (1996) Identification of cyclin A as a molecular target of antinuclear antibodies (ANA) in hepatic and non-hepatic diseases. *J Hepatol* **25**, 859–866.

15 Czaja AJ, Ming C, Shirai M, Nishioka M (1995) Frequency and significance of antibodies to histones in autoimmune hepatitis. *J Hepatol* **23**, 32–38.

16 Czaja AJ, Nishioka M, Morhed SA, Haciya T (1994) Patterns of nuclear immunofluorescence and reactivities to recombinant nuclear antigens in autoimmune hepatitis. *Gastroenterol* **107**, 200–207.

17 Czaja AJ, Cassani F, Cataleta M, Valenti P, Bianchi FB (1996) Frequencies and significance of antibodies to actin in type 1 autoimmune hepatitis. *Hepatol* **24**, 1068–1073.

18 Manns MP, Strassburg CP (2001) Autoimmune hepatitis: clinical challenges. *Gastroenterol.* **120**, 1502–1517.

19 Gregorio GV, Portman B, Reid F, Donaldson PT, Doherty DG, McCartney M, Vergani D, Mieli-Vergai G (1997) Autoimmune hepatitis in childhood: a 20-year experience. *Hepatol.* **25**, 541–547.

20 Toh BH (1997) Smooth muscle autoantibodies and autoantigens. *Clin. Exp. Immunol.* **38**, 621–628.

21 Czaja AJ, Homburger HA (2001) Autoantibodies in liver disease. *Gastroenterol.* **120**, 239–249.

22 Strassburg CP, Manns MP (2002) Autoantibodies and autoantigens in autoimmune hepatitis. *Sem. Liver Dis.* **22**, 39–351.

23 Bottazzo GF., Florin-Christensen A., Fairfax A, Swana G, Doniach D, Groeschel-Stewart U (1979) Classification of smooth muscle autoantibodies detected by immunofluorescence. *J Clin Pathol* **29**, 403–410.

24 Targan SR, Landers C, Vidrich A, Czaja AJ (1995) High-titer antineutrophil cytoplasmic antibodies in type 1 autoimmune hepatitis. *Gastroenterol* **108**, 1159–1166.

25 Zauli D, Ghetti S, Grassi A. Descovich C, Cassani F, Ballardini G, Muratori L, Bianchi FB (1997) Antineutrophil cytoplasmic antibodies in type 1 and type 2 autoimmune hepatitis. *Hepatol* **25**, 1105–1107.

26 Orth T, Gerken G, Kellner R, Meyer zum Büschenfelde KH, Mayet WJ (1997) Actin is a target antigen of antineutrophil cytoplasmic antibodies (ANCA) in autoimmune hepatitis type-1. *J Hepatol* **26**, 37–47.

27 Terjung B, Herzog V, Worman HJ, Gestmann I, Bauer C, Sauerbruch T, Spengler U (1998) Atypical antineutrophil cytoplasmic antibodies with perinuclear fluorescence in chronic inflammatory bowel disease and hepatobiliary disorders colocalize with nuclear lamina proteins. *Hepatol* **28**, 332–340.

28 McFarlane JG, McFarlane BM, Major GN, Tolley P, Williams R (1984) Identification of the hepatic asialo-glycoprotein receptor (hepatic lectin) as a component of liver specific membrane lipoprotein (LSP). *Clin. Exp. Immunol.* **55**, 347–354.

29 Poralla T, Treichel U, Lohr H, Fleischer B (1991) The asialoglycoprotein receptor as a target structure in autoimmune liver disease. *Sem. Liv. Dis.* **11**, 215–222.

30 Treichel U, Poralla T, Hess G, Manns MP, Meyer zum Büschenfelde KH (1990) Autoantibodies to human asialoglycoprotein receptor in autoimmune type chronic hepatitis. *Hepatol.* **11**, 606–612.

31 McFarlane IG, Hegarty JE, McSorley CG, McFarlane BM, Williams R (1984) Antibodies to liver-specific protein predict outcome of treatment withdrawal in autoimmune chronic active hepatitis. *Lancet* **2**, 954–956.

32 Czaja AJ, Pfeifer KD, Decker RH, Vallari AS (1996) Frequency and significance of antibodies to asialoglycoprotein receptor in type 1 autoimmune hepatitis. *Dig. Dis. Sci.* **41**, 1733–1740.

33 Czaja AJ, Manns MP, Homurger HA (1992) Frequency and significance of antibodies to liver/kidney microsome type 1 in adults with chronic active hepatitis. *Gastroenterol.* **103**, 1290–1295.

34 Homberg JC, Abuaf N, Bernard O, Islam S, Alvarez F, Khalil SH, Poupon R, Darnis F, Levy VG, Grippon P (1987) Chronic active hepatitis associated with liver/kidney microsome type 1: a second type of autoimmune hepatitis. *Hepatol.* **7**, 1333–1339.

35 Manns MP, Griffin KJ, Sullivan KF, Johnson EF (1991) LKM-1 autoantibodies recognize a short linear sequence in P450IID6, a cytochrome P-450 monooxygenase. *J. Clin. Invest.* **88**,1370–1378.

36 Strassburg CP, Obermeyer-Straub P, Alex B, Durazzo M, Rizzetto M, Tukey RH, Manns MP (1996) Autoantibodies against glucuronosyltransferases differ between viral hepatitis and autoimmune hepatitis. *Gastroenterol.* **11**, 1582–1592.

37 Strassburg CP, Obermayer-Straub P, Manns MP (1996) Autoimmunity in hepatitis C and D virus infection. *J. Viral. Hepat.* **3**, 49–59.

38 Rizzetto M, Swana G, Doniach D (1973) Microsomal antibodies in active chronic hepatitis and other disorders. *Clin. Exp. Immunol.* **15**, 331–344.

39 Zanger UM, Hauri HP, Loeper J, Homberg JC, Meyer UA (1988) Antibodies against human cytochrome P-450db1 in autoimmune hepatitis type 2. *Proc. Natl. Acad. Sci. USA.* **85**, 8256–8260.

40 Guenguen M, Meunier-Rotival M, Bernard O, Alvarez F (1988) Anti-liver-kidney microsome antibody recognizes a cytochrome P450 from the IID subfamily. *J. Exp. Med.* **168**, 801.

41 Manns M, Meyer zum Büschenfelde KH, Slusarczyk J, Dienes HP (1984) Detection of liver-kidney microsomal antibodies by radioimmunoassay and their relation to antimitochondrial antibodies in inflammatory liver disease. *Clin. Exp. Immunol.* **54**, 600–608.

42 Manns MP, Johnson EF, Griffin KJ, Tan EM, Sullivan KF (1989) Major antigen of liver kidney microsomal antibodies in idiopathic autoimmune hepatitis is cytochrome P450db1. *J. Clin. Invet.* **83**, 1066–1072.

43 Manns MP, Griffin KJ, Sullivan KF, Johnson EF (1991) LKM-1 autoantibodies recognize a short linear sequence in P450IID6, a cytochrome P-450 monooxygenase. *J. Clin. Invest.* **88**, 1370–1378.

44 Manns M, Zanger U, Gerken G, Sullivan KF, Meyer zum Büschenfelde KH, Eichelbaum M (1990) Patients with type II autoimmune hepatitis express functionally intact cytochrome P450 db1 that is inhibited by LkM1 autoantibodies in vitro but not in vivo. *Hepatol.* **12**, 127–132.

45 Löhr HF, Schlaak JF, Lohse AW, Bocher WO, Arenz M, Gerken G, Meyer zum Büschenfelde KH (1996) Autoreactive CD4+ LKM-specific and anticlonotypic T cell response in LKM-1 antibody-positive autoimmune hepatitis. *Hepatol.* **24**, 1416–1421.

46 Duclos-Vallee JC, Hajoui O, Yamamoto AM, Jacqz-Aigrin E, Alvarez F (1995) Conformational epitopes on CYP2D6 are recognized by liver/kidney microsomal antibodies. *Gastroenterol.* **108**, 470–476.

47 Dalekos GN, Wedemeyer H, Obermayer-Straub P, Kayser A, Barut A, Frank H, Manns MP (1999) Epitope mapping of cytochrome P4502D6 autoantigen in patients with chronic hepatitis C during a interferon treatment. *J. Hepatol.* **30**, 366–375.

48 Ma Y, Peakman M, Lobo-Yeo A, Wen L, Lenzi M, Gaken J, Farzaneh F, Mieli-Vergani G, Bianchi FB, Vergani D (1994) Differences in immune recognition of cytochrome P4502D6 by liver kidney microsomal (LKM) antibody in autoimmune hepatitis and chronic hepatitis C virus infection. *Clin. Exp. Immunol.* **97**, 94–99.

49 Muratori L, Parola M, Ripalti A, Robino G, Muratori P, Bellomo G, Corini R, Lenzi M, Laandini MP, Albano E, Bianchi FB (2000) Liver/kidney microsomal antibody type 1 targets CYP2D6 on hepatocyte plasma membrane. *Gut* **46**, 553–561.

50 Loeper J, Descatoire V, Maurice M, Beaune P, Belghiti J, Houssin D, Ballet F, Feldmann G, Guengerich FP, Pessayre D (1993) Cytochromes P450 in human hepatocyte plasma membrane: recognition by several autoantibodies. *Gastroenterol.* **104**, 203–216.

51 Trautwein C, Ramadori G, Gerken G, Meyer zum Büschenfelde KH, Manns MP (1992) Regulation of cytochrome P450 2D by acute phase mediators in C3H7HeJ mice. *Biochem. Biophys. Res. Commun.* **182**, 617–623.

52 Philipp T, Durazzo M, Trautwein C, Alex B, Straub P, Lamb JG, Johnson EF, Tukey RH, Manns MP (1994) Recognition of uridine diphosphate glucuronosyl transferases by LKM-3 antibodies in chronic hepatitis D. *Lancet* **344**, 578–581.

53 Crivelli O, Lavarini C, Chiaberge E, Amoroso A, Farci P, Negro F, Rizzetto M (1983) Microsomal autoantibodies in chronic infection with HbsAg associated delta agent. *Clin. Exp. Immunol.* **54**, 232–238.

54 Strassburg C, Obermayer-Straub P, Alex B, Durazzo M, Rizzetto M, Tukey RH, Manns MP (1996) Autoantibodies against glucuronosyl transferases differ between viral hepatitis and autoimmune hepatitis. *Gastroenterol.* **11**, 1582–1592.

55 Lenzi M, Manotti P, muratori L, Cataleta M, Ballardini G, Cassani F, Bianchi FB (1995) Liver cytosolic 1 antigen-antibody system in type 2 autoimmune hepatitis and hepatitis C virus infection. *Gut* **36**, 749–754.

56 Martini E, Abuaf N, Cavalli F, Durand V, Johanet C, Homberg JC (1988) Antibody to liver cytosol (anti-LC1) in patients with autoimmune chronic active hepatitis type 2. *Hepatol.* **8**, 1662–1666.

57 Lapierre P, Hajoui O, Homberg JC, Alvarez F (1999) Fomiminotransferase cyclodeaminase is an organ specific autoantigen recognized by sera of patients with autoimmune hepatitis. *Gastroenterol.* **116**, 643–649.

58 Manns M, Gerken G, Kyriatsoulis A, Staritz M, Meyer zum Büschenfelde KH (1987) Characterization of a new subgroup of autoimmune chronic active

hepatitis by autoantibodies against a soluble liver antigen. *Lancet* **I**, 292–294.

59 Volkmann MML, Bäurle A, Heid H, Strassburg CP, Tratwein C, Fiehn W, Manns MP (2001) Soluble liver antigen: isolation of a 35 kD recombinant protein (SLA-P35) specifically recognizing sera from patients with autoimmune hepatitis type 3. *Hepatol.* **33**, 591–596.

60 Wies I, Brunner S, Henninger J, Herkel J, Kanzler S, Meyer zum Büschenfelde KH, Lohse AW (2000) Identification of target antigen for SLA/LP autoantibodies in autoimmune hepatitis. *Lancet* **355**, 1510–1515.

61 Kanzler S, Weidemann C, Gerken G, Löhr HF, Galle PR, Meyer zum Büschenfelde KH, Lohse AW (1999) Clinical significance of autoantibodies to soluble liver antigen in autoimmune hepatitis. *J. Hepatol.* **31**, 635–640.

62 Stechemesser E, Klein R, Berg PA (1993) Characterization and clinical relevance of liver-pancreas antibodies in autoimmune heaptitis. *Hepatol.* **18**, 1–9.

63 Manns M, Gerken G, Kyriatsoulis A, Tratwein C, Reske K, Meyer zum Büschenfelde KH (1987) Two different subtypes of antimitochondrial antibodies are associated with primary biliary cirrhosis: identification and characterization by radioimmunoassay and immunoblotting. *Hepatol.* **5**, 893–899.

64 Jones DE, Watt FE, Metcalf FE, Bassendine MF, James OF (1999) Familial primary cirrhosis reassessed: a geographically-based population study. *J Hepatol.* **30**, 402–407.

65 Gershwin ME, Mackay IR (1991) Primary biliary cirrhosis: paradigm or paradox for autoimmunity. *Gastroenterol.* **100**, 822–833.

66 Heathcote J (2000) Update on primary biliary cirrhosis. *Can. J. Gastroenterol.* **14**, 43–48.

67 Ishii H, Saifuku K, Namihisa T (1985) Multiplicity of mitochondrial inner membrane antigens from beef heart reacting with antimitochondrial antibodies in sera of patients with primary biliary cirrhosis. *Immunol. Lett.* **9**, 325–330.

68 Manns MP, Krüger M (1994) Immumogenetics of chronic liver diseases. *Gastroenterol.* **106**, 1676–1697.

69 Nishio A, Keeffe E, Gershwin ME (2002) Immunopathogenesis of primary biliary cirrhosis. *Sem. Liver Dis.* **22**, 291–302.

70 Bandin O, Couvalin J, Poupon R, Dubel L, Homberg JC, Johanet C (1996) Specificity and sensitivity of gp210 autoantibodies detected using an enzyme-linked immunosorbent assay and a synthetic polypeptide in the diagnosis of primary biliary cirrhosis. *Hepatol.* **23**, 1020–1024.

71 Wesierska-Gadek J, Honenauer H, Hitchman E, Penner E (1996) Autoantibodies against nucleoporin p62 constitute a novel marker of primary biliary cirrhosis. *Gastroenterol.* **110**, 840–847.

72 Szostecki C, Krippner H, Penner E, Bautz FA (1987) Autoimmune sera recognize a 100 kD nuclear protein antigen (sp100). *Clin. Exp. Immunol.* **68**, 108–116.

73 Courvalin JC, Lassoued K, Worman HJ, Blobel G (1990) Identification and characterization of autoantibodies against the nuclear envelope lamin B receptor from patients with primary biliary cirrhosis. *J. Exp. Med.* **172**, 961–967.

74 Chazouilleres O, Wendunm D, Serfaty L, Montembault S, Rosmorduc O, Poupon R (1998) Primary biliary cirrhosis – autoimmune hepatitis overlap syndrome: clinical features and response to therapy. *Hepatol.* **28**, 296–301.

75 Czaja AJ (1998) Frequency and nature of the variant syndroms of autoimmune liver disease. *Hepatol.* **28**, 360–365.

14
Autoantibodies in Autoimmune Thyroid Disease

Osvaldo Martinez and Bellur S. Prabhakar

14.1
The Thyroid Gland

The thyroid gland produces the thyroid hormone that is required to maintain normal metabolism of the body. A highly regulated feedback loop controls thyroid function and helps maintain the euthyroid status (Fig. 14.1). Thyroid-stimulating hormone (TSH) is produced in the anterior pituitary in response to stimulation by thyroid-releasing hormone (TRH) produced in the hypothalamus. The TSH binds to the thyrotropin receptor (TSHR), which then activates adenylyl cyclase and phosphatidyl inositol pathways and leads to the production of thyroid hormone. Hormone production begins when tyrosine residues of the thyroglobulin (Tg) are iodinated and then coupled through the catalytic action of the thyroid peroxidase (TPO), leading to the formation of the thyroid hormone precursor T4. The T4 undergoes deiodination and results in the formation of the thyroid hormone triiodothyronine (T3). The T3 binds to its cognate receptor in cells throughout the body and forms a complex, which is translocated to the nucleus. There it binds to the thyroid hormone response elements and exerts its effects by activating transcription of relevant genes. The euthyroid state is maintained by a positive feedback from the thyrotropin-releasing hormone (TRH), which stimulates TSH production and negative feedback from T3, which causes downregulation of TRH and thus TSH production. Deregulation caused by autoimmunity leads to symptoms associated with hyperthyroidism or hypothyroidism through increased or decreased production of thyroid hormone, respectively (Fig. 14.1).

14.2
Autoimmune Diseases of the Thyroid

Autoimmunity to thyroid antigens is the most common cause of thyroid diseases including Hashimoto's thyroiditis (HT), Graves' disease (GD), and primary myxedema (PM). Different autoimmune diseases of the thyroid share similar

Autoantibodies and Autoimmunity: Molecular Mechanisms in Health and Disease. Edited by K. Michael Pollard
Copyright © 2006 WILEY-VCH Verlag GmbH & Co. KGaA, Weinheim
ISBN: 3-527-31141-6

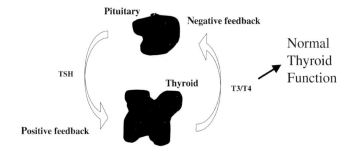

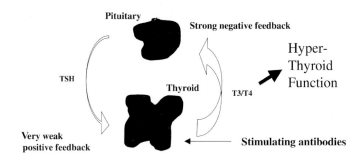

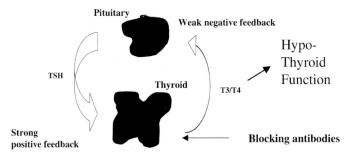

Fig. 14.1 Regulation of thyroid hormone production. The upper panel shows a normal hypothalamus-pituitary-thyroid axis, which maintains hormonal homeostasis and regulates normal thyroid function. The middle panel illustrates the effects of stimulatory Abs (TSAb) as seen in patients with Graves' disease. The lower panel shows the effects of blocking Abs (TSBAb) as seen in patients with primary myxedema.

immunological characteristics and are thought to be interrelated. However, particular thyroid antigens, immunological abnormalities, symptoms, and clinical courses are associated with specific thyroid diseases. For example, it is well known that anti-thyroid antibodies circulate in the serum of patients that suffer from HT and GD, but it is generally accepted that HT is primarily a T cell–mediated disease in which thyroglobulin-specific T cells infiltrate the thyroid and cause glandular destruction that results in hypothyroidism. In contrast,

GD, the most prevalent of the TSHR-mediated autoimmune diseases, is mediated by anti-TSHR autoantibodies that can act as TSH agonists and cause hyperthyroidism. However, if the anti-TSHR antibodies act as TSH antagonists, they can result in primary myxedema (PM), which is characterized by hypothyroidism.

14.3
Autoantibodies in Thyroiditis

Autoimmune thyroid diseases are characterized by the presence of autoantibodies to multiple thyroid antigens [1] including thyroglobulin (TG), thyroid peroxidase (TPO), and the TSHR. As mentioned above, these proteins play essential roles in the production of thyroid hormone. With respect to specific diseases, Over 90% and ~80% of patients with GD have anti-TSHR and anti-TPO autoantibodies, respectively, while over 90% of patients with HT have anti-TPO and/or anti-TG autoantibodies. Unlike anti-TSHR antibodies, anti-TPO and anti-TG antibodies do not play a significant role in the pathogenesis of either HT or GD. However, they are helpful in the differential diagnosis and may serve as predictors of ensuing thyroiditis. The Whickam study, an extensive population-based study, showed that after a 20-year follow-up, the odds ratio (with 95% confidence) of developing thyroiditis in individuals with thyroid autoantibodies and elevated TSH but normal free T4 was 38 (22–65) for men and 173 (81–370) for women [2, 3]. In another study, which followed patients with subclinical hypothyroidism (TSH levels >4 mU L^{-1}) for over nine years, 59% of women with TPO autoantibodies became hypothyroid as compared to 23% of women without TPO autoantibodies [4]. Similarly, the presence of TPO and TG autoantibodies, along with abnormal TSH levels, is associated with a higher incidence of hypothyroidism in juveniles and children, but the evidence is less compelling for pregnant women [1].

A large proportion of women (~20–40%) have thyroid infiltration, and 10–20% of these women are positive for anti-TPO autoantibodies [1, 5]; however, only approximately 3% of women show clinical disease. Together, TPO and TG antibodies are useful in confirming the diagnosis of Hashimoto's thyroiditis. Some contend that TG autoantibodies, which rarely occur on their own, may not be as useful [6], while others claim specific disease associations. For example, presence of TG antibodies, without TPO antibodies, often could be indicative of thyroid hypertrophy and small nodules. However, in patients with HT, it is more common to find both antibodies rather than the anti-Tg antibodies alone [7]. Since the presence of TG-specific antibodies could interfere with the measurement of TG, and the TG levels in the sera serve as very useful markers to detect recurrence of thyroid cancer, testing for anti-TG antibodies to ensure that they are not interfering with the TG assay will aid in the proper diagnosis of thyroid cancers. Therefore, measurement of anti-TPO and anti-TG antibodies could be of significant clinical value. In contrast, anti-TSHR antibodies not only serve as reliable markers for GD and primary myxedema (PM) but also play a very important role in the pathogenesis of these diseases.

14.4
TSHR-mediated Autoimmunity

Pathogenic autoantibodies to the TSHR disturb normal hypothalamus-pituitary-thyroid regulation of thyroid function [8–10] (Fig. 14.1). GD is characterized by hyperthyroidism, which often leads to tachycardia, anxiety, excessive sweating, and acute weight loss. On the other hand, autoimmune PM is characterized by hypothyroidism that can lead to physical and mental lethargy, bradycardia, and weight gain. Pathogenic antibodies (TSAbs) from patients with GD bind to TSHR and stimulate thyroid, but in PM, pathogenic antibodies (TSBAbs) block either the binding of TSH or TSH-mediated activation of thyroid cells. Unlike in HT, the primary cause of thyroid dysfunction in GD and PM is not due to glandular destruction but rather to physiological perturbation of thyroid function mediated by anti-TSHR antibodies. The important question is how one develops pathogenic antibodies against the thyroid. Since self-tolerance prevents development of autoimmune responses, breakdown in self-tolerance must precede the generation of autoantibodies.

14.5
Development of Autoantibodies Against TSHR

The central dogma in immunology is defined by the ability of immune cells to discriminate between self and non-self. The discrimination against self is governed by mechanisms that mediate tolerance to normal antigens in the body. When tolerance is broken, self is recognized as non-self or foreign, and therefore the immune system begins to attack the organ in question. Evidence from transgenic models that use foreign antigen hen egg lysozyme (HEL) expressed on the thyroid cells and HEL antigen-specific B and T cells suggests that a breakdown in T-cell tolerance to a thyroid antigen is required before B cells can produce anti-thyroid antibodies [11, 12]. Specifically, B cells that express transgenic receptors that recognize the HEL expressed on the thyroid as a transgene are not eliminated or inactivated. This means that the pre-immune B-cell repertoire against the thyroid antigen (i.e., HEL) is intact and that the tolerance would have to depend on mechanisms other than B-cell deletion to avoid autoantibody production. Since TSHR (as well as HEL) is a protein antigen, it likely requires T-cell help for both initiation and maintenance of anti-TSHR antibody response. This is clearly illustrated by experiments showing that T cells that carry the transgenic T-cell receptor against thyroid-expressed HEL are hyporesponsive to the HEL antigen. This T-cell tolerance could not only help keep T cells in check but also could prevent T cell–dependent activation of autoreactive B cells. However, in the same study the authors were able to stimulate HEL-specific T cells with a stronger stimulus, suggesting a putative mechanism by which a break in T-cell tolerance to thyroid antigens may occur. Once T-cell tolerance is overcome, the thyroid antigen–specific B cells can be readily activated, leading to antibody production. In Graves' patients, a majority of the stimulatory activity in the serum resides in the IgG fraction of the antibodies [13, 14]. This is consistent with the concept that a breakdown in T-cell tolerance is required for the production of pathogenic autoantibodies because B cells require T-cell help for isotype switching from IgM to IgG and affinity maturation.

Given the right circumstances, a breakdown in tolerance precipitated by thyroid injury (e.g., environmental stress factors) could lead to thyroid autoimmunity. At the site of injury and inflammation, thyroid antigens could be processed by professional antigen-presenting cells (APCs). The APCs will carry the antigen to the draining lymph nodes and present the thyroid antigen in the context of the right MHC class II to an appropriate $CD4^+$ T helper cell, leading to its activation. In the same context, an autoreactive B cell could also acquire the thyroid antigen by binding to it with its IgM receptor and present it to the appropriate T cells. This interaction between T cells and B cells with a common antigen specificity (linked recognition), and in the presence of sufficient amounts of the thyroid antigen, could result in the formation of germinal centers where B-cell differentiation could take place with T-cell help. A continued antigenic stimulation would lead to B-cell isotype switching and somatic hypermutation of the B-cell receptors, resulting in high-affinity antibody production. Interestingly, there is evidence to suggest that anti-thyroid antibody–producing B cells accumulate in the thyroid where they are continuously exposed to the antigen [1]. Once sufficient amounts of anti-TSHR antibodies of high affinity accumulate in the serum, they can continually stimulate the TSHR, resulting in Graves' disease. What predisposes certain individuals to GD and what triggers the initial autoimmune response are not completely understood. However, it is generally accepted that genetic and environmental factors could act in concert to initiate an anti-thyroid autoimmune response.

14.6
The Role of Genetic Factors

The etiology of autoimmune thyroid disease (AITD) is unclear. Similar to other autoimmune diseases, genetic, environmental, and other endogenous factors contribute to the initiation of the disease. Increased incidence of GD among members of a family and a higher degree of disease concordance among identical twins indicate that genetic factors may play an important role in determining susceptibility to GD [15–17]. As in most other autoimmune diseases, the strongest bias in developing GD is gender: women are 5–10 times more likely than men to develop the disease. Two recent reviews on genetic susceptibility to GD have summarized and discussed the implications of a large number of studies [18, 19]. The general conclusions one can draw from studies to date is that multiple genetic factors appear to contribute to the risk of developing GD. Some of the susceptibility gene(s) appear to be associated with the X chromosome, others seem to be specific to GD (e.g., GD-1, GD-2, and GD-3), and yet others such as MHC class II alleles and CTLA4 are involved in the generation of immune responses [20, 21]. The CTLA4 protein exists in multiple isoforms due to genetic polymorphism of AT dimers at the 3'-untranslated region of the third exon. This is often linked with another polymorphism in the first exon [22]. A 106–base pair AT polymorphism is thought to be associated with increased risk of GD [20, 23]. Similarly, other associations with genetic polymorphism in CTLA4 have been reported [24–26]. Earlier studies have shown that patients with GD express HLA-B8 more often than control subjects without the disease [27]. Other studies have shown that the risk of developing the disease is higher among individuals with an MHC class II haplotype of HLA-DR3 [28, 29]. Similarly, the risk is increased in individuals with a DQA1-*0501 haplotype [30, 31]. In contrast, the expression of HLA DR $\beta1*07$ appears to confer protection [32]. There is also a racial variation in the association of MHC haplotypes with an increased risk for the development of GD [32]. However, it is no coincidence that the genetic associations with GD are related to genes involved in immune regulation. Although GD is an autoantibody-mediated disease, as discussed above, genetic factors such as linkage to MHC class II alleles and CTLA4 point to an essential T-cell role in its development. How the autoimmune response is initiated in genetically susceptible individuals is not fully understood, but environmental factors appear to play an important role.

14.7
The Role of Environmental Factors

Like other autoimmune diseases, environmental factors have long been suspected in the etiology of the disease. For example, excess iodine intake is a risk factor for developing autoimmune thyroid diseases in both humans and animal models of AITD [33, 34]. Stress, drugs, and smoking can also contribute to the development of the disease. The common mode of action of all these factors is that they place stress on the thyroid [35]. It is possible that these environmental stresses can lead to thyroid injury, which may in turn release thyroid autoantigens or alter the immunogenicity of the thyroid antigens. Another set of environmental factors linked to AITD [36] and host immune responses is microbial infections, which can cause overexpression (e.g., heat shock proteins, MHC class II molecules, costimulatory molecules, etc.) and/or altered expression of certain self-proteins (altered self). Presentation of these antigens by professional APCs could provide the necessary strength of signal or be perceived as foreign [37] and lead to the activation of T cells. Alternatively, aberrant expression of MHC and/or costimulatory molecules, due to infection and inflammation, can allow thyrocytes to serve as APCs that can restimulate T cells. Superantigens and mitogenic bacterial products could also activate immune cells with a wide range of different antigen specificities, including for self-antigens, in a nonspecific manner and initiate an autoimmune response. Molecular mimicry is yet another mechanism often invoked to explain autoimmune responses that result from activation of T cells or B cells that recognize a microbial antigen and can simultaneously cross-react with an autoantigen. For example, *Y. enterocolitica* has been implicated in GD induction because of its ability to produce superantigens and mitogens and because of the cross-reactivity of its lipoprotein with the TSHR [38].

14.8
Assays for TSHR Autoantibodies

Passive transfer of immunoglobulins from GD patients to experimental animals caused increased thyroid hormone production [39]. The discovery that autoantibodies were the cause of Graves' disease began the quest to detect, quantify, and characterize these antibodies. Two main assays are used to detect and characterize anti-TSHR autoantibodies. One measures the inhibition of TSH binding (TBII) to the TSHR, while the other measures the stimulatory activity (TSAb) of the antibody through cAMP production by TSHR-expressing cells. The latter assay can be readily modified to detect blocking activity (TSBAb) by measuring the ability of a given antibody to prevent cAMP production in the presence of a known amount of TSH. Although there is considerable agreement between results from TBII and TSAb assays, such agreement is lacking between the antibody titer/activity in the serum and the severity of the disease [40–43]. It is interesting to note that the TBII assay can detect both TSAb and TSBAb antibodies, suggesting that antibodies can bind to a number of different sites on the TSHR and prevent TSH binding (perhaps due to stearic hindrance), but their binding to specific epitopes might be required to exert their functional effects. These and other results (reviewed in [44]) show that some of the antibody-binding sites overlap and others are mutually exclusive. The TBIIs found in patients with Hashimoto's thyroiditis or primary myxedema differ from the TBIIs found in GD because they can inhibit the stimulating activity of both TSAbs and TSH [46]. In contrast, many Graves' TBIIs can inhibit TSH binding, but not the TSAb activity. However, this cannot be generalized because some GD patients' sera do contain antibodies that can block both [47]. These observations show the complexity of the autoantibody response against the TSHR. Moreover, they show that it is not simply the presence or absence of stimulating and blocking antibodies, but a balance between the levels of stimulating and blocking activity against the TSHR, that determine the disease outcome.

14.9
Thyrotropin Receptor Down-modulation

The TSHR can be divided into three parts [48]: (1) a long hydrophilic region (aa 1–418), (2) a region with seven hydrophobic, membrane-spanning domains similar in sequence to other G protein–coupled receptors (aa 419–682), and (3) a short (aa 683–764) cytoplasmic domain (Fig. 14.2). TSHR is different from other gonadotropin receptors in that it contains two inserts within the extracellular domain (TSHR ECD): one of 50 amino acids in the region of residues 300–400 of the TSHR and a second of eight residues (aa 38–45) [48–50]. The ectodomain contains six potential N-linked glycosylation sites that are required for proper folding of the receptor and for patient autoantibody binding. The TSHR ECD is the primary region of TSH and TSHR Ab binding [47–50] and can undergo processing to yield two subunits (A and B) that can remain associated through disulfide bonds [50]. Once TSH and TSAB bind to the receptor, they transduce signals to the cell, resulting in G-protein uncoupling and activation of adenylyl cyclase and cAMP production. Once the cAMP is activated, it can bind to its responsive elements and mediate a wide range of signaling and gene activation.

TSHR down-modulation and/or desensitization on thyrocytes provide yet another level of regulation for TSHR function. Following ligand binding to G protein–coupled receptors [51–53], the ligand-receptor complex is internalized, resulting in the termination of cAMP signaling [54, 55], initiation of mitogenic activity [56], dephosphorylation, and re-sensitization or down-modulation of the receptor [57, 58]. However, how the receptor-mediated signaling is down-modu-

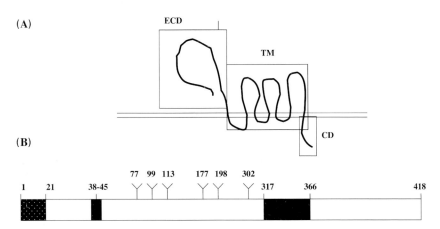

Fig. 14.2 (A) Schematic representation of TSHR. Shown are the extracellular domain (ECD), the transmembrane domain (TM), and the short cytoplasmic domain (CD) of TSHR. (B) The TSHR ECD, consisting of first 21 residues as signal peptide and two regions that are unique to TSHR, between residues 38–45 and 317–366, when compared to other G protein–coupled receptors. Six potential N-linked glycosylation sites at positions 77, 99, 113, 177, 198, and 302 are indicated by "Y" symbols.

lated in the thyroid is not fully understood. Although a great deal of information has been gathered on the internalization of receptors that contain a single transmembrane domain [59], limited data exist on endocytosis of glycoprotein hormone receptors, which contain multiple membrane-spanning domains. This is particularly true of the TSHR protein upon ligand (TSH) binding, and there is no known report on the fate of this receptor upon TSAb or TSBAb binding.

Milgrom's group [60] has studied TSHR trafficking. They found that the receptor was expressed on the plasma membrane and clathrin-coated pits and that a minor fraction of the expressed protein was constitutively localized to endosomes [60]. Upon TSH addition, there was an increase in the endocytosis of the receptor. While the TSH was degraded in the lysosomes, a great majority of the internalized TSHR was recycled to the cell surface, which could be blocked by treatment with monensin. Furthermore, another study [61] provided further evidence for receptor recycling by demonstrating the co-localization of newly internalized TSHR to RhoB-containing early endosomes. Early endosomes are involved in dissociation and sorting of receptor-ligand complexes in an environment that is least damaging [62], whereas the late endosomes and lysosomal vesicles are primarily involved in accumulating and digesting both exogenous and endogenous macromolecules [63]. It appears that one molecule of TSH can bind to one TSHR; however, since the Abs are bivalent it is possible that they could simultaneously bind to two TSHR molecules. It is interesting to speculate whether TSAb binding due to bivalency and larger size (150 kDa) might prevent or slow receptor internalization and allow it to stay on the cell surface longer than after TSH binding, resulting in a prolonged activation of the thyroid. If this were to occur on a continual basis, it could lead to the development of hyperthyroidism [61]. More definitive studies are required to establish a link between perturbations in receptor trafficking and the pathogenesis of GD.

14.10
Functional Domains of TSHR

Several approaches have been used for determining the functionally relevant epitopes bound by autoantibodies on TSHR. One involved construction of TSHR-LH/CGR chimeras, in which select segments of TSHR were replaced with the corresponding segments from the LH/CGR. Studies from this approach resulted in the identification of putative TSH, blocking, and stimulatory antibody-binding regions of TSHR [57, 74, 80, 99]. Another approach has been to use deletion mutants and/or site-directed mutagenesis to identify functionally relevant regions of TSHR. These studies revealed that certain glycosylation sites and cysteine residues are absolutely essential for proper folding of the receptor, as well as for TSH and antibody binding [70, 71, 100]. Because of limitations associated with each of these approaches, no single approach has yielded conclusive results on the overall structure-function relationship of the TSHR. However, collectively, these studies have led to several important conclusions. It appears that both TSH and autoantibodies can primarily bind to the ECD of the TSHR. The TSH-binding epitope consists of discontinuous amino acids that come together due to protein folding. Antibodies against one or more of these epitopes can inhibit TSH binding or TSH-mediated activation of cells by affecting a step subsequent to TSH binding. The stimulatory autoantibody binding sites reside predominantly at the N-terminus of the protein, while the blocking antibodies bind primarily to the C-terminus of the TSHR ECD [50]. Recently, several other studies employing TSHR-LH/CGR chimeras have used significant numbers of patient sera to begin to categorize the autoantibody response in Graves' disease [44, 45].

14.11
TSAb Epitopes in GD

Determining the TSAb epitopes (stimulatory antibody-binding sites) is vital to understanding how they stimulate the receptor and for the development of therapeutic intervention. Many studies have attempted to define TSAb epitopes and have provided significant insights, but they have failed to provide definitive answers. One of the difficulties in performing such studies is that the TSAb binding requires native TSHR conformation. Negative results from assays that use mutational analysis, chimeric constructs, or TSHR fragments are hard to interpret because one cannot distinguish between lack of binding due to the loss of epitope versus improper folding that could make the epitope, although present, inaccessible. Moreover, use of sera from patients who often exhibit a complex and heterogeneous polyclonal autoantibody response also makes it very difficult to define various functional epitopes. Logically, the functional equivalent of TSH would be a stimulatory antibody that can block TSH binding. However, the TBII activity does not always correlate with the TSAb activity and in some cases may represent TSBAbs or functionally inert antibodies. Therefore, the stimulating epitope on TSHR does not appear to be a narrow epitope that is similarly bound by both TSH and TSAbs. Moreover, although TBII antibodies can inhibit TSH binding, they often fail to inhibit TSAbs, again pointing to the complex nature of various binding sites.

Until today, the most valuable approach to determining the TSAb epitopes of TSHR has been the use of chimeric constructs in which pieces of the luteinizing hormone (LH) receptor have been used to replace the corresponding regions of the TSHR (Fig. 14.3). Although these receptors are structurally very similar, they show only ~40% identity. Further, there are unique insertions within the TSHR (Fig. 14.2) not found in other G protein–coupled receptors. Also, glycosylation patterns, known to be important for proper folding of the protein required for TSAb and TSH binding [64], are different in both proteins. Nevertheless, these studies have provided very insightful information on the various binding sites on TSHR. A summary of some of these studies is provided in Fig. 14.3.

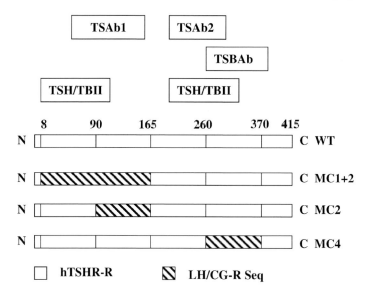

Fig. 14.3 Domain mapping of TSHR regions involved in TSAb, TBII, and TSH activity using TSHR-LH/CGR chimeras. Loss of stimulating (TSAb) and TBII activity in ~70 GD patients' IgGs when tested against three chimeras of the TSHR-LH/CGR: MC2 (residues 90–165 of the TSHR substituted), MC1+2 (residues 8–165 of the TSHR substituted), and MC4 (residues 261–370). Shown are numbers of positive sera against the corresponding construct. ++++ Indicates strongest activity, ++ indicates moderate activity, and – indicates no activity. Depicted above the figure are areas of the TSHR ECD where TSH, stimulatory antibodies (TSAb), TSH-binding inhibitory antibodies (TBII), and blocking antibodies (TSBAb) have been shown to bind. (Modified from [44, 45]).

Receptor	TSH stimulation cAMP activity	TSAb # patient sera tested (cAMP activity)	TBII # patients >20% TBII (TBII activity)
Wild type TSHR	++++	68 (++++)	68 (++++)
Mc2 chimera	++++	65 (-)	65 (+++)
Mc1+2 chimera	++	67 (-)	55 (++)
Mc4 chimera	+	70 (+++)	70 (++++)

Substitution of residues 8–165 of the TSHR with the corresponding region of the LH/CGR (MC1+2) eliminates the ability to respond to TSAbs (i.e., TSAb1), but not to TSH. Furthermore, if only residues 90–165 of the TSHR are substituted (MC2), TSAb activity is still lost or diminished in 96% of Graves' IgGs, but TSH activity is retained [65–67]. Although these results point to the importance of residues 90–165, earlier site-directed mutagenesis studies had identified residues 30–61 as being critical for TSAb activity [48, 49, 68–74]. However, specific epitopes within this 90–165 residues with which TSAbs interact have not yet been elucidated [48, 49, 68–72]. These two sets of results would suggest that the TSAb epitopes might be made of both contiguous and non-contiguous amino acids formed as a consequence of protein folding that results in the three-dimensional conformation of the protein. Recent studies confirmed that TSAb epitopes reside in the N-terminus of the protein within the A subunit of the TSHR ECD [75, 76].

Recently, there have been reports on the generation of stimulating monoclonal antibodies derived from mice and hamsters (reviewed in Ref. [77]). It would be very interesting to determine whether they all bind to the same or similar epitopes. Since the crystal structure of other G protein–coupled receptors have been determined, it is likely that the structure of TSHR will be solved in the near future. A final resolution of TSH and various autoantibody-binding sites will emerge once the crystal structure of TSHR is determined.

14.12
TSBAbs with TBII Activity

The TBII activity present in the sera of patients with GD is most likely due to TSAbs, and they primarily bind to epitopes in the N-terminus of TSHR as demonstrated by using LH/CGR-TSHR chimeras. In contrast, the TBII activity found in the sera of patients with HT or PM most likely represents TSBAb activity, and they predominantly bind to epitopes in the C-terminus of the TSHR ECD. This indicates that the TSBAb activity, however, does not always correlate with the TBII activity and vice versa. Epitopes involved in TSBAb binding are primarily located on the C-terminal portion of the TSHR ECD, probably within residues 261–395. This is in contrast to TSAb epitopes (TSAb1), which are primarily located at the N-terminal portion of the TSHR ECD (Fig. 14.3). Evidence to date suggests that these N-terminal and C-terminal areas come together due to protein folding and that the function of the receptor is critically maintained by proper three-dimensional structure. Another study, in which insect cell–derived fragments of TSHR were used, showed binding of TSBAbs to the C-terminus region of the TSHR [47]. The clinical relevance of these antibodies in PM is evident in that they can block TSH-mediated activation of the thyroid and result in hypothyroidism. However, more recently their importance in modulating GD has become clearer. It had been previously suspected that during pregnancy the amelioration of Graves' disease was due to a decrease in TSAbs; however, Kung et al. showed that disease remission during pregnancy [78] was associated with the appearance of TSBAbs whose epitopes were located in the C-terminus of the TSHR ECD [79].

14.13
The Heterogeneous and Homogeneous TSAbs

There are TSAbs whose activity solely depends on residues 25–165 (TSAb1, homogeneous) or may also depend on sites present more on the C terminal part (TSAb2, heterogeneous). These new studies show a new category of GD pathogenic antibodies that may be relevant to the clinical progression of the disease [67]. In these studies newly diagnosed GD patients' sera were tested against the chimeric LH/CG-TSHR constructs. Consistent with earlier results (see Section 14.11), about 67% of the patient sera lost TSAb activity when they were tested against MC1+2 (aa 8–165 are substituted) and/or MC2 (aa 90–165 are substituted) chimeras. However, in about 33% of sera from newly diagnosed Graves' patients, TSAb activity was not completely lost when tested against these N-terminal chimeras, which indicated that additional TSAb epitopes might be present elsewhere in the receptor. It was suggested [80] that this additional epitope(s) might result from bridging of residues in the N-terminus with the residues in the C-terminus of the TSHR ECD due to folding of the receptor. It was also suggested that the C-terminal region was less critical than the N-terminus, for either TSH or TSAb activity [50, 81–84].

Several studies have revealed an interesting phenomenon where specificity of TSAb to a heterogeneous epitope could be predictive of a more rapid response to longer remission [66, 67, 85]. Specifically, treatment with oral immunosuppressives, methimazole (MMI), or propylthiouracil (PTU) [67] resulted in a 30% increase in disease remission in patients who developed heterogeneous TSAbs. Further, a correlation was shown between the presence of TSAbs against the heterogeneous epitope with faster remission, at lower doses of PTU or MMI [66, 67]. In another study, investigators suggested that the heterogeneous TSAb epitope was also predictive of a successful response to MMI or PTU in 80% of hyperthyroid patients with a small goiter or low TBII values [84].

14.14
Immunomodulation

There are limitations in our ability to monitor the evolution of the immune response against self-antigens in humans before the onset of clinical symptoms; we therefore must rely on studies from animal models. There is no animal model in which GD develops spontaneously. Developing an animal model for GD has been hindered by our inability to purify TSHR in sufficient quantities for the induction and characterization of experimental autoimmune GD (EAGD). Even with the cloning of the receptor, establishing an animal model for GD has been very challenging. Recently, however, several promising models of EAGD have emerged [86]. These animal models have used different immunization protocols and sources of TSHR to induce the disease. Adenovirus vectors that contain TSHR cDNA, DNA vaccination, or cells that overexpress TSHR have been used as immunogens to induce EAGD with varying degrees of success. These animal models have provided an opportunity to understand the evolution of the disease as well as to test different therapeutic approaches.

The discovery of "preferred" cytokine secretion profiles from *in vitro* CD4 T-cell clones nearly two decades ago has led to a great deal of work on T-cell subset differentiation [87]. Generally, based on their ability to produce distinct cytokines, T cells can differentiate into two subsets called Th1 and Th2. Although more complicated, one can functionally categorize Th1 cells as those producing IL-12 and IFN-γ and supporting cell-mediated immune responses, while Th2 cells can be characterized as those producing IL4 and supporting antibody production. Modulation of immune responses where one type of response is enhanced at the expense of the other has had a significant impact on both onset of disease in animal models and our understanding of disease progression. For example, infection of susceptible BALB/c (H-2d) mice with the intracellular parasite *Leishmania major* induces predominantly a Th2-type T-cell response that leads to death, but the resistant B10.D2 (H-2d) strain of mice develops a Th1 response that can control parasite replication and result in its expulsion. Other examples of the protective or susceptible nature of Th1 or Th2 cytokine secretion profiles abound in the literature [87]. Even more interesting is our ability to skew the immune response artificially from a Th1 to a Th2 or vice versa, with life-and-death consequences for the experimental mice. For example, in BALB/c mice, expression of exogenous IL-12 (which skews the response to a Th1 response) can confer protection [88]. In fact, recombinant cytokines that can skew the immune response have been used to ameliorate experimental thyroiditis [89]. In these studies, it was shown that granulocyte-macrophage colony–stimulating factor, but not fms-like tyrosine kinase receptor 3-ligand, was able to skew the immune response toward the Th2 type and prevent development of thyroiditis. These studies provide intriguing glimpses into the possibility of immunomodulating diseases.

The animal models of GD have provided some interesting insights; however, a consensus as to the specific effects of skewing the response towards Th1 or Th2 on GD development or maintenance has not emerged. Studies have shown a dominance of Th1 immune responses in some models of GD [90–92]. Splenocytes from immunized mice secreted either spontaneously or after TSHR addition a Th1 cytokine IFN-γ, but not Th2 cytokine IL-4. In addition, injection of an adenovirus expressing TSHR and IL-4, and not TSHR and IL-12, inhibited the induction of EAGD. Th2 response-inducing adjuvants, alum, and pertussis toxin, but not a Th1 response-inducing adjuvant poly (I:C), suppressed the development of EAGD in BALB/c mice immunized with dendritic cells infected with an adenovirus encoding TSHR [93]. These studies suggested a Th1 response dominance in EAGD.

On the other hand, it is generally believed that GD is characterized by a Th2-dominant response [94]. Several reports have shown an increase in the frequency of EAGD when pertussis toxin and/or alum that skew the immune response towards the Th2 type were used in conjunction with the TSHR [95, 96]. Dogan et al. [97] showed production of IgG1 (Th2) and IgG2a (Th1) antibodies, and secretion of both IL-4 (Th2) and IFN-γ (Th1) cytokines, in TSHR-immunized BALB/c mice with EAGD. However, IFN-$\gamma^{-/-}$ mice, but not IL-4$^{-/-}$ mice, developed hyperthyroidism upon immunization with TSHR and demonstrated that the Th2 response was required for the development of EAGD. In another study [98], EAGD was induced in mice whose signal transducer and activator of transcription-4 (Stat-4) or Stat-6 genes were deleted. While 50% of wild-type BALB/c and Th1-impaired Stat-4(–/–) mice developed hyperthyroidism, none of the Th2-impaired Stat-6(–/–) mice became hyperthyroid. Further, Stat-4(–/–) mice demonstrated strong Th2-type responses such as the production of IL-4 and IgG1 anti-TSHR antibodies, and Stat-6(–/–) mice had a strong Th1 immune response characterized by IFN-γ production and IgG2a antibodies. Together, these observations suggest an important role for Th2-dominant responses. Intuitively, a strong role for Th2 would be consistent with the production of autoantibodies required for disease induction.

The differences seen in the different models of EAGD could be due to the differences in the strain of mice used, environmental factors, TSHR preparations used and route of immunization, and adjuvants used in different studies. Further studies are required to conclusively determine whether there is a dominance of a Th1 or a Th2 response or whether both are required, albeit at different stages of the pathogenesis of the disease. Once the role of specific cytokines is established, cytokine therapies can be tested before, during, and after disease onset to determine efficacy of the regimen to suppress the development of the disease or to treat it.

14.15
Conclusions

Our understanding of the role of autoantibodies in Graves' disease pathogenesis is limited to the assays, which we can use to measure or characterize the autoantibodies. The better the assays are, the more useful they will be in understanding the pathogenesis of GD as well as in predicting the efficacy of various therapeutic regimens. There is also a need to better understand the evolution of the antibody response, because it would be useful in evaluating anti-thyroid antibodies. For example, as alluded to with the discovery of heterogeneous or homologous epitopes, it would be most useful to determine progression towards generation of antibodies required for stimulation of the receptor and the specific epitopes on the TSHR with which they react. If one can determine these epitopes and then measure the amounts of specific antibodies against relevant epitopes and develop methods to modulate the immune response against specific epitopes, one can perhaps coax the immune system away from producing pathogenic antibodies. To this end, several animal models of experimental autoimmune Graves' disease have recently emerged. These models could be used to better understand the evolution and diversity requirements of autoantibodies in Graves' disease.

References

1 Weetman AP. Autoimmune *Autoimmunity* **2004**, 37(4), 337–340.

2 Tunbridge WM, Evered DC, Hall R, Appleton D, Brewis M, Clark F, Evans JG, Young E, Bird T and Smith PA. *Clin Endocrinol* (Oxf). **1977**, 7(6), 481–493.

3 Vanderpump MP, Tunbridge WM, French JM, Appleton D, Bates D, Clark F, Grimley Evans J, Hasan DM, Rodgers H, Tunbridge F, et al. *Clin Endocrinol* (Oxf). **1995**, 43(1), 55–68.

4 Huber G, Staub JJ, Meier C, Mitrache C, Guglielmetti M, Huber P and Braverman LE. *J. Clin. Endocrinol. Metab.* **2002**, 87, 3221–3226.

5 Knudsen N, Jorgensen T, Rasmussen S and Perrild H. *Clin Endocrinol.* **1999**, 51, 361–367.

6 Nordyke RA, Gilbert FI, Miyamoto LA and Fleury KA. *Arch Intern Med* **1993**, 153, 862–865.

7 Takamatsu J, Yoshida S, Yokazawa T, Hirai K, Kuma K, Ohsawa N and Hosoya T. *Thyroid* **1998**, 8, 1101–1105.

8 Smith BR, McLachlan SM and Furmaniak J. *Endocr. Rev.* **1988**, 9, 106–121.

9 McKenzie JM and Zakarija M. *J. Clin. Endocrinol. Metab.* **1989**, 69, 1093–1096.

10 McGregor AM. *Clin. Endocrinol. (Oxf).* **1990**, 33, 683–685.

11 Akkaraju S, Ho WY, Leong D, Canaan K, Davis MM, Goodnow CC. *Immunity* **1997**, 7(2), 255–271.

12 Akkaraju S, Canaan K, Goodnow CC. *J Exp Med.* **1997**, 186(12), 2005–2012.

13 Weetman AP, Yateman ME, Ealey PA, Black CM, Reimer CB, Williams RC Jr, Shine B and Marshall NJ. *J Clin Invest.* **1990**, 86(3), 723–727.

14 MacNeil S, Munro DS, Metcalfe R, Cotterell S, Ruban L, Davies R, Weetman AP. *J Endocrinol.* **1994**, 143(3), 527–540.

15 Bartels ED. *Heredity in Graves' disease.* Copenhagen, Enjnar Munksgaards Forlag **1941**.

16 Brix TH, Christensen K, Holm NV, Harvald B, Hegedus L *Clinical Endocrinol* **1998**, 48, 397–400.

17 Brix TH, Kyvik KO, Christensen K, Hegedus LJ. Clin Endocrinol Metab **2001**, 86, 930–934.

18 Tomer Y, Davies TF. The genetics of familial and non-familial hyperthyroid Graves' disease. In: Rapoport B, McLachlan SM (eds). *Graves' Disease: Pathogenesis and treatment.* Boston: Kluwer Academic Publishers, 19–41, **2000**.

19 Tomer Y, Davies TF. Genetic factors relating to the thyroid with emphasis on complex diseases. In: Waas JAH and Shalet SM (eds). *Oxford Textbook of Endocrinology and Diabetes.* Oxford: Oxford University Press, 351–366, **2002**.

20 Yanagawa T, Hidaka Y, Guimaraes V, Soliman M, DeGroot LJ. *J Clin Endocrinol Metab* **1995**, 80, 41–45.

21 Kotsa K, Watson PF and Weetman AP. *Clinical Endocrinology* **1997**, 46, 551–555.

22 Donner H, Rau H, Walfish PG, Walfish PG, Braun J, Siegmund T, Finke R, Herwig J, Usadel KH, Badenhoop K. *J Clin Endocrinol Metab* **1997**, 82, 143–146.

23 Yanagawa T, Taniyama M, Enomoto S, Gomi K, Maruyama H, Ban Y, Saruta T *Thyroid* **1997**, 7, 843–846.

24 Heward JM, Allahabadia A, Armitage M, Hattersley A, Dodson PM, MacLeod K, Carr-Smith J, Daykin J, Daly A, Sheppard MC, Holder RL, Barnett AH, Franklyn JA, Gough SC. *J Clin Endocrinol Metab* **1999**, 84, 2398–2401.

25 Vaidya B, Imrie H, Perros P, Young ET, Kelly WF, Carr D, Large DM, Toft AD, McCarthy MI, Kendall-Taylor P, Pearce SH. *Human Molecul Genet* **1999**, 8, 1195–1199.

26 Kouki T, Sawai Y, Gardine C, Fisfalen M-E, Alegre M-L, DeGroot LJ. *J Immunol* **2000**, 165, 6606–6611

27 Grumet FC, Payne RO, Konishi J, Kriss JP. *J Clin Endocrinol Metab* **1974**, 39, 1115

28 Farid NR, Stone E, Johnson G. *Clin Endocrinol* **1980**, 13, 535–544.

29 Mangklabruks A, Cox N, DeGroot LJ. *J Clin Endocrinol Metab* **1991**, 73, 236–244.

30 Yanagawa T, Mangklabruks A, Chang Y-B, Okamoto Y, Fisfalen M-E, Curran PG, DeGroot LJ. *J Clin Endocrinol Metab* **1993**, 76, 1569–1574.

31 Yanagawa T, Mangklabruks A, DeGroot LJ. *J Clin Endocrinol Metab* **1994**, 79, 227–229.

32 Chen Q-Y, Huang W, She J-X, Baxter F, Volpe R, MacLaren NK. *J Clin Endocrinol Metab* **1999**, 84, 3182–3186.

33 Weetman AP, McGregor AM. *Endocrine Rev* **1994**, 15, 788–830.

34 Ruwhof C and Drexhage IIA. *Thyroid* **2001**, 11, 427–436.

35 Weetman AP. *European Journal of Endocrinology* **2003**, 148, 1–9.

36 Prabhakar BS, Bahn RS, Smith TJ. *Endocrine Reviews* **2003**, 24(6), 802–835.

37 Notkins AL, Onodera T, Prabhakar BS. Virus-induced autoimmunity. *In Concepts in Viral Pathogenesis* ed, Notkins, AL and Oldstone, MBA. Springer-Verlag, 210–215, **1984**.

38 Gangi E, Kapatral V, El-Azami El-Idrissi M, Martinez O, Prabhakar BS. *Autoimmunity* **2004**, 37, 515–520.

39 McKenzie JM *Physiol Rev* **1968**, 48, 252–309

40 Rapoport B, Chazenbalk GD, Jaume JC, McLachlan SM. *Endocr Rev.* **1998**, 19(6), 673–716.

41 Pinchera A, Fenzi GF, Macchia E, Vitti P, Monzani F, Kohn LD. *Ann Endocrinol (Paris).* **1982**, 43(6), 520–533.

42 Feldt-Rasmussen U, Schleusener H, Carayon P. *Clin Endocrinol Metab.* **1994**, 78(1), 98–102.

43 Di Cerbo A, Di Paola R, Menzaghi C, De Filippis V, Tahara K, Corda D, Kohn LD. *J Clin Endocrinol Metab.* **1999**, 84(9), 3283–3292.

44 Kohn LD, Harii N. *Autoimmunity.* **2003**, 36(6–7), 331–337.

45 Cho BY. *J Korean Med Sci.* **2002**, 17(3), 293–301.

46 Kohn LD, Hoffman WH, Tombaccini D, Marcocci C, Shimojo N, Watanabe Y. *J Clin Endocrinol Metab.* **1997**, 82, 3998–4009.

47 Cundiff JG, Kaithamana S, Seetharamaiah GS, Baker JR, Prabhakar BS. *J Clin Endocrinol Metab.* **2001**, 86, 3998–4009.

48 Kohn LD, Giuliani C, Montani V, Napolitano G, Ohmori M, Ohta M, Saji M, Schuppert F, Shong M-H, Suzuki K, Taniguchi S-I, Yano K and Singer DS. Antireceptor Immunity. In Rayner D and Champion B (Eds): *Thyroid Immunity.* R. G. Landes Biomedical Publishers, Austin/Georgetown, Texas, 115–170, **1995**.

49 Kohn LD, Shimura H, Shimura Y, Hidaka A, Giuliani C, Napolitano G, Litwack G. *Vitam Horm.* **1995**, 50, 287–384.

50 Rapoport B, Chazenbalk GD, Jaume JC, McLachlan SM. *Endocr Rev.* **1998**, 19, 673–716.

51 Ferguson SSG, Zhang J, Barak LS and Caron MG. *Adv.Pharmacol.***1998**, 42, 420–424.

52 Kruupnick JG and Benovic JL. *Annu. Rev. Pharmacol. Toxicol.* **1998**, 38, 289–319.

53 Lefkowitz RJ. *J. Biol. Chem.* **1998**, 273, 18677–18680.

54 Segaloff DL and Ascoli M. *J. Biol. Chem.* **1981**, 256, 11420–11423.

55 Min K-S, Liu X, Fabritz J, Jaquette J, Abell AN and Ascoli M. *J. Biol. Chem.* **1998**, 273, 34911–34919.

56 Daaka Y, Luttrell LM, Ahn S, Della Rocca GJ, Ferguson SSG, Caron MG and Lefkowitz RJ. *J. Biol. Chem.* **1998**, 273, 685–688.

57 Nakamura K, Lazari MFM, Li S, Korgaonka C and Ascoli M. *Mol. Endocrinol.* **1999**, 13(8), 1295–1304.

58 Gagnon AW, Kallal L and Benovic JL. *J. Biol. Chem.* **1998**, 273, 6976–6982.

59 Riezman H, Woodman PG, van Meer G and Marsh M. *Cell.* **1997**, 91, 731–738.

60 Baratti-Elbaz C, Ghinea N, Lahuna O, Loosfelt H, Pichon C, Milgrom E. *Molecular Endocrinology* **1999**, 19, 1751–1765.

61 Singh SP, McDonald D, Hope TJ, Prabhakar BS. *Endocrinology.* **2004**, 145(2), 1003–1010.

62 Mayor S, Presley JF, Maxfield FR. *J Cell Biol* **1993**, 121, 1257–1269.

63 Mellman I. *Annu Rev Cell Dev Biol* **1996**, 12, 575–625.

64 Seetharamaiah GS, Dallas JS, Patibandla SA, Thotakura NR, Prabhakar BS. *J Immunol.* **1997**, 158(6), 2798–2804.

65 Tahara K, Ban T, Minegishi T, Kohn LD. *Biochem Biophys Res Commun.* **1991**, 179, 70–77.

66 Kim WB, Cho BY, Park HY, Lee HK, Kohn LD, Tahara K, Koh CS. *J Clin Endocrinol Metab.* **1996**, 81, 1758–1767.

67 Kim WB, Chung HK, Lee HK, Kohn LD, Tahara K, Cho BY. *J Clin Endocrinol Metab.* **1997**, 82, 1953–1959.

68 Kosugi S, Ban T, Akamizu T, Kohn LD. *Mol Endocrinol.* **1992**, 6, 168–180.

69 Kosugi S, Ban T, Kohn LD. *Mol Endocrinol.* **1993**, 7, 114–130.

70 Kosugi S, Ban T, Akamizu T. *J Biol Chem.* **1991**, 266, 19413–19418.

71 Kosugi S, Ban T, Akamizu T, Kohn LD. *Biochem Biophys Res Commun.* **1991**, 180,1118–1124.

72 Kohn LD, Kosugi S, Ban T, Saji M, Ikuyama S, Giuliani C, Hidaka A, Shimura H, Akamizu T, Tahara K, et al. *Int Rev Immunol.* **1992**, 9, 135–165.

73 Akamizu T, Inoue D, Kosugi S, Ban T, Kohn LD, Imura H, Mori T. *Endocr J.* **1993**, 40, 363–372.

74 Akamizu T, Inoue D, Kosugi S, Kohn LD, Mori T. *Thyroid.* **1994**, 4, 43–48

75 Chazenbalk GD, Pichurin P, Chen CR, Latrofa F, Johnstone AP, McLachlan SM, Rapoport B. *J Clin Invest.* **2002**, 110(2), 209–217.

76 Schwarz-Lauer L, Chazenbalk GD, Mclachlan SM, Ochi Y, Nagayama Y, Rapoport B. *Thyroid.* **2002**, 12(2), 115–120.

77 Costagliola S, Vassart G *Thyroid.* **2002**, 12(12), 1039–1041.

78 Kung AWC, Lau KS, Kohn LD. *J Clin Endocrinol Metab.* **2001**, 86, 3647–3653.

79 Kung AWC, Lau KS, Kohn LD. *Thyroid.* **2000**, 10, 909–917.

80 Tahara K, Ishikawa N, Yamamoto K, Hirai A, Ito K, Tamura Y, Yoshida S, Saito Y, Kohn LD. *Thyroid* **1997**, 7, 867–877.

81 Sugawa H, Akamizu T, Kosugi S, Ueda Y, Ohta C, Okuda J, Mori T. *Eur J Endocrinol.* **1995**, 133, 283–293.

82 Ueda Y, Sugawa H, Akamizu T, Okuda J, Ueda M, Kosugi S, Ohta C, Kihou Y, Mori T. *Eur J Endocrinol.* **1995**, 132, 62–68.

83 Ueda Y, Sugawa H, Akamizu T, Okuda J, Kiho Y, Mori T. *Thyroid* **1993**, 3, 111–117.

84 Ueda Y, Sugawa H, Akamizu T, Okuda J, Ueda M, Kosugi S, Ohta C, Kihou Y, Mori T. *Eur J Endocrinol.* **1995**, 132, 62–68.

85 Kim TY, Park YJ, Park DJ, Chung H-K, Kim WB, Kohn LD, Cho BY. *J Clin Endocrinol Metab.* **2003**, 88, 117–124.

86 Seetharamaiah GS. *Autoimmunity.* **2003**, 36(6–7), 381–387.

87 Mosmann TR, Sad S. *Immunol Today.* **1996**, 17(3), 138–146.

88 Gabaglia CR, Pedersen B, Hitt M, Burdin N, Sercarz EE, Graham FL, Gauldie J, Braciak TA. *J Immunol.* **1999**, 162(2), 753–760.

89 Vasu C, Holterman MJ, Prabhakar BS. *Autoimmunity.* **2003**, 36(6–7), 389–396.

90 Pichurin P, Yan XM, Farilla L, Guo J, Chazenbalk GD, Rapoport B, McLachlan SM. *Endocrinology.* **2001**, 142, 3530–3536.

91 Pichurin P, Pichurina O, Chazenbalk GD, Paras C, Chen CR, Rapoport B, McLachlan SM. *Endocrinology.* **2002**, 143, 1182–1189.

92 Nagayama Y, Mizuguchi H, Hayakawa T, Niwa M, McLachlan SM, Rapoport B. *J Immunol.* **2003**, 170, 3522–3527.

93 Kita-Furuyama M, Nagayama Y, Pichurin P, McLachlan SM, Rapoport B, Eguchi K. *Clin Exp Immunol.* **2003**, 131, 234–240.

94 Elson CJ, Barker RN. *Curr Opin Immunol.* **2000**, 12, 664–669.

95 Kita M, Ahmad L, Marians RC, Vlase H, Unger P, Graves PN, Davies TF. *Endocrinology.* **1999**, 140, 1392–1398.

96 Rao PV, Watson PF, Weetman AP, Carayanniotis G, Banga JP. *Endocrinology.* **2003**, 144, 260–266.

97 Dogan RN, Vasu C, Holterman MJ, Prabhakar BS. *J Immunol.* **2003**, 170(4), 2195–2204.

98 Land KJ, Moll JS, Kaplan MH, Seetharamaiah GS. *Endocrinology.* **2004**, 145(8), 3724–3730.

99 Nagayama Y, Wadsworth HL, Russo D, Chazenbalk GD, Rapoport B. *J Clin Invest.* **1991**, 88, 336–340.

100 Kosugi S, Ban T, Akamizu T, Kohn DL. *Biochem Biophys Res Commun.* **1992**, 189, 1754–1762.

15
Autoantibodies in Diabetes

Sarah M. Weenink and Michael R. Christie

15.1
Introduction

Type 1 diabetes mellitus is an organ-specific autoimmune disease characterized by a deficiency in endogenous insulin, the metabolic hormone responsible for maintaining blood glucose homeostasis. The World Health Organization estimates that more than five million individuals suffer from type 1 diabetes worldwide. Affected individuals develop acute hyperglycemia, exhibiting excessive levels of glucose in the blood stream, while the surrounding tissues of the body are starved of an energy source. Despite extensive research efforts, there is no known cure and treatment options have advanced little since 1922, when Banting and Best first demonstrated the ability to manage type 1 diabetes through regular administration of exogenous insulin [1]. Even with insulin treatment, diabetic complications are common and debilitating and include neuropathy, retinopathy, nephropathy, and increased risk of coronary disease, with a consequent decrease in life expectancy [2].

Type 1 diabetes arises as the result of autoreactive immune cell–mediated destruction of insulin-producing β-cells of the pancreas. Concordance rates for both mono- and dizygotic twins indicate susceptibility to be under complex polygenic control [3], with additional modulation by environmental factors, such as infections or diet [4, 5]. In common with other autoimmune diseases, the primary genetic risk factor for susceptibility to type 1 diabetes is the inheritance of certain MHC alleles, expressed in the form of heterodimeric proteins that present peptides derived from antigens to T cells [6, 7]. Thus, a strong risk association is established between type 1 diabetes and expression of HLA-DR3 and -DR4 alleles. In Caucasians affected by type 1 diabetes, 95% express HLA-DR3 and/or -DR4, compared with an occurrence of just 40–50% in unaffected subjects [8]. More precise characterization of HLA gene variants on the short arm of chromosome 6 has localized the primary genetic association of type 1 diabetes in Caucasian populations to be at the HLA-DQ locus, although there is likely to be an independent contribution from HLA-DR4 alleles. The alleles associated with the highest risk are HLA-DQ8 (*DQB1*0302*) and HLA-

Autoantibodies and Autoimmunity: Molecular Mechanisms in Health and Disease. Edited by K. Michael Pollard
Copyright © 2006 WILEY-VCH Verlag GmbH & Co. KGaA, Weinheim
ISBN: 3-527-31141-6

DQ2 (*DQB1*0201*) [9]. Protective MHC alleles also exist that safeguard an individual against type 1 diabetes. For example, individuals that express HLA-DQ6 (*DQA1*0102/DQB1*0602*) develop type 1 diabetes rarely, even in the presence of DQ8 or DQ2 [9]. Similarly, expression of either of the alleles *DRB1*0406* or *DRB1*0403* reduces the risk conferred by the DQ8 molecule [10, 11]. It is expected that these genes act by regulating the presentation of peptides derived from antigens involved in the diabetes process to effector or regulatory T cells.

A major feature of type 1 diabetes is the infiltration of lymphocytes into the pancreatic islets of Langerhans. This "insulitis" is usually associated with damage to or destruction of the insulin-producing beta cells within the islet. Our understanding of the mechanisms of beta-cell destruction is complicated by the wide variety of immune cells infiltrating the pancreatic islets. These include B lymphocytes, T cells of both CD4$^+$ and CD8$^+$ lineages, macrophages, and dendritic cells [12–14]. In order to unravel the etiology of type 1 diabetes, researchers have made substantial use of spontaneous and induced animal models, including the bio-breeding rat [15] the non-obese diabetic (NOD) mouse [16], and a streptozotocin-induced rodent model [17]. The most extensively studied of these is the NOD mouse, which has provided a valuable resource in which genetic and environmental backgrounds have been manipulated to examine their effects upon the development and progression of type 1 diabetes.

Studies with NOD mice have revealed that lymphocytic infiltration into the pancreatic islets occurs 2–4 months before the development of overt diabetes. Macrophages and dendritic cells are the earliest cell types to infiltrate the islets [12], and this early infiltration is followed by beta-cell damage that may occur directly through the actions of proinflammatory cytokines secreted by these cells [18, 19]. However, T lymphocytes have emerged as the predominant initiator and effector cells of diabetes. This is supported by the high frequency of these cells in the islet infiltrate at disease diagnosis [20]. Furthermore, splenic T cells from diabetic NOD mice induce disease upon transfer to neonatal or sublethally irradiated animals [21, 22]. Similarly, a human case report shows diabetes development following bone marrow transplantation from a diabetic to a non-diabetic individual [23]. Meanwhile, neonatal thymectomy, which impairs T-cell development, significantly reduces the incidence of insulitis and diabetes in NOD mice [24, 25], as does immunosuppressive treatment in humans [26]. Further experimental work has revealed that both CD4$^+$ and CD8$^+$ T-lymphocyte subsets are important to the disease process, but to different extents at distinct stages in its progression [27, 28]. CD8$^+$ T cells may inflict acute cytotoxic damage upon the β-cells, e.g., after recognition of peptides from specific islet-cell β-cell antigens associated with cell-surface class I MHC molecules. Class I MHC expression is upregulated in the inflamed islet in type 1 diabetes [29]. It is the CD8-positive T cells that have been reported as the predominant cell type infiltrating islets in human diabetes, consistent with a role for cytotoxic T cells in beta-cell damage [30]. Together, these studies implicate the T cell as a promising target of therapies aimed at halting autoimmunity to the pancreatic beta cell and, as a consequence, preventing diabetes progression in susceptible individuals.

Despite the prominent role of T cells in type 1 diabetes, it is widely accepted that the development of autoimmune diabetes involves the activation of both the cellular and humoral arms of the adaptive immune response, in that auto-antibodies reactive to islet-cell components are also detected in diabetes. Pancreatic islet-cell antibodies (ICAs) were first detected in the serum of diabetic patients using immunofluorescent techniques 30 years ago [31] and have proved invaluable for the diagnosis of the disease. Moreover, the ability to detect ICAs many years before the onset of overt disease permits the identification of pre-diabetic individuals as candidates for therapeutic intervention.

Whether circulating islet autoantibodies contribute to beta-cell destruction is uncertain. Despite early experiments suggesting that ICAs were capable of lysing islet β-cells [32], further evidence of a direct pathogenic role of antibodies secreted by B cells has not been forthcoming. Humoral reactivity coincides with onset of insulitis in NOD mice [33]. However, neither the initiation of anti-islet autoimmunity nor the subsequent destruction of the β-cells appears to be antibody-mediated, and, unlike T cells, B lymphocytes from a diabetic mouse are not capable of inducing disease in transfer experiments [21]. Furthermore, individuals lacking B cells may still develop type 1 diabetes [34]. Nevertheless, depletion of B lymphocytes early in disease progression in NOD mice delays, and in some animals prevents, subsequent development of disease [35–38]. B cells within islet lesions may provide an important source of antigen-presenting cells during the disease process [39]. Binding of antibodies to specific antigens facilitates their efficient internalization and also enhances their trafficking into the late endosomal compartments for processing. Here, the bound antibody may influence the ultimate T-cell response by altering proteolysis of the antigen [40–42]. Antibodies may enhance the presentation of epitopes by protecting them from proteolysis, facilitating their loading into the binding groove of class II MHC molecules, or reducing competition for MHC binding by suppressing the presentation of other epitopes [43]. Alternatively, the presentation of epitopes to T cells may be suppressed if high-affinity antibodies do not dissociate from the antigen to allow for processing [41, 43]. This modulation of antigen processing through the binding of antibodies has been postulated to play a role in the development of autoimmunity by enhancing the presentation of previously cryptic epitopes to an awaiting repertoire of self-reactive T cells.

Hence, while it is generally accepted that T cells are central to the autoimmune process in type 1 diabetes, the B cell does have a major influence on the development, maintenance, and specificity of the autoimmune response. Circulating antibodies are a readily accessible marker of an ongoing autoimmune response to pancreatic islets that may precede the clinical development of disease. Knowledge of both antibody and T-cell responses to islet antigens, and the relationships between these, is therefore critical for the development of strategies to predict and prevent type 1 diabetes. In this chapter, we review our current understanding of the components of pancreatic islets that are targeted by autoantibodies in type 1 diabetes and the relationship of the B-cell response to T-cell reactivity and disease development in type 1 diabetes.

15.2
Islet-cell Antigens

Autoantibody reactivity to islet-cell antigens was first detected as serum immunoreactivity to pancreatic islets on tissue sections by indirect immunofluorescence [31]. ICA detection subsequently became widely used to demonstrate the presence of islet autoantibodies in a high proportion of type 1 diabetic patients at the time of disease onset. Studies in non-diabetic relatives of patients have demonstrated the appearance of these antibodies many years before disease onset in at-risk individuals [44]. These observations established ICA as an important predictive marker for disease, particularly in first-degree relatives of diabetic patients, and initiated a search for the identity of the antibody targets in islet cells. Studies first by Pav et al. [45] and then by Palmer [46] showed that insulin itself is one potential target of autoantibodies in diabetes. The failure of insulin to completely block serum antibody reactivity to islets on tissue sections indicated the presence of other target islet-cell antigens. Baekkeskov et al. were able to specifically immunoprecipitate radio-labeled proteins of 64 kDa from extracts of isolated human islets with serum antibodies from a majority of diabetic patients at the time of diabetes onset [47]. These "64k-antibodies" were shown to appear years before clinical onset of disease in at-risk relatives [48], as is the case for ICA. Subsequent work has shown that there are at least three distinct protein targets, all of similar molecular weight, for 64k-antibodies: the enzyme glutamic acid decarboxylase (GAD) [49] and proteins of the tyrosine phosphatase family, IA-2 (otherwise known as ICA512) [50] and phogrin (or IA-2β) [51]. Hence, like many other autoimmune disorders, type 1 diabetes is associated with antibody reactivity to multiple antigens in the target tissue.

15.2.1
Insulin as an Autoantigen

It is well established that therapeutic injection of insulin into type 1 diabetic patients leads to the generation of insulin antibodies; in rare cases, such an immune response can lead to immunological insulin resistance. Type 1 diabetes is also associated with the appearance of insulin antibodies before clinical diagnosis and prior to initiation of insulin treatment [46]. Levels of antibodies detected after initiation of insulin treatment do not correlate with those detected at disease onset, so the response to the exogenous insulin is independent of the autoimmune response [52]. Insulin has also been shown to be a target of circulating natural autoantibodies that are generally of low affinity, often polyreactive, and that may play a role in immune regulation. Insulin can therefore be a target of immunity in a range of circumstances, and not all antibody responses are diabetes-associated.

Insulin autoantibodies (IAAs) are commonly detected in diabetic patients who are young at the time of clinical diagnosis and are less common in older patients [53]. The presence of IAAs in diabetes is positively associated with the ex-

pression of HLA-DR4 in the patients [54], providing a link with genes conferring susceptibility to disease. Insulin is also the only antigen that is reproducibly detected as a target of autoantibodies in the NOD mouse. Furthermore, in-
sulin-reactive CD4- and CD8-positive T cells have been isolated from pancreases
of NOD mice, and it has been estimated that T cells to insulin represent a major proportion of the islet-infiltrating T cell population [55]. T cells from diabetic
NOD mice reactive to insulin are capable of transferring diabetes to non-diabetic animals [56] and may therefore contribute to beta-cell destruction in the
animal model. These observations have established insulin as a major target of
the immune response in pre-diabetes.

Further evidence of a role for insulin in the pathogenesis of type 1 diabetes
has come from genetic studies that identify a major diabetes susceptibility locus
that maps to variable number of tandem repeats (VNTR) upstream of the insulin gene on chromosome 11 [57]. Short repeats (class I VNTR) predispose to
diabetes. Long and short VNTR are associated with differences in levels of insulin expression, short repeats being associated with higher insulin expression in
the pancreas but low expression in the thymus [58], a major site of T-cell "education" and immunological tolerance induction. It has been proposed that low
levels of thymic insulin expression associated with class I VNTR may lead to defective induction of immunological tolerance to insulin, thereby predisposing to
an autoimmune response.

Insulin is synthesized by the pancreatic beta cell as a single-chain precursor,
preproinsulin, comprised of the 86-amino-acid proinsulin and preceded by a 24-
residue signal sequence that is cleaved during translation as the protein is translocated into the lumen of the endoplasmic reticulum. Further proteolytic processing of proinsulin occurs within insulin secretory granules, where the hormone is
stored prior to exocytosis. This processing involves cleavage at dibasic amino acids
to yield mature insulin that is comprised of a 21-amino-acid A-chain connected by
intermolecular disulfide bonds to a 30-amino-acid B-chain (Fig. 15.1A). The C-
peptide that connects the A- and B-chains in proinsulin is excised and secreted together with insulin after stimulation of pancreatic beta cells.

Structural features required for IAA reactivity have been investigated by examining the ability of modified insulins, and insulins from other species, to block
autoantibody binding to native human insulin using sera from diabetic patients
or IAA-positive relatives of patients. Autoantibodies associated with diabetes can
bind proinsulin, but antibody reactivity specific to the prohormone is rare, indicating that disease-associated epitopes are exposed on both insulin and its precursor. Guinea pig and fish insulin, which differ substantially in amino acid sequence from the human protein between residues A8–A12 and B1–B3 showed
poor inhibition of IAA binding [59]. Human insulin substituted at position 13
of the A-chain also competed poorly. The studies implicate amino acids B1–B3
and A8–A13 as important for binding of diabetes-associated IAAs (Fig. 15.1A).
A different pattern of binding has been detected for low-affinity IAAs not associated with disease progression [60] that bind well to fish insulin but are dependent on amino acids B28–B30 for binding.

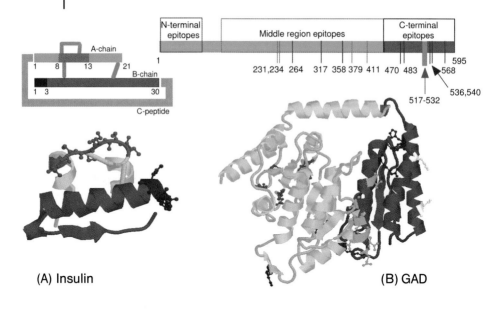

(A) Insulin

(B) GAD

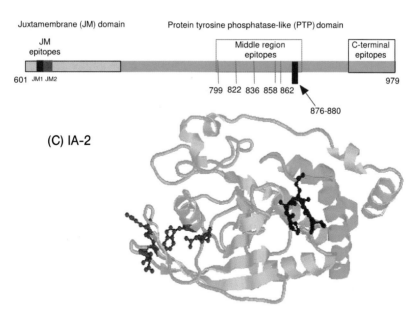

(C) IA-2

Fig. 15.1 Structural modeling of islet autoantigens in type 1 diabetes and localization of major autoantibody epitopes. Linear and three-dimensional representations of major islet-cell antigens and localization of regions important for autoantibody binding.
(A) Insulin is composed of an A-chain (turquoise) linked to a B-chain (purple) by disulfide bonds (orange) after proteolytic removal of a linking C-peptide (pale blue). Epitopes for diabetes-associated IAA are found within residues 8–13 of the A-chain (magenta) and 1–3 of the B-chain (brown).
(B) Three distinct regions for autoantibodies to GAD65 are at the N-terminus, middle, and ~C-terminus of the molecule. The struc-

15.2.2
Glutamic Acid Decarboxylase

Glutamic acid decarboxylase (GAD) was first detected as an autoantigen in stiff-person syndrome [61], a neurological disorder characterized by rigidity of the musculature often accompanied by muscle spasms. The syndrome is the result of impairment of inhibitory neuronal systems operating through the neuro-transmitter γ-amino butyric acid (GABA), and symptoms can be alleviated by drugs that enhance GABA-ergic neurotransmission. It was noted that a propor-tion of patients with stiff-person syndrome have other autoimmune disorders and that these patients have antibodies in both the serum and cerebrospinal fluid that are reactive on brain sections to regions rich in GABA-ergic neurons. The target antigen for these antibodies was shown to be the enzyme that cata-lyzes synthesis of GABA in these neurons, GAD [61].

Approximately 30% of patients with autoimmune stiff-person syndrome pro-gress to insulin-dependent diabetes [62]. As a consequence of this link between stiff-person syndrome and diabetes, it was noted that the molecular weight of GAD, approximately 64 kDa, was equivalent to that of the "64k-antigen" shown to be immunoprecipitated from islet extracts by antibodies in the majority of pa-tients with type 1 diabetes. These observations led to the demonstration that GAD is a major target of autoantibodies, not only in the rare neurological syn-drome but also, and more commonly, in the majority of patients with type 1 diabetes [49]. More recent reports have also implicated GAD as a target of anti-bodies in another neurological disorder, Batten disease [63].

GAD is expressed predominantly in the GABA-ergic neurons, but also in a number of peripheral tissues including the pancreatic islets, the oviduct, ovary, and testis; low levels of GAD enzyme activity have also been detected in liver and kidney [64]. The protein is expressed as two major isoforms, GAD65 and GAD67 (of 65 kDa and 67 kDa, respectively) that are the products of different genes; in humans, the gene for GAD65 is on chromosome 10 and that for GAD67 on chromosome 2 [65]. The two isoforms exhibit considerable sequence

ture shown in (B) represents the middle and C-terminus of GAD65 and has been modeled on the crystal structure of ornithine decar-boxylase [75]. Amino acids in the middle and C-terminal regions of GAD65 implicated in autoantibody binding have been identified with the aid of human monoclonal antibod-ies, and these are distributed throughout the molecule so that much of the GAD surface is recognized by antibodies.

(C) Autoantibody reactivity to IA-2 is con-fined to the cytoplasmic domain of the pro-tein (amino acids 601–979). Epitopes for diabetes-associated antibodies have been localized to the juxtamembrane domain (two linear epitopes, JM1 and JM2, in blue and red on the linear representation of the cytoplasmic domain) and the PTP domain. The three-dimensional structure of the PTP domain has been modeled [102], and the figure shows the position of epitopes in the middle region, identified as two clusters of amino acids (magenta and brown), and at the C-terminus (green), where participating amino acids have not been identified.

diversity over the first 100 amino acids at the amino terminus of the molecule but have approximately 75% sequence homology over the rest. There are two distinct functions for the biosynthesis of GABA. GAD has a metabolic role by allowing energy generation from glutamate through the GABA shunt; it also has a role in signaling through GABA receptors in the nervous system and in pancreatic islets. GABA is synthesized and stored in these tissues in synaptic-like vesicles and subsequently secreted. The existence of two isoforms of GAD may in part reflect these different functions. GAD67 is predominantly cytoplasmic and freely soluble, whereas GAD65 is hydrophobic and, in neuronal cells and pancreatic islets, the smaller GAD isoform associates with the cytoplasmic face of synaptic-like vesicle membranes where GABA is stored [66]. The nature of the membrane anchor for GAD65 is unclear, but palmitoylation of the molecule at cysteine residues at positions 30 and 45 of the molecule appears important for membrane association [67].

GAD65 is the predominant isoform recognized by antibodies in type 1 diabetes [68]. Thus, approximately 70% of type 1 diabetic patients have antibodies to the 65-kDa isoform but only 10–15% to GAD67. This contrasts with the situation in stiff-person syndrome, where the majority of autoimmune patients have antibodies to both GAD isoforms [69]. Much of the GAD67 antibody reactivity in diabetes may be adsorbed by addition of purified GAD65; hence, binding to the larger isoform by antibodies in a minority of patients is likely to be the consequence of common epitopes on the two proteins due to structural similarities.

Epitopes for GAD antibodies (GADA) have been investigated by analysis of antibody binding to deletion mutants and chimeric molecules constructed with different regions of GAD65 and GAD67. Studies with these chimeric molecules in type 1 diabetes have identified three regions of the GAD65 molecule that harbor distinct conformational epitopes for antibodies in type 1 diabetes (Fig. 15.1B). One of these is located towards the amino terminus of the molecule (amino acids 1–83), one in the middle of the molecule (96–444), and one towards the C-terminus (445–585) [69–71].

Further characterization of these GAD epitopes has been facilitated by the generation of a number of human monoclonal GADA, following Epstein-Barr virus transformation of B lymphocytes obtained from peripheral blood of patients with diabetes [72, 73]. Epitopes for these antibodies have been defined by analysis of binding to GAD65/GAD67 chimeric proteins and to single amino acid–substituted GAD65 [74]. Putative antibody contact residues have been mapped onto structural models of GAD65, generated using the crystal structure of ornithine decarboxylase as template [75, 76]. The results of these studies demonstrate a diverse range of epitopes, such that much of the protein surface of GAD65 is recognized by autoantibodies in diabetes. The localization of some of these epitopes is illustrated in Figure 15.1 B. These include conformational epitopes within the middle region of GAD65 with contributing amino acids from different parts of the middle region (residues marked in pink and brown on the blue chain in Fig. 15.1B) and epitopes in the C-terminal region localized on three alpha helices (green, brown, and gray on the purple chain in Fig. 15.1 B).

Competition studies have been performed with recombinant Fab fragments of some of these monoclonal antibodies to estimate the contribution of regions recognized by the monoclonal antibodies to total serum immunoreactivity [77]. A high proportion of antibody reactivity was competed by Fab fragments of monoclonal antibodies recognizing the middle region of the molecule, showing that these regions are commonly recognized in type 1 diabetes. Hence, a pattern is emerging of highly diverse immune reactivity to GAD65, with little evidence of an immunodominant region on the molecule.

There are further differences in the pattern of reactivity of GADA in stiff-person syndrome compared with those in type 1 diabetes. Titers of GADA are considerably higher in stiff-person syndrome than in type 1 diabetes [78]. Furthermore, there are three regions of the GAD65 molecule that are preferentially targeted by autoantibodies in stiff-person syndrome but rarely in type 1 diabetes [78–80]. These include a linear epitope between amino acids 1 and 16 at the amino terminus of the molecule and two conformational epitopes between residues 188 and 442 and 442 and 563. Analysis of epitope specificity may therefore be useful in distinguishing immune responses to antigens common to different autoimmune disorders.

15.2.3
IA-2 (ICA512) and Phogrin (IA-2β)

Following the identification of GAD as a major 64-kDa protein target for antibodies in type 1 diabetes, other evidence demonstrated the existence of distinct proteins of very similar molecular weight that are also recognized by antibodies associated with the disease [81]. Antibodies to these proteins may even be more closely linked to diabetes development than those to GAD itself. The proteins have been identified as two related proteins of the protein-tyrosine phosphatase family, termed IA-2 (or ICA512) and phogrin (or IA-2β), that are products of two distinct genes on human chromosomes 2 and 7, respectively [50, 51]. These genes encode protein precursors of 105 kDa and 110 kDa that are subsequently glycosylated and subject to post-translational processing to generate mature proteins of approximately 64 kDa [82–84]. Both proteins are expressed by a number of neuroendocrine tissues, including regions of the brain, pituitary, and pancreatic islets and, within these tissues, are localized to secretory granules where they are anchored by a single transmembrane domain [83, 84]. Both IA-2 and phogrin have a single tyrosine phosphatase–like domain within the cytoplasmic region of the proteins, but both lack enzyme activity as a result of substitutions at key amino acids that are highly conserved in other active tyrosine phosphatases [85, 86]. The two proteins are highly homologous (>80% sequence similarity) within the cytoplasmic region of the molecule, particularly within the PTP domain, but are more diverse (approximately 50% similarity) in the region localized within the secretory granule lumen. The functions of IA-2 and phogrin in neuroendocrine tissues are not fully defined, but both proteins are found associated with the cytoskeleton, where they may play a role in granule-cytoskeletal interactions in secretory granule storage or exocytosis [87–90]. There are differences, however, in the timing of expression of IA-2 and phogrin, since the latter is expressed in the developing pancreas very early in fetal development, while IA-2 is not detectable until shortly after birth [91, 92]. The timing of IA-2 expression, concomitant with maturation in insulin secretory responses of pancreatic islets to glucose in early life, provides additional evidence for a role of the protein in hormone secretion [93]. The late expression of IA-2 in development may also have implications for the autoimmune response [92], since late fetal and early neonatal life is a critical period in induction of immunological self-tolerance.

The intralumenal domains of IA-2 and phogrin are transiently exposed on the cell surface of islet cells and other neuroendocrine tissues during exocytosis [94]. However, all of the autoantibody reactivity in diabetes is directed to the cytoplasmic regions of the molecules; thus, antibodies cannot normally bind these molecules on the intact beta cell [50]. Of the two proteins, IA-2 is the dominant antibody target, while antibody reactivity to phogrin is likely to be the consequence of cross-reactive epitopes located on the two structurally similar proteins [95]. Analysis of antibody binding to IA-2 deletion mutants and IA-2/phogrin chimeric molecules has identified three distinct regions of antibody reactivity (Fig. 15.1 C): a region within the juxtamembrane domain that contains two non-overlapping linear epitopes, JM1 (amino acids 611–620, blue in Fig. 15.1 C) and JM2 (residues 621–630, red in Fig. 15.1 C) [96]; a region within the central portion of the PTP domain (amino acids 795–889, boxed magenta in Fig. 15.1 C) encompassing conformational epitopes [97–99]; and a region at the C-terminus of the IA-2 molecule (931–979, green in Fig. 15.1 C) [100]. Epitopes that are common to IA-2 and phogrin are located within the middle and C-terminus of the cytoplasmic domain [95].

As is the case for GAD, the availability of human monoclonal autoantibodies from diabetic patients and structural modeling of the IA-2 PTP domain based on crystal structures of other PTPs have assisted the definition of major disease-associated antibody epitopes. A number of human monoclonal antibodies have been obtained by Epstein-Barr virus transformation of B lymphocytes from type 1 diabetic patients, and these bind epitopes within the juxtamembrane and PTP domains of the IA-2 molecule [101]. One of these monoclonal antibodies, termed 96/3, was shown to effectively compete for IA-2 binding with serum antibodies from a majority of patients with type 1 diabetes, and this antibody binds to an epitope within a region (amino acids 795–889) that is frequently targeted by antibodies in type 1 diabetes. Peptide phage display and molecular modeling have identified potential 96/3 antibody contact residues at positions 799, 836, and 858 within the PTP domain of IA-2, and substitution of each of these amino acids was found to inhibit binding of IA-2 antibodies (IA-2A) in sera from type 1 diabetic patients [102]. Substitution of amino acids 822 and 862 also inhibits binding. Fab fragments of 96/3 antibodies also block antibody binding in a majority of patients, in some cases by close to 100% (S. Weenink, unpublished observations). The region of the IA-2 PTP domain recognized by the 96/3 monoclonal antibody therefore contains dominant epitopes for IA-2A in type 1 diabetes. A distinct middle region epitope (marked in brown in Fig. 15.1 C) lies between amino acids 876 and 880 [97].

15.2.4
Other Target Antigens

Antibodies to insulin, GAD65 and IA-2 are well established as distinct and important markers for diabetes diagnosis and prediction and the latter two antigens contribute to ICA reactivity on frozen sections of pancreas [103]. However it is clear that diabetic patients have increased immune reactivity to several other components of pancreatic islets, including proteins and glycolipids (Table 15.1). There is evidence that the sialo-ganglioside GM2-1 may represent a major component of ICA [104] and that antibodies to the glycolipid are associated with progression to diabetes in relatives with ICA. Sulfatides have also been shown to be reactive with antibodies in a high proportion of diabetic patients at disease onset [105]. Other protein antigens, such as ICA69 [106] and Glima 38 [107], have shown some promise as predictive markers for diabetes, but difficulties in establishing reproducible assays for these antibodies have prevented their widespread use in large-scale screening studies. Some antibodies, such as those to Glima 38, may be strongly associated with other established antibody markers, such as IA-2A [108]. It seems likely that, as a consequence of islet damage and antigen release in an inflamed islet, there is increased immune reactivity to a wide range of pancreatic islet components. Some of these immune responses are detected at low frequency in the diabetic population, their target antigens may be widely expressed in tissues, and antibodies may be detected in autoimmune diseases other than diabetes [109, 110]. There is currently little evidence that detection of autoantibodies to antigens other than insulin, GAD, and IA-2 adds significantly to diabetes prediction.

Antibodies that are reactive to heat shock proteins have also been detected in type 1 diabetes [111]. Since heat shock proteins are ubiquitous, it may seem surprising that immune reactivity to heat shock protein should be found in an organ-specific autoimmune disease such as diabetes. Increased T-cell reactivity is also a feature of the NOD mouse [112, 113], and immune responses to heat shock proteins have also been associated with other autoimmune disorders, in-

Table 15.1 Targets for islet-cell autoantibodies in type 1 diabetes.

Antigen	Ref.	Antigen	Ref.
Insulin	46	Glima-38	107
GAD65	49	Ganglioside GM2-1	104
GAD67	68	Sulfatide	105
IA-2 (ICA512)	50	ICA69	106
Phogrin (IA-2b)	51	Heat shock protein	111

cluding rheumatoid arthritis and systemic lupus erythematosus [114]. In some experimental diseases, T cells to heat shock proteins may be pathogenic, but there is considerable evidence that immunity to hsp60 is part of normal immunoregulation [114]. Heat shock proteins are upregulated in inflamed tissues, and the immune system may exploit this as a "danger signal" for the recruitment and regulation of inflammatory cells [115]. Immune regulation may be mediated by the secretion of cytokines that downregulate pathogenic responses; in the case of type 1 diabetes, such bystander suppression could be mediated by Th2 cytokines, IL-4, IL-10, or TGF-*β*. Detection of antibody or T-cell reactivity to heat shock protein may therefore provide a general indication of an ongoing inflammatory response [116] and may explain the association of immune responses to these antigens in a number of chronic autoimmune disorders. If these responses do turn out to participate in immune regulation, then there may be the potential to exploit this as a general therapy for autoimmune disease, and trials of heat shock protein peptide therapy have already been initiated in diabetes [117].

15.3
Islet Autoantibodies and the Prediction of Type 1 Diabetes

15.3.1
Antibody Detection and Standardization

Characterization of serum autoantibodies to the major islet-cell antigens associated with type 1 diabetes has shown that these are of high affinity, but of low capacity, and frequently recognize epitopes that are highly dependent on the native conformation of the molecule. Thus, islet autoantibodies in diabetes tend not to bind antigen on Western blots or fixed tissue sections where antigen conformation is disrupted by ionic detergents or chemical cross-linking [49]. This is in contrast to the situation in stiff-person syndrome, where autoantibodies readily bind GAD on Western blots and epitope characterization has identified major linear epitopes on the molecule. The characteristics of autoantibodies in diabetes place limitations on the type of assays that can be used for autoantibody detection. Procedures where antigen is directly bound to a solid phase, as in a direct ELISA, invariably perform poorly [118]. This is probably the result of conformational changes in the protein on binding to the solid phase, steric hindrance of antibody binding to plate-bound antigen, and low signal relative to background binding as a consequence of low antibody concentration in the test sample. In the research setting, the most successful assays for islet autoantibodies have been radioligand-binding assays, where antigen is synthesized by transcription and translation of specific cDNA *in vitro* in the presence of radiolabeled amino acids and then is incubated in the presence of serum antibodies in liquid phase [118]. Radiolabeled antigen bound to autoantibody is recovered by immunoprecipitation with protein A-Sepharose and quantified by scintillation counting. Such assays for antibodies to GAD and IA-2 have been successfully established in many laboratories worldwide, and reference standards have been made available through the World Health Organization to allow quantification of antibody levels in units that are comparable between laboratories. Diabetes antibody proficiency programs have shown good concordance between participating laboratories in GAD and IA-2 antibody assay performance [119].

The preferred method for detection of IAAs has been by radioimmunoassay using ^{125}I-labeled insulin and separation of antibody-bound antigen with polyethylene glycol or activated charcoal. These procedures have often used long incubation times and relatively large volumes of serum for antibody detection. More recently, IAA microassays using protein A precipitation have been introduced [120], but the performance of these in standardization programs has been poor relative to those for GADA and IA-2A [119]. This may be because insulin is a small molecule that has few epitopes for antibodies and requires radioiodination to generate protein of high enough specific radioactivity for detection; addition of a large iodine group to the molecule may to some extent impair antibody binding. Thus, although insulin has long been recognized as a major target for antibodies, the reliability of procedures for IAA detection lags behind those for GADA and IA-2A.

15.3.2
Development of Islet Autoantibodies in Early Life

A number of large-scale prospective studies have been established with the intention of following the natural history of autoantibody responses to islet-cell autoantigens in early life. These studies have also tried to identify factors important for the initiation of islet autoimmunity and to estimate the risk for later development of diabetes of individuals in whom islet autoantibodies are detected. Three major studies are established. The BABYDIAB Study [121] was started in 1989 and is a multi-center study in Germany following offspring of diabetic parents from birth. In the US, the Diabetes Autoimmunity Study in the Young (DAISY) based in Denver [122] has, since 1993, followed young (<4 years), first-degree relatives of diabetic patients, as well as children with no family history of diabetes, who were identified at birth as having high- or moderate-risk diabetes-susceptibility HLA-DQ genotypes. Thirdly, the Type 1 Diabetes Prediction and Prevention (DIPP) study follows children in the general population in Finland (a country with high diabetes incidence) who have high- and moderate-risk HLA-DQ alleles [123]. The results of each of these studies provide important information about the initiation of autoimmune responses to islet autoantigens in early life in both families with a history of type 1 diabetes and members of the general population expressing diabetes-susceptibility HLA genes.

Although islet autoantibodies can be detected at birth, the majority of these are likely to be the result of transplacental transfer of antibodies from a diabetic mother and are not associated with later detection of islet autoantibodies in the children [124]. Initiation of islet autoimmunity in fetal life is apparently very

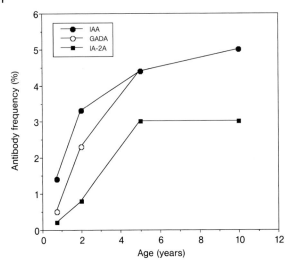

Fig. 15.2 Frequency of autoantibodies to islet-cell antigens in off-spring of diabetic parents followed from birth. The figure shows a graphical representation of islet autoantibodies from the BABYDIAB study. (Data from Hummel et al. [125]).

rare. Islet antibodies do start to appear in the first year of life and are commonly detected by the age of five years (Fig. 15.2); autoantibody frequency starts to plateau at around the age of 10 years [125]. Hence, immune responses to islet antigens are most commonly initiated in the first five years of life, and future screening programs for islet autoantibodies to identify individuals at risk of diabetes development would be best carried out at this time.

In all the prospective studies, IAAs are the most common marker in the first sample in which autoantibodies are detected [125, 126]. In approximately 40% of cases, the detection of a single islet autoantibody in a young child is accompanied or followed by the appearance of other islet autoantibody specificities. In individual patients, the sequential appearance of different antibodies over time periods of many months has been observed [121]. Progression to multiple antibody positivity is most common when the first antibody appears at an early age [125]. Antibodies may persist over time, but there can also be considerable changes in antibody levels, often with peak responses around the age of two years, and individuals may seroconvert from positive to negative over time [127]. Loss of autoantibodies is particularly common for IAA [126]. The results of these prospective studies show that islet autoimmunity can be initiated within the first 1–5 years of life and is often accompanied by spreading of autoimmune responses to other islet antigens, consistent with early destructive autoimmunity with release of islet antigens. However, these early autoimmune responses may be self-regulated, such that antibody levels decline over time.

In addition to the intermolecular spreading of autoimmunity to islet antigens described above, changes in the specificity of the immune response to epitopes on individual antigens are found following the first detection of islet autoimmunity. In the case of GAD, early autoantibody responses are directed predominantly to epitopes in the middle region of the molecule (amino acids 96–444) [71]. Subsequent spreading of antibody reactivity to epitopes in other parts of the molecule is common and is most frequently directed to those in the amino terminal region. IA-2A in early life are often reactive to one of two epitopes in the juxtamembrane domain of the molecule (JM1 and JM2 in Fig. 15.1 C); the specific epitope recognized is dependent on HLA-DR or -DQ genes expressed [96, 97]. Antibodies subsequently develop to epitopes in the PTP domain and include those that are cross-reactive with the closely related phogrin. Antibody reactivity to juxtamembrane epitopes can decline or disappear over time, such that in the established IA-2 response, PTP domain–reactive antibodies predominate [97].

15.3.3
Distribution of Antibodies in Diabetic Patients at Time of Disease Diagnosis

By the time of disease onset, the majority (>90%) of patients with type 1 diabetes possess serum antibodies to at least one of the major islet-cell antigens in type 1 diabetes—GAD65, IA-2, or insulin [128]. The precise specificity of antibodies present in the serum of individual patients is dependent on both the age of the patient and the HLA genes expressed by the individual (Fig. 15.3). The frequency of IAA and IA-2A at the time of diabetes onset is highest among individuals who develop the disease at an early age and is less frequent in older patients [128]. IAAs show a particularly strong negative association with age. Since prospective studies have shown that some islet autoantibodies, particularly IAAs, can decrease in titer to undetectable levels over time [126], the absence of these at the time of disease onset does not necessarily imply a lack of an immune response to that antigen in the pre-diabetic period. In contrast to IAA and IA-2A, GADA are present at moderate to high frequency in young patients, but antibody levels are highest in older patients. GADA have a greater tendency to persist than do antibodies to other islet antigens. GADA have been shown to be still present many years after diabetes onset, despite loss of beta-cell function and the disappearance of other antibody markers [129].

The distribution of IAA, GADA, and IA-2A in representative populations of young and older patients with recent-onset type 1 diabetes is shown in Figure 15.3 (top panels). More than 85% of young (<10 years at onset) diabetic patients possess antibodies to multiple islet-cell antigens, but this frequency decreases in older patients as a consequence of the lower prevalence of IAA and IA-2A.

The presence of autoantibodies to insulin and IA-2, at diabetes onset or in the pre-diabetic period, is associated with the expression of HLA-DR4 or associated DQ alleles (Fig. 15.3, bottom panels) [54, 130]. There are reports that GADA are also associated with the expression of high-diabetes-risk HLA haplo-

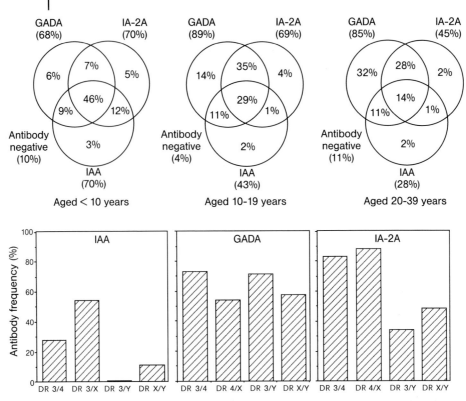

Fig. 15.3 Frequency of autoantibodies at time of onset of type 1 diabetes and influence of age and HLA. Upper panels: Age associations of islet autoantibodies are shown as Venn diagrams, with proportions of diabetic patients within each age group positive for antibodies or antibody combinations given within the circles. Lower panels: frequency of antibodies at time of diabetes onset according to HLA type of patients. (Data are from the Belgian Diabetes registry (I. Weets and F. Gorus, unpublished), modified from Gorus et al. [128]).

types [131], and frequencies are highest in patients with HLA-DR3 (Fig. 15.3), although such an association is not always observed. Since the HLA-DR and -DQ genes encode gene products that participate in immune function by presentation of antigenic peptides to T cells, which regulate antibody production, a link between HLA expression and islet autoantibodies might be expected. However, our understanding of the role of the HLA in the presentation of specific fragments of islet antigens to T cells in type 1 diabetes is at present very limited (see below), and there have been few studies showing a direct correlation between T-cell and antibody responses to specific islet antigens. Interpretation of the HLA data is complicated by the observation that individuals with high-risk HLA alleles, including DR4, have evidence of a more rapid progression to clinical diabetes [132]. The association of HLA-DR4 with IAA and IA-2A may therefore be secondary to more aggressive beta-cell destruction, and consequent antigen release, in DR4-positive individuals.

In addition to the high frequency of islet autoantibodies in type 1 (insulin-dependent) diabetes, it has become apparent that these antibodies are found in a significant proportion of older individuals who are diagnosed as type 2 diabetic and are not initially dependent on insulin treatment. In a study of >3500 patients aged between 25 and 65 years diagnosed with type 2 diabetes, ICA was present in 6% and GADA in 10%, 4% had both markers [133]. IA-2A are also detected, but the frequency is lower (<3%) than for GAD antibodies or ICA. The frequency of autoantibodies was highest in younger type 2 diabetic patients [133]. Although initially treated with oral hyperglycemic agents for months or years, the majority of type 2 diabetic patients with islet autoantibodies eventually become insulin-dependent; more than 80% of patients with both ICA and GADA require insulin treatment within six years of diabetes diagnosis, and IA-2A are a particularly strong marker for insulin dependency. It is suggested that these patients have a slowly progressing form of autoimmune diabetes, called latent autoimmune diabetes in adults (LADA). Detection of islet antibodies may be valuable for the early identification of patients who are diagnosed as type 2 diabetic but who will eventually require insulin treatment.

15.3.4
Islet Autoantibodies and Diabetes Prediction

Subjects participating in prospective studies of islet autoimmunity early in life (e.g., BABYDIAB, DAISY, DIPP) have also been followed for subsequent development of diabetes, and these studies provide an indication of the value of autoantibodies as markers for diabetes development. The vast majority of subjects who developed diabetes at an early age in these studies possessed multiple islet autoantibodies months or years before disease onset [121, 126]. The cumulative risk of developing diabetes within five years of developing one or more islet autoantibodies was estimated to be between 40% and 50% for individuals with multiple antibodies, but only 3% for those positive for only a single antibody specificity (IAA, GADA, or IA-2A).

In these prospective studies of autoimmunity in early childhood, follow-up to disease is necessarily restricted to a narrow time window in the first few years of life, but the vast majority of patients who develop diabetes will do so at an older age. Calculations of disease risk for antibody positivity may be underestimated if based only on observations in these young subjects. Family studies where siblings, parents, and offspring of diabetic patients are screened for islet autoantibodies at older ages, and are subsequently followed for some years for development of disease, can also provide important information on the value of markers in diabetes prediction. Statistical analysis of the data (with life tables) obtained from such studies may be used to obtain estimates of disease risk over the period of follow-up, and the proportion of individuals positive for markers in those who develop disease provides an indication of the sensitivity of a test.

Family studies were initially used to study disease progression in family members who were positive or negative for ICA. Although >80% of relatives who progressed to diabetes were positive for ICA, indicating high sensitivity for the test, a large proportion (around 60%) of relatives with these antibodies did not develop disease, even with long-term follow-up. Once specific target antigens for islet autoantibodies were identified, studies were performed to determine whether testing for these new markers in ICA-positive relatives could improve the specificity of diabetes prediction (studies 1 and 2 in Table 15.2). These showed that the presence of two or more antibody markers in addition to ICA indicated high risk (>80%) for progression to diabetes within 10 years [134, 135]. Subsequent analyses of IAA, GADA, and IA-2A in relatives without prior selection for ICA confirmed the high specificity of multiple islet autoantibodies for diabetes prediction [136–138], while maintaining high sensitivity for identifying pre-diabetic individuals (60–80% of pre-diabetic individuals positive for two or more antibody markers; studies 3–5 in Table 15.2). These studies also showed a more rapid progression to clinical diabetes in individuals positive for IA-2 antibodies compared with similar analyses for other islet antibodies, such that the five-year diabetes risk was particularly high for IA-2A (Table 15.2). The risk for other markers may increase to that for IA-2A with longer periods of follow-up.

Analysis of multiple islet autoantibodies provides a means to identify with some accuracy those relatives of diabetic patients most at risk of diabetes development. However, the vast majority of new cases of diabetes have no family history of disease, and thus strategies for diabetes prediction need to be developed for the general population. Since disease prevalence in the general population is

Table 15.2 Value of islet autoantibodies in diabetes prediction.[a]

| Marker | Five-year diabetes risk (%) | | | | | Sensitivity (%) | | | | |
| | Study | | | | | Study | | | | |
	1 [b]	2 [b]	3	4	5	1	2	3	4	5
IAA	25	28	59	29	12	61	67	76	25	63
GADA	18	56	52	39	19	67	83	90	69	70
IA-2A	76	65	81	55	59	50	83	64	69	70
One antibody	0	0	15	0 [c]	6 [c]	6	11	18	13	22
Two antibodies	0	17	44	26 [c]	23 [c]	17	44	28	66	41
Three antibodies	44	77	100	62 [c]	34 [c]	78	44	52	6	22

a) Estimated percentage of risk and sensitivity conferred by antibody markers in non-diabetic relatives of type 1 diabetes patients for development of diabetes within five years of detection. Values are from published studies as follows: study 1 [134]; study 2 [135]; study 3 [136]; study 4 [137]; study 5 [138].
b) Subjects were pre-selected for positivity for ICA.
c) ICA was included as an additional marker in estimates of risk of multiple antibodies.

considerably lower than that in relatives, very large numbers of individuals need to be followed for long periods of time if precise estimates of risk are to be obtained. Such studies have not yet been performed. Nevertheless, comparison of frequencies and levels of ICA, IAA, GADA, and IA-2A in non-diabetic and newly diagnosed diabetic schoolchildren from a region of the UK has provided estimates of risk that these markers confer for diabetes development in the general population [139]. Individually, risk for diabetes development for individuals with high titers of each of ICA, IA-2A, and GADA was estimated to be 20–24%, while detection of two or more of these markers increased risk to 71% with a sensitivity of 83%. In making these calculations, it was assumed that autoantibodies appear by the age of 10 years and are stable until development of disease. While such assumptions may not be entirely valid, the analysis does suggest that combinations of autoantibodies are able to predict diabetes with reasonable accuracy in the general population.

15.4
Relationship of Islet Autoantibodies to T-cell Responses in Type 1 Diabetes

The analysis of islet autoantibodies provides a means by which individuals may be identified at early stages of pancreatic autoimmunity and gives an indication of the risk of development of type 1 diabetes. T cells are likely to be more directly related to diabetes development than are antibodies, but it is unclear to what extent autoantibody secretion reflects a pathogenic T-cell response. Measures of disease-related T-cell responses in diabetes and an understanding of the relationships of these to autoantibodies are essential for further advances in our understanding of the etiology of type 1 diabetes and to provide an accurate assessment of autoimmune status. Indicators of T-cell autoimmunity will become particularly valuable for monitoring signs of disease recurrence following immune intervention and islet transplantation.

Analysis of T-cell reactivity in diabetes has proven to be an extremely complex task. Assessment of these responses requires that the lymphocyte population be isolated from the host individual and maintained in a viable state in culture while being stimulated with the antigen of interest. The outcome is then measured in some form of readout. The fundamental sensitivity of the T-cell population to external factors may result in disease-specific responses being distorted when attempts are made to assess them *in vitro*. Accordingly, the modulating effects on T-cell responses of nearly every facet of T-cell culture and assay continue to be hotly debated in international T-cell workshops. Factors likely to be important include the source and purity of antigen, serum supplements, culture medium, cell numbers and density in culture, the nature of the antigen-presenting cell (APC), the use of fresh versus cryopreserved cells, and the inclusion of response-potentiating factors [140–146]. Meaningful interpretation of T-cell responses in human diabetes has been hampered by a lack of appropriate controls. An added complication is that the T-cell population of most interest in type 1 diabetes resides in the pancreas, but this population is normally inaccessible. Any reliable method for measuring antigen-specific T-cell responses in diabetes must therefore have sufficient sensitivity to detect those islet-reactive T cells that migrate to the periphery, where they occur at extremely low frequencies, typically one in 10^5 cells [147, 148].

Initial studies to detect islet antigen–specific cells among the peripheral T-cell population from diabetic patients relied on the capacity of these cells to proliferate in response to exogenous antigen. Evidence of mitotic activity was typically provided by assessing changes in cellular DNA content through the incorporation of radiolabeled nucleotides [149]. Knowledge of autoantibody targets led to purified preparations of recombinant GAD65, insulin, and IA-2 (expressed in *E. coli*, yeast, or insect cells) being investigated as potential targets of pathogenic T cells. Increased proliferative responses to these autoantigens were detected in peripheral blood mononuclear cells (PBMC) isolated from type 1 diabetic patients [150–152]. Similarly high T-cell reactivity was detected in PBMC from relatives of diabetic patients identified as being at-risk for diabetes through possession of islet autoantibodies, but not from healthy, islet autoantibody–negative controls. A primary or dominant target of the T-cell response in type 1 diabetes was not identified among these candidates but, as with autoantibody reactivity, those most at risk of developing disease have T-cell autoreactivity to multiple autoantigens [153, 154].

Proliferation assays for T-cell responses to islet-cell antigens also suggested an inverse correlation with autoantibody levels [155, 156], leading to the suggestion that individuals who exhibit higher concentrations of antibodies might be expected to progress more slowly to clinical disease. Such observations have even thrown into question the use of islet autoantibodies as markers for predicting type 1 diabetes [157]. However, the reliability of T-cell response data obtained using recombinant autoantigen preparations, which are probably contaminated with highly antigenic bacterial proteins, has been questioned, and disease-associated responses to such preparations have not been reproduced in T-cell workshops [145, 158]. Furthermore, T-cell proliferation assays yield little information on the nature of the response to the antigen of interest, and results obtained may be clouded by effects of regulatory cells present in the culture [159]. As a result of these problems, the emphasis of T-cell studies has turned to the monitoring of specific cytokines secreted in response to peptide antigen stimulus.

Early assays to detect cytokine secretion by T cells relied upon ELISA of culture supernatants following the incubation of T cells with antigen and APC [160]. While being adequate for assessing strong responses that result from viral or bacterial challenges, these assays unfortunately lack the sensitivity required to detect the activity of rarer autoantigen-specific T cells. Instead, the enzyme-linked immunospot assay (ELISPOT) has become the method of choice for analyzing autoreactive T-cell responses in diabetes. This technique represents a significant advance on standard ELISA methodology in that cytokine production is assessed at the single-cell level and is able to provide an estimate of frequency of individual T cells secreting a specific cytokine in response to antigen or peptide [161]. ELISPOT is currently sensitive to a level of one in 10^5–10^6 cells [162–164]. The assay involves the capture of cytokine directly onto the surface of an antibody-coated microtiter plate as it is secreted. Further treatment with a combination of anti-cytokine antibodies and detection reagents then allows individual cells secreting cytokine to be visualized in the form of spots on the plate, where the size and intensity are proportional to the amount of cytokine secreted per cell.

A number of strategies have been employed to identify the immunodominant T-cell epitopes within the known type 1 diabetes autoantigens for use in these assays. These include the screening of naturally processed peptides eluted from type 1 diabetes–associated HLA [165–168] or synthetic peptides spanning an autoantigen [152, 169–171] for their ability to stimulate responses in either T-cell lines generated against purified antigen or peripheral blood lymphocytes isolated from type 1 diabetes subjects. Using such approaches, T-cell responses have been identified in type 1 diabetes that target the (pro)insulin residues B9–23, B11–C24, B20–C4, C18–A1, C28–A21, and C35–50 [172–174]. For GAD65, a number of T-cell epitopes have been identified spanning residues 115–130, 206–220, 247–285, 481–495, and 555–570 [165, 166, 168–171]. Meanwhile, multiple independent studies have identified a focus of T-cell reactivity to IA-2 against two central regions of the PTP domain, residues 787–817 and 831–869 [152, 167, 175, 176].

Comparison of these T-cell determinants with previously identified autoantibody epitopes (Fig. 15.1) suggests that these may frequently overlap, raising the question as to whether T- and B-cell responses at the epitope level are related [102, 177]. Antigen-specific B cells and the soluble antibodies that they secrete are able to play a major role in shaping T-cell responses through their ability to act as highly efficient APCs [178]. Examples of both B cell–mediated enhancement and suppression of T-cell epitopes in type 1 diabetes have been reported. In one study, stimulation of a T-cell hybridoma recognizing the GAD 274–286 epitope was greatly enhanced when the APCs were exposed to GAD65 protein complexed with anti-GAD serum antibodies, rather than the recombinant antigen alone [179]. In another study, GAD65-specific B cells were able to enhance the processing and presentation of T-cell determinants when they resided outside the antibody epitope region, but any overlap between the antibody and T-cell epitopes led to a dominant suppression of antigen presentation [177]. The possible suppression of diabetogenic T-cell responses by autoantibodies has led to the suggestion that recombinant Fabs may represent a novel tool by which to modulate the disease process [77].

When T-cell responses were determined against proinsulin peptides in antibody-positive, first-degree relatives of type 1 diabetes patients, a significant positive correlation was seen between insulin autoantibody levels and the T-cell response [154]. Further refinement of these experiments revealed that T cells from individuals with increased levels of IAAs prior to the onset of clinical disease characteristically secreted cytokines of a Th2 or regulatory (Tr) phenotype (IL-4, IL-5, and/or IL-10) in response to synthetic proinsulin peptides [180–182]. By contrast, T cells from individuals already undergoing insulin therapy for type 1 diabetes, and therefore responding to exogenous injected insulin, exhibited increased production of the Th1 cytokine IFN-γ [181]. Recent results from our own laboratory also reveal a positive association between T-cell responses to peptides representing residues 831–860 of IA-2 and autoantibodies to the 96/3 epitope region of the molecule (residues 795–889 of the IA-2 PTP; Fig. 15.1) that overlaps this region (S. Weenink, unpublished observations). Diabetic patients with higher levels of autoantibodies to the 96/3 epitope region were found by ELISPOT to have increased frequency of T cells secreting IL-10 in response to synthetic peptides spanning the 831–860 region.

Together, these observations challenge the belief that proinflammatory Th1 cytokine responses (IFN-γ) exclusively drive disease progression in type 1 diabetes, while anti-inflammatory Th2 responses (IL-4, IL-10) offer protection [183]. Instead, the Th2 predominance of T-cell reactivity that is associated with the presence of antibodies strongly linked with diabetes progression suggests that elevated Th2 or regulatory responses continue in the presence of destructive autoimmunity. Similar observations of an early Th2-type response have been reported in pre-diabetic NOD mice and in T cells that protect against diabetes isolated from islet infiltrates from diabetic mice [184, 185]. Such a Th2 environment would account for the activation of the humoral immune response (autoantibody production). However, the critical factor that tips the balance into a Th1 state towards destructive insulitis and overt disease remains unknown.

15.5
Conclusions

Diabetes susceptibility genes, T-cell responses to islet antigens, and the detection of autoantibodies all provide important information on the risk of an individual developing diabetes. While susceptibility genes are still common in the non-diabetic population and analysis of T-cell responses has proved technically difficult, characterization of autoantibodies and their specific targets is now sufficiently advanced to predict type 1 diabetes with reasonable accuracy. Furthermore, associations between autoantibody and T-cell responses are emerging, and we are starting to understand the relationship between autoantibody detection and the underlying T-cell response. Further knowledge of these T-cell responses in diabetes, and the manner in which they are regulated, is now essential for the development of strategies for immune intervention, such that progress in the autoantibody field can be put to practical use to prevent diabetes in those at risk.

Acknowledgments

We thank Dr. Steinunn Baekkeskov for coordinates of a model of the molecular structure of the middle and C-terminal domains of glutamate decarboxylase and Dr. Günther Peters for coordinates of a model for the PTP domain of IA-2. We are grateful to Dr. Frans Gorus for providing data on the frequency of autoantibodies at time of diabetes from the Belgian Diabetes Registry. Studies from our own laboratory were funded by Diabetes UK, the Wellcome Trust, and the European Union.

References

1 F.G. Banting, C.H. Best, and J.J.R. Macleod, *Am J Physiol*, **1922**. 59, 479.

2 K.L. Bate and G. Jerums, *Med J Aust*, **2003**. 179, 498–503.

3 J.I. Rotter and E.M. Landaw, *Clin. Genet.*, **1984**. 26, 529–542.

4 K. Helmke, A. Otten, W.R. Willems, R. Brockhaus, G. Mueller-Eckhardt, T. Stief, J. Bertrams, H. Wolf, and K. Federlin, *Diabetologia*, **1986**. 29, 30–33.

5 H.J. Bodansky, P.J. Grant, B.M. Dean, J. McNally, G.F. Bottazzo, M.H. Hambling, and J.K. Wales, *Lancet*, **1986**. 2, 1351–1353.

6 F. Pociot and M.F. Mcdermott, *Genes Immun*, **2002**. 3, 235–249.

7 E. Thorsby, *The Immunologist*, **1995**. 3, 51–58.

8 E. Wolf, K.M. Spencer, and A.G. Cudworth, *Diabetologia*, **1983**. 24, 224–230.

9 E. Thorsby and K.S. Rønningen, *Diabetologia*, **1993**. 36, 371–377.

10 D.E. Undlien, T. Friede, H.G. Rammensee, G. Joner, K. Dahl-Jørgensen, O. Søvik, H.E. Akselsen, I. Knutsen, K.S. Rønningen, and E. Thorsby, *Diabetes*, **1997**. 46, 143–149.

11 F. Cucca, R. Lampis, F. Frau, D. Macis, E. Angius, P. Masile, M. Chessa, P. Frongia, M. Silvetti, A. Cao, and et al., *Hum. Immunol.*, **1995**. 43, 301–308.

12 A. Jansen, F. Homo-Delarche, H. Hooijkaas, P.J. Leenen, M. Dardenne, and H.A. Drexhage, *Diabetes*, **1994**. 43, 667–675.

13 A. Miyazaki, T. Hanafusa, K. Yamada, J. Miyagawa, H. Fujino-Kurihara, H. Naka-jima, K. Nonaka, and S. Tarui, *Clin. Exp. Immunol.*, **1985**. 60, 622–630.

14 A. Signore, P. Pozzilli, E.A. Gale, D. Andreani, and P.C. Beverley, *Diabetologia*, **1989**. 32, 282–289.

15 A.F. Nakhooda, A.A. Like, C.I. Chappel, C.N. Wei, and E.B. Marliss, *Diabetologia*, **1978**. 14, 199–207.

16 S. Makino, K. Kunimoto, Y. Muraoka, Y. Mizushima, K. Katagiri, and Y. Tochino, *Jikken Dobutsu*, **1980**. 29, 1–13.

17 G.L. Wilson and E.H. Leiter, *Curr Top Microbiol Immunol*, **1990**. 156, 27–54.

18 A. Rabinovitch, W. Sumoski, R.V. Rajotte, and G.L. Warnock, *J. Clin. Endocrinol. Metab.*, **1990**. 71, 152–156.

19 C.A. Delaney, D. Pavlovic, A. Hoorens, D.G. Pipeleers, and D.L. Eizirik, *Endocrinology*, **1997**. 138, 2610–2614.

20 W. Gepts, *Diabetes*, **1965**. 14, 619–633.

21 A. Bendelac, C. Carnaud, C. Boitard, and J.F. Bach, *J Exp Med*, **1987**. 166, 823–832.

22 L.S. Wicker, B.J. Miller, and Y. Mullen, *Diabetes*, **1986**. 35, 855–860.

23 E.F. Lampeter, M. Homberg, K. Quabeck, U.W. Schaefer, P. Wernet, J. Bertrams, H. Grosse-Wilde, F.A. Gries, and H. Kolb, *Lancet*, **1993**. 341, 1243–1244.

24 S. Makino, Y. Harada, Y. Kishimoto, and Y. Hayashi, *Jikken Dobutsu*, **1986**. 35, 495–498.

25 M. Ogawa, T. Maruyama, T. Hasegawa, T. Kanaya, F. Kobayashi, Y. Tochino, and H. Uda, *Biomed. Res.*, **1985**. 6, 103–105.

26 P.F. Bougneres, J.C. Carel, L. Castano, C. Boitard, J.P. Gardin, P. Landais, J. Hors, M.J. Mihatsch, M. Paillard,

J. L. Chaussain, and Et Al., *N Engl J Med,* **1988.** 318, 663–670.

27 T. W. Kay, H. L. Chaplin, J. L. Parker, L. A. Stephens, and H. E. Thomas, *Res. Immunol.,* **1997.** 148, 320–327.

28 F. S. Wong and C. A. Janeway, Jr., *Res. Immunol.,* **1997.** 148, 327–332.

29 I. L. Campbell, G. H. Wong, J. W. Schrader, and L. C. Harrison, *Diabetes,* **1985.** 34, 1205–1209.

30 A. J. Jarpe, M. R. Hickman, J. T. Anderson, W. E. Winter, and A. B. Peck, *Reg Immunol,* **1990.** 3, 305–317.

31 G. Bottazzo, A. Florin Christensen, and D. Doniach, *Lancet,* **1974.** ii, 1279–1283.

32 M. J. Dobersen, J. E. Scharff, F. Ginsberg-Fellner, and A. L. Notkins, *N Engl J Med,* **1980.** 303, 1493–1498.

33 R. Tisch, X.-D. Yang, S. M. Singer, R. S. Liblau, L. Fugger, and H. O. Mcdevitt, *Nature,* **1993.** 366, 72–75.

34 S. Martin, D. Wolf-Eichbaum, G. Duinkerken, W. A. Scherbaum, H. Kolb, J. G. Noordzij, and B. O. Roep, *N Engl J Med,* **2001.** 345, 1036–1040.

35 D. V. Serreze, W. S. Gallichan, D. P. Snider, K. Croitoru, K. L. Rosenthal, E. H. Leiter, G. J. Christianson, M. E. Dudley, and D. C. Roopenian, *Diabetes,* **1996.** 45, 902–908.

36 F. S. Wong, I. Visintin, L. Wen, J. Granata, R. Flavell, and C. A. Janeway, *J. Exp. Med.,* **1998.** 187, 1985–1993.

37 H. Noorchashm, N. Noorchashm, J. Kern, S. Y. Rostami, C. F. Barker, and A. Naji, *Diabetes,* **1997.** 46, 941–946.

38 T. Akashi, S. Nagafuchi, K. Anzai, S. Kondo, D. Kitamura, S. Wakana, J. Ono, M. Kikuchi, Y. Niho, and T. Watanabe, *Int. Immunol.,* **1997.** 9, 1159–1164.

39 D. V. Serreze, S. A. Fleming, H. D. Chapman, S. D. Richard, E. H. Leiter, and R. M. Tisch, *J Immunol,* **1998.** 161, 3912–3918.

40 H. W. Davidson and C. Watts, *J Cell Biol,* **1989.** 109, 85–92.

41 C. Watts and A. Lanzavecchia, *J. Exp. Med.,* **1993,** 178, 1459–1463.

42 F. Manca, D. Fenoglio, A. Kunkl, C. Cambiaggi, M. Sasso, and F. Celada, *J Immunol,* **1988.** 140, 2893–2898.

43 P. D. Simitsek, D. G. Campbell, A. Lanzavecchia, N. Fairweather, and C. Watts, *J. Exp. Med.,* **1995,** 181, 1957–1963.

44 G. F. Bottazzo, B. M. Dean, A. N. Gorsuch, A. G. Cudworth, and D. Doniach, *Lancet,* **1980.** 1, 668–672.

45 J. Pav, Z. Jezkova, and F. Skrha, *Lancet,* **1963.** 2, 221–222.

46 J. Palmer, C. Asplin, P. Clemons, K. Lyen, O. Tapati, P. Raghu, and T. Pauquette, *Science,* **1982.** 222, 1337–1338.

47 S. Baekkeskov, J. H. Nielsen, B. Marner, T. Bilde, J. Ludvigsson, and Lernmark, *Nature,* **1982.** 298, 167–169.

48 L. M. Baekkeskov S, Kristensen J, Srikanta S, Bruining G, Mandrup-Poulsen T, De Beaufort C, Soeldner J, Eisenbarth G, Lindgren F, Sundquist G, Lernmark A, *J Clin Invest,* **1987.** 79, 926–934.

49 S. Baekkeskov, H. Aanstoot, S. Christgau, A. Reetz, M. Solimena, M. Cascalho, F. Folli, H. Richter-Olesen, P. De Camilli, *Nature,* **1990.** 347, 151–156.

50 M. A. Payton, C. J. Hawkes, and M. R. Christie, *J. Clin. Invest.,* **1995.** 96, 1506–1511.

51 C. J. Hawkes, C. Wasmeier, M. R. Christie, and J. C. Hutton, *Diabetes,* **1996.** 45, 1187–1192.

52 J. Karjalainen, M. Knip, A. Mustonen, and H. K. Akerblom, *Diabetologia,* **1988.** 31, 129–133.

53 P. Vardi, A. G. Ziegler, J. H. Mathews, S. Dib, R. J. Keller, A. T. Ricker, J. I. Wolfsdorf, R. D. Herskowitz, A. Rabizadeh, G. S. Eisenbarth, and J. S. Soeldner, *Diabetes Care,* **1988.** 11, 736–739.

54 A. G. Ziegler, E. Standl, E. Albert, and H. Mehnert, *Diabetes,* **1991.** 40, 1146–1149.

55 K. Haskins and D. Wegmann, *Diabetes,* **1996.** 45, 1299–1305.

56 D. Daniel, R. G. Gill, N. Schloot, and D. Wegmann, *Eur J Immunol,* **1995.** 25, 1056–1062.

57 D. E. Undlien, S. T. Bennett, J. A. Todd, H. E. Akselsen, I. Ikaheimo, H. Reijonen, M. Knip, E. Thorsby, and K. S. Ronningen, *Diabetes,* **1995.** 44, 620–625.

58 P. Vafiadis, S. T. Bennett, J. A. Todd, J. Nadeau, R. Grabs, C. G. Goodyer, S. Wickramasinghe, E. Colle, and C. Polychronakos, *Nat. Genet.,* **1997.** 15, 289–292.

59 L. Castano, A. G. Ziegler, R. Ziegler, S. Shoelson, and G. S. Eisenbarth, *Diabetes,* **1993.** 42, 1202–1209.

60 P. Achenbach, K. Koczwara, A. Knopff, H. Naserke, A. G. Ziegler, E. Bonifacio, *J. Clin. Invest.,* **2004.** 114, 589–597.

61 M. Solimena, F. Folli, R. Aparisi, G. Pozza, and P. De Camilli, *New Engl. J. Med.,* **1990.** 322, 1555–1560.

62 M. Solimena, M. H. Butler, and C. P. De, *J.Endocrinol. Invest.,* **1994,** 17, 509–520.

63 S. Chattopadhyay, M. Ito, J. D. Cooper, A. I. Brooks, T. M. Curran, J. M. Powers, and D. A. Pearce, *Hum. Mol. Genet.,* **2002.** 11, 1421–1431.

64 M. R. Christie, T. J. Brown, D. Cassidy, *Diabetologia,* **1992.** 35, 380–384.

65 A. Lernmark, *J. Intern. Med.,* **1996.** 240, 259–277.

66 A. Reetz, M. Solimena, M. Matteoli, F. Folli, K. Takei, and P. De Camilli, *EMBO J.,* **1991.** 10, 1275–1284.

67 Y. Shi, B. Veit, and S. Baekkeskov, *J. Cell Biol.,* **1994,** 927–934.

68 W. A. Hagopian, B. Michelsen, A. E. Karlsen, F. Larsen, A. Moody, C. E. Grubin, R. Rowe, J. Petersen, R. Mcevoy, and . Lernmark, *Diabetes,* **1993.** 42, 631–636.

69 M. H. Butler, M. Solimena, R. J. Dirkx, A. Hayday, and P. De Camilli, *J. Exp. Med.,* **1993,** 178, 2097–2106.

70 N. Ujihara, K. Daw, R. Gianani, E. Boel, L. Yu, and A. C. Powers, *Diabetes,* **1994.** 43, 968–975.

71 E. Bonifacio, V. Lampasona, L. Bernasconi, and A. G. Ziegler, *Diabetes,* **2000.** 49, 202–208.

72 W. Richter, J. Endl, T. H. Eiermann, M. Brandt, R. Kientsch-Engel, C. Thivolet, H. Jungfer, and W. A. Scherbaum, *Proc. Natl. Acad. Sci.,* **1992.** 89, 8467–8471.

73 A. M. Madec, F. Rousset, S. Ho, F. Robert, C. Thivolet, J. Orgiazzi, and S. Lebecque, *J. Immunol.,* **1996.** 156, 3541–3549.

74 W. Richter, Y. Shi, and S. Baekkeskov, *Proc. Natl. Acad. Sci. USA,* **1993,** 2832–2836.

75 H. L. Schwartz, J. M. Chandonia, S. F. Kash, J. Kanaani, E. Tunnell, A. Domingo, F. E. Cohen, J. P. Banga, A. M. Madec, W. Richter, and S. Baekkeskov, *J. Mol. Biol.,* **1999.** 287, 983–999.

76 M. A. Myers, G. Fenalti, R. Gray, M. Scealy, J. C. Tong, O. El-Kabbani, and M. J. Rowley, in *Immunology of Diabetes Ii: Pathogenesis from Mouse to Man.* 2003. pp. 250–252.

77 C. J. Padoa, J. P. Banga, A. M. Madec, M. Ziegler, M. Schlosser, E. Ortqvist, I. Kockum, J. Palmer, O. Rolandsson, K. A. Binder, J. Foote, D. Luo, and C. S. Hampe, *Diabetes,* **2003.** 52, 2689–2695.

78 J. Kim, M. Namchuk, T. Bugawan, Q. Fu, M. Jaffe, Y. Shi, H. J. Aanstoot, C. W. Turck, H. Erlich, V. Lennon, and S. Baekkeskov, *J. Exp. Med.,* **1994.** 180, 595–606.

79 E. Bjork, L. A. Velloso, O. Kampe, and F. A. Karlsson, *Diabetes,* **1994,** 161–165.

80 K. Daw, N. Ujihara, M. Atkinson, and A. C. Powers, *J. Immunol.,* **1996.** 156, 818–825.

81 M. R. Christie, G. Vohra, P. Champagne, D. Daneman, and T. L. Delovitch, *J Exp Med,* **1990.** 172, 789–794.

82 M. S. Lan, J. Lu, Y. Goto, and A. L. Notkins, *DNA Cell Biol,* **1994.** 13, 505–514.

83 M. Solimena, R. Dirkx, J. Hermel, S. Pleasic-Williams, J. Shapiro, and D. Rabin, *Autoimmunity,* **1995.** 21, 38.

84 C. Wasmeier and J. C. Hutton, *J. Biol. Chem.,* **1996.** 271, 18161–18170.

85 M. Streuli, N. X. Krueger, T. Thai, M. Tang, and H. Saito, *EMBO J,* **1990.** 9, 2399–2407.

86 G. Magistrelli, S. Toma, and A. Isacchi, *Biochem. Biophys. Res. Commun.,* **1996.** 227, 581–588.

87 T. Ort, S. Voronov, J. Guo, K. Zawalich, S. C. Froehner, W. Zawalich, and M. Solimena, *EMBO J.,* **2001.** 20, 4013–4023.

88 S. Berghs, D. Aggujaro, R. Dirkx, E. Maksimova, P. Stabach, J.M. Hermel, J. P. Zhang, W. Philbrick, V. Slepnev, T. Ort, and M. Solimena, *J. Cell Biol.,* **2000.** 151, 985–1001.

89 C. Wasmeier and J. C. Hutton, *Diabetologia,* **1999.** 42, 498.

90 C. Wasmeier and J. C. Hutton, *J. Biol. Chem.,* **2001.** 276, 31919–31928.

91 M. K. Chiang and J. G. Flanagan, *Development,* **1996.** 122, 2239–2250.

92 C. Roberts, G. A. Roberts, K. Lobner, M. Bearzatto, A. Clark, E. Bonifacio, and M. R. Christie, *J. Histochem. Cytochem.,* **2001.** 49, 767–775.

93 K. Lobner, H. Steinbrenner, G. A. Roberts, Z. D. Ling, G. C. Huang, S. Piquer,

D.G. Pipeleers, J. Seissler, and M.R. Christie, *Diabetes*, **2002**. 51, 2982–2988.

94 M. Solimena, R. Dirkx, Jr., J.M. Hermel, S. Pleasic Williams, J.A. Shapiro, L. Caron, and D.U. Rabin, *EMBO J.*, **1996**. 15, 2102–2114.

95 E.C.I. Hatfield, C.J. Hawkes, M.A. Payton, and M.R. Christie, *Diabetologia*, **1997**. 40, 1327–1333.

96 M. Bearzatto, H. Naserke, S. Piquer, K. Koczwara, V. Lampasona, A. Williams, M.R. Christie, P.J. Bingley, A.G. Ziegler, and E. Bonifacio, *J. Immunol.*, **2002**. 168, 4202–4208.

97 V. Lampasona, M. Bearzatto, S. Genovese, E. Bosi, M. Ferrari, and E. Bonifacio, *J Immunol*, **1996**. 157, 2707–2711.

98 B. Zhang, M.S. Lan, and A.L. Notkins, *Diabetes*, **1997**. 46, 40–43.

99 J. Seissler, M. Schott, N.G. Morgenthaler, and W.A. Scherbaum, *Clin. Exp. Immunol.*, **2000**. 122, 157–163.

100 L. Farilla, C. Tiberti, A. Luzzago, L.P. Yu, G.S. Eisenbarth, R. Cortese, F. Dotta, and U. Di Mario, *Eur. J. Immunol.*, **2002**. 32, 1420–1427.

101 V. Kolm-Litty, S. Berlo, E. Bonifacio, M. Bearzatto, A.M. Engel, M. Christie, A.G. Ziegler, T. Wild, and J. Endl, *J. Immunol.*, **2000**. 165, 4676–4684.

102 J.A. Dromey, S.M. Weenink, G.H. Peters, J. Endl, P.J. Tighe, I. Todd, and M.R. Christie, *J. Immunol.*, **2004**. 172, 4084–4090.

103 M.A. Myers, D.U. Rabin, and M.J. Rowley, *Diabetes*, **1995**, 1290–1295.

104 F. Dotta, R. Gianani, M. Previti, L. Lenti, S. Dionisi, M. D'erme, G.S. Eisenbarth, and U. Di Mario, *Diabetes*, **1996**. 45, 1193–1196.

105 K. Buschard, K. Josefsen, T. Horn, and P. Fredman, *Lancet*, **1993**. 342, 840.

106 M. Pietropaolo, L. Castano, S. Babu, R. Buelow, Y.-L.S. Kuo, S. Martin, A. Martin, A.C. Powers, M. Prochada, J. Naggert, E.H. Leiter, and G.S. Eisenbarth, *J. Clin. Invest.*, **1993**. 92, 359–371.

107 H.J. Aanstoot, S.M. Kang, J. Kim, L.A. Lindsay, U. Roll, M. Knip, M. Atkinson, P. Mose Larsen, S. Fey, J. Ludvigsson, and Et Al., *J. Clin. Invest.*, **1996**. 97, 2772–2783.

108 F. Winnock, M.R. Christie, M.R. Batstra, H.J. Aanstoot, I. Weets, K. Decochez, P. Jopart, D. Nicolaij, and F.K. Gorus, *Diabetes Care*, **2001**. 24, 1181–1186.

109 V. Lampasona, M. Ferrari, E. Bosi, M.R. Pastore, P.J. Bingley, and E. Bonifacio, *J. Autoimmun.*, **1994**. 7, 665–674.

110 S. Martin, V. Lampasona, M. Dosch, and M. Pietropaolo, *Diabetologia*, **1996**. 39, 747.

111 L. Horvath, L. Cervenak, M. Oroszlan, Z. Prohaszka, K. Uray, F. Hudecz, E. Baranyi, L. Madacsy, M. Singh, L. Romics, G. Fust, and P. Panczel, *Immunol. Lett.*, **2002**. 80, 155–162.

112 O.S. Birk, D. Elias, A.S. Weiss, A. Rosen, R. Vanderzee, M.D. Walker, and I.R. Cohen, *J. Autoimmun.*, **1996**. 9, 159–166.

113 A.G.S. Van Halteren, B. Mosselman, B.O. Roep, W. Van Eden, A. Cooke, G. Kraal, and M.H.M. Wauben, *J. Immunol.*, **2000**. 165, 5544–5551.

114 W. Van Eden, R. Van Der Zee, A.G.A. Paul, B.J. Prakken, U. Wendling, S.M. Anderton, and M.H.M. Wauben, *Immunol. Today*, **1998**. 19, 303–307.

115 S. Gallucci and P. Matzinger, *Curr. Opin. Immunol.*, **2001**. 13, 114–119.

116 S.M. Anderton, R. Vanderzee, and J.A. Goodacre, *Eur. J. Immunol.*, **1993**. 23, 33–38.

117 I. Raz, D. Elias, A. Avron, M. Tamir, M. Metzger, and I.R. Cohen, *Lancet*, **2001**. 358, 1749–1753.

118 C.F. Verge, D. Stenger, E. Bonifacio, P.G. Colman, C. Pilcher, P.J. Bingley, and G.S. Eisenbarth, *Diabetes*, **1998**. 47, 1857–1866.

119 P.J. Bingley, E. Bonifacio, and P.W. Mueller, *Diabetes*, **2003**. 52, 1128–1136.

120 A.J. Williams, P.J. Bingley, E. Bonifacio, J.P. Palmer, and E.A. Gale, *J. Autoimmun.*, **1997**. 10, 473–478.

121 A.G. Ziegler, M. Hummel, M. Schenker, and E. Bonifacio, *Diabetes*, **1999**. 48, 460–468.

122 J.M. Barker, K.J. Barriga, L.P. Yu, D.M. Miao, H.A. Erlich, J.M. Norris, G.S. Eisenbarth, and M. Rewers, *J. Clin. Endocrinol. Metab.*, **2004**. 89, 3896–3902.

123 T. Kimpimaki, A. Kupila, A.M. Hamalainen, M. Kukko, P. Kulmala, K. Savola, T. Simell, P. Keskinen, J. Ilonen, O. Simell, and M. Knip, *J. Clin. Endocrinol. Metab.*, **2001**. 86, 4782–4788.

124 H.M. Stanley, J.M. Norris, K. Barriga, M. Hoffman, L.P. Yu, D.M. Miao, H.A. Erlich, G.S. Eisenbarth, and M. Rewers, *Diabetes Care*, **2004**. 27, 497–502.

125 M. Hummel, E. Bonifacio, S. Schmid, M. Walter, A. Knopff, and A.G. Ziegler, *Ann. Intern. Med.*, **2004**. 140, 882–886.

126 T. Kimpimaki, P. Kulmala, K. Savola, A. Kupila, S. Korhonen, T. Simell, J. Ilonen, O. Simell, and M. Knip, *J. Clin. Endocrinol. Metab.*, **2002**. 87, 4572–4579.

127 E. Bonifacio, M. Scirpoli, K. Kredel, M. Fuchtenbusch, and A.G. Ziegler, *J. Immunol.*, **1999**. 163, 525–532.

128 F. Gorus, P. Goubert, C. Semaluka, C. Vandewalle, J. De Schepper, A. Scheen, M. Christie, D. Pipeleers, and Belgian-Diabetes-Registry, *Diabetologia*, **1997**. 40, 95–99.

129 M.R. Christie, D. Daneman, P. Champagne, and T.L. Delovitch, *Diabetes*, **1990**. 39, 653–656.

130 S. Genovese, R. Bonfanti, E. Bazzigaluppi, V. Lampasona, E. Benazzi, E. Bosi, G. Chiumello, and E. Bonifacio, *Diabetologia*, **1996**. 39, 1223–1226.

131 S.W. Serjeantson, M.R.J. Kohonen-Corish, M.J. Rowley, I.R. Mackay, W. Knowles, and P. Zimmet, *Diabetologia*, **1992**. 35, 996–1001.

132 M. Knip, J. Ilonen, A. Mustonen, and H.K. Akerblom, *Diabetologia*, **1986**, 347–351.

133 R. Turner, I. Stratton, V. Horton, S. Manley, P. Zimmet, I.R. Mackay, M. Shattock, G.F. Bottazzo, and R. Holman, *Lancet*, **1997**. 350, 1288–1293.

134 P.J. Bingley, M.R. Christie, E. Bonifacio, R. Bonfanti, M. Shattock, M.T. Fonte, G.F. Bottazzo, and E. Gale, *Diabetes*, **1994**. 43, 1304–1310.

135 M.R. Christie, U. Roll, M.A. Payton, E.C.I. Hatfield, and A.G. Ziegler, *Diabetes Care*, **1997**. 20, 965–970.

136 C.F. Verge, R. Gianani, E. Kawasaki, L. Yu, M. Pietropaolo, R.A. Jackson, H.P. Chase, and G.S. Eisenbarth, *Diabetes*, **1996**. 45, 926–933.

137 P. Kulmala, K. Savola, J.S. Petersen, P. Vahasalo, J. Karjalainen, T. Lopponen, T. Dyrberg, H.K. Akerblom, M. Knip, *J. Clin. Invest.*, **1998**. 101, 327–336.

138 K. Decochez, I.H. De Leeuw, B. Keymeulen, C. Mathieu, R. Rottiers, I. Weets, E. Vandemeulebroucke, I. Truyen, L. Kaufman, F.C. Schuit, D.G. Pipeleers, and F.K. Gorus, *Diabetologia*, **2002**. 45, 1658–1666.

139 P.J. Bingley, E. Bonifacio, M. Shattock, H.A. Gillmor, P.A. Sawtell, D.B. Dunger, R. Scott, G.F. Bottazzo, and E. Gale, *Diabetes Care*, **1993**, 45–50.

140 B.O. Roep, *Diabetologia*, **1999**. 42, 636–637.

141 B.O. Roep, M.A. Atkinson, P.M. Van Endert, P.A. Gottlieb, S.B. Wilson, and J.A. Sachs, *J Autoimmun*, **1999**. 13, 267–282.

142 H.M. Dosch, J. Karjalainen, J. Vandermeulen, M.A. Atkinson, K.J. Kao, and N.K. Maclaren, *N. Engl. J. Med.*, **1994**, 1616–1617.

143 N.C. Schloot, G. Meierhoff, M.K. Faresjo, P. Ott, A. Putnam, P. Lehmann, P. Gottlieb, B.O. Roep, M. Peakman, and T. Tree, *J. Autoimmun.*, **2003**. 21, 365–376.

144 M. Atkinson, M. Honeyman, M. Peakman, and B. Roep, *Diabetologia*, **2000**. 43, 819–820.

145 M. Peakman, T.I. Tree, J. Endl, P. Van Endert, M.A. Atkinson, and B.O. Roep, *Diabetes*, **2001**. 50, 1749–1754.

146 C.R. Kreher, M.T. Dittrich, R. Guerkov, B.O. Boehm, and M. Tary-Lehmann, *J Immunol Methods*, **2003**. 278, 79–93.

147 C.L. Day, N.P. Seth, M. Lucas, H. Appel, L. Gauthier, G.M. Lauer, G.K. Robbins, Z.M. Szczepiorkowski, D.R. Casson, R.T. Chung, S. Bell, G. Harcourt, B.D. Walker, P. Klenerman, and K.W. Wucherpfennig, *J Clin Invest*, **2003**. 112, 831–842.

148 N.A. Danke and W.W. Kwok, *J Immunol*, **2003**. 171, 3163–3169.

149 P.F. Piguet and P. Vassalli, *Eur J Immunol*, **1973**. 3, 477–483.

150 M. Atkinson, D. Kaufman, L. Campbell, K. Gibbs, S. Shah, D.-F. Bu, M. Erlander, A. Tobin, and N. Maclaren, *Lancet,* **1992.** 339, 458–459.

151 T.M. Ellis, D.A. Schatz, E.W. Ottendorfer, M.S. Lan, C. Wasserfall, P.J. Salisbury, J.X. She, A.L. Notkins, N.K. Maclaren, and M.A. Atkinson, *Diabetes,* **1998.** 47, 566–569.

152 C.J. Hawkes, N.C. Schloot, J. Marks, S.J.M. Willemen, J.W. Drijfhout, E.K. Mayer, M.R. Christie, and B.O. Roep, *Diabetes,* **2000.** 49, 356–366.

153 B. Brooks-Worrell, V.H. Gersuk, C. Greenbaum, and J.P. Palmer, *J Immunol,* **2001.** 166, 5265–5270.

154 I. Durinovic-Bello, M. Hummel, and A.G. Ziegler, *Diabetes,* **1996.** 45, 795–800.

155 L.C. Harrison, M.C. Honeyman, H.J. Deaizpurua, R.S. Schmidli, P.G. Colman, B.D. Tait, and D.S. Cram, *Lancet,* **1993.** 341, 1365–1369.

156 B.O. Roep, G. Duinkerken, G.M. Schreuder, H. Kolb, R.R. De Vries, and S. Martin, *Eur. J. Immunol.,* **1996.** 26, 1285–1289.

157 M. Lowdell and G.F. Bottazzo, *Lancet,* **1993.** 341, 1378–1379.

158 S. Hawke, G. Harcourt, N. Pantic, D. Beeson, N. Willcox, and J. Newson Davis, *Lancet,* **1993.** 342, 246.

159 G. Meierhoff, P.A. Ott, P.V. Lehmann, and N.C. Schloot, *Diabetes Metab Res Rev,* **2002.** 18, 367–380.

160 L.O. Gehman and R.J. Robb, *J Immunol Methods,* **1984.** 74, 39–47.

161 D.D. Anthony and P.V. Lehmann, *Methods,* **2003.** 29, 260–269.

162 T. Helms, B.O. Boehm, R.J. Asaad, R.P. Trezza, P.V. Lehmann, and M. Tary-Lehmann, *J Immunol,* **2000.** 164, 3723–3732.

163 M.D. Hesse, A.Y. Karulin, B.O. Boehm, P.V. Lehmann, and M. Tary-Lehmann, *J Immunol,* **2001.** 167, 1353–1361.

164 A.Y. Karulin, M.D. Hesse, M. Tary-Lehmann, and P.V. Lehmann, *J Immunol,* **2000.** 164, 1862–1872.

165 L.S. Wicker, S.L. Chen, G.T. Nepom, J.F. Elliott, D.C. Freed, A. Bansal, S. Zheng, A. Herman, A. Lernmark, D.M. Zaller, L.B. Peterson, J.B. Rothbard, R. Cummings, and P.J. Whiteley, *J Clin Invest,* **1996.** 98, 2597–2603.

166 J. Endl, H. Otto, G. Jung, B. Dreisbusch, F. Donie, P. Stahl, R. Elbracht, G. Schmitz, E. Meinl, M. Hummel, A.G. Ziegler, R. Wank, and D.J. Schendel, *J. Clin. Invest.,* **1997.** 99, 2405–2415.

167 M. Peakman, E.J. Stevens, T. Lohmann, P. Narendran, J. Dromey, A. Alexander, A.J. Tomlinson, M. Trucco, J.C. Gorga, and R.M. Chicz, *J. Clin. Invest.,* **1999.** 104, 1449–1457.

168 G.T. Nepom, J.D. Lippolis, F.M. White, S. Masewicz, J.A. Marto, A. Herman, C.J. Luckey, B. Falk, J. Shabanowitz, D.F. Hunt, V.H. Engelhard, and B.S. Nepom, *Proc Natl Acad Sci USA,* **2001.** 98, 1763–1768.

169 M.A. Atkinson, M.A. Bowman, L. Campbell, B.L. Darrow, D.L. Kaufman, and N.K. Maclaren, *J. Clin. Invest.,* **1994.** 94, 2125–2129.

170 S.D. Patel, A.P. Cope, M. Congia, T.T. Chen, E. Kim, L. Fugger, D. Wherrett, and G. Sonderstrup-Mcdevitt, *Proc Natl Acad Sci USA,* **1997.** 94, 8082–8087.

171 A.E. Herman, R.M. Tisch, S.D. Patel, S.L. Parry, J. Olson, J.A. Noble, A.P. Cope, B. Cox, M. Congia, and H.O. Mcdevitt, *J Immunol,* **1999.** 163, 6275–6282.

172 G. Semana, R. Gausling, R.A. Jackson, and D.A. Hafler, *J Autoimmun,* **1999.** 12, 259–267.

173 D.G. Alleva, P.D. Crowe, L. Jin, W.W. Kwok, N. Ling, M. Gottschalk, P.J. Conlon, P.A. Gottlieb, A.L. Putnam, and A. Gaur, *J Clin Invest,* **2001.** 107, 173–810.

174 I. Durinovic-Bello, B.O. Boehm, and A.G. Ziegler, *J. Autoimmun.,* **2002.** 18, 55–66.

175 M.C. Honeyman, V. Brusic, N.L. Stone, and L.C. Harrison, *Nat Biotechnol,* **1998.** 16, 966–969.

176 T. Lohmann, T. Halder, J. Engler, N.G. Morgenthaler, U.Y. Khoo-Morgenthaler, S. Schroder, J. Seissler, W.A. Scherbaum, and H. Kalbacher, *Exp Clin Endocrinol Diabetes,* **1999.** 107, 166–171.

177 J.C. Jaume, S.L. Parry, A.M. Madec, G. Sonderstrup, and S. Baekkeskov, *J. Immunol.,* **2002.** 169, 665–672.

178 J.A. Berzofsky, *Surv Immunol Res,* **1983.** 2, 223–229.

179 H. Reijonen, T.L. Daniels, A. Lernmark, and G.T. Nepom, *Diabetes,* **2000.** 49, 1621–1626.

180 I. Durinovic-Bello, N. Maisel, M. Schlosser, H. Kalbacher, M. Deeg, T. Eiermann, W. Karges, and B.O. Boehm, in *Immunology of Diabetes Ii: Pathogenesis from Mouse to Man.* 2003. p. 288–294.

181 I. Durinovic-Bello, M. Schlosser, M. Riedl, N. Maisel, S. Rosinger, H. Kalbacher, M. Deeg, M. Ziegler,

J. Elliott, B.O. Roep, W. Karges, and B.O. Boehm, *Diabetologia,* **2004.** 47, 439–450.

182 I. Durinovic-Bello, M. Riedl, S. Rosinger, N. Maisel, H. Kalbacher, M. Deeg, H.J. Schreckling, M. Schlosser, M. Ziegler, P. Kuehnl, and B.O. Boehm, *Ann N Y Acad Sci,* **2002.** 958, 209–213.

183 S. Arif, T.I. Tree, T.P. Astill, J.M. Tremble, A.J. Bishop, C.M. Dayan, B.O. Roep, and M. Peakman, *J. Clin. Invest.,* **2004.** 113, 451–463.

184 H. Kolb, *Diabetes Metab Rev,* **1997.** 13, 139–146.

185 S.M. Dilts and K.J. Lafferty, *J. Autoimmun.,* **1999.** 12, 229–232.

Part 4

Autoantibodies as Molecular and Cellular Probes

Autoantibodies and Autoimmunity: Molecular Mechanisms in Health and Disease. Edited by K. Michael Pollard
Copyright © 2006 WILEY-VCH Verlag GmbH & Co. KGaA, Weinheim
ISBN: 3-527-31141-6

16
Autoantibody Recognition of Cellular and Subcellular Organelles *

Ivan Raška and Šárka Růžičková

16.1
Introduction

Autoantibodies (autoAbs) targeting cellular molecules, usually proteins, nucleic acids, and nucleoproteins, are recognized with an increasing frequency in a variety of diseases. The prototype category of human autoimmune diseases that exhibit serum autoAbs are systemic rheumatic diseases such as systemic lupus erythematosus (SLE), Sjögren's syndrome, polymyositis/dermatomyositis (PM/DM), scleroderma, rheumatoid arthritis, and mixed connective tissue disease (MCTD) (Tan 1989a, 2001; Chen et al. 2004; Gilburd et al. 2004; Horvath et al. 2001; Garcia de la Pena-Lefebvre et al. 2004; Bridges 2004; Kanazawa et al. 2004; Sherer et al. 2004). The occurrence of autoAbs is also associated with thewell-known organ-specific autoimmune diseases that include autoimmune thyroiditis, Graves's disease, autoimmune gastritis, primary biliary cirrhosis, myasthenia gravis, and various dermatological disorders such as pemphigus and bullous pemphigus, as well as several other disorders (Bach et al. 1998; Monzani et al. 2004; Franic et al. 2004; Bittencourt et al. 2004; Miyachi et al. 2004; Giraud et al. 2004; Ohkura et al. 2004; Latrofa et al. 2004; Schott et al. 2004; Anzai et al. 2004; Mimouni et al. 2004). The production of self-reactive autoAbs also takes place under altered cellular mechanisms involved in tumorigenesis (Imai et al. 1993; Tan 2001; Zhang et al. 2001; Mozo et al. 2002; Hong et al. 2004a), or it can arise during viral infections (Eystathioy et al. 2002a; Strassburg et al. 2003). Finally, autoAbs are seen in drug-induced lupus syndrome (e.g., by procainamide and hydralazine) (Rubin et al. 1985; Rubin et al. 2004; Teodorescu et al. 2004) and in disorders associated with occupational or diet hazards (Rom et al. 1983; Haustein and Ziegler 1985; Black et al. 1985; Bell et al. 1992, 1995; Hultman et al. 1995, 1996; Chen et al. 2002a).

Similar autoAbs can be found in currently used animal models of autoimmunity, particularly rodent models (Pollard et al. 2003). In these models, produc-

---

* A list of abbreviations used is located at the end of this chapter.

Autoantibodies and Autoimmunity: Molecular Mechanisms in Health and Disease. Edited by K. Michael Pollard
Copyright © 2006 WILEY-VCH Verlag GmbH & Co. KGaA, Weinheim
ISBN: 3-527-31141-6

tion of autoAbs can be spontaneous, such as that observed in animals ensuing from crosses between New Zealand black and white mice strains (Reimer et al. 1987a; Jacob et al. 1987; Finck et al. 1994). It can also be induced by exogenous agents such as mercuric chloride (Hultman et al. 1996), by direct immunization with antigens such as thyroglobin and acetylcholine receptors (von Westarp et al. 1977; Lindstrom 1976; Scott et al. 2004), or by gene mutations encountered in mice with gene specific knockouts (Pollard et al. 2003).

The presence of autoAbs in patients' sera has its straightforward clinical importance. In turn, target structures of autoAbs, often autoAbs associated with systemic rheumatic diseases, regularly represent key players in fundamental cellular processes such as DNA replication and repair or RNA synthesis and processing as well as in processes involved in cell cycle progression, endoplasmic reticulum transport, and apoptosis signalling. Here, we shall provide an overview of the importance of autoAbs as probes in molecular cell biology, with emphasis on a role of autoAbs in microscopy investigations of cells and tissues.

16.2
Autoantibodies Are Important in Clinical and Basic Research

Early studies led to the observation of autoAbs in serum of patients with SLE; subsequently, the DNA and the deoxyribonucleoprotein were identified as the cognate autoAgs (Hargraves et al. 1948; Tan and Kunkel 1966). Later on, these findings were followed by a large series of clinical investigations demonstrating the relationship between autoAbs and clinical syndromes (Scofield 2004). Whereas the mechanisms leading to the occurrence of serum autoAbs in various autoimmune diseases are unknown (Zinkernagel 2000), the clinical tests establishing the occurrence of autoAbs belong to important standard diagnostic tests. Importantly, the determination of target structures for autoAb binding sometimes has a definite diagnostic value. For instance, anti-DNA, anti-histone, and anti-Smith (Sm) autoAbs are highly characteristic for SLE, anti-DNA topoisomerase I autoAbs for systemic scleroderma, and anti-centromeric autoAbs for the CREST (*c*alcinosis, *R*aynaud's syndrome, *e*sophageal dysmotility, *s*clerodactyly, and *t*elangiectasia) subset of scleroderma (Tan and Kunkel 1966; Mattioli and Reichlin 1973; Pinnas et al. 1973; Moroi et al. 1980; Chung and Utz 2004; Scofield 2004). However, anti-U1 RNP autoAbs reflect a diversity, as they are associated with both SLE and MCTD (von Mühlen and Tan 1995; Pollard 2004; Utz et al. 1997; Overzet et al. 2000). Along this line, certain autoAb responses are consistently associated with one another. Thus, the profile of serum autoAbs may have a prognostic value (Love et al. 1991; DeGiorgio et al. 2001; van Gaalen et al. 2004) and facilitates the clinical treatment follow-up in many cases (Vencovsky et al. 2003; Berglin et al. 2004; von Mühlen and Tan 1995).

The mechanism by which cellular components become autoimmunogenic remains unknown. Moreover, both the mechanism of the autoAb production and the nature of antigenic stimuli are enigmatic. However, it has been shown that induction of non-apoptotic cell death by exposure of cells to mercury *in vitro* resulted in mercury-protein (e.g., fibrillarin) interaction. This leads to the altered proteolysis and production of unique cleavage fragments that represent a source of antigenic determinants for self-reactive T cells (Pollard et al. 2000). Furthermore, the accumulation of 20S and 26S proteasomes and their colocalization with fibrillarin within the nucleus were demonstrated under subtoxic concentrations of mercuric chloride (Chen et al. 2002b). Proteasomes generate oligopeptides, and a fraction of oligopeptides escapes complete destruction. They are subsequently transported through the endoplasmic reticulum and then subjected to antigen presentation in context of the major histocompatibility class I (MHC I) molecules; thus, the self-intracellular antigens can be recognized as foreign by T cells (Chen et al. 2002b).

The autoAbs are assumed to form immune complexes with autoAgs in extracellular fluids. This does not affect the function of their target autoantigens (autoAgs) (Tan 1989b). However, if autoAbs can enter the cells, as described previously (Alarcón-Segovia et al. 1978; Ma et al. 1991; Koscec et al. 1997), they could act as the inhibitors of biological functions of their cognate autoAgs. It would mean the inhibition of functions such as DNA replication, transcription, mRNA splicing, and translation, i.e., functions essential for survival and replication of the cell.

A major breakthrough in autoAb research came 25 years ago. Surprisingly, it was not in the clinical field, but in basic research. Lerner and Steitz (1979) showed that the Sm autoantigen (autoAg) and nuclear ribonucleoprotein (U1 RNP) autoAg were RNP particles that were in complexes with small nuclear RNAs (snRNAs), called uridylate (U) snRNAs, and different proteins. Enigmatic snRNAs, which are abundant nuclear RNA species, had then been known for years (Busch and Smetana 1970; Reddy and Busch 1981). Specifically, using Sm and U1 RNP autoAbs, U1, U2, U4, U5, and U6 snRNAs were involved. The breakthrough came with the result that these autoantibodies blocked the splicing reactions *in vitro* (Lerner et al. 1980). This result not only established the function in splicing for a subset of snRNPs but also provided a new way of studying the mechanism of the splicing process. Most recently, the novel complex of proteins containing the U1 snRNP-A protein (U1A) was found in serum of a patient with SLE. In this case, the inhibition of splicing and of *in vitro* polyadenylation was also shown; moreover, the serum component displaying the specificity for U1A protein recognized the identical epitope as the monoclonal antibody and identified a new protein complex within the cell (Faig and Lutz 2003).

Along these lines, today's concept is that the most prominent autoAgs, particularly those defined through the systemic rheumatic diseases, are ubiquitous nuclear proteins involved in fundamental cellular events (Tan 1989a; von Mühlen and Tan 1995; Mahler et al. 2003). The important feature of autoAgs arising from their biological functions is their evolutionary conservation across the species. In this regard, the autoAbs represent an important diagnostic tool for autoimmune diseases, and moreover their reaction with respective autoAg provides the possibility to analyze the nature, properties, and function(s) of autoAg itself (Tan 1989a; von Mühlen and Tan 1995; Mahler et al. 2003; Pollard 2004).

16.3
Epitopes Recognized by Autoantibodies

The autoAbs can serve as biological probes to detect their cognate autoAgs using standard approaches such as immunoblotting, immunoprecipitation, enzyme-linked immunosorbent assay (ELISA), and microscopy, particularly fluorescence microscopy (Tan 1989a; von Mühlen and Tan 1995; Mahler et al. 2003; Pollard 2004). With the help of antigenic material from different species, the use of these approaches allows for a determination of the presence of simple or complex auto-epitopes and autoepitope conservation across species. An emphasis will be put on the use of microscopy techniques in this review, and immunocytochemical (IC) approaches will be described in detail separately in Section 16.4.

The cloning of cDNAs of expressed proteins from cDNA libraries from a variety of species represents another possibility of how to study the nature of auto-Ags that contain in common, across species, conserved sequences and conformational protein elements (Pollard 2004). However, this method is used mostly in the characterization of the primary structure of a variety of human cytoplasmic and nuclear proteins, which is important for the determination of autoantigenic epitopes.

The inhibition experiments using either peptide libraries and/or autoAbs represent an effective tool complementing the techniques combining site-directed mutagenesis and expression vector constructs to study the molecular base and biological function of autoAgs (Mahler et al. 2003).

Recently, the progress of proteomics in the field of autoimmune diseases (Robinson et al. 2002a) led to the development of novel strategies such as multiplex assay systems based on microarray technology (Robinson et al. 2002b), using recombination proteins, peptides, and nucleic acids as antigens for detection of autoAbs, or fluorescent microsphere immunoassays, using antigen-coated beads (Pickering et al. 2002; Pollard 2004). These techniques allow screening and characterization of autoAgs and epitopes of all types in a very short time simultaneously in a single array. The process from the identification of autoAb and its relevant autoantigen/autoepitope to the development of detecting/diagnostic reagent could thus be remarkably shortened.

The structure of autoepitopes is diverse (Fig. 16.1) (Mahler et al. 2003). Their nature comprises primary, secondary, tertiary, and quaternary structures as well as modified epitopes. In addition, epitopes can be hidden in the structure of the native autoAg or can mimic the structure of an antigen of a different nature. Primary epitope (Fig. 16.1A) comprises a linear stretch of up to 10 amino acids (AAs) and can be detected by almost all methods (e.g., in the centromeric protein CENP-A). The secondary epitope (Fig. 16.1B), represented by simple three-dimensional α-helices (α-helical epitope region in protein PM/Scl-100) or β-turns, can be

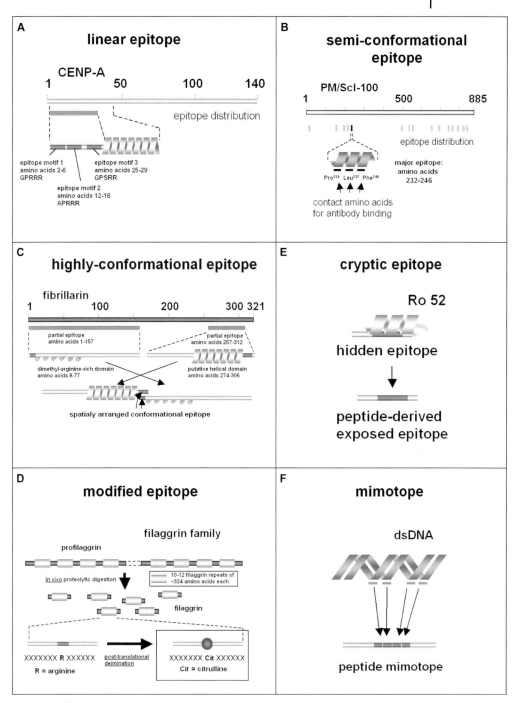

Fig. 16.1 Different epitope types. The general nature of autoepitopes includes primary (A), secondary (B), and tertiary (C). Moreover, the existence of modified (D) and hidden (E) autoepitopes as well as epitopes mimicking the autoepitopes (F) has been established. (Reproduced from Mahler et al. (2003) with permission from Elsevier Ltd.).

determined by epitope-mapping strategies combined with computer-based analyses. The most complicated is the analysis of tertiary (Fig. 16.1 C) (the epitope is spatially organized as in the molecule of fibrillarin) and quaternary structures (e.g., histone H2A-H2B-DNA complex) (Burlingame et al. 1994) due to the distribution of AAs forming the epitope over distant parts of the protein's primary sequence or due to a combination of different components in the complex autoAg. The identification of post-translationally modified AAs (Fig. 16.1 D) by dimethylation (Brahms et al. 2000) or citrullination (Schellekens et al. 2000) of arginine residues in a set of human nuclear proteins such as the Sm D (Brahms et al. 2000), fibrillarin (Aris and Blobel 1991), and nucleolin (Lapyere et al. 1986) requires the development of assays using the modified amino acid. All of the above-mentioned autoAg epitopes may be hidden (Fig. 16.1 E) (Deshmukh et al. 1999) in the native form of antigen due to formation of secondary, tertiary, or quaternary structure, as it is seen in Ro52 protein. The accessibility of the cryptic binding site to (auto)antibody is established after disruption of the three-dimensional structure by denaturation or proteolytic cleavage. AutoAbs against cryptic autoepitopes rising from cleaved or modified autoAgs are associated with a variety of human autoimmune diseases (Greidinger et al. 2000). Structures mimicking the epitopes, so-called mimotopes (Fig. 16.1 F), can display sequence homology to the autoAg of interest or the structural homology lacking such sequence identity. Such mimotopes can be represented by a short peptide that is recognized by anti-dsDNA autoAbs, as was recently shown (Sun et al. 2001). These mimotopes can be analyzed using recombinant proteins for immunoblotting, immunoprecipitation, and ELISA and by random peptide phage display and peptide scans (Mahler et al. 2003; Zhang and Davidson 1999; Sun et al. 2001). The set of overlapping synthetic peptides covering the entire sequence of human histone H1 was used to identify the immunodominant epitope, and its immune reactivity was correlated with disease activity in human SLE patients (Schett et al. 2002). Another application of the library of synthetic peptides to determine the exact structure and amino acid sequence of target autoepitopes is the inhibition of autoreactivity of autoAbs *in vitro*. Such an approach allowed the detection of the decapeptide that inhibits the binding of anti-dsDNA and antibody deposition in kidneys, which suggests possible implications in the therapy of human autoimmune diseases (Sharma et al. 2003; Mahler et al. 2003).

Although not established with the help of autoAbs, we wish to provide the reader with the results that document the most sophisticated possibilities of epitope characterization (Fig. 16.2) (Conway et al. 2003). Surprisingly, this result came from the field of structural biology and was achieved by the application of cryo-electron microscopy (cryo-EM) and three-dimensional image reconstruction to hepatitis B virus (HBV) capsid labeled with a Fab fragment. The Fab fragment binds specifically to the quaternary epitope shared by a dimer of core capsid protein. This example of epitope mapping demonstrates a highly conformational epitope. The individual core proteins are not arranged in an equivalent way in the capsid, but through quasi-equivalence principles governing the architecture of self-assembly structures, i.e., icosahedral viruses in this case (Caspar and Klug 1962). Thus, the dimer of the core protein may be, within the capsid,

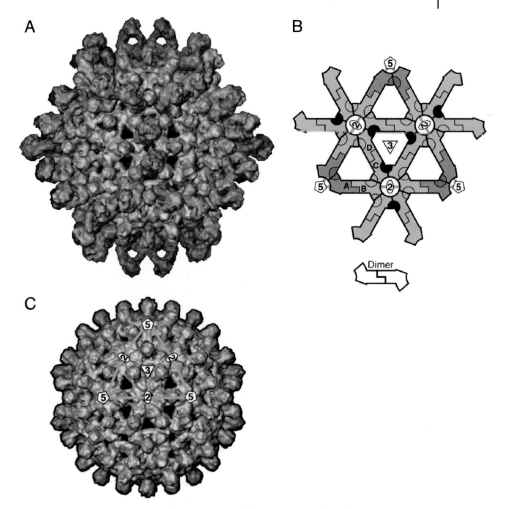

Fig. 16.2 Cryo-EM reconstruction of HBV capsid labeled with Fab fragment targeting the quaternary epitope between the subunit dimer (A) and the control capsid (C). The capsid protein is blue, and the Fab density is pink. (B) Lattice diagram of a single triangular facet, which is also marked on the control capsid, and a single dimer. In the lattice diagram, the packing of dimers, the positions of symmetry axes, and the placement of four quasi-equivalent subunits, A, B, C, and D, are marked. Rings marking the positions of the epitopes are shaded according to occupancy: the C-D site is dark, representing 100% occupancy; the A-A sites around the fivefold vertex are gray, representing 20–40% occupancy; the unoccupied D-B and B-C sites have empty rings. (Reproduced from Conway et al. (2003) with permission from the American Society for Microbiology).

exposed to different traction and torque forces. The epitope, depending on its position on the capsid surface, thus shows, after the labeling, from 0% to 100% occupancy with the Fab fragment. This example, which could not be demonstrated through other approaches, represents the power of today's structural biology.

We wish to finish this subsection with the following comment. We believe that the actual scientific challenge of today's molecular and cell biology is not the sheep Dolly or stem cells, but the complexity of the functional organization of chromatin. Now that the proteome of various cell parts and/or organelles has become clearly defined, many new autoAbs to cell components will be easily defined. Autoimmune sera and particularly (high-titer) SLE sera target chromatin structures (Sherer et al. 2004). We are of the opinion that such anti-chromatin sera will be shown to contain autoAbs directed to all kinds of "epiproteome" epitopes such as histone and chromatin non-histone protein modifications.

16.4
Immunocytochemistry and Autoantibodies

Fluorescence microscopy demonstration of autoAbs in patients' sera is a routine procedure performed in clinical laboratories. In research laboratories, autoAbs serve as molecular and cellular probes in the detection of their cognate antigens using fluorescence, confocal, and electron microscopy (EM). AutoAbs are commonly more useful IC probes than specific sera raised in immunized animals against the same "autoantigen" and, similarly, "autoimmune" monoclonal antibodies are usually more useful than hybridomas in which lymphocytes from standardly immunized animals were used for hybridoma fusion (Tan 1989a; Tan et al. 1994; von Mühlen and Tan 1995; Mahler et al. 2003; Pollard 2004). For such "autoimmune" hybridomas, either lymphocytes from patients or, more commonly, rodent lymphocytes in animal models of autoimmunity were used. This is apparently due to the fact that autoAbs frequently target functionally important autoAgs, and thus epitopes that are conserved across species, and even epitopes associated with the active domain in the autoAg (Tan 1989a; Tan et al. 1994; von Mühlen and Tan 1995; Mahler et al. 2003; Pollard 2004).

The principles of microscopic approaches used in immuno(cyto)chemistry mapping are explained in Figures 16.3 to 16.5. We emphasize that the approach used should allow the autoAbs to "find" their target autoAg (also, in the second step of the procedure, the secondary antibodies bearing a marker should "find" the bound autoAbs) in the cell, but, at the same time, they should not allow the cellular macromolecules to move away from their genuine location. The first condition is usually met through the use of detergent or acetone, or through the mechanical opening of cells by sectioning. The second condition is fulfilled through (more-or-less stringent) fixation of cells and tissues (Raška 2003).

In Figure 16.6, we provide the reader with an example of the commercial monoclonal antibody to actin with which we have elucidated a new phenomenon of

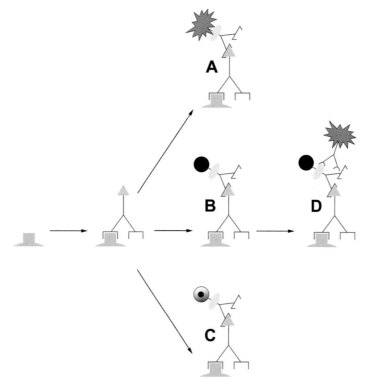

Fig. 16.3 LM and EM approaches used in IC mapping. In the most common two-step IC procedure, the primary antibody molecules bind the target (blue) within a sample. Consequently, secondary antibodies, bound to a detectable (fluorescent, electron-dense) marker, are used to locate the primary antibody molecules. In LM, fluorophores (A) of different colors can be used simultaneously to map several different epitopes. Moreover, the IC fluorescence pattern can be complemented with common fluorescence dyes (in the case of nucleus DAPI, Hoechst, YOYO-1, and others), phase contrast, or differential interference contrast. The contrast of the EM image is generated by the scattering of the electron beam on nuclei of heavy atoms. Thin-sectioned cells, consisting of light atoms (carbon, hydrogen, oxygen, nitrogen, etc.), are stained with salts of heavy atoms such as uranyl acetate to generate a contrast of cell structures. IC approaches employ the colloidal gold particles (5–15 nm) bound to secondary antibodies (B). In monochrome EM image, the size of the gold particle, rather than its color, can distinguish among different epitopes. In a special case of the EM IC procedure – pre-embedding, in-volume labeling (Fig. 16.5) – a secondary antibody is bound to a very small gold particle (1 nm in diameter) to be able to penetrate the sample. Consequently, the small gold particles, which cannot produce a sufficient contrast, are silver intensified (C) *in situ*, and enlarged silver particles are observed. The concomitant visualization of the LM and EM labeling in a thin-sectioned cell can be performed. To obtain such a result, a standard two-step labeling with colloidal gold adducts is performed (B) on thin sections placed on the supporting EM grid, and a third antibody, with an affinity to the secondary antibodies, conjugated to a fluorophore, is applied (D). The thin sections are counterstained with a dye and observed in the fluorescence microscope. The thin sections are then stained with uranyl acetate and the image of the same nucleolar section is taken in EM. (Reproduced from Raška (2003) with permission from Elsevier Ltd.).

BrUTP   **Biotin-UTP**

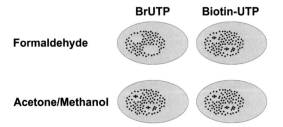

Formaldehyde

Acetone/Methanol

Fig. 16.4 Accessibility of cell structures to IC probes. In this particular case, the mapping of nucleolar transcription sites is documented (Koberna et al. 2000; Raška 2003).
If mapped using BrUTP incorporation into newborn RNA, nucleolar transcription sites are not revealed after the standard formaldehyde fixation procedure. Other nucleotide analogues, such as biotinylated UTP, have to be used to localize the nucleolar transcription events. Bromine epitopes in nucleoli are not accessible for IC probes. Physical sectioning of the nucleolus, as in the case of post-embedding, on-section labeling (see Fig. 16.5), can help to uncover them. In this case, only the epitopes exposed to the section surface are visualized. Another approach leading to the detection of brominated RNA in nucleolus is the use of acetone/methanol fixation. One has to keep in mind that such an approach severely alters the ultrastructure of the specimen. Indeed, while aldehydic fixatives cross-link macromolecules, acetone/methanol treatment rather precipitates them. Thus, the use of acetone/methanol fixation may be correct only within the frame of LM resolution. (Reproduced from Raška (2003) with permission from Elsevier Ltd.).

cold-dependent *in situ* epitope detectability (Fidlerova et al. 2005). In contrast to generally known fixation-dependent changes in epitope detectability (or temperature-dependent changes in the kinetics of antigen-antibody reactions), we demonstrate specific, cold-dependent detection of an epitope in a new *in situ* location that, depending on the temperature during which the fixed cells are labeled, produces a different fluorescent pattern. At room temperature, the cytoplasmic cytoskeleton is revealed, and at 4 °C, nuclear labeling is put into evidence as well (Fidlerova et al. 2005). This example complements Figure 16.1 and testifies that with immuno(cyto)chemistry, which represents the fundamental tool in molecular and cell biology, we have to be, as with every experimental approach, cautious.

With autoimmune sera, we may face a major drawback. They can be polyspecific (typically SLE sera) even though highly monospecific sera (e.g., some scleroderma sera) can be found. Thus, if indicated, specific autoAbs have to be affinity-purified from polyspecific autoimmune sera (Olmstead 1981; Pollard 2004). The existence of high-titer monospecific sera or high-titer sera with a highly restricted profile of antinuclear autoAbs targeting functionally important nuclear macromolecules made possible the breakthroughs achieved with autoAbs in the nuclear research.

Even though a given IC approach may reveal itself to be inadequate for detection of a particular autoAg, suitable means for the permeabilization-fixation protocol can be usually found. This is why we always begin in light microscopy

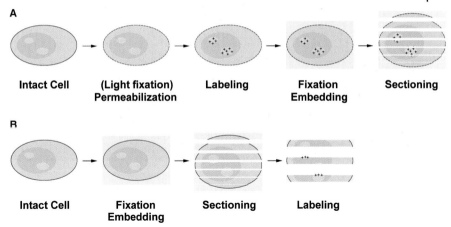

Fig. 16.5 Comparison between pre- and post-embedding labeling approaches. (A) Post-embedding, on-section labeling: Cells or pieces of tissue are first fixed, embedded in plastic resin, or frozen, and hard, tiny blocks containing the biological material are (thin)-sectioned. The labeling on plastic sections, or thawed cryosections, is then performed. For LM, the sections are mounted. For EM, the sections are stained by uranyl acetate. In the post-embedding approach, only target macromolecules exposed on the surface of plastic sections are detectable, and the labeling efficiency is thus usually lower than in the pre-embedding approach. The penetration of IC probes into thawed cryosections is limited and depends on the extent of fixation. On the other hand, the sectioning itself may help to expose otherwise hidden epitopes. (B) Pre-embedding, in-volume labeling: Cultured and/or isolated cells or cells in the small pieces of tissue are made permeable (e.g., detergent treatment, thawed thick cryosections, and vibratome sections are used). Fixation impedes the penetration of the labeling probes such as antibodies into the cell interior, and the specimen is therefore either unfixed or, at most, lightly fixed. After the labeling, the specimen is mounted in LM, or thoroughly fixed, resin-embedded, thin-sectioned, and stained with uranyl acetate in EM. The target macromolecules can be potentially labeled throughout the cell interior, but the penetration problem of IC probes into the cell interior may occur. In the pre-embedding EM approach, the cell structures may not be well preserved. In summary, if used, the pre-embedding EM procedure requires a correlation with the parallel post-embedding EM approach. (Reproduced from Raška (2003) with permission from Elsevier Ltd.).

(LM) with two entirely different fixation-permeabilization procedures, formaldehyde/triton and methanol/acetone procedures. Formaldehyde generates a truly chemical fixation, while methanol/acetone fixation results in dehydration/precipitation of macromolecules. In Figure 16.4, we provide an interesting example in which, in contrast to methanol/acetone treatment, formaldehyde fixation results in inaccessibility of the epitope and thus generates a bias (Koberna et al. 2000; Raška 2003).

We emphasize that EM has a resolution power almost three orders of magnitude higher than that of LM (see Fig. 16.8). Thus, while the methanol/acetone procedure is convenient for LM applications, the cell structure looks ruined in the EM if methanol/acetone fixation has been used. Also, EM IC is more diffi-

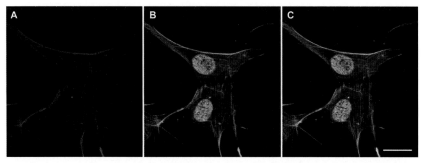

Fig. 16.6 Cold-dependent epiC labeling. Fixed human primary fibroblasts were incubated with anti-actin monoclonal antibody (detecting epi1 epitope of actin) for 2 h at room temperature (RT), followed by incubation with Cy3-conjugated goat anti-mouse secondary antibody (A) for 40 min at RT. After wash, the cells were incubated again with the same anti-actin antibody overnight at +4 °C, followed by incubation with Alexa Fluor 488 goat anti-mouse secondary antibody (B). Merging of both channels is shown (C). If labeled at RT, only cytoplasm is labeled. If labeled at +4 °C, both cytoplasm and nucleus are labeled (bar: 20 μm). This figure was kindly provided by Dr. H. Fidlerová.

cult than LM mapping. Indeed, the success in EM mappings represents only the subset of successful LM mappings. An important corollary ensues: one should avoid EM IC if the parallel fluorescence LM IC, performed on either whole cells or sectioned material, has failed.

16.5
Autoantibodies as Probes for Cytoplasmic Antigens

Historically, clinical and basic research has focused on antinuclear autoAbs and on nuclear autoAgs (von Mühlen and Tan 1995). In the last few years, considerably more attention is being given to the study of cytoplasmic autoAgs (Stinton et al. 2004). These are represented by organelles or macromolecular assemblies such as mitochondria, lysosomes, endosomes, cytoskeleton, centrosomes, the Golgi complex, and translation machinery. Recently, a novel cytoplasmic organelle termed the GW body was described with the help of the autoantibody (Stinton et al. 2004).

Some of these autoAbs are exclusively associated with particular diseases or with distinct forms of autoimmune diseases, such as autoAbs recognizing mitochondrial antigens of the inner mitochondrial membrane (Bogdanos et al. 2003). This type of autoAbs, termed anti-M2, is regarded as specific for primary biliary cirrhosis (Bogdanos et al. 2003; Zuber and Recktenwald 2003). Other cytoplasmic organelles detected by autoAbs, especially by sera from patients with SLE, include endosomes – respectively, their components such as early endosome antigen 1, cytoplasmic linker protein-170, and lysobisphosphatidic acid – and lysosomes and their autoAg h-LAMP2 (Selak et al. 1999; Griffith et al. 2002; Stinton et al. 2004).

Special cytoplasmic autoAbs occurring in sera of patients with Wegener's granulomatosis, vasculitis, and inflammatory bowel disease (Peter and Schoenfeld 1996) are termed anti-neutrophil cytoplasmic antibodies (ANCAs). They are divided according to the labeling pattern into two groups, C-ANCAs, which label the cytoplasm of neutrophils and monocytes, and P-ANCAs, which display a perinuclear labeling pattern (Wiik and van der Woude 1989). Proteinase 3 – a protein involved in proteolytic degradation of such proteins as elastin, lamin, and collagen – and myeloperoxidase, an enzyme abundantly expressed in neutrophils, are the major C-ANCA and P-ANCA antigens, respectively (Goldschmeding et al. 1989; Falk and Jennette 1988; Peter and Schoenfeld 1996). Recently, new autoAgs of anti-neutrophil autoAbs in neutrophils and their immature stages were identified in sera of patients with SLE (Chen et al. 2004).

As mentioned above, cytoplasmic autoAbs can be specific for particular forms of autoimmune disease. This is also the case of autoAbs directed against microtubule-associated protein 2, which is a neuron-specific protein that maintains the integrity of the neuronal cytoskeleton (Maccioni and Cambiazo 1995). These autoAbs were specific for patients with neuropsychiatric SLE (Williams et al. 2004). AutoAbs targeting actin, myosin, and other cytoskeletal proteins were also observed in sera of patients with rheumatoid arthritis (Shrivastav et al. 2002). Besides these, there is a heterogeneous group of anti-cytoskeletal autoAbs that occur in liver disease, cardiomyopathy, and pemphigus vulgaris and that target actin, tubulin, keratin, desmin, or vimentin (Johnson et al. 1965; Raška et al. 1991b; Gregor et al. 1987; Whitehouse et al. 1974; Kurki et al. 1977; Leibovitch et al. 1995; Pelacho et al. 2004).

A number of autoAgs in centrioles/centrosomes (cytoplasmic organelles that in interphase are located not far from the nuclear envelope and that in metaphase establish opposite poles of the mitotic spindle) were identified with sera from patients with Raynaud's syndrome, scleroderma, or CREST syndrome (S. Sato et al. 1994; Tuffanelli et al. 1983; Bao et al. 1995; Hayakawa et al. 2004a; Sager et al. 1989). The autoAgs of centrioles and centrosomes are represented by a wide spectrum of proteins including centractin; γ-tubulin; tektin A, B, and C; p34^{cdc2}; cyclins A, B1, and B2; mitotin; PCM1; ninein; Cep 250; and pericentrin-B (Bao et al. 1995, 1998; Peter and Schoenfeld 1996; Mack et al. 1998; Li et al. 2001).

Another cytoplasmic organelle, the Golgi complex, was also shown to be recognized by autoAbs known as anti-Golgi complex antibodies (AGAs) (Stinton et al. 2004). Since 1993 there have been many studies identifying individual autoAgs that are integral parts of the Golgi complex. Among such proteins are golgin-95 and -160 (Fritzler et al. 1993; Eystathioy et al. 2000; Nozawa et al. 2004; Hong et al. 2004b; Stinton et al. 2004) as well as golgin-245 and giantin (Nozawa et al. 2004). The AGAs have been found in several systemic autoimmune diseases such as SLE, RA, MCTD, and Wegener's granulomatosis (Fritzler et al. 1984, 1993; Mayet et al. 1991; Hong et al. 1992, 2004b; Rossie et al. 1992; Eystathioy et al. 2000; Nozawa et al. 2004; Stinton et al. 2004).

Various autoimmune diseases are associated with the occurrence of autoAbs to translation machinery. The autoAbs specific for patients with primary myositis recognize the enzyme histidyl-tRNA synthetase (Jo-1) (Nishikai and Reichlin 1980). This autoAg catalyzes the esterification of histidine to its respective tRNA, and its localization in both nucleus and cytoplasm has been described (Shi et al. 1991). Recently, it was shown that histidyl-tRNA synthetase tagged with a green fluorescent protein (GFP) localizes mainly in cytoplasm and that occasionally it is colocalized with a nuclear pore complex. This apparently indicates the influx of histidyl-tRNA synthetase–GFP fusion protein into the nucleus (Kamei 2004). In addition, autoAbs specific for other aminoacyl tRNA synthetases such as alanyl-, threonyl-, glycyl-, and isoleucyl-tRNA synthetase were also observed (Peter and Schoenfeld 1996). Many of the anti-cytoplasmic autoAbs found especially in SLE patients are directed against ribosomal components, e.g., the phosphoproteins P0, P1, and P2 (Francoeur et al. 1985); the L5/5S protein complex (Steitz et al. 1988); the S10 protein of the 40S ribosomal subunit (T. Sato et al. 1991); and L12 and P proteins (T. Sato et al. 1990, 1994). In a recent study, it was shown that especially anti-P autoAbs are strongly related to the various forms of central nervous disturbances in patients with SLE (Reichlin 2003). Other examples of autoAbs encountered first in myositis patients are those targeting SRP54 (Reeves et al. 1986; Kao et al. 2004). The SRP (signal recognition particle) is composed of six polypeptides and a small RNA molecule (Zwieb and Larsen 1994), and these play a role during translocation of newly synthesized protein from the ribosome into the endoplasmic reticulum (Rapoport 1990).

The most exciting finding among cytoplasmic structures was the discovery of GW bodies (GWBs) with the help of the autoantibody (Eystathioy et al. 2002b, 2003a; Stinton et al. 2004). These GWBs, in the form of a few fluorescent cytoplasmic bodies, were detected using serum from a patient with motor and sensory neuropathy that was preceded by Sjögren's syndrome and SLE (Eystathioy et al. 2003a). The characteristic marker for this structure is the protein termed GW182 (Eystathioy et al. 2002b). The GWs do not colocalize with Golgi complex, endosomes, lysosomes, or peroxisomes, suggesting that GWBs represent a novel cytoplasmic structure of human cells. GW182 represents a new class of RNP autoAg, and GWBs are apparently involved in mRNA decapping and degradation (Eystathioy et al. 2003b).

16.6
Autoantibodies as Probes for Nuclear Antigens

In contrast to autoAbs targeting cytoplasmic autoAgs, autoAbs identifying nuclear autoAgs frequently played a decisive role in fuelling the scientific progress of nuclear cell biology. The nucleus does not possess internal membranes, and for many years studies on the cell biology of the nucleus were limited by a relative lack of distinctive substructures that were amenable to biochemical purification.

The same applies to cell biology studies, since the nucleus lacks distinctive substructures revealed by microscopy. When a typical mammalian nucleus is seen even in the EM, clumps of heterochromatin are visible at the nuclear periphery and the nucleolus is readily identified by virtue of its electron-dense nature, but otherwise the nucleoplasm appears rather featureless and amorphous. However, during the second part of the 1980s and particularly in the 1990s, a very different view (Fig. 16.7) became evident when antibody probes, commonly autoantibody probes, were used to detect specific nuclear factors (or, in the case of chromosome territories, to detect through *in situ* hybridization the specific nucleic acid sequences). Many nuclear proteins localize to distinct regions, domains or bodies of the nucleus (Fig. 16.7) that can be recognized in the fluorescence microscope. We say that the nucleus is subcompartmentalized[1].

The high-titer autoAbs in human autoimmune diseases such as SLE are directed against chromosome/chromatin structures. Their target is frequently the complex of double-stranded DNA and histones (Burlingame and Rubin 1996) that forms a higher-order structure, the nucleosome. In this structure the DNA wraps around an octamer composed of two copies of histones H2A, H2B, H3, and H4 that form the core of the nucleosome (Wolffe 1992). Histone H1 connects nucleosomal cores and locks two helical turns around the histone core, forming a more highly organized chromatin structure resembling beads on a string (Boulikas 1993). The higher orders of chromatin/chromosome organization are unknown, including the structure of the next order, the 30-nm chromatin filament. Moreover, the structure of the nucleosome is now the center of interest of the whole scientific community. We speak today not just about the genome but also about the epigenome (Jenuwein 2002; McNairn and Gilbert 2003). The histones are post-translationally modified by acetylation, phosphorylation, and methylation, and these changes, together with the methylation of DNA within CpG islands of cytosine and guanine, are key players in the chromatin activity, respectively inactivity (silencing). A large number of histone modifications are known, and, for instance, if "yesterday" we were considering whether a given lysine residue in histones H3 and H4 is or is not methylated, "today" we also have to consider whether the lysine residue bears a mono-, di-, or trimethyl group (Jenuwein 2002; Novik et al. 2002). In this context, the histones represent one category of important factors influencing the regulation of gene expression, and it has been shown that in drug-induced SLE, the main target of autoAbs is the (H2A-H2B)-DNA complex (Burlingame and Rubin 1996). Recently, the histone H1 was identified as a highly specific autoAg for SLE (Schett et al. 2002). Thus, anti-chromatin autoAbs targeting histones as well as a very high number of identified non-histone chromatin and chromatin-associated factors (including RNA polymerases I, II, and III; myriads of transcription factors; replication factors; and heterogeneous nuclear RNP proteins) con-

---

1) We shall omit the enumeration of the very high number of autoAgs associated with chromatin, nuclear speckles, and nucleolus and refer the reader to more specific review articles by von Mühlen and Tan (1995), Mahler et al. (2003), and Sherer et al. (2004).

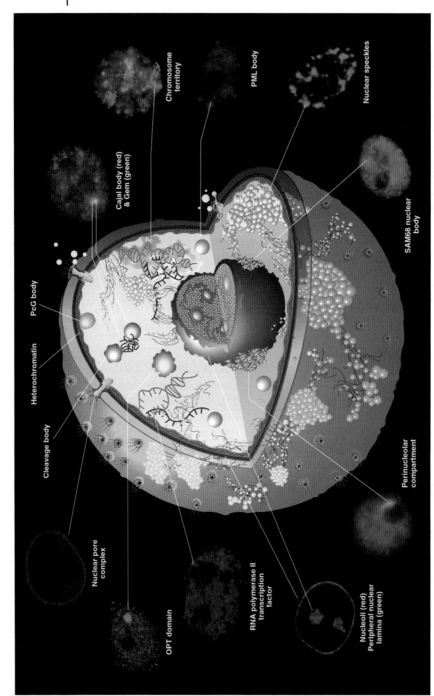

Fig. 16.7 Illustration of a mammalian cell nucleus and fluorescence patterns corresponding to various nuclear domains that have been identified. Chromosome territories have been identified with the *in situ* hybridization approach, but patterns of most remaining domains could be also obtained with the help of autoAbs. This figure was kindly provided by Dr. D. Spector. (Reproduced from Spector (2001) with permission from The Company of Biologists).

tinue to play an important role in the elucidation of the chromatin structure (Stanek et al. 1997; Pollard 2004). Just to remind the reader, another autoAg, DNA topoisomerase II, is a major structural component of the chromosomal scaffold (Hoffmann et al. 1989; Hayakawa et al. 2004b; Chang et al. 2004).

A distinct chromatin structure recognized by autoAbs is the centromere (kinetochore), which is the integral part of human chromosomes and is required for cell division (Hoffmann et al. 1989; Mitchell 1996). The centromere contains alphoid repetitive satellite DNA associated with a set of centromeric proteins (CENPs). The CENPs were discovered by using the serum of patients with CREST syndrome (Moroi et al. 1980), and anti-centromeric autoAbs were also detected in other human diseases such as Raynaud's syndrome, telangiectasia, gastric antral vascular ectasia, etc. (Fritzler 1993; Rattner et al. 1998; He et al. 1998). With the help of anti-centromeric autoAbs and autoAbs to some other nuclear autoAgs (e.g., mitotic spindle apparatus autoAgs, lamin autoAgs), a breakthrough in our knowledge of chromosomal regions and chromosome loci positioning as well as mitosis has been achieved (Hoffmann et al. 1989; Warburton et al. 1997; Andrade et al. 1996).

AutoAbs are potent tools in expanding our knowledge on the nuclear pore complex (NPC) and the nuclear lamina (Enarson et al. 2004). They are targets of the autoimmune response in patients with autoimmune liver disease, SLE, and related conditions (Enarson et al. 2004; Miyachi et al. 2004). The pore complex, which is one of the largest macromolecular complexes of the cell, allows for the transport of molecules in and out of the nucleus. Nuclear lamina is a structure near the inner nuclear membrane and the perinuclear chromatin. It is composed of lamins B and A/C (lamins A and C being just the splice variants of a single gene), which are also present in the nuclear interior, and lamin-associated proteins (LAMs). The nuclear lamina is an essential component of cells and is involved in most nuclear activities including DNA replication, RNA synthesis, nuclear and chromatin organization, cell cycle regulation, cell development and differentiation, nuclear migration, and apoptosis (Enarson et al. 2004). Many autofigs are associated with nuclear envelope (NE) and lamina. AutoAg targets include the lamins A, B, and C of the nuclear lamina; gp210, p62, Nup153, and Tpr within the NPC; and lamin B receptor (LBR), MAN1, and the lamin-associated proteins LAP1 and LAP2, which are integral proteins of the internal nuclear membrane in which more than 50 proteins have been identified (Enarson et al. 2004). AutoAbs to these NE targets have been shown to be correlated with various autoimmune diseases such as primary biliary cirrhosis, other autoimmune liver diseases, and systemic rheumatic diseases. Interestingly, some autoimmune sera label both centromeres and NPCs in interphase cells (Enarson et al. 2004; Miyachi et al. 2004).

The nuclear speckles are enriched in splicing factors and in the factors of the transcription machinery, but the transcription does not occur in the speckles (Spector 2003). If growing mammalian cells are labeled with autoAbs to splicing components, 20–50 shining nuclear domains, i.e., speckles, are usually observed. At the EM level, the speckles consist of morphologically well-defined interchromatin granule clusters (ICGs) and of domains of perichromatin fibrils, some of which are believed to represent precursor mRNAs (pre-mRNAs) (Puvion et al. 1984; Fakan 1994; Melcak et al. 2000). Most mammalian pre-mRNAs contain introns and usually have to be spliced before being transported to the cytoplasm. It has been shown biochemically that the spliceosome formation and splicing may be co-transcriptional events (Wuarin and Schibler 1994). It has been demonstrated that speckles serve as pools of splicing factors that are recruited to the transcription sites (Huang and Spector 1996; Misteli et al. 1997). Speckles are apparently sites of active splicing, as unspliced and released transcripts diffuse from transcription sites into speckles (Huang and Spector 1996; Ishov et al. 1997; Dirks et al. 1997; Snaar et al. 1999; Melcak et al. 2000, 2001).

Cajal bodies (CBs) are small nuclear organelles that contain the three eukaryotic RNA polymerases and a variety of factors involved in transcription and processing of all types of RNA (Raška et al. 1990, 1991a; Gall 2001; Stanek and Neugebauer 2004). It is suggested that pol I, pol II, and pol III transcription and processing complexes are pre-assembled in the CBs before transport to the sites of transcription on the chromosomes and in the nucleoli. The protein marker of Cajal bodies, p80-coilin, was identified with an autoantibody and enabled the investigation of this nuclear organelle. In this way, another nuclear subcompartment could be characterized: the Gemini of cajal bodies, termed the Gems (Liu and Dreyfuss 1996), which contain the survival of motor neurons (SMN) protein. This protein is the product of the disease-determining gene of the neurodegenerative disorder spinal muscular atrophy (SMA) (Liu and Dreyfuss 1996; Gubitz et al. 2004).

The promyelocytic leukemia nuclear body (PML nuclear body) is another nuclear subcompartment discovered with the help of autoAbs targeting P-100 and PML protein (Ascoli and Maul 1991; Szostecki et al. 1990; André et al. 1996). Interest in these bodies was increased upon finding that a fusion protein resulting from a t(15;17) translocation between the PML protein and the retinoid acid receptor alpha, in acute promyelocytic leukemia, resulted in the disruption of these bodies (Puvion-Dutilleul et al. 1995; Koken et al. 1994). Treatment of the leukemia patients with retinoic acid or arsenic trioxide allowed their remission, and, concomitantly, the reformation of PML bodies was observed (Puvion-Dutilleul et al. 1995; Dyck et al. 1994; Koken et al. 1994). A clear function of PML bodies was, however, not established.

A distinct class of autoAgs recognized by sera of patients with autoimmune diseases such as scleroderma and polymyositis (Reimer et al. 1987b; Lee and Craft 1995; Mahler et al. 2003) is associated with the nucleolus. The nucleolus is a subnuclear compartment of eukaryotic cells in which the intense synthesis of ribosomal rRNA and biogenesis of ribosomes take place (Raška 2004). Human diploid cells contain about 400 ribosomal genes organized in the form of several tens of head-to-tail tandem repeats at well-described positions within five pairs of chromosomes, termed nucleolar organizer regions (NORs). The transcription of ribosomal genes is driven by the nucleolar RNA polymerase I, which synthesizes the long precursor rRNA (pre-rRNA) containing 18S, 5.8S, and 28S rRNA sequences (Raška 2004). The biogenesis of mature ribosomal RNA necessitates the presence of non-ribosomal proteins and ribonucleoproteins (RNPs) containing large varieties of small nucleolar RNAs (snoRNAs) (Fatica and Tollervey 2002; Tschochner and Hurt 2003). Ribosomal RNA associates with about 70 ribosomal proteins in the nucleolus. The numerous autoAgs of this subcellular compartment also include several key proteins: RNA polymerase I that transcribes the ribosomal DNA and is enriched in the nucleolar fibrilar centers (FC), but also maps to the dense fibrilar components (DFC) (Fig. 16.8) (Reimer et al. 1987 b; Raška 2004); an important transcription factor termed the NOR90 protein/upstream binding factor that maps to both the DFC and the FC (Rodriguez-Sanchez et al. 1987); DNA topoisomerase I, which is involved in the transcription and maps to the DFC and, to a lesser extent, to the FC (Fig. 16.8; Raška et al. 1995); fibrillarin that plays a role in 18S rRNA processing and maps to the DFC (Figs. 16.8 and 16.9; Ochs et al. 1985; Reimer et al. 1987 a; Dragon et al. 2002); and a subset of ribosomal proteins that maps to the DFC and the GC (Fig. 16.10; Raška et al. 1995). With these autoAb examples (Figs. 16.8 to 16.10.) and with the help of other autoAbs, the nucleolar ultrastructure could be dissected as various autoAgs could be confined to various nucleolar domains. The nucleolus represents the prototype nucleolar organelle that could be, with the help of auto-Abs, described in functional terms such as sites of active or inactive ribosomal DNA, sites of early or late rRNA processing, or sites of ribosome assembly (e.g., Reimer et al. 1987 b; Raška et al. 1989; Raška 2005). Thus, together with the parallel implementation of the functional proteomics (Tschochner and Hurt 2003), enormous progress has been made in understanding how the nucleolar substructures are related to the pathway of ribosome biogenesis.

16.7
Conclusions

The purpose of this chapter was to document the dual significance of autoantibody research, in clinical medicine on one hand and in basic research on the other. Initially, the detection of autoantibodies in human sera became a routine and important test in clinical laboratories. Later on, it became apparent that more detailed characterization of autoantibodies may have a prognostic value and may facilitate clinical treatment follow-up in many cases. Despite such progress, the etiopathogenesis of autoimmune diseases is still unknown. In contrast, autoantibodies have become powerful tools in molecular and cell biology. With the help of autoantibodies, the function of snRNAs was discovered 25 years ago and the mechanism of the splicing process could be described later. These observations opened a new era in basic research, and autoantibodies became "reporter molecules" or molecular probes useful in the identification of autoantigens that are usually evolutionarily conserved and are crucial players in fundamental cellular processes such as DNA replication, transcription, translation, protein transport, and cell cycle progression. In many instances, the func-

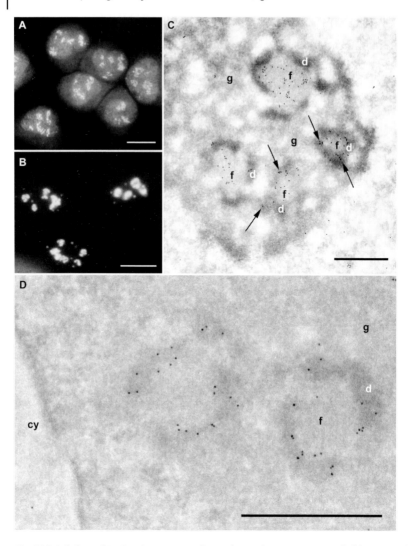

Fig. 16.8 Labeling of RNA polymerase I and fibrillarin. LM (A, B) and EM (C, D) labeling of RNA polymerase I (A, C) and fibrillarin (B, D) in a HeLa cell. Autoimmune serum highly enriched in anti-RNA polymerase I autoAbs (A, C) and "autoimmune" monoclonal antibody to fibrillarin were used. Note the large difference in resolution power between LM (A, B) and EM (C, D). The nucleolar fluorescence pattern is well distinguished and appears to be composed of finer (A) and coarser (B) fluorescent dots. Thin cryosections were used for EM in which the three basic nuclear substructures are seen: electronlucent FC surrounded by DFC and nuclear granular components (GC). Labeling due to RNA polymerase I in C (10-nm gold particles) is enriched in FC but is also present in the DFC (arrows). Fibrillarin (10-nm gold particles) is specifically enriched in the DFC (D). ch: chromatin; cy: cytoplasm; f: nucleolar fibrillar center; d: nucleolar dense fibrillar component; g: nucleolar granular components; the same designations are used in Figs. 16.9. and 16.10 (bar in A and B: 10 μm; bar in C and D: 500 nm). (Reproduced from Raška et al. (1989) with permission from Elsevier Ltd.).

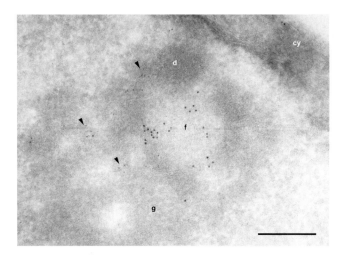

Fig. 16.9 Double labeling of RNA polymerase I and DNA topoisomerase I. In this thin cryo-sectioned RV cell, the RNA polymerase I label (10-nm gold particles) is within the nucleolus found more in the FC, whereas the DNA topoisomerase I label (5-nm gold particles; arrows) is found more in the DFC (bar: 500 nm). (Reproduced from Raška et al. (1989) with permission from Elsevier Ltd.).

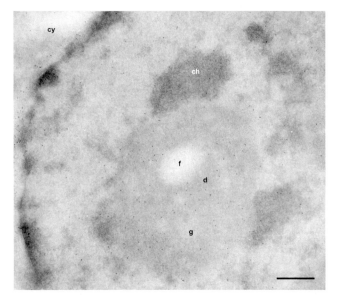

Fig. 16.10 Labeling of ribosomal proteins. The cryo-sectioned HeLa cell was labeled (10-nm gold particles) with autoAbs to ribosomal proteins. The label is enriched in the cytoplasm and in the nucleolar DFC and FC (bar: 500 nm). (Reproduced from Raška et al. (1995) with permission from Elsevier Ltd.).

tion of these autoantigens was determined. The progress was particularly apparent with regard to the cell nucleus. Autoantibodies have enabled us to expand our knowledge about chromatin, nuclear speckles, the nuclear pore complex, nuclear lamina, the nucleolus, Cajal bodies, Gems, and PML bodies. Today, more attention is also being given to the study of cytoplasmic autoantigens. This trend is probably best documented by the discovery of novel cytoplasmic organelles: GW bodies, the plausible site of mRNA degradation. Finally, new multiplex technologies such as proteomics, peptide microarrays, and fluorescent microsphere immunoassays represent powerful approaches to characterize the autoantigens in detail. This may lead to new therapeutic possibilities and a better understanding of the nature of autoimmune diseases.

Acknowledgments

The authors thank Jan Malínský for preparation of the figures and Dr. Z. Cvackova and Ms. S. Rysava for the preparation of the manuscript. This work was supported by Czech grants MSM0021620806 and LC535, AV0Z50110509, 304/04/0692, IAA5039103, 00023728, NK7922, and the Wellcome Trust grant 075834.

Abbreviations

AA	amino acid	GFP	green fluorescent protein
autoAbs	autoantibodies	GWBs	GW bodies containing
autoAgs	autoantigens		multiple glycine (G)/
AGA	anti-Golgi complex auto-antibody		tryptophan (W) repeats
		IC	immunochemistry
ANCA	anti-neutrophil cytoplasmic autoantibody	LM	light microscopy
		MCTD	mixed connective tissue disease
CBs	Cajal bodies		
CREST	calcinosis, Raynaud's syndrome, esophageal motility, sclerodactyly, and telangiectasia	mRNA	messenger RNA
		NE	nuclear envelope
		NOR	nucleolar organizer region
		rRNA	ribosomal RNA
DFC	dense fibrilar component	RNP	ribonucleoprotein
dsDNA	double-stranded DNA	SLE	systemic lupus erythematosus
EM	electron microscopy		
FC	nucleolar fibrilar center	snRNA	small nuclear RNA
GC	nucleolar granular component	tRNA	transfer RNA

References

Alarcón-Segovia, D.; Ruíz-Argüelles, A.; Fishbein, E. *Nature* **1978**; *271*, 67–69

Andrade, L. E.; Chan, E. K.; Peebles, C. L. *Arthritis Rheum.* **1996**; *39*,1643–1653

André, C.; Guillemin, M. C.; Zhu J. *Exp. Cell. Res.* **1996**; *229*, 253–260

Anzai, H.; Fujii, Y.; Nishifuji, K. *J. Dermatol Sci.* **2004**; *35*, 133–142

Aris, J. P.; Blobel, G. *Proc. Natl. Acad. Sci. USA* **1991**; *88*, 931–935

Ascoli, C. A.; Maul, G. G. *J. Cell. Biol.* **1991**; *112*, 785–795

Bach, J. F.; Koutouzov, S.; van Endert, P. M. *Immunol. Rev.* **1998**; *164*, 139–155

Bao, L.; Varden, C. E.; Zimmer, W. E. *Mol. Biol. Rep.* **1998**; *25*, 111–119

Bao, L.; Zimmer, W. E.; Balczon, R. *Autoimmunity* **1995**; *22*, 219–228

Bell, S. A.; Du Clos, T. W.; Khursigara, G. *J. Autoimmun.* **1995**; *8*, 293–303

Bell, S. A.; Hobbs, M. V.; Rubin, R. L. *J. Immunol.* **1992**; *148*, 3369–7336

Berglin, E.; Padyukov, L.; Sundin, U. *Arthritis Res. Ther.* **2004**; *6*, 303–308

Bittencourt, P. L.; Farias, A. Q.; Abrantes-Lemos, C. P. *J. Gastroenterol. Hepatol.* **2004**; *19*, 873–878

Black, D. L.; Chabot, B.; Steitz, J. A. *Cell* **1985**; *42*, 737–750

Bogdanos, D. P.; Baum, H.; Vergani, D. *Clin. Liver. Dis.* **2003**; *7*, 759–777

Boukilas, T. *Toxicol. Lett.* **1993**; *67*, 129–150

Brahms, H.; Raymackers, A.; Union, F. *J. Biol. Chem.* **2000**; *275*, 17122–17129

Bridges, S. L. *Curr. Rheumatol. Rep.* **2004**; *6*, 343–350

Burlingame, R. W.; Boey, L. M.; Starkebaum, G. *J. Clin Invest.* **1994**; *94*, 184–192

Burlingame, R. W.; Rubin, R. L. *Mol. Biol. Rep.* **1996**; *23*, 159–166

Busch, H.; Smetana, K. *The Nucleolus*, ACADEMIC PRESS, New York, London, **1970**

Caspar, D. L. D.; Klug, A. *Physical Principles in the Construciton of Regular Viruses*, Cold Spring Harbor Symposia on Quantitative Biology, **1962**; *27*, 1–24

Chang, Y. H.; Shiau, M. Y.; Tsai, S. T. *Biochem. Biophys. Res. Commun.* **2004**; *320*, 802–809

Chen, M.; Hemmerich, P.; von Mikecz, A. *Immunobiology.* **2002a**; *206*, 474–483

Chen, M.; Rockel, T.; Steinweger, G. *Mol. Biol. Cell.* **2002b**; *13*, 3576–3587

Chen, M.; Zhao, M. H.; Zhang, Y. *Lupus* **2004**; *13*, 584–589

Chung, L.; Utz, P. J. *Curr. Rheumatol. Rep.* **2004**; *6*, 156–163

Conway, J. F.; Watts, N. R.; Belnap, D. M. *J. Virol.* **2003**; *77*, 6466–6473

DeGiorgio, L. A.; Konstantinov, K. N.; Lee, S. C. *Nat. Med.* **2001**; *7*, 1189–1193

Deshmukh, U. S.; Lewis, J. E.; Gaskin, F. *J. Exp. Med.* **1999**; *189*, 531–540

Dirks, R. W.; de Pauw, E. S. D.;Rapp, A. K.; *J. Cell Sci.* **1997**; *110*, 191–201

Dragon, F.; Gallagher, J. E.; Compagnone-Post P. A. *Nature* **2002**; *417*, 505–513

Dyck, J. A.; Maul, G. G.; Miller, W. H. Jr. *Cell* **1994**; *76*, 333–343

Enarson, P.; Rattner, J. B.; Ou, Y. *J. Mol. Med.* **2004**; *82*, 423–433

Eystathioy, T.; Peebles, C. L.; Hamel, J. C. *Arthritis Rheum.* **2002a**; *46*, 726–734

Eystathioy, T.; Chan, E. K. L.; Tenebaum, S. A. *Mol. Biol. Cell* **2002b**; *13*, 1338–1351

Eystathioy, T.; Jakymiw, A.; Fujita, D. J. *J. Autoimmun.* **2000**; *14*, 179–187

Eystathioy, T.; Jakymiw, A.; Chan, E. K. *J Mol Med.* **2003a**; *81*, 811–818

Eystathioy, T.; Jakymiw, A.; Chan, E. K. L. *RNA* **2003b**; *9*, 1171–1173

Faig, O. Z.; Lutz, C. S. *Scand. J. Immunol.* **2003**; *57*, 79–84

Fakan, S. *Trends. Cell. Biol.* **1994**; *4*, 86–90

Falk, R. J.; Jennette, J. C. N. *J. Med.* **1988**; *318*, 1651–1657

Fatica, A.; Tollervey, D. *Curr. Opin. Cell. Biol.* **2002**; *14*, 313–318

Fiedlerová, H.; Masata M.; Malinsky J. *J. Cell. Biochem.* **2005**, *94*, 899–916

Finck, B. K.; Chan, B.; Wofsy, D. *J. Clin. Incest.* **1994**; *94*, 585–591

Francoeur, A. M.; Peebles, C. L.; Heckman, K. J. *J. Immunol.* **1985**; *135*, 2378–2384

Franic, T. V.; Judd, L. M.; Nguyen, N. V. *Am. J. Physiol. Gastroivest. Liver. Physiol.* **2004**; *287*, 910–918

Fritzler, M. J.; Etherington, J.; Sokoluk, C. *J. Immunol.* **1984**; *132*, 2904–2908

Fritzler, M. J.; Hamel, J. C.; Ochs, R. L. *Exp. Med.* **1993**; *178*, 49–62

Gall, J. G. *FEBS Lett.* **2001**; *498*, 164–167

Garcia de la Pena-Lefebvre, P.; Chanseaud, Y.; Tamby, M. C. *Clin. Immunol.* **2004**; *111*, 241–251

Gilburd, B.; Abu-Shakra, M.; Shoenfeld, Y. *Clin. Dev. Immunol.* **2004**; *11*, 53–56

Giraud, M.; Beaurain, G.; Eymard, B. *Genes. Immun.* **2004**; *5*, 398–404

Goldschmeding, R.; van der Schoot, C. E.; ten Bokkel Huinink, D. *J. Clin. Invest.* **1989**; *84*, 1577–1587

Gregor, P.; Jira, M.; Raška, I. *Eur. Heart J.* **1987**; *8*, 773–778

Greidinger, E. L.; Casciola-Rosen, L.; Morris, S. M. *Arthritis Rheum.* **2000**; *43*, 881–888

Griffith, K. J.; Ryan, J. P.; Senécal, J. L. *Clin. Exp. Immunol.* **2002**; *127*, 533–538

Gubitz, A. K.; Feng, W.; Dreyfuss, G. *Exp. Cell. Res.* **2004**; *296*, 51–56

Hargraves, M. M.; Richmond, H.; Morton, R. *Mayo Clin. Proc.* **1948**; *27*, 25–28

Haustein, U. F.; Ziegler, V. *Int. J. Dermatol.* **1985**; *24*, 147–151

Hayakawa, I.; Sato, S.; Hasegawa, M. *Clin. Rheumatol.* **2004a**; *23*, 266–268

Hayakawa, I.; Hasegawa, M.; Takehara, K. *Arthritis Rheum.* **2004b**; *50*, 227–232

He, D.; Zeng, C.; Woods, K. *Chromosoma* **1998**; *107*, 189–197

Hoffmann, A.; Heck, M. M.; Bordwell, B. *J. Exp. Cell. Res.* **1989**; *180*, 409–418

Hong, H. S.; Misek, D. E.; Wang, H. *Cancer Res.* **2004a**; *64*, 5504–5510

Hong, H. S.; Chung, W. H.; Hung, S. I. *Scand. J. Immunol.* **2004b**; *59*, 79–87

Hong, H. S.; Morshed, S. A.; Tanaka, S. *Scand. J. Immunol.* **1992**; *36*, 785–792

Horvath, L.; Czirjak, L.; Telete, B. *Immunol. Lett.* **2001**; *75*, 103–109

Huang, S.; Spector, D. L. *J. Cell Biol.* **1996**; *133*, 719–732

Hultman, P.; Turley, S. J.; Enestrom, S. *J. Autoimmun.* **1996**; *9*, 139–149

Hultman, P.; Ganowiak, K.; Turley, S. J. *Clin. Immunol. Immunopathol.* **1995**; *77*, 291–297

Imai, H.; Nakano, Y.; Kiosawa, K. *Cancer* **1993**; *71*, 26–36

Ishov, A. M.; Stenberg, R. M.; Maul, G. G. *J. Cell. Biol.* **1997**; *138*, 5–16

Jakob, C. O.; van der Meide, P. H.; McDevitt, H. O. *J. Exp. Med.* **1987**; *166*, 798–803

Jenuwien, T. *Science* **2002**; *297*, 2215–2218

Johnson, G. D.; Holborow, E. J.; Glynn, L. E. *Lancet* **1965**; *2*, 878–879

Kamei, H. *J. Autoimmun.* **2004**; *22*, 201–210

Kanazawa, M.; Wada, Y.; Ohno, T. *Clin. Rheumatol.* **2004**; *23*, 456–459

Kao, A. H.; Lacomis, D.; Lucas, M. *Rheumatol.* **2004**; *50*, 209–215

Koberna, K.; Stanek, D.; Malinsky, J. *Acta Histochem.* **2000**; *102*, 15–20

Koken, M. H.; Puvion-Dutilleul, F.; Guillemin, M. C. *EMBO J.* **1994**; *13*, 1073–1083

Koscec, M.; Koren, E.; Wolfson-Reichlin, M. *J. Immunol.* **1997**; *159*, 2033–2041

Kurki, P.; Linder, E.; Virtanen, I. *Nature* **1977**; *268*, 240–241

Lapeyre, B.; Amalric, F.; Ghaffari, S. H. *J. Biol. Chem.* **1986**; *261*, 9167–9173

Latrofa, F.; Chazenbalk, G. D.; Pochutin, P. *J. Clin. Endocrinol. Metab.* **2004**; *89*, 4734–4745

Lee, B.; Craft, J. E. *Int. Rev. Immunol.* **1995**; *12*, 129–144

Leibovitch, L.; George, J.; Levi, Y. *Immunol. Lett.* **1995**; *48*, 129–132

Lerner, M. R.; Boyle, J. A.; Mount, S. M. *Nature* **1980**; *283*, 220–224

Lerner, M. R.; Steitz, J. A. *Proc. Natl. Acad. Sci. USA* **1979**; *76*, 5495–5499

Li, Q.; Hansen, D.; Killilea, A. *J. Cell. Sci.* **2001**; *114*, 797–809

Lindstrom, J. *J. Supramol. Struct.* **1976**; *4*, 389–403

Liu, Q.; Dreyfuss, G. *EMBO J.* **1996**; *15*, 3555–3565

Love, L. A.; Leff, R. L.; Fraser, D. D. *Medicine* **1991**; *70*, 360–374

Ma, J.; Chapman, G. V.; Chen, S. L. *Immunol.* **1991**; *84*, 83–91

Maccioni, R. B.; Cambiazo, V. *Physiol. Rev.* **1995**; *75*, 835–864

Mack, G. J.; Rees, J.; Sandblom, O. *Arthritis Rheum.* **1998**; *41*, 551–558

Mahler, M.; Blüthner, M.; Pollard, K. M. *Clinical. Immunology* **2003**; *107*, 65–79

Mattioli, M.; Reichlin, M. *J. Immunol.* **1973**; *110*, 1318–1324

Mayet, W. J.; Herman, E.; Csermok, E. *J. Immunol. Methods* **1991**; *143*, 57–68

McNairn, A. J.; Gilbert, D. M. *Bioessays.* **2003**; *25*, 647–656

Melcak, I.; Cermanova, S.; Jirsova, K. *Mol. Biol. Cell* **2000**; *11*, 189–204

Melcak, I.; Melcakova, S.; Kopsky, V. *Mol. Biol. Cell* **2001**; *12*, 393–406

Mimouni, D.; Foedinger, D.; Kouba, D. J. *J. Am. Acad.Dermatol.* **2004**; *51*, 62–67

Misteli, T.; Cáceres, J. F.; Spector, D. *Nature* **1997**; *387*, 523–527

Mitchell, A. R. *Mut. Res.* **1996**; *372*, 153–162

Miyachi, K.; Hirano, Y.; Horigome T. *Clin. Exp. Immunol.* **2004**; *136*, 568–573

Monzani, F.; Caraccio, N.; Dardano, A. *Clin. Exp. Med.* **2004**; *3*, 199–210

Moroi, Y.; Peebles, C.; Fritzler, M. J. *Proc. Natl. Acad. Sci. USA* **1980**; *77*, 1627–1631

Mozo, L.; Simo A.; Suarez A. *Eur. J. Gastroenterol. Hepatol.* **2002**; *14*, 771–774

Nishikai, M.; Reichlin, M. *Arthrim Rheum.* **1980**; *23*, 881–888

Novik, K. L.; Nimmrich, I.; Genc, B. *Curr. Issues. Mol. Biol.* **2002**; *4*, 111–128

Nozawa, K.; Fritzler, M. J.; von Muhlen, C. A. *Arthritis Res. Ther.* **2004**; *6*, 95–102

Ohkura, T.; Taniguchi, S.; Yamada K. *Biochem. Biophys. Res. Commun.* **2004**; *321*, 432–440

Ochs, R. L.; Lischwe, M. A.; Spohn, W. H. *Biol. Cell* **1985**; *54*, 327–336

Olmsted, J. B. *J. Biol. Chem.* **1981**; *256*, 11955–11957

Overzet, K.; Gensler, T. J.; Kim, S. J. *Arthritis Rheum.* **2000**; *43*, 1327–1336

Pelacho, B.; Natal, C.; Espana, A. *FEBS Lett.* **2004**; *566*, 6–10

Peter, J. B., and Shoenfeld, Y., *Autoantibodies,* ELSEVIER, Amsterdam, **1996**

Pickering, J. W.; Martins, T. B.; Greer, R. W. *Am. J. Clin. Pathol.* **2002**; *117*, 589–596

Pinnas, J. L.; Northway, J. D.; Tan, E. M. *J. Immunol.* **1973**; *111*, 996–1004

Pollard, K. M., Autoantibodies and Autoimmunity in *Encyclopedia of Molecular Cell Biology and Molecular Medicine*, p. 459–479, R. A. Meyers (ed.), WILEY-VCH, Weinheim, **2004**

Pollard, K. M.; Hultman, P.; Kono, D. H. *Ann. N. Y. Acad. Sci.* **2003**; *987*, 236–239

Pollard, K. M.; Pearson, D. L.; Bluthner, M. *J. Immunol.* **2000**; *165*, 2263–2270

Puvion, E.; Viron, A.; Xu, F. X. *Exp. Cell. Res.* **1984**; *152*, 357–367

Puvion-Dutilleul, F.; Chelbi-Alix, M. K.; Koken, M. *Exp. Cell. Res.* **1995**; *218*, 9–16

Rapoport, T. A. *Trends Biochem. Sci.* **1990**; *15*, 355–358

Raška, I.; Koberna, K.; Malinsky, J. *J. Biol. Cell.* **2004**; *96*, 579–564

Raška, I. *Trends Cell. Biol.* **2003**; *13*, 517–525

Raška, I.; Andrade, L. E.; Ochs, R. L. *Exp. Cell. Res.* **1991 a**; *195*, 27–37

Raška, I.; Petrasovicova, V.; Jarnik, M. *Czech Med.* **1991 b**; *14*, 135–145

Raška, I.; Dundr, M.; Koberna, K. *J. Struct. Biol.* **1995**; *114*, 1–22

Raška, I.; Ochs, R. L.; Andrade, L. E. *J. Struct. Biol.* **1990**; *104*, 120–127

Raška, I.; Reimer, G.; Jarnik, M. *Biol. Cell* **1989**; *65*, 79–82

Rattner, J. B.; Mack, G. J.; Friutzel, M. *J. Mol. Biol. Rep.* **1998**; *25*, 143–155

Reddy, R., Busch, H., U snRNAs of Nuclear snRNPs in *The Cell Nucleus*, Vol. III, H. Bush (Ed.), ACADEMIC PRESS, New York, **1981**

Reeves, W. H.; Nigam, S. K.; Blobel, G. *Proc. Natl. Acad. Sci. USA* **1986**; *83*, 9507–9511

Reichlin, M.; *Lupus* **2003**; *12*, 916–918

Reimer, G.; Pollard, K. M.; Penning, C. A. *Athritis Rheum.* **1987a**; *30*, 793–800

Reimer, G.; Raška, I.; Tan, E. M.; et al. *Virchows. Arch. B.* **1987b**; *54*, 131–134

Robinson, W. H.; Steinman, L.; Utz, P. J. *Arthritis Rheum.* **2002a**; *46*, 885–893

Robinson, W. H.; DiGennaro, C.; Hueber, W. *Nature Med.* **2002b**; *8*, 295–301

Rodriguez-Sanchez, J. L.; Gelpi, C.; Juarez, C. *J. Immunol.* **1987**; *123*, 2579–2584

Rom, W. N.; Turner, W. G.; Banner, R. E. *Chest* **1983**; *83*, 515–819

Rossie, K. M.; Piesco, N. P.; Charley, M. R. *Scand. J. Rheumatol.* **1992**; *21*, 109–115

Rubin, R. L.; McNally, E. M.; Nusinow, S. R. *Clin. Immunol. Immunopathol.* **1985**; *36*, 49–59

Rubin, R. L.; Teodorescu, M.; Beutner E. H. *Lupus* **2004**; *13*, 249–256

Sager, P. R.; Rothfield, N. L.; Oliver, J. M. *J. Cell. Biol.* **1989**; *103*, 1–77

Sato, S.; Fujimoto, M.; Ihn, H. *Dermatology* **1994**; *189*, 23–26

Sato, T.; Uchiumi T.; Kominami, R. *Biochem. Biophys. Res. Commun.* **1990**; *172*, 496–502

Sato, T.; Uchiumi, T.; Arakawa, M. *Clin. Exp. Immunol.* **1994**; *98*, 35–39

Sato, T.; Uchiumi, T.; Ozawa, T. *J. Rheumatol.* **1991**; *18*, 1681–1684

Schellekens, G. A.; Visser, H.; de Jong, B. A. *Arthritis Rheum.* **2000**; *43*, 155–163

Schett, G.; Smolen, J.; Zimmermann, C. *Lupus* **2002**; *11*, 709–715

Schott, M.; Morgenthaler, N. G.; Fritzen, R. *Horm. Metab. Res.* **2004**; *36*, 92–96

Scofield, R. H. *Lancet* **2004**; *363*, 1544–1546

Scott, B. G.; Yang, H.; Tuzun, E. *J. Neuroimmunol.* **2004**; *153*, 16–25

Selak, S.; Schoeroth, L.; Senécal, J. L. *J. Invest. Med.* **1999**; *47*, 311–318

Sharma, A.; Isenberg, D.; Diamond, B. *Rheumatology* **2003**; *42*, 453–460

Sherer Y.; Gorstein A.; Fritzler M. *Semin. Arthritis Rheum.* **2004**; *34*, 501–537.

Shi, M. H.; Tsui, F. W.; Rubin, L. A. *J. Rheumatol.* **1991**; *18*, 252–258

Shrivastav, M.; Mittal, B.; Aggarwal, A. *Clin. Rheumatol.* **2002**; *21*, 505–510

Snaar, S. P.; Vincent, M.; Dirks, R. W. *J. Histochem. Cytochem.* **1999**; *47*, 245–524

Spector, D. L. *J. Cell Sci.* **2001**; *114*, 2891–2893

Spector, D. L. *Annu. Rev. Biochem.* **2003**; *72*, 573–608

Stanek, D.; Neugebauer, K. M. *J. Cell. Biol.* **2004**; *166*, 1015–1025

Stanek, D.; Vencovsky, J.; Kafkova, J. *Arthritis Rheum.* **1997**; *40*, 2172–2177

Steitz, J. A.; Berg, C.; Hendrik, J. P. *J. Cell. Biol.* **1988**; *106*, 545–556

Stinton, L. M.; Eystathioy, T.; Selak, S. *Clin. Immunol.* **2004**; *110*, 30–44

Strassburg, C. P.; Vogel, A.; Manns, M. P. *Autoimmun. Rev.* **2003**; *2*, 322–331

Sun, Y.; Fong, K. Y.; Chung, M. C. *Int. Immunol.* **2001**; *13*, 223–232

Szostecki, C.; Guldner, H. H.; Netter, H. J. *J. Immunol.* **1990**; *145*, 4338–4347

Tan, E. M. *Adv. Immunol.* **1989a**; *44*, 93–151

Tan, E. M. *J. Clin. Invest.* **1989b**; *84*, 1–6

Tan, E. M. *J. Clin. Invest.* **2001**; *101*, 1411–1415

Tan, E. M. and Kunkel, H. G. *J. Immunol.* **1966**; *96*, 464–471

Tan, E. M.; Muro, Y.; Pollard, K. M. *Clin. Exp. Rheumatol.* **1994**; *12 (Suppl 11)*, 27–31

Teodorescu, M.; Ustiyan, V.; Russo, K. *Clin. Immunol.* **2004**; *110*, 145–153

Tschochner, H.; Hurt, E. *Trends Cell Biol.* **2003**; *13*, 255–263

Tuffanelli, D. L.; McKeon, F.; Kleinsmith, D. M. *Arch. Dermatol.* **1983**; *119*, 560–566

Utz, P. J.; Hottelet, M.; Schul, P. H.; et al. *J. Exp. Med.* **1997**; *185*, 843–854

van Gaalen, F. A.; van Aken, J.; Huizinga, T. W. *Arthritis Rheum.* **2004**; *50*, 2113–2121

Vencovsky, J.; Machacek, S.; Sedova, L. *Ann. Rheum. Dis.* **2003**; *62*, 427–430

von Mühlen, C. A.; Tan, E. M. *Semin. Arthritis Rheum.* **1995**; *24*, 323–358

von Westarp, C.; Knox, A. J.; Row, V. V. *Acta. Endocrinol.* **1977**; *84*, 759–767

Warburton, P. E.; Cooke, C. A.; Bourassa S. *Curr. Biol.* **1997**; *7*, 901–904

Whitehouse, J. M.; Fergusson, N.; Currie, G. A. *Clin. Exp. Immunol.* **1974**; *17*, 227–235

Wiik, A.; van der Woude, F. J. *APMIS* **1989**; *97 (Suppl 6)*, 6–7

Williams, R. C. Jr.; Sugiura, K.; Tan, E. M. *Arthritis Rheum.* **2004**; *50*, 1239–1247

Wolffe, A. *Chromatin structure*, Academic Press, London, **1992**

Wuarin, J.; Schibler, U. *Mol. Cell. Biol.* **1994**; *14*, 7219–7225

Zhang, J. Y.; Chan, E. K.; Peng, X. X. *Clin. Immunol.* **2001**; *100*, 149–156

Zhang, M.; Davidson, A. *Autoimmunity* **1999**; *30*, 131–142

Zinkernagel, R. *Nat. Immunol.* **2000**; *1*, 181–185

Zuber, M. A.; Recktenwald, C. *Eur. J. Med. Res.* **2003**; *8*, 61–70

Zwieb, C.; Larsen, N. *Nucleic Acid Res.* **1994**; *22*, 3483–3484

17

Autoantibody Recognition of Macromolecular Structures and Their Subunits

Erica A. Champion and Susan J. Baserga

17.1
Autoantibodies Used to Probe the Function of Macromolecular Structures

Typically, molecular biology is used as a tool to study the pathogenesis of disease. Though this was the original intention of using autoantibodies to probe the cell, it soon became clear that patient-derived autoantibodies would be a useful tool in molecular biology. Indeed, a great deal of information has been gained in the field of basic research. This chapter is about the macromolecular structures of the cell and how autoantibodies have been used to discover them or their functions. Although there are many macromolecular assemblies targeted by autoantibodies inside the cell (Table 17.1), they have been most useful in the study of ribonucleoproteins (RNPs), complexes of RNA, and protein.

The identification of small RNAs in the nucleus of eukaryotic cells spawned from studies of ribosomal RNA (rRNA) processing in the 1960s and 1970s. At this time, the central dogma of DNA to RNA to protein was being expanded upon by the discovery that mRNA must be processed (capped, appended with a poly-A tail, and often spliced) in order to be used as a template for protein translation. Likewise, tRNA processing and rRNA processing were of considerable interest [1].

Methods at that time were such that one could isolate RNA from various subcellular compartments via phenol extraction, separate them according to size by ultracentrifugation on a sucrose gradient, and measure base composition using electrophoresis and chromatography [1]. Therefore, when RNA was extracted from mammalian nuclei, the only way to identify the different species was by size and base composition. Two groups found that in addition to the large (18S-45S, rRNAs) RNAs found in the nucleus, there were a number of small (4-6S) RNA species that were rich in uridylic acid and therefore designated U RNAs [2, 3]. Cellular fractionation indicated that U3 was the major species in the nucleolus, while the others were primarily found in the nucleus [3]. Little was learned about the function of these new small nuclear RNAs until the application of autoantibodies as molecular probes and additional methods became available.

Autoantibodies and Autoimmunity: Molecular Mechanisms in Health and Disease. Edited by K. Michael Pollard
Copyright © 2006 WILEY-VCH Verlag GmbH & Co. KGaA, Weinheim
ISBN: 3-527-31141-6

Table 17.1 Macromolecular structures commonly targeted by autoantibodies.

Macro-molecular complex	Localization	Major autoantigenic component(s)	Clinical association [a]	Function	Ref.
Spliceosome	Nucleus	Sm proteins; U1, U2, U4, U5, U6-specific proteins	SLE, RA, Scl, MCTD	Pre-mRNA splicing	Section 17.2, Table 17.2, and references therein
SSU processome	Nucleolus	Fibrillarin, Mpp10, hU3-55K	SLE, RA, Scl, RP	Pre-18S rRNA processing	Section 17.3, Table 17.3, and references therein
Box C/D snoRNPs	Nucleolus	Fibrillarin	SLE, RA, Scl, RP	rRNA methylation	Section 17.3 and references therein
Box H/ACA snoRNPs	Nucleolus	Unknown	Arthritis	rRNA pseu-douridylation	148
Ro and La RNPs	Nucleus, cytoplasm	Ro 52 kDa, Ro 60 kDa, La 48 kDa	SLE, SS	Unknown	Section 17.4 and references therein
RNase P/MRP (Th/To)	Nucleolus	Rpp30, Rpp38, hPop1, Rpp14, hPop5, Rpp40, hPop4, Rpp21	Scl, RP, SLE	MRP: cleavage A3 of rRNA; M → G1 transition? P: 5′ end processing of tRNA	Section 17.5, Table 17.4, and references therein
Exosome	Nucleolus	PM-Scl 100, PM-Scl 75, hRrp4, hRrp40, hRrp41, hRrp42, hRrp46, hCsl4	PM, Scl, PM/Scl	5.8S rRNA 3′ end formation	Section 17.6, Table 17.5, and references therein
RNA polymerases I, II, and III	Nucleus, nucleolus	NOR-90/hUBF, RPC62, RPC155	Scl, SLE, PM/Scl	DNA transcription	Section 17.7, references therein, 149
Ribosome	Cytoplasm	P proteins, 28S rRNA, S10, L12	SLE	Protein synthesis	150–152
Proteasome	Nucleus, cytoplasm	C9, C2, C8, C5	Myositis, SLE, MS	Protein degradation	153–156
Centromere/kinetochore	Nucleus	CENPs A, B, C	CREST, SLE	Mitotic spindle	157

Table 17.1 (continued)

Macro-molecular complex	Localization	Major autoantigenic component(s)	Clinical association [a]	Function	Ref.
PCNA/Cyclin	Nucleus/ nucleolus in proliferating cells	Cyclin A, 45 kDa, 50 kDa	SLE, AIH, RA, MCTD	Cell cycle control	158–160
SRP	Cytoplasm	54 kDa	PM, SLE	Protein targeting to ER	161, 162
Histidyl tRNA synthetase (Jo-1)	Cytoplasm	HRS	Myositis	Peptide synthesis	163
Ku	Nucleus	70 kDa, 86 kDa	SLE, SS, Scl, PM/Scl, myositis	ATP-dependent DNA helicase	164–167
Topo-isomerase I	Nucleus	Scl-70	CREST, Sc, RP	DNA supercoiling	168
Histones	Nucleus	H1, H2a, H2b, H3, H4	SLE	Chromatin scaffold	169
Nucleic acids	Nucleus	ssDNA, dsDNA, ssRNA, dsRNA	SLE	Genetic information carrier	170

a) Abbreviations: SLE=systemic lupus erythematosus; RA=rheumatoid arthritis; Scl=scleroderma; RP=Raynaud's phenomenon; PM=polymyositis; PM/Scl=polymyositis-scleroderma overlap syndrome; SS=Sjögren's syndrome; AIH=autoimmune hepatitis; MCTD=mixed connective tissue disorder; CREST=calcinosis, Raynaud's phenomenon, esophageal dysfunction, sclerodactyly, and telangiectasia; MS=multiple sclerosis. Details on clinical associations can be found in [148, 171–173].

Initially, the specificity of autoimmune sera was used as a marker for different autoimmune diseases. This was possible using double immunodiffusion in agar gel (Ouchterlony) or by immunostaining [4, 5]. But when autoantibodies were used to probe cell extracts and isolate particular RNAs, it was apparent that this would be a powerful tool to study the small RNAs in terms of their associated proteins and to determine a function for the RNPs.

Since then, autoantibodies have been valuable for the study of RNPs in a number of ways. Often, it has been possible to identify a number of RNAs that could be grouped by a common set of proteins, suggesting a common function. The function of an RNP could also be tested *in vitro*, using autoantibodies to inhibit the proposed function. Additionally, autoantibodies were essential for the discovery of non-abundant RNAs and their associated proteins by allowing the enrichment of a particular RNP. From these first studies, a new discipline in molecular biology was established.

17.2
Autoantibodies as Probes for the Mechanism of Pre-mRNA Splicing

It was an M.D./Ph.D. student at Yale University, Michael Lerner, working under the mentorship of Joan Steitz in the Department of Molecular Biophysics and Biochemistry, who made the leap that birthed the field of small RNP biology. They were the first to use autoantibodies as probes for understanding macromolecular structures, and the structures that they described were small nuclear ribonucleoproteins (snRNPs).

17.2.1
Patients with Systemic Lupus Erythematosus (SLE) Make Antibodies to snRNPs

The occasion of the discovery of snRNPs was a convergence of medicine and molecular biology. Anti-Sm autoantibodies were first described in Stephanie Smith, a lupus patient of Drs. Henry Kunkel and Eng Tan at Rockefeller Hospital in the 1950s and 1960s [5]. The Sm antigen was shown to be nuclear in localization and conserved across species [6]. The antigen of anti-RNP sera (also designated anti-Mo) in patients with SLE and mixed connective tissue disease (MCTD) [7] was sensitive to trypsin and RNase, indicating that it was likely to be an RNP. It localized to the nucleus of mouse cells in a speckled pattern by indirect immunofluorescence. The Sm and RNP antigens were subsequently shown to be molecularly associated [8].

To define precisely the molecular targets of these SLE autoantibodies, Lerner and Steitz performed immunoprecipitations with anti-Sm and anti-RNP sera on extracts made from mouse cells labeled with ^{32}P [9]. They analyzed the resulting labeled small RNAs in the precipitate by denaturing polyacrylamide gel electrophoresis (Fig. 17.1). Following autoradiography, they identified the previously sequenced U1 and U2 snRNAs as well as three other snRNAs, which they called U4, U5, and U6, to be immunoprecipitated by anti-Sm sera. In contrast, they found, with two different anti-RNP sera, that only U1 was immunoprecipitated by anti-RNP sera and suggested that it be renamed anti-U1 RNP. The bands on the gel were indeed U1 and U2 snRNAs because the T1 RNase fingerprint matched that of the previously sequenced U1 and U2 from rat cells. They also carried out important controls such as immunoprecipitation with normal human serum, showing that it did not co-immunoprecipitate these snRNAs. In addition, neither anti-Sm nor anti-U1 RNP could immunoprecipitate deproteinized RNA. Thus, Lerner and Steitz asserted that the autoimmune sera were immunoprecipitating RNA-protein complexes, and called them snRNPs (pro-

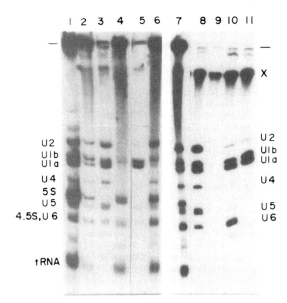

Fig. 17.1 Gel fractionation of snRNAs from nuclear preparations and immune precipitates. ^{32}P-labeled RNAs were extracted with phenol from: lane 1, whole nuclei; lane 2, nuclear soni- cate; lane 3, Pansorbin precipitate with anti-Sm serum; lane 4, remaining supernatant from lane 3; lane 5, Pansorbin precipitate with anti-RNP serum; lane 6, supernatant from lane 5; lane 7, nuclear sonicate; lane 8, anti-Sm Pansorbin precipitate; lane 9, Pansorbin precipitate with normal serum; lane 10, Pansorbin precipitate with serum characterized as mostly RNP; lane 11, anti-RNP Pansorbin precipitate. Lanes 1–6 and 7–11 represent two different experi- ments. (Reprinted from [9]).

nounced "snurps"). Furthermore, to examine the nature of the protein constitu- ents of snRNPs, immunoprecipitations on extracts from ^{35}S methionine-labeled mouse cells were carried out, and it was evident that both anti-U1 RNP and anti-Sm immunoprecipitate the same seven proteins in the same amounts. They rightly concluded, in their own words, that "we have established the bio- chemical identity of the nuclear antigens designated RNP and Sm in the rheu- matic disease literature."

What did we learn about the macromolecular structure of snRNPs from these first experiments? First, that the snRNAs were not free in the cell, but stably as- sociated with proteins. Second, that there were antigenic proteins common to all snRNPs (though this was slightly revised later; see below and Table 17.2). Third, that there is a strong possibility that each snRNP is in a separate com- plex. Fourth, that the technique of using autoimmune sera to detect snRNPs might be used to investigate whether snRNPs are required for the RNA proces- sing of nuclear pre-mRNAs and to discover additional macromolecular assem- blies. These were two predicted applications of the newly developed methodolo- gy that were realized.

Table 17.2 Autoantibodies to spliceosome components.

Autoantibody	Antigen	Function	Ref.
Anti-Sm	Sm proteins B/B' and D_{1-3} common to major spliceosome U1, U2, U4, U5 snRNPs; LSm proteins of U6	Sm proteins required for trimethyl guanosine cap modification on snRNA; nuclear localization of snRNPs	28, 174
Anti-U1 RNP	70K, A and C U1 snRNP-specific proteins	U1 snRNP base pairs with 5' splice site	28, 43, 175
Anti-U2	A' and B' U2 snRNP-specific proteins	U2 snRNP base pairs with branch point	43, 175, 176
Anti-U4/U6	150 kDa protein of U4/U6 snRNP	U4 snRNP escorts U6 snRNP to the spliceosome via base-pairing; U6 base pairs with 5' splice site after U1 is released	37, 175
Anti-U5	U5 snRNP-specific proteins	U5 snRNP interacts with both exons in spliceosome	38, 39, 175

17.2.2
Are snRNPs Involved in Splicing?

Pre-mRNA splicing was first described in viral systems based on the discontinuity of viral genes and their mature mRNAs [10, 11]. It was soon clear that this was not some unusual consequence of the compact nature of viral genomes, as it was also described soon after in mammalian cells. The protein-coding portion of genes from higher eukaryotes was interrupted by DNA sequence that would not be in frame if an RNA bearing these sequences were translated. However, the mature cytoplasmic mRNA lacked these sequences and was thus perfectly translatable. The pre-mRNA must, therefore, be spliced before it is translated. The translatable portion of the pre-mRNA came to be known as exons, and the portion to be spliced out as introns.

Two groups [12, 13] proposed that snRNPs are involved in pre-mRNA splicing. Lerner et al. made a multifaceted argument backed up by experimental evidence. They reasoned that if the U1, U2, U4, U5, and U6 snRNPs were involved in pre-mRNA splicing, they would be conserved in all species where splicing was known to occur. This was demonstrated to be so by immunoprecipitations with autoimmune sera in extracts representing human, mouse, and insect. In addition, snRNPs would be present in the highest abundance in metabolically active cells, such as the liver, and reduced in silenced cells, such as chicken erythrocytes. This was also verified. Gradient fractionation of nuclear extract indicated that the snRNPs could be found in fractions bearing the pre-mRNAs, providing evidence that they are indeed associated. Most importantly, both Lerner et al. and Rogers and Wall observed that the U1 snRNA had potential base-pairing interactions with the pre-mRNA splice sites. This provided a framework for thinking about how snRNPs might function in splicing by using snRNA complementarity to pre-mRNA. In addition, if snRNPs were involved in pre-mRNA splicing, then adding autoantibodies to splicing reactions should be inhibitory, generating a critical, testable hypothesis.

17.2.3
A Useful Tool: Anti-Sm Monoclonal Antibodies Derived from an SLE Mouse Model

With the knowledge that MRL/l mice, afflicted with a lupus-like syndrome, also make anti-Sm antibodies [14], the laboratories of Charles Janeway and Joan Steitz collaborated on the production of an anti-Sm hybridoma cell line using the spleen of the MRL/l mouse as a source of antibody [15]. Ethan Lerner, also an M.D./Ph.D. student at Yale, working with his brother, Michael, recovered monoclonal antibodies to the Sm proteins (hybridoma cell line Y12) and to rRNA and DNA. The anti-Sm monoclonal antibody performed identically to patient sera in co-immunoprecipitation of U1, U2, U4, U5, and U6 snRNAs from ^{32}P-labeled HeLa cell extracts. This renewable resource of anti-Sm antibodies was a valuable tool for investigating the assembly and function of snRNPs, and both the antibody and the hybridoma cell line have been shared (and continue to be shared) with laboratories around the world. As a result, the anti-Sm monoclonal antibody developed in 1981 has been cited so frequently that the publications are too numerous to mention here.

In Joan Steitz's laboratory the anti-Sm monoclonal antibody was used by a graduate student, Karen Montzka (now Wassarman), to detect new low-abundance Sm protein-containing snRNPs, which they called U11 and U12 [16]. Having hypothesized that there were snRNPs that could not be resolved on denaturing polyacrylamide gels, they searched for them on 2D gels following large-scale anti-Sm immunoprecipitations from HeLa cell extracts. The function of U11 and U12 remained a mystery until eight years later, when it was proven that they were involved in pre-mRNA splicing of AT-AC introns, a previously undetected minor class of introns found in eukaryotic cells [17–21].

17.2.4
Autoantibodies Are Used to Test Whether snRNPs Are Involved in Pre-mRNA Splicing

To investigate whether snRNPs are involved in pre-mRNA splicing using autoantibodies, the development of pre-mRNA splicing assays was essential. The assays evolved between 1981 and 1985, and at each step in their development, when autoantibodies were used to probe the mechanism of splicing, it was clear that snRNPs were necessary for the splicing reactions to occur.

The first experimental evidence that snRNPs were required for pre-mRNA splicing was derived from analysis of splicing in isolated nuclei from adenovirus-infected HeLa cells [22]. Pre-incubation of the nuclei with both anti-Sm and anti-U1 RNP inhibited splicing of adenovirus early mRNAs. In contrast, normal human serum or other autoantibodies (anti-Ro and anti-La) had no effect. Further evidence that snRNPs were involved in splicing came from a coupled transcription-processing system where anti-Sm (patient sera and monoclonal antibody) and anti-U1 RNP sera inhibited splicing of transcripts from the adenovirus major late promoter [23]. Similarly, injection of SV40 viral DNA with anti-Sm and anti-U1 RNP sera into *Xenopus* oocytes indicated inhibition of splicing of SV40 late viral transcripts [24]. Consistent with the perception that the splicing machinery must be conserved, they thus demonstrated that "human antibodies inhibit splicing of monkey viral RNA in frog oocytes." The laboratories of Walter Keller and Reinhard Lührmann used anti-Sm autoimmune sera conjugated to protein A-Sepharose to *deplete* splicing extracts of snRNPs, which has some biochemical advantages over adding the sera to the splicing reactions [25]. They found that depletion of only 50% of the snRNPs resulted in splicing inhibition of adenovirus major late mRNA. Grabowski et al. [26] coined the term "spliceosome" (splicing body) to describe the multicomponent RNA-protein complex where pre-mRNA splicing takes place. They showed, using anti-Sm and anti-U1 RNP sera, that the spliceosome contains snRNPs. Indeed, snRNPs are involved in splicing.

17.2.5
The Protein Components of snRNPs

Investigators have long been interested in the protein components of the snRNPs and, with autoimmune sera in hand, they began to define them. At first this was carried out in a cumbersome manner using immunoprecipitations on extracts from ^{35}S methionine–labeled cells (e.g., [9]) and later using immunoblots or Western blots (e.g., [27]). Much work in a number of different laboratories has contributed to the conclusion that the anti-Sm sera reacts with the B'/B and D_{1-3} components of the Sm proteins (defined as B/B', D_{1-3}, E, F, and G) and that the anti-U1 RNP sera reacts with the U1 snRNP-specific proteins U1-70K, A, and C to varying extents (reviewed in [28]). With the advent of cDNA expression library screening, autoantibodies were also used to clone the genes coding for the antigenic proteins, as is detailed in Chapter 18 of this book.

17.2.6
Subcellular Localization of Splicing Components

The subcellular localization of the anti-Sm and anti-U1 RNP antigens was studied as part of the initial characterization and identification of the autoantibodies.
They were found to be nuclear, in a distinctive speckled pattern that excluded
the nucleoli [7, 29]. Similarly, the anti-Sm monoclonal antibody yielded a
speckled nuclear pattern in indirect immunofluorescence [15]. Thus, snRNPs
were localized to discrete areas of the nucleus in speckles.

As microscopy techniques and microscopes improved, it was possible to ask
whether the anti-Sm and anti-U1 RNP patient antibodies were recognizing the
same set of nuclear speckles. Double immunofluorescence staining followed by
digital image analysis indicated that both antigens were without a doubt found
together in nuclear speckles [30]. This prompted the tantalizing hypothesis that
the speckles represent sites of transcription and pre-mRNA processing. After
many years of experimentation, it is now clear that the speckles contain little
DNA and are therefore not the sites of transcription and splicing, but are instead thought to be assembly/modification sites that deliver snRNPs to actively
transcribed genes. Furthermore, the nuclear speckles are dynamic entities, as
RNA and protein components can move among them and other parts of the nucleus (reviewed in [31]).

17.2.7
Specific Autoantibodies to Each Spliceosomal snRNP

Since they were first used to probe the structure of snRNPs, extensive work
with the anti-Sm and anti-U1 RNP autoantibodies has demonstrated that many
times they are of mixed specificity. For example, Western blot analysis of purified U5 snRNPs with anti-Sm and anti-U1 RNP sera indicated that they also
contained antibodies to U5-specific proteins [32]. However, antibodies specific to
the U2, U4, U5, and U6 snRNPs have proved to be much more rare in occurrence (see Table 17.2).

Antibodies specific for the U2 snRNP were first detected in a Japanese patient
with scleroderma-polymyositis overlap syndrome (1/500 sera screened) and subsequently in several other screens [33–36]. Similarly, autoantibodies to the U4/
U6 particle have been detected in a screen of 400 sera from patients with systemic sclerosis [37]. (The U4 and U6 snRNAs can be found in a single particle
because of the extensive base pairing between the snRNAs.) Anti-U5-specific autoantibodies have been described in sera from patients with systemic sclerosis-
polymyositis overlap syndrome (1/1171 patients with connective tissue diseases
and 1/281 patients with systemic sclerosis) [38, 39].

Most recently, it has become clear that the U6 snRNA is associated with a different set of proteins than the Sm proteins but that they form the same structure [40, 41]. They are called LSm (Like Sm) proteins. IgM autoantibodies to the
LSm4 protein associated with the U6 snRNA have been found in a patient with

infectious mononucleosis, and IgG anti-LSm4 antibodies have been found to co-exist in many anti-Sm sera [42]. Thus, Sm autoantigens likely include both Sm and LSm complexes.

17.2.8
SLE Led the Way to Our Current Understanding of the Mechanism of Pre-mRNA Splicing

The discovery in 1979 that autoantibodies from patients with SLE recognize snRNPs was fundamental to the elucidation of their function in pre-mRNA splicing. With the knowledge that snRNPs are involved in splicing but lacking the understanding of how, in the 1980s investigators turned increasingly to biochemical exploitation of *in vitro* splicing extracts and then to yeast genetics upon the identification of snRNPs in *S. cerevisiae*. Our current knowledge is that in the major spliceosome, the U1 snRNP interacts with the 5′ splice site on the pre-mRNA and the U2 snRNP with the branch point in the intron, both via base-pairing interactions (Fig. 17.2; reviewed in [43, 44]). The tri-snRNP of U4/U5/U6 then joins the pre-mRNA, and a dynamic series of RNA rearrangements occurs, resulting in the release of the U1 and U4 snRNPs. In the minor spliceo-

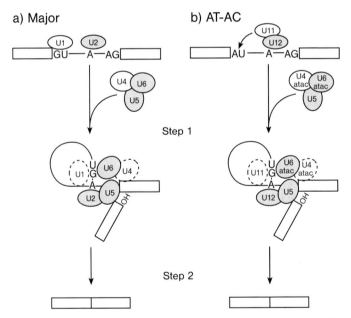

Fig. 17.2 Spliceosome assembly and action. (a) The major spliceosome and (b) the AT-AC spliceosome are pictured at an early stage of spliceosome assembly and after the first reaction step (formation of the lariat intermediate) has occurred. U11 and U12 are pictured as entering the spliceosome as a two-snRNP complex. After joining of the U4-U6-U5 or U4atac-U6atac-U5 tri-snRNP, a conformational change occurs that loosens the association of U1 or U11 and U4 or U4atac with the spliceosome. (Reprinted from [43]).

some (Fig. 17.2), U11 and U12 replace U1 and U2, and the U4 and U6 analogues, U4atac and U6atac, replace their counterparts. There is evidence that RNA splicing is an RNA-catalyzed reaction, with the U6 snRNP playing the central role. Recently we learned that RNA splicing requires many more factors than originally envisioned (reviewed in [44]) and that transcription, splicing, and mRNA export are interconnected (reviewed in [45]).

17.3
U3 and the Box C/D Small Nucleolar RNAs (snoRNAs)

The box C/D family of snoRNAs was discovered as an unexpected result of using autoantibodies to study the protein components of the U3 snoRNP. U3 was the first of this family to be identified because it is very abundant in the cell and therefore easily visualized without stringent purification. Through early studies, it was determined that U3 is part of a ribonucleoprotein complex that has a function in pre-rRNA processing, but the protein components of that RNP remained elusive. Autoantibodies identified the first U3-associated protein, fibrillarin. But perhaps more importantly, immunoprecipitation of RNA using the fibrillarin autoantibodies revealed additional fibrillarin-associated RNAs that were less abundant than U3. These RNAs were found to share the box C/D motif and a set of common proteins and were found to function in methylation of pre-rRNA. Interestingly, U3 does not share the common box C/D function, but rather is required for cleavage of the small subunit pre-rRNA.

17.3.1
The U3 snoRNA in Ribosome Biogenesis

Early studies of the large rRNAs and their precursors revealed that rRNA was processed prior to incorporation into the mature ribosome. While mature rRNAs of 18S and 28S were found in the cytoplasm of mammalian cells, larger precursors could be found in the nucleolus. The kinetics of radioactively labeled precursor rRNAs showed a stepwise series of cleavage events that derived the mature 18S and 28S rRNAs from a single 45S precursor. As shown in Figure 17.3, it was known that the 45S precursor is transcribed as a single unit and cleaved at four sites: (1) separating the 5′ external transcribed spacer (ETS) from the 18S rRNA, (2) separating the 18S from the first internal transcribed spacer (ITS1), (3) separating ITS1 from the 5.8S and 28S rRNAs, and (4) separating the 5.8S rRNA from the 28S rRNA. Except for the alternation of cleavages 2 and 3 depending on species and conditions, these cleavages were observed to occur in order [1]. Since then, many *trans*-acting factors have been discovered to assist in the processing of rRNA, and the sites of cleavage have been defined more precisely, but the major cleavages remain the same [46].

It was generally hypothesized and accepted by the early 1980s that U3 had a role in rRNA maturation [47], but evidence to define this role was lacking. U3

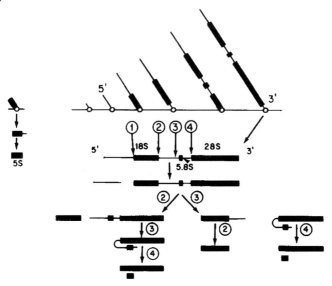

Fig. 17.3 Scheme for processing mammalian ribosomal RNA. The primary product of rRNA synthesis is a 45S molecule of about 12.5 kb. The first cleavage at site 1 removes the 5′-terminal leader sequence. The second cleavage can be at either site 2 or site 3, depending on the species of cell and to some extent on environmental conditions; the predominant pathway apparently is determined by the conformational state of the first intermediate. The final trimming near site 4 is usually the rate-limiting step in the processing pathway, thus causing a substantial accumulation of the proximal intermediate, the 32S component. This trimming involves at least two cuts in the polynucleotide backbone, one at the 5′ end of the 28S component and another at the 3′ end of the 5.8S component. The 5.8S component, 140 nucleotides in length, is a stretch in the 5′ region of the 32S component that remains bound to 28S component by base paring after the final cleavage. (Reprinted from [1]).

had been colocalized with rRNA in the nucleolus [3], and chemical association of the U3 RNA with rRNA had been demonstrated [48]. Furthermore, it was shown that the U3 RNA could be found in ribonucleoprotein particles that associate with the 32S pre-rRNA via RNA-RNA and RNA-protein interactions [49]. When immunoprecipitation of the U1 and U2 snRNAs by human autoimmune sera implicated these RNPs in processing of pre-mRNA in the nucleus, it was further hypothesized that U3 performed an analogous function in the nucleolus: processing of pre-rRNA [50]. Still, the question remained: how?

17.3.2
Fibrillarin Is the First U3-associated Protein

Protein components of RNPs are critical for their function, yet the proteins associated with the U3 snoRNA could not be identified until the 1980s, when it was determined that human autoantibodies could precipitate the U3 snoRNA.

When scleroderma patient sera were used in protein immunoprecipitation, a protein of 34 kDa was isolated. Conversely, antibodies raised against this 34-kDa protein were able to immunoprecipitate the U3 snoRNA. Because the protein was visualized in the fibrillar regions of the nucleolus, it was named fibrillarin [51, 52].

Further studies using both patient sera and various anti-U3 RNP antibodies identified at least five potential additional U3-associated proteins [53]. Indeed, genetic and biochemical studies uncovered 11 additional U3-associated proteins in 15 years (Table 17.3 and references therein). Still, additional uncharacterized proteins remained. With the application of mass spectrometry and affinity purification techniques to study peptide fragments from purified cell extracts, nucleolar proteins were identified in bulk: a proteomic analysis of the yeast nucleolus found 271 proteins, 30% encoded by previously uncharacterized genes [54–56]. It is currently understood that the U3 snoRNA exists in two RNPs: a small nucleolar RNP (snoRNP) that sediments at 12S on a sucrose gradient (see Table 17.3) and a large RNP termed the SSU processome that sediments at 80-90S and is described below.

Purifications of the yeast U3 RNP yielded a total of 40 U3-associated proteins (Table 17.3) [55–57]. Each of these proteins was localized to the nucleolus and shown to associate specifically with the U3 snoRNA [55, 57]. Previous experiments *in vitro* in mouse cell extracts and *in vivo* in yeast and *Xenopus* oocytes had proven that the U3 snoRNA was required for 18S pre-rRNA processing [58–60]. Therefore, these proteins were genetically depleted and shown to be required for maturation of the small subunit (18S) rRNA, indicating that each individual protein is integral to the function of the U3 RNP in pre-rRNA processing. The entire ~2.2-MDa complex, named the SSU processome for its role in small subunit processing, most likely corresponds to the >60S complex observed in earlier gradients [49]. Additionally, the SSU processome likely corresponds to the terminal knobs observed decorating the ends of pre-rRNA transcripts in Miller chromatin spreads (Fig. 17.4) [61], because upon depletion of any SSU processome protein, the terminal knobs do not form [55].

Knowing the identity of the proteins involved in pre-rRNA processing is the first step to understanding how mature rRNA is produced. Currently, work is being done to determine why and how each of the 40 proteins is necessary for rRNA maturation. It is remarkable that a complex as large as the ribosome itself is required for just a small portion of ribosome assembly. Furthermore, none of the 40 proteins yet identified is predicted to be an endonuclease, which could perform the cleavages that release the small subunit rRNA from the 45S precursor. This suggests that the SSU processome may function structurally in ribosome biogenesis, by coordinating the orientation of the pre-rRNA to allow cleavage by a yet unidentified endonuclease. To begin to explore this hypothesis, studies are underway to determine the structure of the U3 snoRNA and its associated proteins.

It is interesting to note that among the 40 U3-associated proteins, only fibrillarin was identified using patient sera. One would expect such a large particle

Table 17.3 Components of the SSU processome. [a]

Yeast protein	ORF name	Human homologue(s)	Size (kDa)	Sub-complex	Comments	Ref.
Utp5	YDR398w	WDR36, KIAA0007	71.9	A/tUtp	WD repeats; Utp15-interacting	55, 177, 178
Utp4	YDR324c	CIRH1A, FLJ10458, REC14	87.8	A/tUtp	WD repeats	55, 56, 177–179
Utp8	YGR128c		80.1	A/tUtp		55, 56, 177–179
Utp9	YHR196w		65.1	A/tUtp	Coiled-coils	55, 56, 177–179
Utp10	YJL109c	FLJ10359	199.9	A/tUtp	HEAT repeats	55, 56, 177–179
Utp15	YMR093w	FLJ12787, HPRP8BP, TUWD12	57.5	A/tUtp	WD repeats; Utp5-interacting	55, 177–179
Utp17/ Nan1/ Lph1	YPL126w	FLJ12519, TLE4, PF20	101.1	A/tUtp	WD repeats; exit from mitosis	55, 56, 177–179
Utp1/ Pwp2	YCR057c	PWP2H, FLJ25955	103.9	B	WD repeats	55, 56, 177, 179
Utp6	YDR449c	HCA66, CRNKL1	52.3	B	cl-TPR	55, 56, 177, 179
Utp12/ Dip2	YLR129w	WDR3, FLJ25955, REC14	106.3	B	WD repeats	55, 56, 177, 179
Utp13/ Cst29	YLR222c	TBL3, WDR5, FLJ25955	91.0	B	WD repeats	55, 56, 177, 179
Utp18	YJL069c		66.4	B	WD repeats	56, 57, 177, 179
Utp21	YLR409c	CGI-48, TBL3, LOC123169	104.8	B	WD repeats	56, 57, 177, 179
Utp22	YGR090w	NOL6	140.5	C		56, 57, 177, 179
Nop1	YDL014w	Fibrillarin (FIB)	34.4	U3 snoRNP	Common box C/D, methyl-transferase	177, 180, 181
Nop5/ Nop58/ Luc9	YOR310c	Nop5/Nop58, NOL5A, PRPF31	56.8	U3 snoRNP	Common box C/D, KKE/D	177, 181–184
Nop56/ Sik1	YLR197w	Nop56, NOL5A, PRPF31	56.7	U3 snoRNP	Common box C/D, KKE/D	56, 177, 181, 185
Rrp9	YPR137w	hU3-55K, TAF5, TAF5L	64.9	U3 snoRNP	WD repeats	55, 56, 177, 181, 186, 187
Snu13	YEL026w	15.5K, RPL7A, NOLA2	13.4	U3 snoRNP	Common box C/D, U4 snRNA	177, 181
Dhr1/ Ecm16	YMR128w	DHX37, DHX29, DHX36	144.8	Un-classified	DEAH box heli-case	56, 177, 188
Imp3	YHR148w	C15ORF12 (hImp3), RPS9	21.8	Un-classified	S4 RBD; inter-acts with Mpp10	55, 56, 177, 189, 190

Table 17.3 (continued)

Yeast protein	ORF name	Human homologue(s)	Size (kDa)	Sub-complex	Comments	Ref.
Imp4	YNL075w	IMP4, RPF1, BRIX	33.5	Un-classified	RNA binding superfamily; interacts with Mpp10	55, 56, 177, 189, 190
Mpp10	YJR002w	MPHOSPH10 (hMpp10), LOC123169	66.8	Un-classified	Coiled-coils; interacts with Imp3, Imp4, U3	55, 56, 177, 191
Rrp5	YMR229c	PDCD11, CRNKL1, CSTF3	193	Un-classified	S1 RBD, cl-TPRs	55, 56, 177, 192
Sof1	YLL011w	DKFZP564-O0463, FLJ25955	56.8	Un-classified	WD repeats	55, 56, 177, 193
Utp2/ Nop14	YDL148c	C4ORF9	94.3	Un-classified	Coiled-coils	55, 56, 177
Utp3/ Sas10	YDL153c	SAS10	70.1	Un-classified	Nap family; silencing; Mpp10-interacting	55, 177
Utp7/ Kre31	YER082c	C6ORF11, PRP19	62.3	Un-classified	WD repeats; adenylate binding site	55, 56, 177
Utp11	YKL099c	CGI-94	30.3	Un-classified	Coiled-coils	55, 177
Utp14	YML093w	UTP14A, DMP1, RBM28	102.9	Un-classified	Coiled-coils; ATP/GTP bind-ing site (P-loop)	55, 177
Utp16/ Bud21	YOR078w		24.2	Un-classified	Coiled-coils; non-essential (cs)	55, 56, 177
Utp19/ Noc4	YPR144c	MGC3162	63.6	Un-classified		56, 57, 177, 194
Utp20/ Yba4	YBL004w	DRIM	287.6	Un-classified	Coiled-coils	56, 57, 177
Krr1	YCL059c	HRB2	37.2	Un-classified	KH domain	56, 57, 177, 195
Emg1/ Nep1	YLR186w	C2F	27.9	Un-classified		56, 57, 177, 196, 197
Rps4	YJR145c	RPS4X, RPS4Y1, RPS4Y2	293.0	Un-classified	Ribosomal protein	56, 57, 177
Rps6	YPL090c	RPS6	270.2	Un-classified	Ribosomal protein	56, 57, 177
Rps7	YOR096w	RPS7	215.3	Un-classified	Ribosomal protein	56, 57, 177

17.4
The La and Ro Autoantigens

Prior to the use of autoantibodies as molecular probes, only the most abundant RNA molecules could be detected. When patient-derived autoantibodies were found to immunoprecipitate proteins associated with novel RNAs, new avenues were opened to the study of RNPs and a new set of non-coding RNAs was identified, including those associated with the Ro and La autoantigens. The La autoantigen is transiently associated with RNA polymerase III transcripts and has been shown to be essential for proper 3′ end maturation of tRNAs in the nucleus. The Ro autoantigens bind a subset of the La-associated RNAs, the Y RNAs, and the Ro particles are proposed to function in quality control of snRNAs in the cytoplasm. Autoimmune sera initially related the La and Ro proteins because they both associate with Y RNAs, but it is becoming evident that they perform distinct functions within the cell.

17.4.1
Ro and La Are Related Autoantigens

After 25 years of using autoantibodies as molecular probes, it is clearer than ever that a direct relationship does not exist between an autoantigenic target and the clinical manifestation of the autoimmune disease. As shown in Table 17.1, patients with SLE may carry autoantibodies to any number of macromolecular complexes. This information was only beginning to come to light in the early 1980s, when an array of patient sera was readily available and the proteins or RNA species targeted could be easily fractionated on a gel. It was at this time that the Ro and La autoantigens were discovered.

When SLE patient sera were used to immunoprecipitate radiolabeled RNA from mouse cell homogenate, discrete sets of bands were observed. Distinct from the set of small U RNAs precipitated by anti-Sm sera, anti-Ro sera immunoprecipitated two novel small cytoplasmic RNAs, and anti-La sera precipitated a highly banded pattern of small RNAs (Fig. 17.5) [70]. It was further determined that the autoantigenicity of these particles depended on a protein component, indicating that the La autoantigen is a snRNP and the Ro autoantigen is a scRNP (small cytoplasmic ribonucleoprotein, pronounced "scyrp") [70].

It appeared that the La snRNPs and Ro scRNPs were quite different, due to their distinct intracellular localizations, but fingerprint analysis of the RNAs suggested that this was not so. In addition to the previously identified 5S rRNA, the La-associated RNAs included one that had an identical fingerprint to the Ro-associated hY5 [71]. Additional reconstruction experiments confirmed the association by showing that the Ro particles contain the La autoantigen, and the two RNPs were united by their association with the Y RNAs [71].

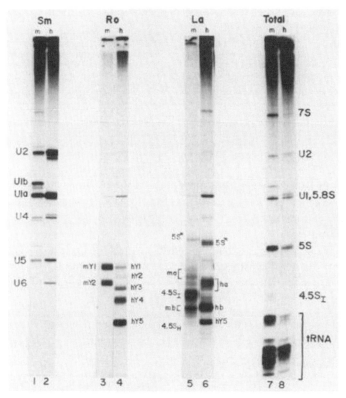

Fig. 17.5 RNA species immunoprecipitated by anti-Sm, anti-Ro, and anti-La antibodies. Immune precipitates from ^{32}P-labeled mouse and human cells. Small RNAs included in antibody precipitates from extracts of ^{32}P-labeled human HeLa (h) and mouse Ehrlich ascites (m) cells were fractionated on a 10% polyacrylamide gel as described in the text. An anti-Sm precipitate is shown in lanes 1 and 2, anti-Ro is shown in lanes 3 and 4, and anti-La is shown in lanes 5 and 6. Lanes 7 and 8 show total small RNAs from mouse Ehrlich ascites cells and HeLa cells, respectively. All lanes shown are from the same gel, although different amounts of precipitates and different exposure times were utilized to maximize visualization of the various small RNA spectra. (Normally, relative to anti-Sm, we utilized twice as many cells for a La precipitate and 10 times as many for a Ro precipitate.) Note that U1 and U2 RNAs appear in low amounts in Ro and La precipitates; the levels of binding (exaggerated because of the large amounts of cells used) can be demonstrated to be non-specific by comparison with non-immune serum (not shown). (Reprinted from [71]).

17.4.2
The La snRNPs

La was known to associate with a number of small non-coding RNAs, including the Y RNAs [71], viral RNAs [71], 5S rRNA and its precursors [72], and tRNAs [72], all established RNA polymerase III transcripts. Indeed, when α-amanitin was used to inhibit transcription by other RNA polymerases, the levels of La-associated RNAs were not affected [71, 72]. This is in fact a necessary correlation, as it was subsequently shown that the 50-kDa La autoantigen binds an oligouridylate stretch that is found at the 3' end of all RNA polymerase III transcripts [73, 74]. Though it has been proposed that La functions in the initiation and termination of polymerase III transcription [75–77], it has also been shown that La acts as a chaperone for pre-tRNAs [78] and likely for other polymerase III transcripts [79].

17.4.3
The Ro scRNPs

In humans, four distinct Y (cytoplasmic) RNAs exist: Y1, Y3, Y4, and Y5 (Y2 is a degradation product of Y1), whereas only two Y RNAs can be found in mice [80]. These poorly conserved RNAs are predicted to form a secondary structure that includes a stem that is required for Ro protein binding [81]. Besides the La 50-kDa protein, two Ro proteins, Ro60 and Ro52, named for their molecular weights, have been found to constitute the Ro scRNP [81, 82]. The function of these RNPs is not known, but it is hypothesized that they associate with misfolded snRNAs as a quality-control mechanism [83].

17.5
RNase P and RNase MRP

The use of autoantibodies has made an exceptional impact on the identification and characterization of the two endoribonucleases RNase P and RNase MRP. Although both had been previously identified based on their nucleolytic activities, their protein and RNA compositions, as well as their functions, could not be determined until the application of autoantibodies revealed that nuclear RNase P and RNase MRP are closely related ribonucleoproteins. Both particles are responsible for specific cleavages in pre-RNAs: RNase P cleaves the 5' end of precursor tRNA, and RNase MRP has been shown to cleave pre-rRNA, though other functions for each have not been ruled out. Remarkably, despite their differing functions, RNases P and MRP share at least eight identical protein components and differ only in their RNA sequence and one additional protein each (Table 17.4).

17.5.1
RNase P and RNase MRP Are Structurally Related

The specific precursor tRNA cleavage activity of RNase P was partially purified over 30 years ago from *E. coli* extract [84], and the activity required one protein and one RNA component [85]. However, methods of identifying these components were not available at that time. Similarly, when RNase MRP was identified in mammalian cells by its function in cleavage of mitochondrial RNA, it

Table 17.4 Components of RNase P and RNase MRP.

Human protein	Yeast homologue	RNase P	RNase MRP	Ref.
RNA	RNA	RPR1	NME1/RRP2	
hPop1	Pop1	+	+	96, 98
	Pop3	+	+	99
Rpp29	Pop4	+	+	100, 106
hPop5	Pop5	+	+	103, 198
	Pop6	+	+	103
Rpp20/Pop7 [a]	Pop7/Rpp2	+	+	103, 105
	Pop8	+	+	103
Rpp30	Rpp1	+	+	102, 104
	Snm1	–	+	101
Rpp21	Rpr2	+	–	103, 108
Rpp38		+	+	104
Rpp14		+	n.d.	106
Rpp25		+	+	107
Rpp40		+	+	105

a) Human Rpp20 is also called Pop7, although its protein sequence shares no significant homology to yeast Pop7. (Adapted from [93]).

was shown to include both protein and RNA components [86, 87], but the identity of these components remained unknown.

Meanwhile, the use of patient-derived autoantibodies allowed the identification of two RNPs with unknown function. The sera of patients with the autoimmune disease scleroderma contain antibodies targeting several intracellular macromolecules. A subset of these sera contains antibodies that precipitate the Th and To antigens, named for the patients from whom the sera were derived. In 1983, Th and To antigens were both found to be associated with RNAs named for their size: 7-2 and 8-2 [88, 89]. Interestingly, these RNAs could not be precipitated in the absence of protein, and each serum could precipitate both RNPs, indicating that the RNPs are likely to share at least one protein component: the Th/To antigen.

Based on the success of using autoantibodies to study the spliceosome, a connection was made between the autoantigenic RNPs and the endonucleolytic RNPs. When serum containing Th antibodies was used to deplete HeLa cell extracts of the Th antigen, the remainder no longer had RNase P activity, indicating that the Th antigen was associated with RNase P [90]. Furthermore, when RNase P was purified from cell extracts, the 8-2 RNA (also known as H1) co-purified [90, 91]. In the same manner, 7-2 was shown to be the RNA component of RNase MRP. That is to say, the anti-Th serum was also able to deplete cell extracts of RNase MRP activity. Additionally, sequence analysis revealed that the RNA that purified with RNase MRP is identical to the 7-2 RNA [92].

The newfound relationship between RNase P and RNase MRP spurred numerous hypotheses regarding their components and functions. For instance, these RNPs probably have at least one common protein component, since they are precipitated by the same sera. If they do share a common protein, they are likely to share a common secondary structural feature to which this common protein may bind. Indeed, though their primary sequences are poorly conserved, recent studies suggest a common secondary structure [93]. Finally, perhaps the most important achievement of this relationship was the identification of the MRP function in the nucleolus.

17.5.2
A New Function of RNase MRP

Initially, the function of MRP was believed to be the cleavage of mitochondrial RNA to create primers for mtDNA replication. This was supported by purification of MRP from discrete cellular compartments, which localized MRP to the mitochondria and nucleus [87]. However, the function of MRP in the nucleus was unknown. Because anti-Th sera stained the granular region of the nucleolus [94], a function in processing of rRNA was suggested. Employing yeast as a genetic tool, Schmitt and Clayton tested this hypothesis [95]. They metabolically depleted the RNA component of MRP, *NME1*, and examined the resulting effects on rRNA processing. In wild-type yeast, the mature 5.8S rRNA is found in two forms, $5.8S_S$ (short) and $5.8S_L$ (long), with $5.8S_S$ being the major species. However, when *NME1* is depleted, $5.8S_L$ becomes predominant, indicating a loss of cleavage at site A_3 [95].

The involvement of MRP in this processing step was also shown to occur *in vitro* [96]. In this case, RNase P and RNase MRP were purified based on a common associated protein, Pop1, and the two RNPs were biochemically separated and assayed for the ability to cleave either pre-tRNA or pre-rRNA. As expected, the RNase P fraction was able to specifically cleave the pre-tRNA but not the pre-rRNA. In contrast, the RNase MRP fraction could cleave pre-rRNA at site A_3, but it could not cleave pre-tRNA.

It is currently understood that the major function of RNase MRP is in rRNA processing. However, cleavage of the pre-rRNA at site A_3 is not essential in yeast, nor is cleavage of mitochondrial RNA. This begs the question of why the RNA component and all the protein components of the RNase MRP are essential in yeast. Perhaps MRP has an additional function that remains to be discovered. Recent studies of mutations in the gene encoding Snm1, the protein unique to RNase MRP, imply a role for MRP in cell cycle control. Specifically, mutations in the gene encoding Snm1 lead to a delay in transition from mitosis to G1 [97].

17.5.3
The Structure and Architecture of RNase P and RNase MRP

In addition to functional studies of the RNPs, numerous structural investigations have been undertaken, specifically the identification of the proteins associated with eukaryotic RNase P and RNase MRP (summarized in Table 17.4). In yeast, four of these proteins were found via genetic screens: Pop1 [98], Pop3 [99], Pop4 [100], and Snm1 [101]. A fifth protein, Rpp1, was identified by its sequence homology to hRpp30, a human component of RNase P [102]. While Pop1, Pop3, Pop4, and Rpp1 were found to associate with both RNase P and RNase MRP by co-immunoprecipitation, antibodies directed against Snm1 only co-immunoprecipitated RNase MRP, identifying Snm1 as the first protein unique to RNase MRP [101]. Five additional proteins were identified in a purification of RNase P: Pop5, Pop6, Pop7, and Pop8 were shown to be associated with both RNPs, and Rpr2 is unique to RNase P [103].

So far 10 proteins have been identified as components of human RNase P (summarized in Table 17.4), though an association with RNase MRP has not been confirmed for all of them. HPop1 was identified by its homology to yeast Pop1, and it was shown to associate with both RNPs by co-immunoprecipitation of both RNPs and RNase P activity [96]. HPop5 was identified by homology to yeast Pop5 and was also shown to be associated with both RNPs [93]. A purification of human RNase P yielded six additional proteins, including Rpp30 and Rpp38, which are recognized by sera from scleroderma patients [104]. The same purification also yielded Rpp20, Rpp40, Rpp14, and Rpp29/hPop4, which were not recognized by tested patient sera, but antibodies raised against each can be used to precipitate RNase P [105, 106]. Rpp25 was also found in a purification of human RNase P [107], and Rpp21 was found by homology to yeast Rpr2 [108], though their association with RNase MRP has not been determined.

Now that at least nine protein components of each RNP have been identified, the focus of current research has shifted to the organization of the RNPs and how that organization leads to function. Both the RNase MRP RNA (NME1/ RRP2) and the RNase P RNA (RPR1) are proposed to form a cage-shaped structure [109, 110] with various sites for protein binding. Protein-RNA interactions have been investigated using yeast three-hybrid assays and UV cross-linking for RNase MRP [111] and RNase P [112]. Interactions between protein components have also been investigated, using yeast two-hybrids and GST pull-down assays [113–115]. As yet, no crystal structure has been published of either RNP. However, in vitro reconstitution experiments indicate that the 8-2 RNA, Rpp21, and Rpp29 alone are adequate for efficient cleavage of tRNA substrates [116]. Though these studies have yielded a wealth of information regarding direct interactions within each RNP, much remains to be learned in order to construct a complete structure of either complex.

17.5.4
Current and Future Uses for Autoantibodies in the Study of RNase P and RNase MRP

In addition to the invaluable discovery that RNase P and RNase MRP are structurally related, autoantibodies continue to contribute to the study of these RNPs, and the information we learn about these RNPs is likely to aid in the study of

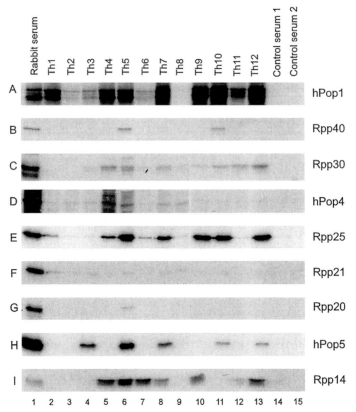

Fig. 17.6 Immunoprecipitation of RNase MRP proteins by anti-Th/To⁺ patient sera. ^{35}S-labeled *in vitro*–translated hPop1 (panel A), Rpp40 (panel B), Rpp30 (panel C), hPop4 (panel D), Rpp25 (panel E), Rpp21 (panel F), Rpp20 (panel G), hPop5 (panel H), and Rpp14 (panel I) were subjected to immunoprecipitation with patient sera Th1–Th12 (lanes 2–13), two control patient sera (lanes 14 and 15), and rabbit antisera that were raised against each of these proteins (lane 1). Co-precipitating proteins were analyzed by sodium dodecyl sulfate-polyacrylamide gel electrophoresis and autoradiography. (Reprinted from [117]).

autoantigenic diseases such as scleroderma. Following identification of the protein components of human RNase P, it became possible to determine which protein components were the autoantigenic targets of scleroderma patient sera. In one study, two different patient sera detected RNase P components Rpp30 and Rpp38 [104]. A larger sample of 12 patient sera expanded the number of proteins identified as Th/To antigens. As shown in Figure 17.6, of 12 anti-Th/To sera tested, most recognized hPop1; about half recognized Rpp30, hPop5, or Rpp14; and only a few recognized Rpp40, hPop4, or Rpp21 [117]. Additional studies comparing antigenic targets and patient prognosis may be valuable in the diagnosis of scleroderma and other autoimmune diseases targeting RNase P and RNase MRP.

17.6
The Exosome

Our understanding of the human exosome developed from the convergence of three separate investigations, each in a different organism. Initially, autoantibodies identified a human complex of nucleolar proteins with unknown function. Once the two major autoantigens were cloned, sequence comparison identified them as homologues of *E. coli* exoribonucleases, suggesting a nucleolytic function in ribosomal RNA processing. The precise function of the human exosome and each of its subunits is currently being elucidated through studies of the yeast exosome, a complex of 11 $3' \rightarrow 5'$ exoribonucleases that is responsible for $3'$ processing of the 5.8S rRNA.

17.6.1
A Molecular Marker for Polymyositis-Scleroderma Overlap Syndrome

A primary goal for the initial studies using human autoimmune sera was to identify common antigens that could be used as diagnostic markers for the various autoimmune diseases. For instance, antibodies against DNA were found in patients with SLE [118], and a ribonucleoprotein (U1) was known to be an antigenic target in mixed connective tissue disease [119, 120]. In routine studies of sera from patients with polymyositis, an autoantigen was identified that was resistant to RNase and DNase treatment, indicating that it is distinct from those previously identified autoantigens [121]. Antibodies to this antigen were found in a high percentage of patients with polymyositis, scleroderma, or polymyositis-scleroderma overlap syndrome, but not in patients with other autoimmune diseases or in normal individuals, encouraging its use as a marker for these diseases and prompting the antigen to be named PM-Scl [122].

By immunofluorescence, patient sera were shown to stain primarily the granular component of the nucleolus, where the later steps of rRNA processing occur, stimulating speculation about a function for the PM-Scl antigen in ribosome biogenesis [123]. However, this speculation could not be confirmed, because no RNA was found to associate with the PM-Scl antigen. Indeed, immunofluorescence was not affected by treatment with RNase, and no RNA was pulled down by immunoprecipitation. Instead, 11–16 proteins with apparent molecular weights of 20–110 kDa were found when patient sera were used to immunoprecipitate radiolabeled HeLa cell extracts (Fig. 17.7) [124]. The function of the PM-Scl antigen, therefore, could not be assigned.

As determined by immunoblotting, the most commonly targeted antigens by autoantibodies in the PM-Scl complex are PM-Scl 100 and PM-Scl 75 [123, 124]. Utilizing anti-PM-Scl patient sera, phage cDNA libraries were screened and the genes for both proteins were cloned [125–128]. Though PM-Scl 75 was predicted to have a molecular weight of 39 kDa, it migrates anomalously at 75 kDa [125]. Without gaining a clue as to the function of either protein from their sequences, the focus of the field shifted from determining their function to identifying their autoantigenic epitopes [126].

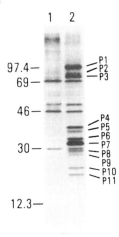

Fig. 17.7 Exosome proteins identified by anti-PM/Scl antibodies. Autoradiogram of [^{35}S]methionine-labeled HeLa cell proteins immunoprecipitated by anti-PM-Scl antibodies (S125) and resolved in 17.5% SDS-polyacrylamide gel. Lane 1 shows proteins precipitated by normal control serum. Lane 2 demonstrates in detail the radiolabeled proteins from HeLa cells that are selectively brought down by anti-PM-Scl antibodies and are named P1–P11. (Reprinted from [123]).

17.6.2
The Exosome Is a Conserved Complex

At the same time, the study of ribosome biogenesis in yeast was flourishing, thanks to its ease in genetic manipulation. Genetic screens could be used to identify gene products involved in various steps of rRNA processing. By this approach Rrp4 was found and was shown to be required for proper processing of the 5.8S rRNA species [129]. Yeast carrying a temperature-sensitive mutation in *rrp4* accumulate a 3′ extended form of 5.8S rRNA at restrictive temperature, due to the loss of Rrp4 3′ → 5′ exonuclease activity [129]. Gradient centrifugation reveals that Rrp4 is just one in a complex of essential exonucleases, and its human homologue, hRrp4, is also found in a similar complex [130].

The yeast exosome was finally linked to the human PM-Scl complex by sequence analysis in 1997. A database search for homologues of the *E. coli* ribonucleases identified PM-Scl 75 as a member of the RNase PH family and PM-Scl 100 as a member of the RNase D family, giving the first hint to their function [131]. Soon thereafter, additional members of the yeast exosome were cloned, including Rrp6, the yeast homologue of PM-Scl 100 [132].

Purification of the yeast exosome uncovered a nuclear complex of 11 proteins, 10 of which (all except Csl4) are predicted by high sequence homology to be 3′ → 5′ exoribonucleases (Table 17.5) [133]. Of these 11 proteins, 10 (all except Rrp6) are essential in yeast [133], and all 11 are required for proper 3′ end formation of the 5.8S rRNA [134]. Most of the yeast exosome components have human homologues (including PM-Scl 100 and PM-Scl 75) that are found in a similar complex in the human nucleus, implying that the PM-Scl complex is the human exosome and is therefore responsible for 3′ end formation of the human 5.8S rRNA.

Additional functions have recently been found for the yeast exosome in RNA processing, such as 3′ end formation of small RNAs, pre-mRNA quality control in the nucleus, and mRNA degradation in the cytoplasm [135]. Interestingly, Rrp6 is not associated with the cytoplasmic exosome [133], and the RNA-binding core exosome protein Csl4/Ski4 appears to be required for mRNA degradation but not for rRNA maturation [136]. It has therefore been suggested that the specificity and activity of the exosome are determined not by its core exonucleolytic components but by additional proteins such as Rrp6 and Csl4/Ski4 that may determine its localization and substrates [135].

17.6.3
Autoantibody Targets in the Human Exosome

The components of the human exosome have been identified largely by their homology to the components of the yeast exosome [133, 137]. Now that these proteins have been identified, they can be evaluated for their autoantigenicity in patients. Although PM-Scl 100 and PM-Scl 75 are the proteins most commonly targeted by autoantibodies, all other exosome components tested were also found to be autoantibody targets (Table 17.5) [137]. This information contributes to our understanding of disease progression. It has been suggested that in the course of autoimmune disease, PM-Scl 100 or PM-Scl 75 is initially targeted and that during cell death, peptides derived from additional exosome components are presented as antigens, and epitope spreading causes these other antigens to be targeted by autoantibodies [137].

17.7
NOR-90/hUBF and RNA Polymerases I, II, and III

In eukaryotes, the nucleolus is the site of ribosome assembly, including transcription of rDNA, processing of the pre-rRNA, and association of many ribosomal proteins with the rRNA. In humans the first step, rDNA transcription, requires the cooperative binding of hUBF and the SL1 complex to the rDNA promoter. Once bound, these proteins activate RNA polymerase I transcription. Together with the chromatin containing the rDNA, these proteins comprise the nucleolar-organizing region (NOR), which was primarily characterized by its distinct speckled pattern when stained with silver salts. Early immunofluorescence experiments using autoimmune patient sera revealed a similar staining pattern, presenting the possibility that the proteins required for rDNA transcription may be autoantigens.

17.7.1
RNA Polymerases I, II, and III

In the early 1980s, patient-derived autoantibodies were known to decorate a number of nuclear and nucleolar components, as determined by a variety of nuclear and nucleolar staining patterns [4]. At the same time, biochemists had pu-

Table 17.5 Components of the exosome.

Human protein	Yeast protein	Function	Auto-antigenicity	Ref.
hRrp4	Rrp4	3′ → 5′ hydrolytic exonuclease	Yes	129, 130, 133, 135, 137
PM-Scl 100	Rrp6	RNase D family; 3′ → 5′ hydrolytic exonuclease; only in nuclear exosome	Yes, a lot	131–133, 137, 199
PM-Scl 75	Rrp45	RNase PH family; 3′ → 5′ phosphorolytic exonuclease	Yes, a lot	131, 133, 135, 137, 199, 200
hRrp40	Rrp40	S1 RNA BD; 3′ → 5′ hydrolytic exoribonuclease	Yes	133, 135, 137, 201
hRrp41	Rrp41/Ski6	RNase PH family; 3′ → 5′ phosphorolytic exonuclease	Yes	130, 133, 135, 137, 201
hRrp42	Rrp42	RNase PH family; 3′ → 5′ phosphorolytic exonuclease	Yes	130, 133, 135, 137
OIP2?	Rrp43	RNase PH family; 3′ → 5′ phosphorolytic exonuclease	Not tested	130, 133, 135
hRrp44/ hDis3	Rrp44/Dis3	RNase R (II) family; 3′ → 5′ hydrolytic exonuclease; human protein not in exosome	Not tested	130, 133, 135, 202
hRrp46	Rrp46	RNase PH family; 3′ → 5′ phosphorolytic exonuclease	Yes	133, 135, 137, 201
hMtr3?	Mtr3	RNase PH family; 3′ → 5′ phosphorolytic exonuclease	Not tested	133, 135
hCsl4	Csl4/Ski4	S1 RNA BD	Yes	133, 136, 137

rified RNA polymerase I activity to homogeneity [138]. The purified complex contained eight proteins and was known to be nucleolar. Upon finding that autoimmune patient sera recognize unidentified antigens in the nucleolus, the hypothesis emerged that one or more subunits of RNA polymerase I could be an autoantigen. Indeed, when patient sera were used to immunoprecipitate purified or native RNA polymerase I, it was clear that several subunits were bound by the autoantibodies; furthermore, injection of patient-derived autoantibodies into *Xenopus* oocytes inhibited rDNA transcription [139, 140].

Interestingly, although purified RNA polymerase I was shown to retain enzymatic activity with only eight polypeptides, the patient sera immunoprecipitated 13 distinct proteins (Fig. 17.8) [140]. Upon further study, the additional polypep-

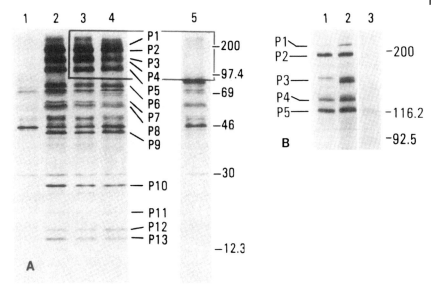

Fig. 17.8 RNA polymerase proteins identified by scleroderma patient sera. (A) Autoradiogram of immunoprecipitated [^{35}S]methionine-labeled HeLa cell proteins resolved in a 17.5% SDS-polyacrylamide gel. Normal human serum (lane 1); representative antinucleolar scleroderma sera (S18 and S124) with speckled staining pattern (lanes 2 and 3, respectively); rabbit anti-RNA polymerase I antibodies (lane 4); normal rabbit serum (lane 5). The rabbit anti-RNA polymerase I and antinucleolar scleroderma antibodies from two representative patients precipitated the same 13 polypeptides (P1–P13) of 210,000 to 14,000 mol wt that were distinct from polypeptides of 70,000, 46,000, and 30,000 mol wt precipitated by normal human serum. In addition, control rabbit serum also brought down a protein of 80,000 mol wt. The 46,000 mol wt protein is actin; the other polypeptides precipitated by normal sera are unknown. (B) Autoradiogram of immunoprecipitated [^{35}S]methionine-labeled HeLa proteins resolved in a 5% SDS-polyacrylamide gel. Antinucleolar scleroderma serum S18 (lane 1); rabbit anti-RNA polymerase I antibodies (lane 2); normal human serum (lane 3). This low-percent gel system was used to demonstrate that distinct high-molecular-weight polypeptides of mol wt 210,000 (P1), 190,000 (P2), 155,000 (P3), 130,000 (P4), 120,000 (P5), and 80,000 (P6) were immunoprecipitated with the rabbit and the human antinucleolar serum. (Reprinted from [140]).

tides were identified as subunits of RNA polymerases II or III. It was determined that the autoantibodies recognized a component of polymerase I that is common to all three polymerases and therefore immunoprecipitated the components of all three [141].

17.7.2
The Nucleolar-organizing Region

Among the three nucleolar patterns observed when cells were stained with patient-derived autoantibodies, the speckled pattern was recognized as staining of the nucleolar-organizing region (NOR). In order to identify the NOR autoantigen, these sera were used to immunoprecipitate a novel protein of 90 kDa, which was accordingly named NOR-90 [142]. Using the autoantibodies to screen a cDNA library, NOR-90 was identified as hUBF, an rDNA transcription factor [143, 144].

Further studies of hUBF show that it is a TATA box–binding protein that binds to the upstream control element (UCE) promoter region of the rDNA [144a]. In concert with the binding of the SL1 complex, hUBF is phosphorylated and subsequently activates rDNA transcription [145]. Because rDNA transcription is active in all stages of the cell cycle except mitosis, hUBF is a basal transcription factor that is inactive only during the M phase and is reactivated during G1 progression [146]. Recent investigations into anti-hUBF autoimmunity suggest that this immune response is antigen driven and that MHC presentation of hUBF generates autoimmunity [147].

References

1 R.P. Perry, RNA processing comes of age. *J Cell Biol*, **1981**. 91, 28s–38s.

2 J.L. Hodnett and H. Busch, Isolation and characterization of uridylic acid-rich 7 S ribonucleic acid of rat liver nuclei. *J Biol Chem*, **1968**. 243, 6334–6342.

3 R.A. Weinberg and S. Penman, Small molecular weight monodisperse nuclear RNA. *Journal of Molecular Biology*, **1968**. 38, 289–304.

4 R.M. Bernstein, J.C. Steigerwald, and E.M. Tan, Association of antinuclear and antinucleolar antibodies in progressive systemic sclerosis. *Clin Exp Immunol*, **1982**. 48, 43–51.

5 W.H. Reeves, S. Narain, and M. Satoh, Henry Kunkel, Stephanie Smith, clinical immunology and split genes. *Lupus*, **2003**. 12, 213–217.

6 E.M. Tan and H.G. Kunkel, Characteristics of a soluble nuclear antigen precipitating with sera of patients with systemic lupus erythematosus. *J. Immunol.*, **1966**. 96, 464–471.

7 M. Mattioli and M. Reichlin, Characterization of a soluble nuclear ribonucleoprotein antigen reactive with SLE sera. *J. Immunol.*, **1971**. 107, 1281–1290.

8 M. Mattioli and M. Reichlin, Physical association of two nuclear antigens and mutual occurence of their antibodies: the relationship of the Sm and RNA protein (Mo) systems in SLE sera. *J. Immunol.*, **1973**. 110, 1318–1324.

9 M.R. Lerner and J.A. Steitz, Antibodies to small nuclear RNAs complexed with proteins are produced by patients with systemic lupus erythematosus. *Proceedings of the National Academy of Sciences of the United States of America*, **1979**. 76, 5495–5499.

10 L.T. Chow, et al., An amazing sequence arrangement at the 5′ ends of adenovirus 2 messenger RNA. *Cell*, **1977**. 12, 1–8.

11 S.M. Berget, C. Moore, and P.A. Sharp, Spliced segments of the 5′ terminus of adenovirus 2 late mRNAs. *Proc Natl Acad Sci USA*, **1977**. 74, 3171–3175.

12 M.R. Lerner, et al., Are snRNPs involved in splicing? *Nature*, **1980**. 283, 220–224.

13 J. Rogers and R. Wall, A mechanism for pre-mRNA splicing. *Proc Natl Acad Sci USA*, **1980**. 77, 1877–1879.

14 R.A. Eisenberg, E.M. Tan, and F.J. Dixon, Presence of anti-Sm reactivity in autoimmune mouse strains. *J. Exp. Med.*, **1978**. 147, 582–587.

15 E.A. Lerner, et al., Monoclonal antibodies to nucleic acid-containing cellular constituents: probes for molecular biology and autoimmune disease. *Proceedings of the National Academy of Sciences of the United States of America*, **1981**. 78, 2737–2741.

16 K.A. Montzka and J.A. Steitz, Additional low-abundance human small nuclear ribonucleoproteins: U11, U12, etc. *Proc Natl Acad Sci USA*, **1988**. 85, 8885–8889.

17 S. L. Hall and R. A. Padgett, Conserved sequences in a class of rare eukaryotic introns with non-consensus splice sites. *J. Mol. Biol.*, **1994**. 239, 351–365.

18 S. L. Hall and R. A. Padgett, Requirement of U12 snRNA for in vivo splicing of a minor class of eukaryotic nuclear pre-mRNA introns. *Science*, **1996**. 271, 1716–1718,

19 W. Y. Tarn and J. A. Steitz, A novel spliceosome containing U11, U12, and U5 snRNPs excises a minor class (AT-AC) intron in vitro. *Cell*, **1996**. 84, 801–811.

20 W. Y. Tarn and J. A. Steitz, Highly diverged U4 and U6 small nuclear RNAs required for splicing rare AT-AC introns. *Science*, **1996**. 273, 1824–1832.

21 W. Y. Tarn, T. A. Yario, and J. A. Steitz, U12 snRNA in vertebrates: evolutionary conservation of 5′ sequences implicated in splicing of pre-mRNAs containing a minor class of introns. *RNA*, **1995**. 1, 644–656.

22 V. W. Yang, et al., A small nuclear ribonucleoprotein is required for splicing of adenoviral early RNA sequences. *Proc Natl Acad Sci USA*, **1981**. 78, 1371–1375.

23 R. A. Padgett, et al., Splicing of messenger RNA precursors is inhibited by antisera to small nuclear ribonucleoprotein. *Cell*, **1983**. 35, 101–107.

24 A. Fradin, et al., Splicing pathways of Sv40 mRNAs in X. laevis occytes differ in their requirements for snRNPs. *Cell*, **1984**. 37, 927–936.

25 A. Kramer, et al., The 5′ terminus of the RNA moiety of U1 small nuclear ribonucleoprotein particles is required for the splicing of messenger RNA precursors. *Cell*, **1984**. 38, 299–307.

26 P. J. Grabowski, S. R. Seiler, and P. Sharp, A multicomponent complex is involved in the splicing of messenger RNA precursors. *Cell*, **1985**. 42, 345–353.

27 I. Pettersson, et al., The structure of mammalian small nuclear ribonucleoproteins. *J. Biol. Chem.*, **1984**. 259, 5907–5914.

28 W. van Venrooij and G. J. Pruijn, Ribonucleoprotein complexes as autoantigens. *Curr Biol*, **1995**. 7, 819–824.

29 J. D. Northway and E. M. Tan, Differentiation of antinuclear antibodies giving speckled staining patterns in immunofluorescence. *Clin. Immun. Immunopath.*, **1972**. 1, 140–154.

30 U. Nyman, et al., Intranuclear localization of snRNP antigens. *J. Cell Biol.*, **1986**. 102, 137–144.

31 A. I. Lamond and D. L. Spector, Nuclear speckles: a model for nuclear organelles. *Nat Rev Mol Cell Biol*, **2003**. 4, 605–612.

32 M. Bach, G. Winkelmann, and R. Luhrmann, 20S small nuclear ribonucleoprotein U5 shows a surprisingly complex protein composition. *Proc Natl Acad Sci USA*, **1989**. 86, 6038–6042.

33 W. H. Reeves, et al., Psoriasis and Raynaud's phenomenon associated with autoantibodies to U1 and U2 small nuclear ribonucleoprotein. *N. Engl. J. Med.*, **1986**. 315, 105–111.

34 I. Pettersson, et al., The use of immunoblotting and immunoprecipitations of (U) small nuclear ribonucleoproteins in the analysis of sera of patients with mixed connective tissue disease and systemic lupus erythematosus. *Arthritis and Rheum.*, **1986**. 29, 986–995.

35 T. Mimori, et al., Autoantibodies to the U2 small nuclear ribonucleoprotein in a patient with scleroderma-polymyositis overlap syndrome. *J. Biol. Chem.*, **1984**. 259, 560–565.

36 W. Habets, et al., Autoantibodies to ribonucleoprotein particles containing U2 small nuclear RNA. *EMBO J.*, **1985**. 4, 1545–1550.

37 Y. Okano and T. A. Medsger, Newly identified U4/U6 snRNP-binding proteins by serum autoantibodies form a patient with systemic sclerosis. *J. Immunol.*, **1991**. 146, 535–542.

38 M. Kubo, et al., Anti-U5 snRNP antibody as a possible serological marker for scleroderma-polymyositis overlap. *Rheumatology*, **2002**. 41, 531–534.

39 Y. Okano, et al., Anti-U5 small nuclear ribonucleoprotein (snRNP) antibodies: a rare anti-U snRNP specificity. *Clin. Immun. Immunopath.*, **1996**. 81, 41–47.

40 T. Achsel, et al., A doughnut-shaped heteromer of human Sm-like proteins binds to the 3′-end of U6 snRNA, thereby facilitating U4/U6 duplex formation in vitro. *EMBO J*, **1999**. 18, 5789–5802.

41 J. Salgado-Garrido, et al., Sm and Sm-like proteins assemble in two related complexes of deep evolutionary origin. *EMBO J*, **1999**. 18, 3451–3462.

42 T. Eystathioy, et al., Autoantibody to hLSm4 and the heptameric LSm complex in Anti-Sm sera. *Arth. Rheum.*, **2002**. 46, 726–734.

43 W. Y. Tarn and J. A. Steitz, Pre-mRNA splicing: the discovery of a new spliceosome doubles the challenge. *TIBS*, **1997**. 22, 132–137.

44 M. S. Jurica and M. J. Moore, Pre-mRNA splicing: awash in a sea of proteins. *Mol. Cell*, **2003**. 12, 4–14.

45 R. Reed, Coupling transcription, splicing and mRNA export. *Curr. Opin. Cell Biol.*, **2003**. 15, 326–331.

46 J. Venema and D. Tollervey, Ribosome synthesis in *Saccharomyces cerevisiae*. *Annu. Rev. Genet.*, **1999**. 33, 261–311.

47 R. Reddy, D. Henning, and H. Busch, Nucleotide sequence of nucleolar U3B RNA. *J Biol Chem*, **1979**. 254, 11097–11105.

48 A. W. Prestayko, M. Tonato, and H. Busch, Low molecular weight RNA associated with 28S nucleolar RNA. *Journal of Molecular Biology*, **1970**. 47, 505–515.

49 P. Epstein, R. Reddy, and H. Busch, Multiple states of U3 RNA in Novikoff hepatoma nucleoli. *Biochemistry*, **1984**. 23, 5421–5425.

50 R. Reddy, D. Henning, and H. Busch, Substitutions, insertions, and deletions in two highly conserved U3 RNA species. *J Biol Chem*, **1980**. 255, 7029–7033.

51 R. L. Ochs, et al., Fibrillarin: a new protein of the nucleolus identified by autoimmune sera. *Biol Cell*, **1985**. 54, 123–133.

52 M. A. Lischwe, et al., Purification and partial characterization of a nucleolar scleroderma antigen (Mr = 34,000; pI, 8.5) rich in N^G, N^G-dimethylarginine. *Journal of Biological Chemistry*, **1985**. 260, 14304–14310.

53 K. A. Parker and J. A. Steitz, Structural analyses of the human U3 ribonucleoprotein particle reveal a conserved sequence available for base-pairing with pre-rRNA. *Molecular and Cellular Biology*, **1987**. 7, 2899–2913.

54 J. S. Andersen, et al., Directed proteomic analysis of the human nucleolus. *Curr. Biol.*, **2002**. 12, 1–11.

55 F. Dragon, et al., A large nucleolar U3 ribonucleoprotein required for 18S ribosomal RNA biogenesis. *Nature*, **2002**. 417, 967–970.

56 P. Grandi, et al., 90S pre-ribosomes include the 35S pre-rRNA, the U3 snoRNP, and 40S subunit processing factors but predominantly lack 60S synthesis factors. *Mol Cell*, **2002**. 10, 105–115.

57 K. A. Bernstein and S. J. Baserga, The small subunit processome is required for cell cycle progression at G1. *Mol Biol Cell*, **2004**. 15, 5038–5046.

58 S. Kass, et al., The U3 small nucleolar ribonucleoprotein functions in the first step of pre-ribosomal RNA processing. *Cell*, **1990**. 60, 897–908.

59 J. M. X. Hughes and M. Ares, Jr., Depletion of U3 small nucleolar RNA inhibits cleavage in the 5′ external transcribed spacer of yeast pre-ribosomal RNA and prevents formation of 18S ribosomal RNA. *EMBO Journal*, **1991**. 10, 4231–4239.

60 R. Savino and S. A. Gerbi, In vivo disruption of Xenopus U3 snRNA affects ribosomal RNA processing. *EMBO Journal*, **1990**. 9, 2299–2308.

61 O. L. Miller, Jr. and B. R. Beatty, Visualization of nucleolar genes. *Science*, **1969**. 164, 955–957.

62 J. M. Yang, et al., Human scleroderma sera contain autoantibodies to protein components specific to the U3 small nucleolar RNP complex. *Arthritis Rheum*, **2003**. 48, 210–217.

63 G. Reimer, et al., Monoclonal antibody from a (New Zealand black X New Zealand white) F1 mouse and some human scleroderma sera target an Mr 34,000 nucleolar protein of the U3 RNP particle. *Arthritis and Rheumatism*, **1987**. 30, 793–800.

64 K. Tyc and J. A. Steitz, U3, U8 and U13 comprise a new class of mammalian snRNPs localized to the cell nucleolus. *EMBO Journal*, **1989**. 8, 3113–3119.

65 S. J. Baserga, X. W. Yang, and J. A. Steitz, An intact Box C sequence is required for binding of fibrillarin, the protein common to the major family of nucleolar snRNPs. *EMBO Journal*, **1991**. 10, 2645–2651.

66 B. Sollner-Webb, Novel intron-encoded small nucleolar RNAs. *Cell*, **1993**. 75, 403–405.

67 Z. Kiss-Laszlo, et al., Site-specific ribose methylation of preribosomal RNA: a novel function for small nucleolar RNAs. *Cell*, **1996**. 85, 1077–1088.

68 B. E. H. Maden, The numerous modified nucleotides in eukaryotic ribosomal RNA. *Progress in Nucleic Acid Research and Molecular Biology*, **1990**. 39, 241–303.

69 V. Atzorn, P. Fragapane, and T. Kiss, U17/snR30 is a ubiquitous snoRNA with two conserved sequence motifs essential for 18S rRNA production. *Mol Cell Biol*, **2004**. 24, 1769–1778.

70 M. R. Lerner, et al., Two novel classes of small ribonucleoproteins detected by antibodies associated with lupus erythematosus. *Science*, **1981**. 211, 400–402.

71 J. P. Hendrick, et al., Ro small cytoplasmic ribonucleoproteins are a subclass of La ribonucleoproteins: further characterization of the Ro and La small ribonucleoproteins from uninfected mammalian cells. *Mol Cell Biol*, **1981**. 1, 1138–1149.

72 J. Rinke and J. A. Steitz, Precursor molecules of both human 5S ribosomal RNA and transfer RNAs are bound by a cellular protein reactive with anti-La lupus antibodies. *Cell*, **1982**. 29, 149–159.

73 M. B. Mathews and A. M. Francoeur, La antigen recognizes and binds to the 3'-oligouridylate tail of a small RNA. *Mol Cell Biol*, **1984**. 4, 1134–1140.

74 J. E. Stefano, Purified lupus antigen La recognizes an oligouridylate stretch common to the 3' termini of RNA polymerase III transcripts. *Cell*, **1984**. 36, 145–154.

75 E. Gottlieb and J. A. Steitz, The RNA binding protein La influences both the accuracy and the efficiency of RNA polymerase III transcription in vitro. *Embo J*, **1989**. 8, 841–850.

76 E. Gottlieb and J. A. Steitz, Function of the mammalian La protein: evidence for its action in transcription termination by RNA polymerase III. *Embo J*, **1989**. 8, 851–861.

77 R. J. Maraia, Transcription termination factor La is also an initiation factor for RNA polymerase III. *Proc Natl Acad Sci USA*, **1996**. 93, 3383–3387.

78 C. J. Yoo and S. L. Wolin, The yeast La protein is required for the 3' endonucleolytic cleavage that matures tRNA precursors. *Cell*, **1997**. 89, 393–402.

79 B. K. Pannone, D. Xue, and S. L. Wolin, A role for the yeast La protein in U6 snRNP assembly: evidence that the La protein is a molecular chaperone for RNA polymerase III transcripts. *Embo J*, **1998**. 17, 7442–7453.

80 S. L. Wolin and J. A. Steitz, Genes for two small cytoplasmic Ro RNAs are adjacent and appear to be single-copy in the human genome. *Cell*, **1983**. 32, 735–744.

81 S. L. Wolin and J. A. Steitz, The Ro small cytoplasmic ribonucleoproteins: identification of the antigenic protein and its binding site on the Ro RNAs. *Proc Natl Acad Sci USA*, **1984**. 81, 1996–2000.

82 E. Ben-Chetrit, et al., A 52-kD protein is a novel component of the SS-A/Ro antigenic particle. *J Exp Med*, **1988**. 167, 1560–1571.

83 X. Chen and S. L. Wolin, The Ro 60 kDa autoantigen: insights into cellular function and role in autoimmunity. *J Mol Med*, **2004**. 82, 232–239.

84 H. D. Robertson, S. Altman, and J. D. Smith, Purification and properties of a specific Escherichia coli ribonuclease which cleaves a tyrosine transfer ribonucleic acid presursor. *J Biol Chem*, **1972**. 247, 5243–5251.

85 B. C. Stark, et al., Ribonuclease P: an enzyme with an essential RNA component. *Proc Natl Acad Sci USA*, **1978**. 75, 3717–3721.

86 D. D. Chang and D. A. Clayton, A novel endoribonuclease cleaves at a priming site of mouse mitochondrial DNA replication. *Embo J*, **1987**. 6, 409–417.

87 D. D. Chang and D. A. Clayton, A mammalian mitochondrial RNA processing activity contains nucleus-encoded RNA. *Science*, **1987**. 235, 1178–1184.

88 C. Hashimoto and J. A. Steitz, Sequential association of nucleolar 7-2 RNA with two different autoantigens. *Journal of Biological Chemistry*, **1983**. 258, 1379–1382.

89 R. Reddy, et al., Detection of a nucleolar 7-2 ribonucleoprotein and a cytoplasmic 8-2 ribonucleoprotein with autoantibodies from patients with scleroderma. *Journal of Biological Chemistry*, **1983**. 258, 1383–1386.

90 H. A. Gold, et al., Antibodies in human serum that precipitate ribonuclease P. *Proceedings of the National Academy of Sciences USA*, **1988**. 85, 5483–5487.

91 M. Bartkiewicz, H. Gold, and S. Altman, Identification and characterization of an RNA molecule that copurifies with RNase P activity from HeLa cells. *Genes Dev*, **1989**. 3, 488–499.

92 H. A. Gold, et al., The RNA processing enzyme RNase MRP is identical to the Th RNP and related to RNase P. *Science*, **1989**. 245, 1377–1380.

93 H. van Eenennaam, et al., Architecture and function of the human endonucleases RNase P and RNase MRP. *IUBMB Life*, **2000**. 49, 265–272.

94 G. Reimer, et al., Immunolocalization of 7-2-ribonucleoprotein in the granular component of the nucleolus. *Exp Cell Res*, **1988**. 176, 117–128.

95 M. E. Schmitt and D. A. Clayton, Nuclear RNase MRP is required for correct processing of pre-5.8S rRNA in *Saccharomyces cerevisiae*. *Molecular and Cellular Biology*, **1993**. 13, 7935–7941.

96 Z. Lygerou, et al., Accurate processing of a eukaryotic precursor ribosomal RNA by ribonuclease MRP in vitro. *Science*, **1996**. 272, 268–270.

97 T. Cai, et al., Mutagenesis of SNM1, which encodes a protein component of the yeast RNase MRP, reveals a role for this ribonucleoprotein endoribonuclease in plasmid segregation. *Mol Cell Biol*, **1999**. 19, 7857–7869.

98 Z. Lygerou, et al., The POP1 gene encodes a protein component common to the RNase MRP and RNase P ribonucleoproteins. *Genes Dev*, **1994**. 8, 1423–1433.

99 B. Dichtl and D. Tollervey, Pop3p is essential for the activity of the RNase MRP

and Rnase P ribonucleoproteins in vivo. *EMBO Journal*, **1997**. 16, 417–429.

100 S. Chu, J. M. Zengel, and L. Lindahl, A novel protein shared by RNase MRP and RNase P. *Rna*, **1997**. 3, 382–391.

101 M. E. Schmitt and D. A. Clayton, Characterization of a unique protein component of yeast RNase MRP: an RNA-binding protein with a zinc-cluster domain. *Genes Dev*, **1994**. 8, 2617–2628.

102 V. Stolc and S. Altman, Rpp1, an essential protein subunit of nuclear RNase P required for processing of precursor tRNA and 35S precursor rRNA in Saccharomyces cerevisiae. *Genes Dev*, **1997**. 11, 2926–2937.

103 J. R. Chamberlain, et al., Purification and characterization of the nuclear RNase P holoenzyme complex reveals extensive subunit overlap with RNase MRP. *Genes and Dev.*, **1998**. 12, 1678–1690.

104 P. S. Eder, et al., Characterization of two scleroderma autoimmune antigens that copurify with human ribonuclease P. *Proc Natl Acad Sci USA*, **1997**. 94, 1101–1106.

105 N. Jarrous, et al., Autoantigenic properties of some protein subunits of catalytically active complexes of human ribonuclease P. *Rna*, **1998**. 4, 407–417.

106 N. Jarrous, et al., Rpp14 and Rpp29, two protein subunits of human ribonuclease P. *Rna*, **1999**. 5, 153–157.

107 C. Guerrier-Takada, et al., Purification and characterization of Rpp25, an RNA-binding protein subunit of human ribonuclease P. *Rna*, **2002**. 8, 290–295.

108 N. Jarrous, et al., Function and subnuclear distribution of Rpp21, a protein subunit of the human ribonucleoprotein ribonuclease P. *Rna*, **2001**. 7, 1153–1164.

109 M. E. Schmitt, et al., Secondary structure of RNase MRP RNA as predicted by phylogenetic comparison. *Faseb J*, **1993**. 7, 208–213.

110 A. C. Forster and S. Altman, Similar cage-shaped structures for the RNA components of all ribonuclease P and ribonuclease MRP enzymes. *Cell*, **1990**. 62, 407–409.

111 H. Pluk, et al., RNA-protein interactions in the human RNase MRP ribonucleoprotein complex. *Rna*, **1999**. 5, 512–524.

112 T. Jiang, C. Guerrier-Takada, and S. Altman, Protein-RNA interactions in the subunits of human nuclear RNase P. *Rna*, **2001**. 7, 937–941.

113 T. J. Welting, W. J. van Venrooij, and G. J. Pruijn, Mutual interactions between subunits of the human RNase MRP ribonucleoprotein complex. *Nucleic Acids Res*, **2004**. 32, 2138–2146.

114 T. Jiang and S. Altman, Protein-protein interactions with subunits of human nuclear RNase P. *Proc Natl Acad Sci USA*, **2001**. 98, 920–925.

115 F. Houser-Scott, et al., Interactions among the protein and RNA subunits of Saccharomyces cerevisiae nuclear RNase P. *Proc Natl Acad Sci USA*, **2002**. 99, 2684–2689.

116 H. Mann, et al., Eukaryotic RNase P: role of RNA and protein subunits of a primordial catalytic ribonucleoprotein in RNA-based catalysis. *Mol Cell*, **2003**. 12, 925–935.

117 H. Van Eenennaam, et al., Identity of the RNase MRP- and RNase P-associated Th/To autoantigen. *Arthritis Rheum*, **2002**. 46, 3266–3272.

118 G. C. Sharp, et al., Association of autoantibodies to different nuclear antigens with clinical patterns of rheumatic disease and responsiveness to therapy. *J Clin Invest*, **1971**. 50, 350–359.

119 R. W. Hoffman and E. L. Greidinger, Mixed connective tissue disease. *Curr Opin Rheumatol*, **2000**. 12, 386–390.

120 G. C. Sharp, et al., Association of antibodies to ribonucleoprotein and Sm antigens with mixed connective-tissue disease, systematic lupus erythematosus and other rheumatic diseases. *N Engl J Med*, **1976**. 295, 1149–1154.

121 J. F. Wolfe, E. Adelstein, and G. C. Sharp, Antinuclear antibody with distinct specificity for polymyositis. *J Clin Invest*, **1977**. 59, 176–178.

122 M. Reichlin, et al., Antibodies to a nuclear/nucleolar antigen in patients with polymyositis overlap syndromes. *J Clin Immunol*, **1984**. 4, 40–44.

123 G. Reimer, et al., Immunolocalization and partial characterization of a nucleolar autoantigen (PM-Scl) associated with polymyositis/scleroderma overlap syndromes. *J Immunol*, **1986**. 137, 3802–3808.

124 C. Gelpi, et al., Identification of protein components reactive with anti-PM/Scl autoantibodies. *Clin Exp Immunol*, **1990**. 81, 59–64.

125 F. Alderuccio, E. K. Chan, and E. M. Tan, Molecular characterization of an autoantigen of PM-Scl in the polymyositis/scleroderma overlap syndrome: a unique and complete human cDNA encoding an apparent 75-kD acidic protein of the nucleolar complex. *J Exp Med*, **1991**. 173, 941–952.

126 M. Bluthner, E. K. Bautz, and F. A. Bautz, Mapping of epitopes recognized by PM/Scl autoantibodies with gene-fragment phage display libraries. *J Immunol Methods*, **1996**. 198, 187–198.

127 Q. Ge, et al., Cloning of a complementary DNA coding for the 100-kD antigenic protein of the PM-Scl autoantigen. *J Clin Invest*, **1992**. 90, 559–570.

128 Q. Ge, et al., Analysis of the specificity of anti-PM-Scl autoantibodies. *Arthritis Rheum*, **1994**. 37, 1445–1452.

129 P. Mitchell, E. Petfalski, and D. Tollervey, The 3′ end of yeast 5.8S rRNA is generated by an exonuclease processing mechanism. *Genes Dev*, **1996**. 10, 502–513.

130 P. Mitchell, et al., The exosome: a conserved eukaryotic RNA processing complex containing multiple 3′ to 5′ exonucleases. *Cell*, **1997**. 91, 457–466.

131 I. S. Mian, Comparative sequence analysis of ribonucleases HII, III, II PH and D. *Nucleic Acids Res*, **1997**. 25, 3187–3195.

132 M. W. Briggs, K. T. Burkard, and J. S. Butler, Rrp6p, the yeast homologue of the human PM-Scl 100-kDa autoantigen, is essential for efficient 5.8 S rRNA 3′ end formation. *J Biol Chem*, **1998**. 273, 13255–13263.

133 C. Allmang, et al., The yeast exosome and human PM-Scl are related complexes of 3′ → 5′ exonucleases. *Genes Dev*, **1999**. 13, 2148–2158.

134 C. Allmang, et al., Degradation of ribosomal RNA precursors by the exosome. *Nucleic Acids Res*, **2000**. 28, 1684–1691.

135 R. Raijmakers, G. Schilders, and G.J. Pruijn, The exosome, a molecular machine for controlled RNA degradation in both nucleus and cytoplasm. *Eur J Cell Biol*, **2004**. 83, 175–183.

136 A. van Hoof, et al., Function of the ski4p (Csl4p) and Ski7p proteins in 3′-to-5′ degradation of mRNA. *Mol Cell Biol*, **2000**. 20, 8230–8243.

137 R. Brouwer, et al., Autoantibodies directed to novel components of the PM/Scl complex, the human exosome. *Arthritis Res*, **2002**. 4, 134–138.

138 K.M. Rose, D.A. Stetler, and S.T. Jacob, Protein kinase activity of RNA polymerase I purified from a rat hepatoma: probable function of Mr 42,000 and 24,600 polypeptides. *Proc Natl Acad Sci USA*, **1981**. 78, 2833–2837.

139 D.A. Stetler, et al., Antibodies to distinct polypeptides of RNA polymerase I in sera from patients with rheumatic autoimmune disease. *Proc Natl Acad Sci USA*, **1982**. 79, 7499–7503.

140 G. Reimer, et al., Autoantibody to RNA polymerase I in scleroderma sera. *J Clin Invest*, **1987**. 79, 65–72.

141 M. Kuwana, et al., Autoantibody reactive with three classes of RNA polymerases in sera from patients with systemic sclerosis. *J Clin Invest*, **1993**. 91, 1399–1404.

142 J.L. Rodriguez-Sanchez, et al., Anti-NOR 90. A new autoantibody in scleroderma that recognizes a 90-kDa component of the nucleolus-organizing region of chromatin. *J Immunol*, **1987**. 139, 2579–2584.

143 H.M. Jantzen, et al., Nucleolar transcription factor hUBF contains a DNA-binding motif with homology to HMG proteins. *Nature*, **1990**. 344, 830–836.

144 E.K. Chan, et al., Human autoantibody to RNA polymerase I transcription factor hUBF. Molecular identity of nucleolus organizer region autoantigen NOR-90 and ribosomal RNA transcription upstream binding factor, **1991**. 174, 1239–1244.

144a H. Kwon and M.R. Green, The RNA polymerase I transcription factor, upstream binding factor, interacts directly with the TATA box-binding protein. *J Biol Chem*, **1994**, 269, 30140–30146.

145 R. Voit and I. Grummt, Phosphorylation of UBF at serine 388 is required for interaction with RNA polymerase I and activation of rDNA transcription. *Proc Natl Acad Sci USA*, **2001**. 98, 13631–13636.

146 J. Klein and I. Grummt, Cell cycle-dependent regulation of RNA polymerase I transcription: the nucleolar transcription factor UBF is inactive in mitosis and early G1. *Proc Natl Acad Sci USA*, **1999**. 96, 6096–6101.

147 J.H. Dagher, et al., Autoantibodies to NOR 90/hUBF: longterm clinical and serological followup in a patient with limited systemic sclerosis suggests an antigen driven immune response. *J Rheumatol*, **2002**. 29, 1543–1547.

148 H. Van Eenennaam, et al., Autoantibodies against small nucleolar ribonucleoprotein complexes and their clinical associations. *Clin Exp Immunol*, **2002**. 130, 532–540.

149 M. Kuwana, K. Kimura, and Y. Kawakami, Identification of an immunodominant epitope on RNA polymerase III recognized by systemic sclerosis sera: application to enzyme-linked immunosorbent assay. *Arthritis Rheum*, **2002**. 46, 2742–2747.

150 K.B. Elkon, E. Bonfa, and N. Brot, Antiribosomal antibodies in systemic lupus erythematosus. *Rheum Dis Clin North Am*, **1992**. 18, 377–390.

151 K.B. Elkon, A.P. Parnassa, and C.L. Foster, Lupus autoantibodies target ribosomal P proteins. *J Exp Med*, **1985**. 162, 459–471.

152 K. Elkon, et al., Identification and chemical synthesis of a ribosomal protein antigenic determinant in systemic lupus erythematosus. *Proc Natl Acad Sci USA*, **1986**. 83, 7419–7423.

153 E. Feist, et al., Proteasome alpha-type subunit C9 is a primary target of autoantibodies in sera of patients with myositis and systemic lupus erythematosus. *J Exp Med*, **1996**. 184, 1313–1318.

154 E. Feist, et al., Autoantibodies in primary Sjogren's syndrome are directed against proteasomal subunits of the alpha and beta type. *Arthritis Rheum*, **1999**. 42, 697–702.

155 I. Mayo, et al., The proteasome is a major autoantigen in multiple sclerosis. *Brain*, **2002**. 125, 2658–2667.

156 C. R. Wilkinson, et al., Localization of the 26S proteasome during mitosis and meiosis in fission yeast. *Embo J*, **1998**. 17, 6465–6476.

157 M. Mahler, R. Mierau, and M. Bluthner, Fine-specificity of the anti-CENP-A B-cell autoimmune response. *J Mol Med*, **2000**. 78, 460–467.

158 J. E. Celis and A. Celis, Cell cycle-dependent variations in the distribution of the nuclear protein cyclin proliferating cell nuclear antigen in cultured cells: subdivision of S phase. *Proc Natl Acad Sci USA*, **1985**. 82, 3262–3266.

159 Y. Takasaki, J. S. Deng, and E. M. Tan, A nuclear antigen associated with cell proliferation and blast transformation. *J Exp Med*, **1981**. 154, 1899–1909.

160 C. P. Strassburg, et al., Identification of cyclin A as a molecular target of antinuclear antibodies (ANA) in hepatic and non-hepatic autoimmune diseases. *J Hepatol*, **1996**. 25, 859–866.

161 W. H. Reeves, S. K. Nigam, and G. Blobel, Human autoantibodies reactive with the signal-recognition particle. *Proc Natl Acad Sci USA*, **1986**. 83, 9507–9511.

162 A. H. Kao, et al., Anti-signal recognition particle autoantibody in patients with and patients without idiopathic inflammatory myopathy. *Arthritis Rheum*, **2004**. 50, 209–215.

163 O. M. Howard, et al., Histidyl-tRNA synthetase and asparaginyl-tRNA synthetase, autoantigens in myositis, activate chemokine receptors on T lymphocytes and immature dendritic cells. *J Exp Med*, **2002**. 196, 781–791.

164 M. Yaneva and F. C. Arnett, Antibodies against Ku protein in sera from patients with autoimmune diseases. *Clin Exp Immunol*, **1989**. 76, 366–372.

165 Y. Takeda and W. S. Dynan, Autoantibodies against DNA double-strand break repair proteins. *Front Biosci*, **2001**. 6, D1412–1422.

166 T. Mimori and J. A. Hardin, Mechanism of interaction between Ku protein and DNA. *J Biol Chem*, **1986**. 261, 10375–10379.

167 R. Tuteja and N. Tuteja, Ku autoantigen: a multifunctional DNA-binding protein. *Crit Rev Biochem Mol Biol*, **2000**. 35, 1–33.

168 G. G. Maul, et al., Determination of an epitope of the diffuse systemic sclerosis marker antigen DNA topoisomerase I: sequence similarity with retroviral p30gag protein suggests a possible cause for autoimmunity in systemic sclerosis. *Proc Natl Acad Sci USA*, **1989**. 86, 8492–8496.

169 Y. Shoenfeld and O. Segol, Anti-histone antibodies in SLE and other autoimmune diseases. *Clin Exp Rheumatol*, **1989**. 7, 265–271.

170 R. J. DeHoratius, et al., Anti-nucleic acid antibodies in systemic lupus erythematosus patients and their families. Incidence and correlation with lymphocytotoxic antibodies. *J Clin Invest*, **1975**. 56, 1149–1154.

171 N. Bizzaro, et al., Variability between methods to determine ANA, anti-dsDNA and anti-ENA autoantibodies: a collaborative study with the biomedical industry. *J Immunol Methods*, **1998**. 219, 99–107.

172 B. S. Reisner, J. DiBlasi, and N. Goel, Comparison of an enzyme immunoassay to an indirect fluorescent immunoassay for the detection of antinuclear antibodies. *Am J Clin Pathol*, **1999**. 111, 503–506.

173 L. Chung and P. J. Utz, Antibodies in scleroderma: direct pathogenicity and phenotypic associations. *Curr Rheumatol Rep*, **2004**. 6, 156–163.

174 C. L. Will and R. Luhrmann, Spliceosomal UsnRNP biogenesis, structure and function. *Curr Opin Cell Biol*, **2001**. 13, 290–301.

175 J. P. Staley and C. Guthrie, Mechanical devices of the spliceosome: motors, clocks, springs, and things. *Cell*, **1998**. 92, 315–326.

176 J. Craft, et al., The U2 small nuclear ribonucleoprotein particle as an autoantigen. Analysis with sera from patients with overlap syndromes. *J Clin Invest*, **1988**. 81, 1716–1724.

177 A. C. Gavin, et al., Functional organization of the yeast proteome by systematic analysis of protein complexes. *Nature*, **2002**. 415, 141–147.

178 J. E. Gallagher, et al., RNA polymerase I transcription and pre-rRNA processing are linked by specific SSU processome components. *Genes Dev*, **2004**. 18, 2506–2517.

179 N. J. Krogan, et al., High-definition macromolecular composition of yeast RNA-processing complexes. *Mol Cell*, **2004**. 13, 225–239.

180 T. Wiederkehr, R. F. Pretot, and L. Minvielle-Sebastia, Synthetic lethal interactions with conditional poly(A) polymerase alleles identify *LCP5*, a gene involved in 18S rRNA maturation. *RNA*, **1998**. 4, 1357–1372.

181 N. J. Watkins, et al., A common core RNP structure shared between the small nucleolar box C/D RNPs and the spliceosomal U4 snRNP. *Cell*, **2000**. 103, 457–466.

182 S. K. Lyman, L. Gerace, and S. J. Baserga, Human Nop5/Nop58 is a component common to the box C/D small nucleolar ribonucleoproteins. *RNA*, **1999**. 5, 1597–1604.

183 D. L. J. Lafontaine and D. Tollervey, Nop58p is a common component of the box C+D snoRNPs that is required for snoRNA stability. *RNA*, **1999**. 5, 455–467.

184 D. L. Lafontaine and D. Tollervey, Synthesis and assembly of the box C+D small nucleolar RNPs. *Mol Cell Biol*, **2000**. 20, 2650–2659.

185 D. R. Newman, et al., Box C/D snoRNA-associated proteins: two pairs of evolutionarily ancient proteins and possible links to replication and transcription. *Rna*, **2000**. 6, 861–879.

186 B. Lubben, et al., Isolation of U3 snoRNP from CHO cells: a novel 55 kDa protein binds to the central part of U3 snoRNA. *Nucleic Acids Research*, **1993**. 21, 5377–5385.

187 J. Venema, et al., Yeast Rrp9p is an evolutionarily conserved U3 snoRNP protein essential for the early pre-rRNA processing cleavages and requires box C for its association. *RNA*, **2000**. 6, 1660–1671.

188 A. Colley, et al., Dhr1p, a putative DEAH-box RNA helicase, is associated with the box C+D snoRNP U3. *Mol Cell Biol*, **2000**. 20, 7238–7246.

189 S. J. Lee and S. J. Baserga, Imp3p and Imp4p: two specific components of the U3 small nucleolar ribonucleoprotein that are essential for pre-18S rRNA processing. *Molecular and Cellular Biology*, **1999**. 19, 5441–5452.

190 S. Granneman, et al., The human Imp3 and Imp4 proteins form a ternary complex with hMpp10, which only interacts with the U3 snoRNA in 60-80S ribonucleoprotein complexes. *Nucleic Acids Res*, **2003**. 31, 1877–1887.

191 J. M. Westendorf, et al., M phase phosphoprotein 10 is a human U3 small nucleolar ribonucleoprotein component. *Mol Biol Cell*, **1998**. 9, 437–449.

192 J. Venema and D. Tollervey, Rrp5 is required for formation of both 18S and 5.8S rRNA in yeast. *EMBO J.*, **1996**. 15, 5701–5714.

193 R. Jansen, D. Tollervey, and E. C. Hurt, A U3 snoRNP protein with homology to splicing factor PRP4 and G beta domains is required for ribosomal RNA processing. *EMBO Journal*, **1993**. 12, 2549–2558.

194 P. Milkereit, et al., A Noc complex specifically involved in the formation and nuclear export of ribosomal 40 S subunits. *J Biol Chem*, **2003**. 278, 4072–4081.

195 R. Gromadka and J. Rytka, The KRR1 gene encodes a protein required for 18S rRNA synthesis and 40S ribosomal subunit assembly in Saccharomyces cerevisiae. *Acta Biochim Pol*, **2000**. 47, 993–1005.

196 P. C. Liu and D. J. Thiele, Novel stress-responsive genes EMG1 and NOP14 encode conserved, interacting proteins required for 40S ribosome biogenesis. *Mol Biol Cell*, **2001**. 12, 3644–3657.

197 D. Eschrich, et al., Nep1p (Emg1p), a novel protein conserved in eukaryotes and archaea, is involved in ribosome biogenesis. *Curr Genet,* **2002**. 40, 326–338.

198 H. van Eenennaam, et al., hPop5, a protein subunit of the human RNase MRP and RNase P endoribonucleases. *J Biol Chem,* **2001**. 276, 31635–31641.

199 R. Raijmakers, et al., PM-Scl-75 is the main autoantigen in patients with the polymyositis/scleroderma overlap syndrome. *Arthritis Rheum,* **2004**. 50, 565–569.

200 R. Raijmakers, et al., The association of the human PM/Scl-75 autoantigen with the exosome is dependent on a newly identified N terminus. *J Biol Chem,* **2003**. 278, 30698–30704.

201 R. Brouwer, et al., Three novel components of the human exosome. *J Biol Chem,* **2001**. 276, 6177–6184.

202 R. Brouwer, G.J. Pruijn, and W.J. van Venrooij, The human exosome: an autoantigenic complex of exoribonucleases in myositis and scleroderma. *Arthritis Res,* **2001**. 3, 102–106.

18
Autoantibodies and the Cloning and Characterization
of Cellular Constituents *

Edward K. L. Chan

18.1
Introduction

Autoantibodies directed against intracellular antigens are characteristic features of a number of human diseases such as Sjögren's syndrome (SjS), systemic lupus erythematosus (SLE), scleroderma, certain malignancies, and paraneoplastic syndromes [1–5]. Studies in systemic rheumatic diseases have provided strong evidence that autoantibodies are maintained by antigen-driven responses [1, 6, 7] and that autoantibodies can be reporters from the immune system revealing the identity of antigens involved in the disease pathogenesis [2]. Some of these autoantibodies serve as disease-specific markers and are directed against intracellular macromolecular complexes or particles such as nucleosomes, nucleoli, small nuclear ribonucleoproteins (snRNPs), centromere antigens, and cytoplasmic RNPs (hY-RNP) [1, 2, 8]. In the last two decades, tremendous progress has been made in identifying the many intracellular autoantigen systems. Antibodies to DNA and histones have been extensively studied and their specificity and disease associations are well characterized [9, 10]. The attention of many investigators has focused on the heterogeneous group of antigens known collectively as non-histone proteins; one of the first to be described was Sm [11]. Antibodies to the Sm antigen are highly diagnostic of SLE, are present in 15–30% of unselected SLE populations, and are found in a subset of patients with chronic hypocomplementemia and nervous system disease [2]. The identification of Sm antigens as well-defined proteins bound to U-rich small nuclear RNAs (snRNAs) has been considered a significant advance, and autoantibodies have served as useful probes to help investigate the important process of pre-mRNA splicing [12].

The study of human autoantibodies and their use as probes of cell structure and function have had an important impact on the disciplines of molecular and cell biology [3]. First, the majority of autoantibodies studied have been shown to

---

* A list of abbreviations used is located at the end of this chapter.

Autoantibodies and Autoimmunity: Molecular Mechanisms in Health and Disease. Edited by K. Michael Pollard
Copyright © 2006 WILEY-VCH Verlag GmbH & Co. KGaA, Weinheim
ISBN: 3-527-31141-6

bind to highly conserved determinants on ubiquitous cellular proteins [1, 2]. Second, many of the autoantibodies associated with systemic rheumatic diseases are often directed to functional macromolecules rather than to structural components [1, 2]. These include histones, DNA and HMG of the nucleosome, the snRNP complex, various centromere and kinetochore components (CENPs), components of the nucleolus, and other subcellular structures. Third, where systems are amenable to testing, it has been shown that the autoantibodies are able to inhibit the cellular functions served by the antigens [1, 2]. Examples include the inhibition of aminoacylation of transfer RNAs by anti-tRNA synthetase antibodies, the relaxation of supercoiled DNA by anti–topoisomerase I antibodies, inhibition of precursor mRNA splicing by anti-Sm/RNP antibodies, and the transcription of RNA by anti-RNA polymerases. Taken together, these observations suggest that the conserved epitopes recognized by human autoantibodies are often the functional or active sites of these intracellular proteins [1, 2]. For immunologists, one of the interesting objectives is the identification of macromolecules and organelles – such as the nucleolus [13, 14], Golgi complex [15], and coiled bodies/Cajal bodies [16] – as targets of autoimmune responses and how this may explain pathogenesis in autoimmune diseases. For cell biologists, attempts to unravel cellular events can be enhanced by the availability of specific autoantibody probes.

18.2
cDNA Expression Cloning as a Tool to Identify Autoantigens

Two of the first reports on the cloning of antigens using human autoantibodies were the La (SS-B) antigen by Chambers and Keene [17] and the CENP-B antigen by Earnshaw et al. [18]. Cloning of autoantigens using human autoantibody probes is a well-established technology in the author's laboratory, which performed the original cloning and analysis of many autoantigens as summarized in Table 18.1 and Figure 18.1. These include ribonucleoproteins SS-B/La [19], 60-kDa [20], and 52-kDa SS-A/Ro [21]; lamin B [22]; the 75-kDa protein of the PM-Scl nucleolar protein complex [13]; the nucleolar autoantigen NOR-90/hUBF [14]; a specific marker protein of the nuclear coiled body known as p80-coilin [16]; the 64-kDa putative mRNA splicing factor HCC1 [23]; autoantigens associated with the Golgi complex known as golgin-95, golgin-160 [24], golgin-245 [25], and golgin-97 [26]; and, more recently, the marker protein GW182 for the cytoplasmic compartment known as GW bodies [27].

The general methodology for cDNA expression cloning in the author's laboratory is outlined in Figure 18.2. In brief, λgt11 or λZap human cDNA libraries are plated at 50,000 plaques per 15-cm plate and 10 large plates are used at a time to screen 500,000 recombinants for low abundant autoantigens. Next, overlay plates with nitrocellulose (NC) circles are presoaked in 10 mM isopropyl Thio-β-D-galactoside (IPTG) to induce the expression of recombinant proteins. Each NC circle is overlaid onto a plate when plaques are visible, usually 4 h at

Table 18.1 Autoantigens identified via cDNA expression cloning during a 15-year period at the W.M. Keck Autoimmune Diseases Center, at the Scripps Research Institute, and at the collaborating laboratory of Dr. Marvin J. Fritzler, University of Calgary.

Antigen type	Ref.	Antigen type	Ref.
Nuclear antigens		**Nuclear and cytoplasmic antigens**	
Lamin B	22	SS-B/La	112
p80-coilin	16	SS-A/Ro 60 kDa	20
HCC1	23	SS-A/Ro 52 kDa	21
SG₂NA	113		
HP1 Hsβ 25 kDa	114	**Cytoplasmic antigens**	
hnRNP R	115	Golgin-95/GM130	24
MPP1	116	Golgin-160	24
DFS70 / p75	117	Golgin-245	25
		Golgin-97	26
Nucleolar antigens		EEA1	78
hUBF/NOR-90	14	p62	36
PM-Scl 75	13	p90	118
No55	119	GW182	27
		Kinectin	120

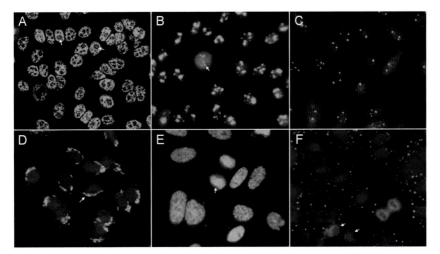

Fig. 18.1 Immunofluorescence analysis of autoantigens identified in expression cloning using HEp-2 cells. (A) 60-kDa SS-A/Ro showing predominantly nuclear speckled staining in all cells and discrete nucleolar localization in some cells (arrows). (B) NOR-90/hUBF localized to the interphase nucleoli and mitotic NOR (arrow). (C) p80-coilin staining of Cajal nuclear bodies, previously known as coiled bodies. (D) GM130 (golgin-95) staining of the Golgi complex often appearing adjacent to the nucleus (arrow). (E) DFS70 showing nuclear fine speckled staining; note that condensed chromatins are also staining (arrow). (F) GW182 staining of GW bodies. Mitotic cells do not have GW bodies (arrows). Original magnification ×400–600.

Successful cloning is enhanced when multiple high-titer sera of the same reactivity are available. We recommend screening with two to three characterized autoimmune sera rather than a single serum to cover the initial total of 500,000 recombinant clones. For example, using two selected sera and the 15-cm circular plate system, each serum is used to screen 250,000 clones in five plates. There are at least two main advantages in selecting more than one serum for screening. First, sera may have different epitope specificity, and apparently equally high-titer sera may detect different clones from a given cDNA library. Our experience is that initial screenings with no positive candidates may later become successful when a different, and sometimes higher-titer, serum is used to repeat the screening. Second, the need for the total amount of a valuable serum is substantially reduced at least by a factor of two to three and may free up reagents for screening of other cDNA libraries.

Selected high-titer autoimmune sera for antibody screening must be analyzed for background reactivity to bacterial and phage proteins. Sera with high background reactivity should be adsorbed with NC filters that are coated with wild-type phage proteins or an unrelated recombinant clone simulating the actual library-screening step. Repeated depletion of anti-bacteria and/or anti-phage antibodies may be necessary depending on the specific sera chosen. The depletion protocol should be monitored to ensure that the depletion is specific for the anti-bacteria and/or anti-phage particle antibodies, and the titer to the auto-antigen of interest should remain unaffected. Adsorbed sera are then ready for screening of the cDNA library.

18.2.2
Selection of cDNA Libraries is Another Critical Factor of Successful Cloning

There are at least three considerations in the selection of appropriate cDNA libraries. First, the expression level of the autoantigen of interest has to be evaluated to determine the optimal source for the cDNA library. Second, the availability of high-quality cDNA libraries is a practical consideration. Thus, when it was reported that the human lymphoid cell line MOLT-4 had one of the highest expression levels of PCNA among those analyzed at the time, a high-quality λgt11 cDNA library was generated from MOLT-4 mRNA by our group for the cloning of PCNA. The library was later used in the cloning of a number of autoantigens that are expressed in this library, including SS-B/La [19], lamin B [22], PM-Scl-75 [13], p80-coilin [16], SS-A/Ro 52-kDa [21] and SS-A/Ro 60-kDa proteins, and NOR-90/hUBF [14]. During the past 10 years, most of the expression cloning utilized λZAP, λZAP II, and ZAP Express libraries representing newer generations of cDNA library vectors constructed at Stratagene (La Jolla, CA). The main important advantage of the λZAP vectors is that the cDNA selected can be rescued directly into the plasmid vector using the helper phage system. ZAP Express has the added advantage of immediate expression of cloned cDNA in a eukaryotic system. The ZAP Express library contains over two million independent clones, and many cDNA inserts are over 3 kb.

The final consideration is that screening of multiple cDNA libraries may be necessary for successful expression cloning. There are many examples in our experience indicating that the lower quality of certain cDNA libraries made it necessary to screen other libraries for a given cDNA. One interesting example contrary to this was the screening of SS-A/Ro 52 kDa, first using the MOLT-4 cDNA library, wherein no positive clone was initially identified, although it was apparent that the MOLT-4 library was superior in quality to other cDNA libraries available in the laboratory at the time. Switching to screening of the HepG2 cell cDNA library yielded one partial cDNA clone for SS-A/Ro 52 kDa protein. As it turned out, the MOLT-4 cDNA library was "too high in quality" because all of the SS-A/Ro 52-kDa protein cDNAs were full-length in size, as demonstrated later with DNA hybridization using the partial cDNA obtained from the HepG2 library [21]. The apparent problem was that the full-length cDNA had an in-frame upstream stop codon preventing protein translation, and thus none of the SS-A/Ro 52-kDa cDNAs from the MOLT-4 library expressed protein and no cDNA clone was detected by the same human serum in the earlier screening experiment.

18.2.3
Useful Controls in Expression Cloning

Given that expression cloning has multiple steps, as outlined in Figure 18.2, successful cloning needs to be monitored by incorporating a number of controls. One of the most frustrating experiences is the absence of positive signals in a large-scale screening experiment. Thus, screening with a prototype anti-SS-B/La serum has served as a positive control to ensure that the overall efficiency in expression cloning is achieved. The typical control experiment is set up by screening 50,000 recombinants of a cDNA library plated in a single 15-cm diameter plate. We routinely observed one to four SS-B/La positive clones when using the prototype serum Ca screened at 1:500 dilution and a cDNA library with >1 million recombinants. For inexperienced investigators in expression cloning, the initial positive SS-B/La clones will be useful as an exercise for the library screening as well as positive controls for the subcloning steps.

A second control that deserves some discussion is the recommended use of duplicate NC filters in the initial screening step (Fig. 18.3). Theoretically, it is possible that only a single NC filter is overlaid per plate and that the signals detected are followed up by subcloning. There are some advantages of using only one NC filter, including the simplification of only one NC filter per plate resulting in a reduction of processing time in both the overlay of NC and the subsequent immunoblotting step. The major disadvantage of using only one NC filter per plate in the initial screening step is the significant number of false positives. The amount of work involved later in subcloning many single-positive plaques can be prohibitively large. With the current use of chemiluminescence, which has a sensitivity many times greater than the radioactivity or colorimetric dyes used in older protocols, as the preferred detection method, random, nonspecific signals can be a significant problem in the interpretation of true signals. The use of a second filter becomes necessary since the number of positive signals in both filters is reduced to a manageable number (Fig. 18.3).

18.2.4
Methods in Verification of Candidates in Expression Cloning

Most initial positive clones require two to three plaque purifications in the subcloning steps [28]. After the first successful subcloning, the purity of the clone often ranges from 1–10% depending on the initial density of plaques in the screening plates (~50,000 plaques per 15-cm diameter plate) and on the size of the agar plug recovered, initially obtained using the large end of a glass Pasteur pipette. After the second subcloning, the purity increases to 20–50% depending on the plaque density in the first subcloning plate (~500–1000 plaques per 90-mm diameter plate) and by using the small end of a glass Pasteur pipette. The third subcloning usually generates 100% purity when picked from a well-isolated plaque. It is obvious that significant time and effort can be saved if one focuses on the true positives while eliminating the false positives as soon as possible during subcloning. The first step in the early verification of the authenticity of a candidate cDNA is to examine whether other human sera with the same autoantibody specificity as the screening serum also recognize the candidate clone. In the example illustrated in Figure 18.4, the experiment was carried

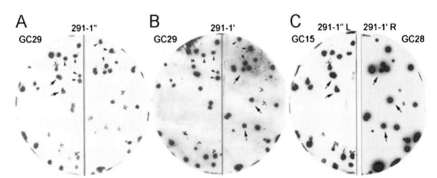

Fig. 18.4 Early verification of a candidate p90 cDNA clone by reactivity with independent autoimmune sera during the plaque-purification step. Panels (A) and (B) show the second step of plaque purification for clone 291 when ~25% of clones gave positive signals (arrowheads, ~150 clones per plate) by serum GC29 in both nitrocellulose filters lifted from the same plate. (C) When the filters were stripped of antibodies, cut into two halves, and re-probed with GC15 (291-1″ L) or GC28 (291-1′ R), both sera recognized the same plaques as GC29 (arrows). Control halves (291-1″ R and 291-1′ L, not shown) probed with a normal human serum or the secondary antibody alone gave no reaction, showing that the stripping procedure was complete (not shown). Clone 291 was recognized by all three anti-p90 human sera, and thus it represented a strong candidate for p90 cDNA.

out during the second subcloning step to confirm that the clone was recognized by other patient sera with the same autoantibody specificity. Candidate clones that are recognized by multiple patient sera, but not normal human sera, have a higher likelihood of being true positives and are selected for further analysis. However, clones that are positive only for the screening serum may also be important and are processed further at least to the stage of the DNA sequencing step (see below).

After a selected cDNA clone is plaque purified to homogeneity, a useful next step is to affinity-purify antibodies from recombinant plaque proteins for early verification of the authenticity of the cDNA clone [13, 21]. The affinity-purified antibodies can be analyzed in immunoblotting and immunofluorescence to determine whether they show reactivity with the putative antigens. Our experience in the cloning of autoantigens suggests that it is important to rule out artifacts or unrelated cDNAs at this stage using this affinity-purification criterion.

An equally important step is to start DNA sequencing determination for the candidate clones as early as possible, because the immunological-based data can sometimes be misleading. The advantage of using a λZAP or ZAP Express–type cDNA library from Stratagene becomes important when the recombinant phages can be quickly subcloned *in vivo* with helper phage into a pBluescript or pBK-CMV plasmid that can be used as DNA templates for initial DNA end sequencing. The determined nucleotide sequences are directly analyzed by the Web-based NCBI BLAST program (http://www.ncbi.nlm.nih.gov/blast/) to identify the cDNA inserts [29]. The sequence identity will help to group the candidates into subgroups for further characterization as discussed in subsequent sections.

18.2.5
Further Characterization of cDNA Clones

The next step in the characterization of cDNA clones for a given candidate autoantigen is to determine the size of the cDNA inserts. Using polymerase chain reaction (PCR), it is feasible to determine consistently the size of cDNA inserts using custom primers corresponding to the λgt11 phage arms flanking the cDNA insert or the T3 and T7 primers flanking the cDNA insert in the λZAP family of vectors. Alternatively, the plasmids used for sequencing can be digested with selected restriction enzymes to determine insert size. Recombinant fusion proteins can be produced directly from subcloned plasmids without further manipulation of the ZAP vectors. These fusion proteins will be analyzed by immunoblotting to determine the approximate size of the protein-coding regions. Reactivity of recombinant protein can be examined by several methods. As discussed earlier in Figure 18.4, phage-encoded recombinant proteins can be used to examine reactivity with other positive sera and negative controls. Recombinant proteins can be produced in *E. coli* using expression vectors such as those driven by the promoter for T7 polymerase, and the recombinant protein can be tagged with 6× His tag, GST, or maltose-binding protein for affinity purification using respective solid-phase affinity columns. Similarly, expression vectors are available for expression in mammalian cells, yeast cells, and insect cells, depending on a variety of factors governing the need for each of these systems. An alternative is to express recombinant protein using an *in vitro* transcription and translation system with the incorporation of a radiolabeled amino acid such as [^{35}S]-methionine. The reactivity of the labeled translation product is examined by immunoprecipitation using a number of positive sera and negative controls. The latter strategy was used in the characterization of cDNAs described in Table 18.1.

Independent Verification That a cDNA Encodes the Respective Autoantigen
Two-dimensional Gel Analysis

The electrophoretic migration of the full-length recombinant protein can be compared to the corresponding cellular protein. This methodology was employed to characterize the full-length cDNA clone for the 52-kDa SS-A/Ro protein [21] and lamin B [22]. This method is not applicable to cDNA clones that do not encode the complete protein or where the cellular protein may undergo significant post-translational modifications.

Partial Protease Mapping

This method is based on the fact that peptides generated from a partial protease digestion are highly characteristic of the protein. The specificity increases when more than one protease is used in the comparison. This method was used in the comparison of the recombinant and cellular 60-kDa SS-A/Ro proteins [20]. This method is more powerful when it is combined with a second dimensional gel analysis [20] or with immunoblotting analysis looking at the reactivity of the fragments.

Biochemical Purification and Amino Acid Sequence Determination for Autoantigens

We used this method to confirm SS-B/La cDNAs; the N-terminal amino acid sequence of peptides of purified bovine SS-B/La was obtained and was shown to be identical with the predicted protein sequence derived from cDNA cloning [19]. This method is not feasible unless the protein is relatively abundant and can be purified readily to homogeneity.

Production of Polyclonal Antibodies

Another method to provide independent verification that the candidate cDNA encodes the relevant autoantigen is to generate polyclonal antibodies by immunizing rabbits or mice with the purified recombinant protein. For example, the recombinant protein corresponding to the putative C-terminal fragment of p80-coilin was used to generate rabbit polyclonal antiserum R288, which demonstrated that it recognized the same protein in cell lysates and gave the same staining of nuclear bodies in IIF [16]. An alternative strategy was to use synthetic peptide antigen corresponding to the C-terminus of p80-coilin for immunization to generate the rabbit polyclonal serum R508, which had similar properties to serum R288 [30]. The production and use of polyclonal antibodies provided convincing evidence in the cloning of PM-Scl-75 [13], all of the Golgi autoantigens [24–26], and GW182 [27].

18.3
Autoantibodies to IGF-II mRNA-binding Protein p62 and Overexpression of p62 in Human Hepatocellular Carcinoma

Autoantibodies have been reported in many human cancers. Hepatocellular carcinoma (HCC) is unique among cancers in that it is possible to identify a cohort of pre-cancer patients who are likely to develop HCC after a period of 10 or more years. It has been observed that about one-third of patients with HCC have circulating autoantibodies to certain intracellular antigens [31–33] and that in some of these patients, transition from chronic liver disease to HCC is associated with the appearance of novel autoantibodies [32, 34]. It has been proposed that these novel antibodies are immune responses to antigens participating in the malignant transformation process [35]. In the author's laboratory, immunoscreening with antibodies in HCC sera has resulted in the identification of several interesting intracellular proteins, but this section will focus on findings primarily associated with the autoantigen p62.

18.3.1
Cloning of IGF-II mRNA-binding Autoantigen p62 in HCC

While analyzing a group of HCC sera originating from China, it was observed that ~20% recognized a cytoplasmic protein of 62 kDa (p62) in immunoblotting analysis. This p62 protein was expressed in high abundance in the liver cancer cell line HepG2 and the bladder carcinoma line T24 but was low or absent in MOLT-4 cells. Serum from a patient with high antibody titer to p62 was used to immunoscreen HepG2 and T24 cDNA expression libraries, and a full-length clone was isolated [36]. When the nucleotide sequence for p62 was first identified, it was shown to be a novel unreported gene. Of great interest was the finding that the deduced amino acid sequence of p62 was highly homologous to a small protein family of mRNA-binding proteins [36].

Figure 18.5 illustrates the features of p62 and two related proteins, ZBP1 [37] and Koc [38], showing their distinct RNA-binding domains. Members of this protein family have RNA recognition motifs (RRM) in the N-terminal region and four hnRNP K homology (KH) domains in the mid- to C-terminal region of the proteins. In our original publication on p62, only a single N-terminal RRM and four KH domains were reported [36], but it is now clear that there are two RRMs in the N-terminal regions based on results from updated sequence analysis programs including BLASTP [29]. Nielsen and coworkers [39] have reported the identification of three related human gene products that are binding proteins for the 5' untranslated region (UTR) of insulin-like growth factor II (IGF-II) leader 3 mRNA. The IGF-II *m*RNA-binding *p*roteins IMP-1, IMP-2, and IMP-3 were identified during studies to isolate proteins binding to IGF-II mRNA in a rhabdosarcoma cell line. The expression of IMPs is developmentally regulated and expressed in the fetus but is undetectable in normal adult tissues. IMP-1, -2, and -3 are clearly derived from separate functional genes on human

p62 and related IMP proteins

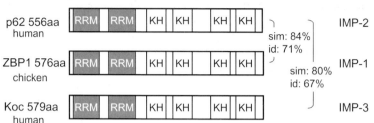

Fig. 18.5 Similarity between p62 and related RRM-KH proteins ZBP1 and Koc. These proteins contained two RNA recognition motifs (RRM) at the N-terminal domain and four hnRNP K homology (KH) domains extending from the mid-region to the C-terminus. These proteins are respective members of the three IGF-II mRNA-binding proteins IMP-1, IMP-2, IMP-3, which are distinct genes on human chromosome 17, 3, and 7, respectively. The sequence similarity (% sim) and identity (% id) between these proteins range from 60–70% and 80–85%, respectively.

chromosome 17, 3, and 7, respectively. IMP-2 is identical to p62 except for a 43-amino-acid insert between the KH2 and KH3 domains derived by differential mRNA splicing from the common precursor gene transcript. IMP-3 is identical to the protein Koc (*K*H domain–containing protein *o*verexpressed in *c*ancer), which was originally identified by differential display analysis of pancreatic cancer versus normal tissues [38]; Koc is not expressed in most normal tissues. IMP-1 is the human homologue of chicken ZBP1 [37] and the murine CRD-BP [40, 41]. ZBP1 (zip code–binding protein) was originally defined as one of the proteins bound to the conserved 54-nucleotide RNA zip-code element in the 3' UTR of beta-actin mRNA, which is required for its localization to the leading edge of fibroblasts [37]. The implication is that ZBP1 is important for cell migration, which plays a significant role in carcinogenesis, although the role for ZBP1 in cancer remains unclear. CRD-BP was identified as the *c*oding *r*egion instability *d*eterminant *b*inding *p*rotein that binds and protects c-*myc* mRNA from endonucleolytic cleavage and therefore extends the *in vivo* half-life of c-*myc*, which has an important consequence in cell proliferation and cancer [40, 41]. Thus, a feature in common to all members of this family is that they are all mRNA-binding proteins and they bind to the 5' UTR (IMPs), the coding region (CRD-BP), or the 3' UTR (ZBP1) of different mRNAs. It should be noted that these IMPs are likely to bind to additional mRNA species.

All three IMPs have some relationship to cancer. The probable links of IMP-1/CRD-BP and IMP-3/Koc to cancer are addressed briefly above. IMP-2/p62 was shown to be an autoantigen, and antibodies were present in 21% of patients with HCC but not in the precursor conditions chronic hepatitis and liver cirrhosis [36]. Immunohistochemical studies have shown ectopic expression of p62 and Koc in cancer nodules of human HCC tissues [42, 43]. IGF-II has been shown to be overexpressed in many cancers, and one of the earliest demonstrations was its overexpression in human HCC [44, 45]. There are transgenic models of IGF-II overexpression that have resulted in carcinogenesis in the transgenic animals [46–48]. In hepatitis B virus transgenic mice, chronic hepatocellular injury led to HCC in some animals, and in examining for abnormalities in structure and expression of a large number of oncogenes and tumor-suppressor genes – including *ras, myc, fos, abl, src,* Rb, and p53 – only IGF-II overexpression was found [49].

18.3.2
Humoral Response to p62 During Transition from Chronic Liver Disease to HCC

A feature of HCC is the well-documented observation that HBV- or HCV-related chronic hepatitis and liver cirrhosis are frequent precursor conditions that predispose its development [50–53]. In many countries where HBV and HCV infections are widely prevalent, patients with resultant chronic liver disease are followed regularly in outpatient clinics for treatment and for early detection of liver malignancy. In some of these patients, serial serum samples over a period of several years have been collected, and in previously reported studies it was shown that novel antibodies appeared during conversion to malignancy that were not present in the pre-malignant chronic liver disease phase [32]. In HCC, where novel autoantibody responses are detected during conversion to malignancy, characterization of the autoantigens associated with the novel immune responses might provide insights into intracellular proteins participating in pathways leading to malignant transformation. The analysis of a group of serial serum samples from 17 Japanese patients with HCC showed the *de novo* appearance of antibodies to p62 during transition from chronic liver disease to HCC (Fig. 18.6) [34]. This prospective study indicates that transition to malignancy can be associated with autoantibody responses to certain cellular proteins that might have roles in the transformation process [34].

18.3.3
Autoantibodies to p62 and Koc Are Widely Present in HCC and Other Cancers

As mentioned above, antibodies to p62 were found in 21% of patients with HCC but not in the precursor conditions chronic hepatitis and liver cirrhosis [36]. Of interest was that Koc has been shown to be transcriptionally overexpressed in pancreatic and other cancers [38]. The domain structure and sequence similarity of the two proteins and their association with cancer prompted a study to determine the humoral immune responses to p62 and Koc in different malignancies and to analyze the similarities and differences of antigenic determinants on p62 and Koc recognized by these autoantibodies. Our study determined the extent and frequency of autoantibodies to p62 and Koc in diverse malignancies, the epitopes on the antigens, and the presence or absence of cross-reactive antibodies [54]. Recombinant polypeptides were expressed from full-length and partial cDNA constructs and used as antigens in Western blotting, ELISA, and immunoprecipitation. After identifying the epitopes, cross-ab-

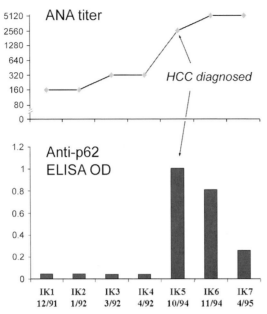

Fig. 18.6 New appearance of autoantibodies to p62 and CENP-F coincides with the detection of HCC in a liver cirrhosis patient associated with positive HCV serology. Four serial serum samples collected from the patient before the diagnosis of HCC had low ANA titers ($\geq 1:320$). When the diagnosis of HCC was made at time point IK5, the ANA titer had increased to $1:2560$ and persisted at high titers ($1:5120$) for six months until the last blood sample was drawn. The new ANA detected was anti-CENP-F antibody, confirmed by an immunoprecipitation assay using the *in vitro*-translated fragment of CENP-F [34]. The lower panel shows the p62 autoantibody concentration semi-quantitated with ELISA against purified recombinant protein.

sorption with recombinant polypeptides was used to determine specificity. Sera from 777 patients with 10 different types of malignancy were analyzed. In sum, autoantibodies to p62 were found in 11.6% and to Koc in 12.2% and cumulatively to one or the other antigen in 20.5% of patient sera, with significant difference from the control populations consisting of normal subjects and autoimmune disease patients ($P<0.01$). The immunodominant epitopes were at the N-termini of both antigens, and absorption studies showed that the majority of autoantibodies were not cross-reactive [54]. Autoantibodies to p62 and Koc were present in approximately similar frequencies in a variety of malignancies, and the immune responses appeared to be independent of each other.

Many investigators have shown that autoantibody responses are predominantly antigen-driven in systemic rheumatic diseases [2]. The reason that intracellular antigens result in the elicitation of autoimmune responses has not been completely elucidated, but one reason might be genetic mutations resulting in production of abnormal proteins or dysregulation of gene expression, such as ectopic expression of oncofetal proteins. It is possible that some of these features may be responsible for the production of autoantibodies to p62 and Koc. The frequency and wide distribution of anti-p62 and anti-Koc antibodies are in line with the frequency and distribution of anti-p53 in different tumors [55]. If this phenomenon is related to aberrant expression of these mRNA-binding proteins, a pathway contributing to tumorigenesis could be by way of dysregulation of IGF-II expression. Further studies such as production of p62 and Koc transgenic mice should provide insights into how these proteins might be involved in malignancy

18.3.4
Aberrant Expression of p62 in HCC

Using immunohistochemistry to examine a group of archival paraffin-embedded HCC tissue blocks, we confirmed that approximately one-third of the patients showed high expression of p62 protein in HCC nodules, whereas adjacent non-malignant parenchymal liver cells had no detectable staining [42, 43]. In addition, normal adult liver tissue did not have detectable p62. We also showed that p62 expression was demonstrated in human fetal liver at the mRNA and protein levels but was undetectable or barely detectable in adult liver. These data are consistent with characteristics of IMP expression reported in fetal and adult tissues [39]. p62 expression was also detected in scattered cells in cirrhotic nodules in contrast to uniform expression in all cells in HCC nodules. These studies show that p62 is developmentally regulated, is expressed in fetal but not in adult liver, and is aberrantly expressed in HCC and could be playing a role in abnormal cell proliferation in HCC and cirrhosis by modulating expression of growth factors such as IGF-II.

The importance of this finding with its relationship to cancer is the fact that IGF-II has been shown to be overexpressed in human cancer [44, 56–58] and that mice transgenic for IGF-II have been shown to develop malignancy and organomegaly of different tissues [46, 47]. Cariani et al. showed that there was increased expression of IGF-II mRNA in human primary liver cancers [44]. Rogler et al. produced IGF-II transgenic mice and showed that some of these mice had altered body composition and increased frequency of a number of different malignancies [47]. Christofori et al. induced tumors in SV40 large T antigen transgenic mice and showed that the mice which developed tumors were those which concomitantly showed expression of IGF-II in the tumors [59]. They postulated that IGF-II was a second signal that enhanced the carcinogenic potential of SV40 large T antigen. Bates et al. also showed the induction of mammary cancer in IGF-II transgenic mice [46]. It should be noted that aberrant expression of IGF-II might not be the only gene that is abnormally regulated by the IMP proteins. Disordered regulation of mRNAs might lead to different phenotypic expressions, depending upon the type of mRNA that is bound by these proteins.

Our studies and those of others [60] have provided evidence that autoantibodies to some cancer-related antigens such as p62/IMP-2, koc/IMP-3, IMP-1, p53, and c-*myc* might be used as markers in cancer. The reservation is that antibodies to individual cancer-specific antigens do not reach levels of sensitivity that could become routinely useful in diagnosis. It is conceivable that autoantibody profiles involving different arrays of "cancer antigens" might be developed in the future and that the procedure could be useful for cancer diagnosis [61, 62].

18.4
Unique Features of Golgi Complex Autoantigens

The Golgi complex is a conserved cytoplasmic organelle localized in the perinuclear region of eukaryotic cells and is characterized by membrane stacks spatially and functionally organized as distinct *cis-*, *medial-*, and *trans*-Golgi networks. The Golgi complex has prominent functions in the processing, transporting, and sorting of newly synthesized proteins derived from the rough endoplasmic reticulum. Anti–Golgi complex antibodies (AGAs) were first identified in the serum of a SjS patient with lymphoma [63]. This was followed by other reports describing AGAs in various systemic autoimmune diseases including SjS [64] and SLE [65]. AGAs were also reported in 10% of patients with HIV infection [66] and 35.7% of HIV carriers [67]; however, in the more recent report of Massabki et al. [68], AGAs were not found in 100 HIV-infected patients. Bizzaro and coworkers reported that the presence of high-titer AGAs might constitute an early sign of systemic autoimmune diseases even in the absence of clinical manifestations [69]. Although there is as yet no clear correlation of AGAs to specific disease or clinical manifestations, recent advances in clinical and research studies of these cytoplasmic autoantigens may provide better understanding in the future.

18.4.1
Cloning of Golgi Autoantigens (Golgins)

Immunoblotting and immunoprecipitation analyses show that proteins recognized by human AGA are heterogeneous [70]. Within the past 10 years, our laboratories and others have cloned and identified a family of novel Golgi autoantigens. These have been achieved primarily by cDNA expression cloning using human autoantibody probes. These Golgi autoantigens are referred to as giantin/macrogolgin/GCP372, golgin-245/p230, GMAP-210, golgin-160/GCP170, golgin-95/GM130, and golgin-97 [24–26, 66, 71]. These proteins have relatively high molecular weights that range from 100 kDa to 370 kDa. Golgins were originally described as autoantigens identified in the Golgi complex recognized by autoantibodies from patients with systemic autoimmune diseases [24]. They share common structural features that include long coiled-coil alpha helical rod-like domains throughout the entire protein except for the amino and carboxyl termini [72]. Recent evidence suggests that golgins are necessary for tethering events in membrane fusion during vesicular transport and as structural supports for Golgi cisternae [73]. More recently, several other Golgi proteins — such as golgin-84, an 84-kDa transmembrane Golgi protein [74] — have been categorized as golgins because of the presence of coiled-coil domains, despite the fact they have not been identified as autoantigens [72].

The other common feature shared by Golgi autoantigens is that biochemical evidence and immunoelectron microscopy data show that they are peripheral or transmembrane proteins localized to the cytoplasmic face of the Golgi complex. It has been reported that several golgins, such as golgin-245 and golgin 97, are attached to Golgi membranes through a GRIP domain in the carboxyl termini [75]. In contrast to other Golgi autoantigens, giantin has a single short transmembrane domain in the carboxyl termini, while the bulk of the protein extends into the cytoplasm [66]. These common features of Golgi autoantigens lead us to propose that these Golgi autoantigens may have common biochemical characteristics and functions that make them preferred autoimmune targets among the ~100 Golgi complex proteins described to date [76].

18.4.2
Prevalence of Human AGA

Although human AGAs have been reported to recognize a number of Golgi proteins, the individual Golgi autoantigen that is the most common target was not identified until recently, when we reported the prevalence of human AGAs to five of the most common Golgi autoantigens [77]. A total of 80 AGA human sera were used to investigate the prevalence of these autoantibodies using immunoprecipitation and ELISA with purified recombinant antigens. The prevalence of reactivity of the 80 human AGA sera is summarized in Table 18.2. The most common Golgi complex autoantigen target was giantin (50%) and the second most common target was golgin-245 (24%). The lowest frequency reactivity was to golgin-97 (3.8%). There were 25 AGA sera (31.3%) that did not react with any of the five Golgi autoantigens used in this study, indicating that there are other, unidentified Golgi autoantigens. Interestingly, the frequency of sera reactive with the five Golgi autoantigens was numerically correlated with the molecular masses of the native Golgi autoantigens (Table 18.2). In addition, we

Table 18.2 Frequency of autoantibodies to specific Golgi autoantigens in 80 human anti-Golgi autoimmune sera.

Golgi autoantigen	Molecular weight (kDa)	Positive sera (%)
Giantin	370	50.0
Golgin-245	245	23.8
Golgin-160	160	13.6
Golgin-95/GM130	130	7.5
Golgin-97	97	3.8
Uncharacterized Golgi antigens		31.3

showed that none of the sera had AGAs to more than three of these five Golgi autoantigens. There were six, 15, and 34 sera with antibodies to three, two, and one of the five Golgi autoantigens, respectively. Interestingly, the sera containing the autoantibodies to more than one Golgi autoantigen reacted with either giantin or golgin-245. In other words, serum autoantibodies that bound golgin-160, GM130, and golgin-97 did not overlap with each other, although the number of sera with these three autoantibodies was small [77]. These results also suggest that the human autoimmune response to Golgi autoantigens appears to be highly specific because many AGA sera react with only one (42.5%) or two (18.8%) of the five autoantigens. Since giantin was the most common Golgi autoantigen, epitope mapping was performed using six overlapping partial-length giantin constructs, confirming that epitopes of giantin are located throughout the length of the protein, with the major epitope localized to the carboxyl-terminal domains [77].

18.4.3
Mechanism of AGA Production and Relation to Other Large Coiled-coil Protein Autoantigens

The Golgi autoantigens identified to date are related in that they have similar overall secondary structures, as evidenced by their extensive coiled-coil rod domains in the central region of the protein. As stated in the previous section, it is interesting that a significant difference in the frequency of autoantibodies to the Golgi autoantigens examined was observed. For example, the frequency of antibody to giantin was 13-fold greater than that to golgin-97. To consider the mechanism of AGA production, it is important to address why giantin has a higher frequency of reactivity than any other Golgi protein. Differences between giantin and other golgins include the fact that giantin is the largest Golgi protein and contains a greater number of coiled-coil subunits compared to the other golgins; in addition, only giantin possesses a transmembrane domain, which may ensure its tighter association with the Golgi complex membranes even when it is released during cell lysis.

It is important to note that autoimmune responses to Golgi autoantigens appear to be highly specific and not merely directed to cross-reactive epitopes of the coiled-coil domains, which is the most obvious common feature of Golgi autoantigens [77]. It is interesting that large coiled-coil-rich proteins (≥ 100 kDa) have been reported as autoantigens in other cytoplasmic compartments (Fig. 18.7). For example, in the endosomal compartment, the two known autoantigens are early endosomal protein EEA1 (180 kDa) [78] and CLIP-170 (170 kDa) [79]. There is also a series of centrosomal autoantigens identified as coiled-coil-rich proteins including pericentrin, a 220-kDa protein [80]; ninein, a protein with alternatively spliced products of 245 kDa and 249 kDa [81]; Cep250 (250 kDa); and Cep110 (110 kDa) [82]. Centromere autoantigens have been described, but the two interesting ones related to this discussion are CENP-E [83] and CENP-F [84], both of which are high-molecular-weight proteins

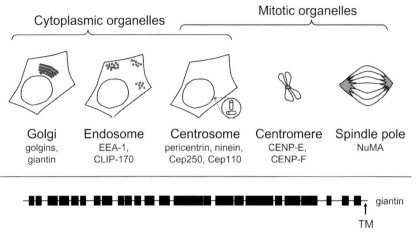

Fig. 18.7 Cytoplasmic compartments with coiled-coil-rich autoantigens. Golgi autoantigens such as giantin, illustrated here with a transmembrane domain (TM), are typically rich in coiled-coil domains. A number of human autoantigens that are rich in coiled-coils have overall similarity to the Golgi autoantigens described to date. These anti-gens are primarily localized to cytoplasmic and mitotic organelles. It is interesting to note that many other cytoplasmic compart-ments known to be targets in autoimmune diseases, such as ribosomes, mitochondria, lysosomes, and GW bodies, do not contain coiled-coil-rich, high-molecular-weight autoantigens.

(312–400 kDa) and have the same type of overall structure as discussed above. NuMA is another large coiled-coil protein located at the mitotic spindle pole and is the most common target autoantigen in sera with mitotic spindle appara-tus staining [85]. Non-muscle myosin (~200 kDa) is a cytoskeletal autoantigen [86] qualified in the same group of high-molecular-weight and coiled-coil-rich autoantigens. It is noteworthy that coexisting autoantibodies to these other coiled-coil-rich organelles were not observed in our analysis of AGA sera [77]. These endosomal, centrosomal, mitotic apparatus, and intracellular autoanti-gens are, like the golgins, proteins with high molecular weights and an overall high content of coiled-coil domains. The combination of these two physical fea-tures in autoantigens may contribute to the induction and production of auto-immune antibodies in certain disease states. One exception to the rule are the lower-molecular-weight nuclear envelope–associated lamins, which are also auto-antigens that are rich in coiled-coiled domains [87].

18.4.4
Modification of Golgi Autoantigens During Cell Death

It has been observed that many autoantigens are parts of multi-protein–nucleic acid complexes [1], although it remains unclear why and how the immune system is able to recognize or target these intracellular autoantigens. It has been proposed that some intracellular autoantigens such as SS-A/Ro and SS-B/La are translocated to apoptotic blebs during apoptosis and that these apoptotic blebs may trigger autoantibody production [88]. Interestingly, Golgi autoantigens were not localized to apoptotic blebs, as shown in our previous study [89]. Immunofluorescence analysis in our studies showed that the Golgi complex was altered and developed distinctive characteristics during apoptosis and necrosis [89]. Our data suggest that, unlike SS-A/Ro and certain other autoantigens, the expression of autoantigens on surface blebs of apoptotic cells is clearly not a universal requirement for autoantibody production. One possible explanation is that they may be recognized as surface structures on cytoplasmic organelles that are released to the immune system in aberrant disease states associated with unregulated apoptosis, or necrosis, resulting from injury or infection. An emerging view is that modified forms of autoantigens generated during cell death might stimulate autoantibody responses if they are presented to the immune system in a proinflammatory context [90]. Casciola-Rosen and coworkers have also proposed that modification of autoantigens during cell death, particularly proteolytic cleavage, may be crucial for the generation of autoantibodies in autoimmune diseases [90]. Indeed, Casiano and coworkers have shown that a variety of intracellular autoantigens are cleaved into fragments during apoptosis and necrosis [91]. Recently, our laboratory and others have shown that some Golgi autoantigens gave distinct cleavage fragments during apoptosis and necrosis [89, 92]. It has been speculated that these modified forms of autoantigens may have enhanced immunogenicity because of exposed cryptic epitopes that are not generated during antigen processing [93, 94]. These epitopes may be recognized as surface structures on cytoplasmic organelles such as the Golgi complex released to, or processed by, the immune system in aberrant disease states. This may explain why giantin has the highest frequency, because during cell death it may be more stably associated with the remaining Golgi surface membrane than other golgins by virtue of its transmembrane domain. Autoantibody responses may be amplified and sustained upon repeated stimulation if the exposure of intracellular antigens to the immune system is associated with defective clearance of apoptotic cells, prolonged primary or secondary necrosis, T-cell cytotoxicity associated with chronic infection, or even antigen mutation or overexpression. It would be important not only to assess the immunogenic potential of subcellular particles and proteolytic fragments released during cell death but also to continue investigating possible defects leading to aberrant apoptosis or phagocyte function and/or aberrant antigen expression in systemic autoimmune diseases.

18.5

Cloning of GW182 Autoantigen and Identification of GW Bodies

In 2002, we reported the cloning of a cDNA for the novel cytoplasmic protein GW182 localized primarily in discrete bodies in the cytoplasm of tissue-cultured cells by using a patient serum to immunoscreen a HeLa cell cDNA library [27]. GW182 contains multiple glycine/tryptophan (GW) repeats and a classical RRM near the C-terminus. Analysis of the full-length cDNA for this novel autoantigen showed that the open reading frame encodes a protein with 1709 amino acids with a calculated molecular mass of 182 kDa. Throughout the protein there are 60 (3.5%) tryptophan residues, 39 of which are adjacent to glycine residues; exceptions are the RRM and a region relatively free of GW. Many of the tryptophans are in regions that appear to be repetitive and are comprised primarily of glycine/tryptophan (GW) or tryptophan/glycine (WG) repeat amino acid sequences, and less often of a variation when tryptophan was followed by an amino acid other than glycine. Although the significance of these repeats is not known, based on this unusual motif and its predicted molecular mass, we have elected to name the protein GW182 and the associated cytoplasmic structures GW bodies (GWBs).

18.5.1

GW Bodies Are Distinct Cytoplasmic Foci

Figure 18.1 F shows the immunostaining of the prototype serum on HEp-2 cell substrate. The brightly stained GWBs appear to vary during the cell cycle — few or no staining in early G1 cells and more numerous and intense staining in late S or G2 cells [95]. GWBs are conserved across species and are detectable at least in chicken fibroblasts, mouse 3T3 cells, and *Xenopus* tissue culture cells. Based on our experience, GWBs are potentially novel structures not previously described. To confirm that these structures are not components of previously described cytoplasmic organelles, we have used the available markers of cytoplasmic organelles including the Golgi complex, endosome, peroxisome, lysosome, proteasome, etc., to show that GWBs are unrelated structures [27]. Using immuno-EM on ultra-thin cryosections of HeLa cells, antibodies to GW182 labeled electron-dense cytoplasmic bodies that range in size from 100 nm to 300 nm and are not bound by a bilayer lipid membrane [27]. Distinct from any known organelle, GWBs appear as cytoplasmic clusters of electron-dense fibrils or strands of 8–10 nm in diameter (Fig. 18.8). Most of the gold particles were observed on clusters of electron-dense fibrils that appear to form a matrix.

Recombinant protein derived from this GW182 cDNA was used to immunize a rabbit, and the resultant rabbit antiserum recognized the same cytoplasmic foci as the human prototype serum, as demonstrated in a double immunofluorescence staining experiment. A second independent proof that the cloned cDNA encodes a protein of GWBs is provided from the green fluorescent protein (GFP)-fusion construct showing that the GFP-fusion protein localized to the

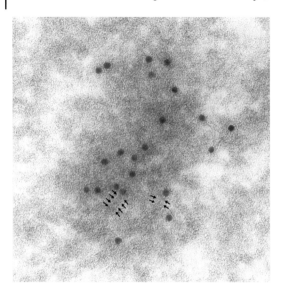

Fig. 18.8 Immunogold electron microscopy localization of GWBs in the cytoplasm of HeLa cells during interphase. Frozen sections of fixed and gelatin-embedded HeLa cells were incubated with the index human anti-GW182 serum diluted 1:400 and then post-immunolabeled with Protein A-gold (10 nm). The gold labels are clustered on electron-dense fibrils or strands 8–10 nm in diameter (arrows). These fibrils appear to form the matrix where the gold labels decorate. Original magnification ×105,000.

same cytoplasmic compartment. Furthermore, we showed in a real-time, live-cell experiment that the GFP-labeled domains are not static entities but show vectoral movement; fusion of GFP-labeled GWBs was also documented using time-lapse microscopy [95].

18.5.2
GWBs Are Foci for mRNA Storage and Degradation

The detection of a well-defined RNA-binding domain in the carboxyl-terminal domain of GW182 led us to investigate the type of cellular RNA that may be associated with GW182. Using an immunoprecipitation assay and extracts from [^{32}P]-phosphate-labeled HeLa cells, we could not show any association between GW182 and small RNAs such as those associated with Sm, SS-A/Ro, and SS-B/La ribonucleoproteins. Through a collaboration with Scott A. Tenenbaum and Jack D. Keene at Duke University, GW182 was shown to be associated with a subset of mRNA [27]. In brief, immunoprecipitation of cell extracts was carried out using specific anti-GW182 antibodies, and the putative mRNA bound to GW182 was extracted and reverse-transcribed to cDNA that was then labeled as probes for cDNA array analysis. This led to the hypothesis that GW182 is involved in pathways of metabolism of mRNA subsets and thus regulates their gene expression. The mRNAs associated with GW182 represent a clustered set of transcripts that are presumed to reside within GWBs [27].

GWB-like, discrete cytoplasmic foci that contained hLSm complex proteins 1–7 as well as the hDcp1 protein have been described by other groups [96, 97]. Both the hLSm1-7 complex [98–100] and hDcp [97, 101, 102] are involved in mRNA decapping and other processes of mRNA degradation. In mammalian cells, decapping has been suggested to be an important step in the process of mRNA decay [103, 104]. Recently, we demonstrated that the hLSm4 protein, a component of the hLSm1-7 complex, and the hDcp1 protein both colocalize with GW182 in GWBs, supporting the hypothesis that GWBs are involved in mRNA degradation [105].

The immuno-EM data (Fig. 18.8) showing that GW182 localized to 8–10-nm strands suggest that GW182 may be an important component of GWBs. *In vitro* gene knockdown of GW182 using specific siRNA led to the disappearance of GWBs, demonstrating that GW182 is a critical component of GWBs [95]. The incremental expression of the GW182 protein in cells induced to proliferate and the cyclic formation and breakdown of GWBs during mitosis are intriguing in view of the notion that GWBs are specialized centers involved in maintaining stability and/or controlling degradation of mRNA. More recent work from our laboratory has demonstrated that GWBs are also foci associated with and required for siRNA function (submitted).

18.5.3
GW182 and Sjögren's Syndrome

Anti-GW182 autoantibodies are relatively rare among human sera from patients with systemic rheumatic diseases examined to date. However, the data showed that 9/18 anti-GW182 positive patients (50%) with available clinical data were diagnosed with SjS [106]. Interestingly ~50% of the patients with anti-GW182 also have antibodies to 52 kDa SS-A/Ro. Our preliminary data showed that increased expression of GW182 is seen in selected foci of salivary gland ducts from SjS patients. Furthermore, it appears that the same foci have elevated expression of SS-B/La, as demonstrated by staining of adjacent section (unpublished data). Our working hypothesis is that local or focal changes in tissue gene expression that lead to overexpression of a subset of macromolecules are the continuous stimuli for the autoimmune responses seen in SjS diseases. The increased expression of self-proteins such as SS-B/La and GW182, which may be complexed with foreign agents or oncofetal macromolecules, may enhance the autoimmune responses. We propose that studying the events in tissue overexpression of self-antigens may provide a useful means to understand the immunopathogenesis of SjS.

18.6
Future Perspectives

The complete sequencing of the human genome has had a significant impact on the identification of autoantigens. Together with the high sensitivity of mass spectrometry-MALDI, complete gene data lead to enhancement in the ability to identify proteins. Undoubtedly, expression cloning of antigens will remain important by providing a means to identify unknowns, given that MS-MALDI also has its limitations. In the identification of autoantigens, there are other challenges in using cDNA expression cloning. For example, expression cloning using the phage-*E.coli* system will not detect autoepitopes that require certain post-translational modifications that are present in the mammalian system. Phosphorylation of the C-terminal domain of the high-molecular-weight subunit of RNA Pol II has been shown to be required for reactivity to human autoantibodies [107, 108]. Some Sm epitopes are known to require dimethyl Arg residues in SmD proteins [109]. The recent finding that autoantibody to citrullinated peptides (anti-CCP) is an important marker for RA [110] as well as early RA [111] has opened a renewed interest in the role of post-translational modification in autoimmune diseases. Nevertheless, cDNA expression cloning may remain important, as demonstrated by the three recent examples presented here, and has led to further exploration of the role of these autoantigens in disease pathogenesis.

Abbreviations

AGA	anti-Golgi complex antibody
ANA	antinuclear antibody
CB	Cajal bodies or coiled bodies
CENP-F	centromere protein F
DAPI	4′,6-diamidino-2-phenylindole
ELISA	enzyme-linked immunosorbent assay
GFP	green fluorescent protein
GWB	GW182-containing cytoplasmic body
HCC	hepatocellular carcinoma
HRPO	horseradish peroxidase
IEM	immunoelectron microscopy
IGF-II	insulin-like growth factor II
IIF	indirect immunofluorescence
IMP	IGF-II mRNA-binding protein
KH	hnRNP K homology domain
Koc	KH domain protein overexpressed in cancer
MCTD	mixed connective tissue disorders
NC	nitrocellulose
NOR	nucleolar organizer region

PBS	phosphate buffered saline
PCNA	proliferating cell nuclear antigen
RRM	RNA recognition motif
SLE:	systemic lupus erythematosus
SjS	Sjögren's syndrome
UTR	untranslated region

References

1 E.M. Tan, E.K.L. Chan, K.F. Sullivan, and R.L. Rubin, *Clin. Immunol. Immunopathol.* **1988**, *47*, 121–141.

2 E.M. Tan, *Adv. Immunol.* **1989**, *44*, 93–151.

3 E.M. Tan, *Cell* **1991**, *67*, 841–842.

4 M.J. Fritzler, *J. Dermatol.* **1993**, *20*, 257–268.

5 E.K.L. Chan and L.E.C. Andrade, *Rheum. Dis. Clin. North Am.* **1992**, *18*, 551–570.

6 D.M. Tillman, N.T. Jou, R.J. Hill, and T.N. Marion, *J. Exp. Med.* **1992**, *176*, 761–779.

7 M.Z. Radic and M. Weigert, *Annu Rev Immunol* **1994**, *12*, 487–520.

8 J.A. Hardin, *Arthritis Rheum.* **1986**, *29*, 457–460.

9 B.D. Stollar, *FASEB J.* **1994**, *8*, 337–342.

10 R.L. Rubin, *Antihistone antibodies*. In *Systemic Lupus Erythematosus*, Vol. 2. (Ed. R.G. Lahita) pp. 247–271, Churchill Livingstone, New York 1992.

11 E.M. Tan and H.G. Kunkel, *J. Immunol.* **1966**, *96*, 464–471.

12 M.R. Lerner and J.A. Steitz, *Proc. Natl. Acad. Sci. USA* **1979**, *76*, 5495–5499.

13 F. Alderuccio, E.K.L. Chan, and E.M. Tan, *J. Exp. Med.* **1991**, *173*, 941–952.

14 E.K.L. Chan, H. Imai, J.C. Hamel, and E.M. Tan, *J. Exp. Med.* **1991**, *173*, 1239–1244.

15 E.K.L. Chan and M.J. Fritzler, *Autoantibodies to Golgi Apparatus antigens*. In *Pathogenic and diagnostic relevance of autoantibodies*. (Ed. K. Conrad, R.L. Humbel, M. Meurer, Y. Shoenfeld and E.M. Tan) pp. 85–100, Pabst Science Publishers, Lengerich, Germany 1998.

16 L.E.C. Andrade, E.K.L. Chan, I. Raska, C.L. Peebles, G. Roos, and E.M. Tan, *J. Exp. Med.* **1991**, *173*, 1407–1419.

17 J.C. Chambers and J.D. Keene, *Proc. Natl. Acad. Sci. USA* **1985**, *82*, 2115–2119.

18 W.C. Earnshaw, K.F. Sullivan, P.S. Machlin, C.A. Cooke, D.A. Kaiser, T.D. Pollard, N.F. Rothfield, and D.W. Cleveland, *J. Cell Biol.* **1987**, *104*, 817–829.

19 E.K.L. Chan, K.F. Sullivan, and E.M. Tan, *Nucleic Acids Res.* **1989**, *17*, 2233–2244.

20 E. Ben-Chetrit, B.J. Gandy, E.M. Tan, and K.F. Sullivan, *J. Clin. Invest.* **1989**, *83*, 1284–1292.

21 E.K.L. Chan, J.C. Hamel, J.P. Buyon, and E.M. Tan, *J. Clin. Invest.* **1991**, *87*, 68–76.

22 K.M. Pollard, E.K.L. Chan, B.J. Grant, K.F. Sullivan, E.M. Tan, and C.A. Glass, *Mol. Cell. Biol.* **1990**, *10*, 2164–2175.

23 H. Imai, E.K.L. Chan, K. Kiyosawa, X.-D. Fu, and E.M. Tan, *J. Clin. Invest.* **1993**, *92*, 2419–2426.

24 M.J. Fritzler, J.C. Hamel, R.L. Ochs, and E.K.L. Chan, *J. Exp. Med.* **1993**, *178*, 49–62.

25 M.J. Fritzler, C.C. Lung, J.C. Hamel, K. Griffith, and E.K.L. Chan, *J. Biol. Chem.* **1995**, *270*, 31262–31268.

26 K.J. Griffith, E.K.L. Chan, C.C. Lung, J.C. Hamel, X. Guo, K. Miyachi, and M.J. Fritzler, *Arthritis Rheum.* **1997**, *40*, 1693–1702.

27 T. Eystathioy, E.K.L. Chan, S.A. Tenenbaum, J.D. Keene, K. Griffith, and M.J. Fritzler, *Mol. Biol. Cell* **2002**, *13*, 1338–1351.

28 Current protocols in molecular biology, John Wiley & Sons, Inc., New York 2004.

29 S.F. Altschul, T.L. Madden, A.A. Schaffer, Z. Zhang, W. Miller, and D.J. Lipman, *Nucleic Acids Res.* **1997**, *25*, 3389–3402.

30 E. K. L. Chan, S. Tanako, L. E. C. Andrade, J. C. Hamel, and A. G. Matera, *Nucleic Acids Res.* **1994**, *22*, 4462–4469.

31 G. Covini, C. A. von Mühlen, S. Pacchetti, M. Colombo, E. K. L. Chan, and E. M. Tan, *J Hepatol* **1997**, *26*, 1255–1265.

32 H. Imai, Y. Nakano, K. Kiyosawa, and E. M. Tan, *Cancer* **1993**, *71*, 26–35.

33 H. Imai, R. L. Ochs, K. Kiyosawa, S. Furuta, R. M. Nakamura, and E. M. Tan, *Am. J. Pathol.* **1992**, *140*, 859–870.

34 J. Y. Zhang, W. Zhu, H. Imai, K. Kiyosawa, E. K. L. Chan, and E. M. Tan, *Clin. Exp. Immunol.* **2001**, *125*, 3–9.

35 E. M. Tan, *J. Clin. Invest* **2001**, *108*, 1411–1415.

36 J. Y. Zhang, E. K. L. Chan, X. X. Peng, and E. M. Tan, *J. Exp. Med.* **1999**, *189*, 1101–1110.

37 A. F. Ross, Y. Oleynikov, E. H. Kislauskis, K. L. Taneja, and R. H. Singer, *Mol. Cell Biol.* **1997**, *17*, 2158–2165.

38 F. Mueller-Pillasch, U. Lacher, C. Wallrapp, A. Micha, F. Zimmerhackl, H. Hameister, G. Varga, H. Friess, M. Buchler, H. G. Beger, M. R. Vila, G. Adler, and T. M. Gress, *Oncogene* **1997**, *14*, 2729–2733.

39 J. Nielsen, J. Christiansen, J. Lykke-Andersen, A. H. Johnsen, U. M. Wewer, and F. C. Nielsen, *Mol. Cell Biol.* **1999**, *19*, 1262–1270.

40 G. A. Doyle, N. A. Betz, P. F. Leeds, A. J. Fleisig, R. D. Prokipcak, and J. Ross, *Nucleic Acids Res.* **1998**, *26*, 5036–5044.

41 P. Leeds, B. T. Kren, J. M. Boylan, N. A. Betz, C. J. Steer, P. A. Gruppuso, and J. Ross, *Oncogene* **1997**, *14*, 1279–1286.

42 M. Lu, R. M. Nakamura, E. D. Dent, J. Y. Zhang, F. C. Nielsen, J. Christiansen, E. K. L. Chan, and E. M. Tan, *Am. J. Pathol.* **2001**, *159*, 945–953.

43 T. Himoto, S. Kuriyama, J. Y. Zhang, E. K. L. Chan, M. Nishioka, and E. M. Tan, *Int. J. Oncol.* **2005**, *26*, 311–317.

44 E. Cariani, C. Lasserre, D. Seurin, B. Hamelin, F. Kemeny, D. Franco, M. P. Czech, A. Ullrich, and C. Brechot, *Cancer Res.* **1988**, *48*, 6844–6849.

45 T. S. Su, W. Y. Liu, S. H. Han, M. Jansen, T. L. Yang-Fen, F. K. P'eng, and C. K. Chou, *Cancer Res.* **1989**, *49*, 1773–1777.

46 P. Bates, R. Fisher, A. Ward, L. Richardson, D. J. Hill, and C. F. Graham, *Br. J. Cancer* **1995**, *72*, 1189–1193.

47 C. E. Rogler, D. Yang, L. Rossetti, J. Donohoe, E. Alt, C. J. Chang, R. Rosenfeld, K. Neely, and R. Hintz, *J. Biol. Chem.* **1994**, *269*, 13779–13784.

48 P. Schirmacher, W. A. Held, D. Yang, F. V. Chisari, Y. Rustum, and C. E. Rogler, *Cancer Res.* **1992**, *52*, 2549–2556.

49 C. Pasquinelli, K. Bhavani, and F. V. Chisari, *Cancer Res.* **1992**, *52*, 2823–2829.

50 R. G. Simonetti, C. Camma, F. Fiorello, F. Politi, G. D'Amico, and L. Pagliaro, *Dig. Dis. Sci.* **1991**, *36*, 962–972.

51 K. Kiyosawa, T. Sodeyama, E. Tanaka, Y. Gibo, K. Yoshizawa, Y. Nakano, S. Furuta, Y. Akahane, K. Nishioka, and R. H. Purcell, *Hepatology* **1990**, *12*, 671–675.

52 B. S. Blumberg, *Proc. Natl. Acad. Sci. USA* **1997**, *94*, 7121–7125.

53 J. Y. Zhang, M. Dai, X. Wang, W. Q. Lu, D. S. Li, M. X. Zhang, K. J. Wang, L. P. Dai, S. G. Han, Y. F. Zhou, and H. Zhuang, *Int. J Epidemiol.* **1998**, *27*, 574–578.

54 J. Y. Zhang, E. K. L. Chan, X. X. Peng, M. Lu, X. Wang, F. Mueller, and E. M. Tan, *Clin. Immunol.* **2001**, *100*, 149–156.

55 T. Soussi, *Cancer Res.* **2000**, *60*, 1777–1788.

56 A. E. Reeve, M. R. Eccles, R. J. Wilkins, G. I. Bell, and L. J. Millow, *Nature* **1985**, *317*, 258–260.

57 J. Scott, J. Cowell, M. E. Robertson, L. M. Priestley, R. Wadey, B. Hopkins, J. Pritchard, G. I. Bell, L. B. Rall, and C. F. Graham, *Nature* **1985**, *317*, 260–262.

58 C. K. Osborne, E. B. Coronado, L. J. Kitten, C. I. Arteaga, S. A. Fuqua, K. Ramasharma, M. Marshall, and C. H. Li, *Mol. Endocrinol.* **1989**, *3*, 1701–1709.

59 G. Christofori, P. Naik, and D. Hanahan, *Nature* **1994**, *369*, 414–418.

60 U. Sahin, O. Tureci, H. Schmitt, B. Cochlovius, T. Johannes, R. Schmits, F. Stenner, G. Luo, I. Schobert, and M. Pfreundschuh, *Proc. Natl. Acad. Sci. USA* **1995**, *92*, 11810–11813.

61 J. A. Koziol, J. Y. Zhang, C. A. Casiano, X. X. Peng, F. D. Shi, A. C. Feng, E. K. L. Chan, and E. M. Tan, *Clin. Cancer Res.* **2003**, *9*, 5120–5126.

62 J. Y. Zhang, C. A. Casiano, X. X. Peng, J. A. Koziol, E. K. L. Chan, and E. M. Tan, *Cancer Epidemiol. Biomarkers Prev.* **2003**, *12*, 136–143.

63 J. L. Rodriguez, C. Gelpi, T. M. Thomson, F. J. Real, and J. Fernandez, *Clin. Exp. Immunol.* **1982**, *49*, 579–586.

64 M. A. Blaschek, Y. L. Pennec, A. M. Simitzis, P. Le Goff, A. Lamour, G. Kerdraon, J. Jouquan, and P. Youinou, *Scand. J. Rheumatol.* **1988**, *17*, 291–296.

65 M. J. Fritzler, J. Etherington, C. Sokoluk, T. D. Kinsella, and D. W. Valencia, *J. Immunol.* **1984**, *132*, 2904–2908.

66 H. P. Seelig, P. Schranz, H. Schroter, C. Wiemann, and M. Renz, *J. Autoimmun.* **1994**, *7*, 67–91.

67 A. Gentric, M. Blaschek, C. Julien, J. Jouquan, Y. Pennec, J. M. Berthelot, D. Mottier, R. Casburn-Budd, and P. Youinou, *Clin. Immunol. Immunopathol.* **1991**, *59*, 487–494.

68 P. S. Massabki, C. Accetturi, I. A. Nishie, N. P. da Silva, E. I. Sato, and L. E. Andrade, *AIDS* **1997**, *11*, 1845–1850.

69 N. Bizzaro, P. Pasini, A. Ghirardello, and B. Finco, *Clin. Rheumatol.* **1999**, *18*, 346–348.

70 J. Kooy, B. H. Toh, and P. A. Gleeson, *Immunol. Cell Biol.* **1994**, *72*, 123–127.

71 C. Infante, F. Ramos-Morales, C. Fedriani, M. Bornens, and R. M. Rios, *J. Cell Biol.* **1999**, *145*, 83–98.

72 F. A. Barr and B. Short, *Curr. Opin. Cell Biol.* **2003**, *15*, 405–413.

73 A. K. Gillingham and S. Munro, *Biochim. Biophys. Acta* **2003**, *1641*, 71–85.

74 R. A. Bascom, S. Srinivasan, and R. L. Nussbaum, *J. Biol. Chem.* **1999**, *274*, 2953–2962.

75 S. Munro and B. J. Nichols, *Curr. Biol.* **1999**, *9*, 377–380.

76 R. S. Taylor, S. M. Jones, R. H. Dahl, M. H. Nordeen, and K. E. Howell, *Mol. Biol. Cell* **1997**, *8*, 1911–1931.

77 K. Nozawa, M. J. Fritzler, C. A. von Mühlen, and E. K. L. Chan, *Arthritis Res. Ther.* **2004**, *6*, R95–R102.

78 S. Selak, E. K. L. Chan, L. Schoenroth, J. L. Senécal, and M. J. Fritzler, *J Investig. Med.* **1999**, *47*, 311–318.

79 K. J. Griffith, J. P. Ryan, J. L. Senécal, and M. J. Fritzler, *Clin. Exp. Immunol.* **2002**, *127*, 533–538.

80 S. J. Doxsey, P. Stein, L. Evans, P. D. Calarco, and M. Kirschner, *Cell* **1994**, *76*, 639–650.

81 V. Bouckson-Castaing, M. Moudjou, D. J. Ferguson, S. Mucklow, Y. Belkaid, G. Milon, and P. R. Crocker, *J. Cell Sci.* **1996**, *109*, 179–190.

82 G. J. Mack, J. Rees, O. Sandblom, R. Balczon, M. J. Fritzler, and J. B. Rattner, *Arthritis Rheum.* **1998**, *41*, 551–558.

83 J. B. Rattner, J. Rees, F. C. Arnett, J. D. Reveille, R. Goldstein, and M. J. Fritzler, *Arthritis Rheum.* **1996**, *39*, 1355–1361.

84 J. B. Rattner, J. Rees, C. M. Whitehead, C. A. Casiano, E. M. Tan, R. L. Humbel, K. Conrad, and M. J. Fritzler, *Clin Invest Med.* **1997**, *20*, 308–319.

85 C. M. Price, G. A. McCarty, and D. E. Pettijohn, *Arthritis Rheum.* **1984**, *27*, 774–779.

86 C. A. von Mühlen, E. K. L. Chan, C. L. Peebles, H. Imai, K. Kiyosawa, and E. M. Tan, *Clin. Exp. Immunol.* **1995**, *100*, 67–74.

87 C. H. Chou and W. H. Reeves, *Mol. Immunol.* **1992**, *29*, 1055–1064.

88 L. A. Casciola-Rosen, G. Anhalt, and A. Rosen, *J. Exp. Med.* **1994**, *179*, 1317–1330.

89 K. Nozawa, C. A. Casiano, J. C. Hamel, C. Molinaro, M. J. Fritzler, and E. K. L. Chan, *Arthritis Res.* **2002**, *4*, R3.

90 L. Casciola-Rosen, F. Andrade, D. Ulanet, W. B. Wong, and A. Rosen, *J Exp. Med.* **1999**, *190*, 815–826.

91 C. A. Casiano, R. L. Ochs, and E. M. Tan, *Cell Death. Differ.* **1998**, *5*, 183–190.

92 M. Mancini, C. E. Machamer, S. Roy, D. W. Nicholson, N. A. Thornberry, L. A. Casciola-Rosen, and A. Rosen, *J Cell Biol.* **2000**, *149*, 603–612.

93 P. J. Utz and P. Anderson, *Arthritis Rheum.* **1998**, *41*, 1152–1160.

94 F. Andrade, S. Roy, D. Nicholson, N. Thornberry, A. Rosen, and L. Casciola-Rosen, *Immunity* **1998**, *8*, 451–460.

95 Z. Yang, A. Jakymiw, M. R. Wood, T. Eystathioy, R. L. Rubin, M. J. Fritzler, and E. K. L. Chan, *J. Cell Sci.* **2004**.

96 D. Ingelfinger, D.J. Arndt-Jovin, R. Luhrmann, and T. Achsel, *RNA* 2002, *8*, 1489–1501.

97 E. Van Dijk, N. Cougot, S. Meyer, S. Babajko, E. Wahle, and B. Séraphin, *EMBO J.* 2002, *21*, 6915–6924.

98 E. Bouveret, G. Rigaut, A. Shevchenko, M. Wilm, and B. Séraphin, *EMBO J.* 2000, *19*, 1661–1671.

99 S. Tharun, W. He, A.E. Mayes, P. Lennertz, J.D. Beggs, R. Parker, *Nature* 2000, *404*, 515–518.

100 S. Tharun and R. Parker, *Mol. Cell* 2001, *8*, 1075–1083.

101 T. Dunckley and R. Parker, *EMBO J.* 1999, *18*, 5411–5422.

102 T. Dunckley and R. Parker, *Methods Enzymol.* 2001, *342*, 226–233.

103 M. Gao, C.J. Wilusz, S.W. Peltz, and J.Wilusz, *EMBO J.* 2001, *20*, 1134–1143.

104 P. Couttet, M. Fromont-Racine, D. Steel, R. Pictet, and T. Grange, *Proc. Natl. Acad. Sci. USA* 1997, *94*, 5628–5633.

105 T. Eystathioy, A. Jakymiw, E.K.L. Chan, B. Séraphin, N. Cougot, and M.J. Fritzler, *RNA* 2003, *9*, 1171–1173.

106 T. Eystathioy, E.K.L. Chan, K. Takeuchi, M. Mahler, L.M. Luft, D.W. Zochodne, and M.J. Fritzler, *J Mol. Med.* 2003, *81*, 811–818.

107 M. Satoh, A.K. Ajmani, T. Ogasawara, J.J. Langdon, M. Hirakata, J. Wang, and W.H. Reeves, *J. Clin. Invest* 1994, *94*, 1981–1989.

108 M. Satoh, M. Kuwana, T. Ogasawara, A.K. Ajmani, J.J. Langdon, D. Kimpel, J. Wang, and W.H. Reeves, *J. Immunol.* 1994, *153*, 5838–5848.

109 M. Mahler, M.J. Fritzler, and M. Bluthner, *Arthritis Res. Ther.* 2005, *7*, R19–R29.

110 W.J. van Venrooij and G.J. Pruijn, *Arthritis Res.* 2000, *2*, 249–251.

111 S. Rantapaa-Dahlqvist, B.A. de Jong, E. Berglin, G. Hallmans, G. Wadell, H. Stenlund, U. Sundin, and W.J. van Venrooij, *Arthritis Rheum.* 2003, *48*, 2741–2749.

112 E.K.L. Chan and E.M. Tan, *J. Exp. Med.* 1987, *166*, 1627–1640.

113 Y. Muro, E.K.L. Chan, G. Landberg, and E.M. Tan, *Biochem. Biophys. Res. Commun.* 1995, *207*, 1029–1037.

114 K. Furuta, E.K.L. Chan, K. Kiyosawa, G. Reimer, C. Luderschmidt, and E.M. Tan, *Chromosoma* 1997, *106*, 11–19.

115 W. Hassfeld, E.K.L. Chan, D.A. Mathison, D. Portman, G. Dreyfuss, G. Steiner, and E.M. Tan, *Nucleic Acids Res.* 1998, *26*, 439–445.

116 M.J. Fritzler, S.M. Kerfoot, T.E. Feasby, D.W. Zochodne, J.M. Westendorf, J.O. Dalmau, and E.K.L. Chan, *J. Investig. Med.* 2000, *48*, 28–39.

117 R.L. Ochs, Y. Muro, Y. Si, H. Ge, E.K.L. Chan, and E.M. Tan, *J Allergy Clin Immunol* 2000, *105*, 1211–1220.

118 L. Soo Hoo, J.Y. Zhang, and E.K.L. Chan, *Oncogene* 2002, *21*, 5006–5015.

119 R.L. Ochs, T.W. Stein, Jr., E.K.L. Chan, M. Ruutu, and E.M. Tan, *Mol. Biol. Cell* 1996, *7*, 1015–1024.

120 Y. Lu, P. Ye, S.-L. Chen, E.M. Tan, and E.K.L. Chan, *Arthritis Res. Ther.* 2005, *7*, R1133–1139.

19
Tolerance and Immunity to the Ro/La RNP Complex [*]

Catherine L. Keech, Tom P. Gordon, and James McCluskey

19.1
Introduction

The presence of high-titer, affinity-matured autoantibodies directed against ubiquitous nuclear components is a common and useful tool in the diagnosis of systemic autoimmune diseases. The correlation of the autoantibody specificity with disease patterns and the clustering of the autoimmune response to specific groups of antigens provide a valuable diagnostic clue to the nature of particular systemic autoimmune diseases [1]. These autoantibodies do not appear to be due to nonspecific B-cell activation; rather, the presence of isotype-switched, persistent, high-titer, multi-determinant antibodies argues for the activation of antigen-specific B cells by the autoantigen itself. In this chapter we review our work on the nature of tolerance and immunity to a single autoantigen La(SS-B) in experimental systems. Over the past 14 years we have examined the immune responses to the nuclear antigen La in both patients and mouse models in order to better understand the targeting of such nuclear autoantigens in systemic autoimmunity. Here we explore the main findings and their implications for understanding the generation of autoantibodies in systemic autoimmunity.

19.2
The Nature of the Autoimmune Response to La

The systemic autoimmune diseases are defined by a combination of clinical and laboratory-based criteria [2]. One of the most useful criteria in assisting diagnosis has been the analysis of antinuclear autoantibodies (ANAs). Analysis of the pattern of ANA staining and identification of the protein or nucleic acid targets of these autoantibodies in many cases provide a highly specific diagnosis of disease, which has argued for the importance of B cells in pathogenesis of these

---

[*] A list of abbreviations used is located at the end of this chapter.

Autoantibodies and Autoimmunity: Molecular Mechanisms in Health and Disease. Edited by K. Michael Pollard
Copyright © 2006 WILEY-VCH Verlag GmbH & Co. KGaA, Weinheim
ISBN: 3-527-31141-6

syndromes. For example, the antigens Ro(SS-A) and La(SS-B) were identified in 1961 as the target of the autoantibody response in primary Sjögren's syndrome (pSS) [3]. Patients were found to develop high-titer IgG responses to La and Ro with a characteristic speckled pattern of ANA activity by indirect immunofluorescence. Unlike many autoantibodies, although the presence of the autoantibody correlates strongly with disease, a direct role for antibodies of these specificities in disease is less clear. In addition, a lower-titer, clustered immune response to Ro and La is also found in about 30% of patients with systemic lupus erythematosus (SLE). Primary Sjögren's syndrome is further characterized by lymphocytic infiltration and exocrine failure of salivary and lachrymal glands and is usually associated with polyclonal hypergammaglobulinemia and production of rheumatoid factor. Patients with pSS can also present with a diversity of lymphocyte abnormalities including lymphocytic infiltrates of the lung and kidneys, purpura, and an increase incidence of B-cell lymphomas.

19.3
The Ro/La Ribonucleoprotein Complex

The strong clustering of the autoantibody response to the Ro and La proteins reflects an autoimmune response to the multi-molecular particle, known as the Ro/La ribonucleoprotein (RNP) complex (Fig. 19.1 A). The Ro/La RNP is composed of a 60-kDa Ro protein (Ro60) associated with the stem region of the small cytoplasmic (Y) RNAs and a 48-kDa La protein bound to the poly U tail of the hY RNA. The physical evidence for the association of a 52-kDa Ro protein (Ro52) with Ro/La RNP remains more controversial, and this is believed to be associated via protein-protein interaction with the Ro60 polypeptide [4]. The function of this particle remains unknown, as do the functions of the Ro60 and Ro52 proteins. The association of La with poly U tails of RNA is believed to be a result of the role La protein plays in the initiation [5, 6] and termination [7, 8] of RNA polymerase III transcription, as all these transcripts have polyuridylated tails. Thus, only a small proportion of La is associated with the Ro/La RNP, with a significant pool of La associated with other RNA polymerase III transcripts. However, the activity of La as an RNA polymerase III transcription factor has recently been questioned [9]. La has now been shown to have wider functions in the cell protecting nascent RNAs from 3′ exonuclease activity (reviewed in Ref. [10]). This La-mediated stabilization of RNAs facilitates RNA-protein complex formation, as well as the maturation of pre-tRNA and nuclear retention of some RNAs and shuttling between distinct niches within the nucleus and the cytoplasm [10, 11]).

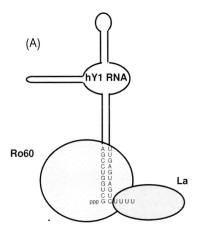

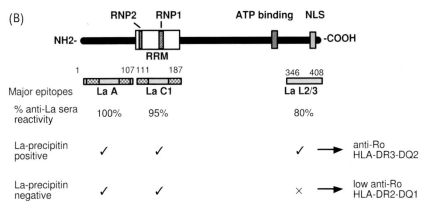

Fig. 19.1 (A) Model of the Ro/La ribonucleo-protein complex. La interacts via its RNA recognition motif (RRM) with the poly-U tail of the small cytoplasmic (Y) RNAs. Ro60 associates with the stem of the Y RNAs (adapted from [4]). (B) The major structural features and immunodominant epitopes of the La autoantigen. Discontinuous epitopes are located within the NH$_2$-terminal fragment (La A; checked regions) and the RRM (La C1, checked regions) that contains consensus sequences for RNP1 and RNP2 RNA-binding protein. The proportion of La-positive sera reactive with each fragment is shown. La precipitin–positive sera react with the three major epitopes shown (La A, La C1, and the carboxy-terminal region La L2/3), while La precipitin–negative sera do not react with the carboxy-terminal fragment (La L2/3).

19.4
Autoimmune Findings in Humans

The advent of recombinant protein technology in the late 1980s led to extensive study on the nature and specificity of the autoantibody response to many auto-antigen targets (including response to La) in the belief that this would illuminate the underlying mechanism driving this autoantibody response in patients.

Three theories were examined: firstly that the autoantibodies arise from polyclonal B-cell activation, secondly that autoantibodies arise as a result of an antigen mimic, and thirdly that the autoantigen itself was the driver of the autoantibody response. As outlined below, the specificity of the anti-La response favors the latter hypothesis, namely, that the Ro/La ribonucleoprotein complex drives the autoimmune response. Thus, detailed B-cell epitope mapping of La has been carried out by several groups (reviewed in [12]) and is illustrated in Figure 19.1 B. Autoantibody epitopes are located at the amino terminus (La A; aa 1–107) and within the central region of La that contains the RNA recognition motif (RRM)(La C1; aa 112–242) and in the carboxy-terminal region (La L2/3; aa 346–408), and up to seven distinct epitopes have been demonstrated across these regions [13] as well as a number of linear determinants [14]. The dominant determinant within the amino terminus (La A) is detectable at the earliest stages in disease and is a complex conformational or discontinuous epitope dependent upon both aa 12–28 and aa 82–99 for expression [15]. A further conformational determinant within the functional RNA recognition motif has been defined, and this epitope is specific for the human La protein [16]. This latter determinant spanned the RNA recognition elements of La; however, antibodies did not inhibit the RNA-binding capacity of La or the subsequent physical association with the Ro60 protein [17]. Thus, the two dominant determinants of the La polypeptide appear to be complex conformational epitopes, suggesting that the native human autoantigen itself is the driver of the diverse autoantibody response in patients. Although potential epitope mimics have been identified in infectious agents, the conformational and species-specific nature of the major determinants of La argues against their origin through cross-reactive B-cell mimicry of linear determinants.

The third major B-cell determinant in La is of particular interest as it provides some insight into the control of autoantibody diversification in patients. The presence of autoantibodies to the carboxy terminus of the La protein (La L2/3) appears late in the immune response, and in a subset of patients, this specificity does not develop at all. Interestingly, the lack of reactivity to this determinant, as detected by ELISA, correlates with an overall weaker anti-La and anti-Ro60 antibody titer and with the inability to form precipitating antibody-antigen lattices. This precipitin-negative anti-La activity is observed in approximately 20% of pSS patients [18]. The clinical features of these patients, including the duration of established disease, were essentially identical in those patients with anti-La precipitins. However, analysis of the HLA class II phenotype identified a strong association of HLA-DR3-DQ2 (DR3-DQA1*0501-DQB1*02) haplotype with the more diversified anti-La precipitin–positive group and HLA-DR2-DQ1 (DR2-DQA1*0102-DQB1*0602) with the restricted, anti-La precipitin–negative subset [19] (Table 19.1). The DR3-DQA1*0501-DQB1*02 haplotype has been implicated in diversified precipitating anti-La/Ro autoimmunity in other patient cohorts ([20] and references therein). These findings suggest that the HLA class II haplotypes control T-helper responses that in turn influence the magnitude of antibody determinant spreading [21]. We have proposed the following model to

Table 19.1 The degree of autoantibody diversity is controlled by HLA class II haplotype.

	HLA genetics in Australian cohort	Autoantibodies detected by ELISA					Precipitins	
		LaA	LaC	LaL2/3	Ro60	Ro52	Anti-La	Anti-Ro
Diverse Ab response	DR3-DQ2	✓	✓	✓	✓	✓	✓	✓
Limited Ab response	DR2-DQ1	✓	✓	✗	✓	✓	✗	✓

explain our findings (Fig. 19.2). B cells with auto-specificity for Ro or La polypeptides normally circulate and are not deleted or anergic because of the high threshold required for self-tolerance in the B compartment. Following uptake and processing of the Ro/La RNP by the Ro-specific B-cell receptor, anti-Ro antibody responses in autoimmune patients are driven by cognate interactions between Ro-specific B cells and helper T cells. Both HLA DR3-DQ2 and DR2-DQ1 haplotypes are able to efficiently present peptides derived from Ro (Fig. 19.2 A, B; upper panels). However, HLA DR3-DQ2 is more efficient at presenting peptides from the La protein than is DR2-DQ1 (Fig. 19.2 A, B; lower panels). Thus, we hypothesize that while DR3-DQ2 efficiently presents peptide determinants from La to La-specific T cells, the HLA DR2-DQ1 haplotype is inefficient at directly driving an anti-La response. As a result, anti-La B cells do not receive the same magnitude of specific helper signals where the HLA-presenting haplotype is DR2-DQ1- compared with DR3-DQ2-presenting elements. As a result, only a lower-titer and limited anti-La response is generated following presentation of Ro-derived peptides by the La-specific B cells. The limited help signal received from Ro-specific CD4$^+$ helper T cells (T$_h$) interacting with La-specific B cells may be the result of dissociation of La from the Ro/La RNP such that uptake of free La does not result in any presentation of Ro epitopes to T cells.

These studies in humans have enabled us to make some generalizations regarding the development of autoantibodies to the Ro/La complex. Firstly, although there may be intrinsic B-cell defects in these patients, the presence of high-titer autoantibodies does not appear to arise from nonspecific B-cell activation; rather, the antibody response is antigen-specifically directed predominantly to conformational determinants of the Ro/La RNP complex. Secondly, these autoantibodies appear to diversify over time, although by the time of diagnosis, the pattern of reactivity is generally fixed. In addition, fine mapping has revealed the role of HLA class II genes in controlling the degree of diversification of the autoantibody response. However, our data do not explain what activates T$_h$ cells that drive B-cell differentiation and autoantibody production. Perhaps intrinsic B-cell defects in pSS render B cells capable of priming T-cell responses, a task usually ascribed to dendritic cells.

(A)

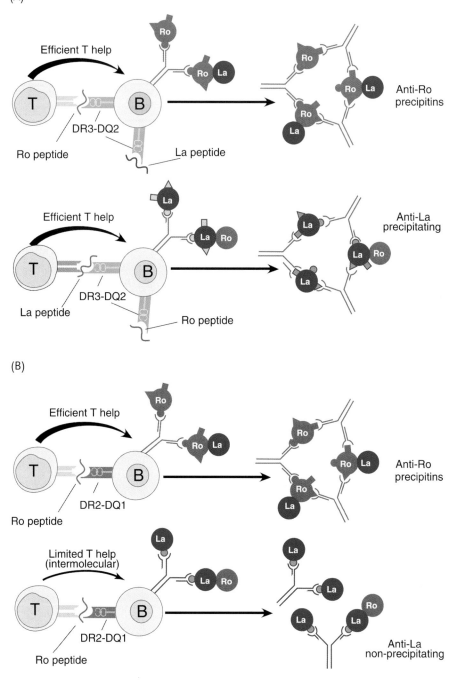

(B)

Fig. 19.2 (legend see page 453)

19.5
Autoimmunity to La in Experimental Models

The examination of the autoantibody response in mouse models allows a detailed analysis of the development of antinuclear antibodies in the context of a non-autoimmune-prone mammalian immune system. Thus, in the absence of any predisposition or perturbation of the immune system we are able to analyze (1) the degree of natural tolerance to these antigens, (2) the immunogenicity of nuclear proteins, and (3) the nature of any antibody diversification.

In mice, the diversification of the immune response was readily demonstrated following immunization of mice with either self- or heterologous recombinant La protein, sub-fragments of La, and peptides derived from the La molecule (reviewed in [21]). As illustrated in Figure 19.3 A, immunization of normal, non-autoimmune mouse strains of mice with sub-fragments of the La molecule led to a strong antibody response to that fragment, followed by the development of antibodies to a number of distinct determinants on the La polypeptide [22]. This intramolecular spreading is attributed to the generation of CD4$^+$ T cells and B cells to the immunizing fragment. T-cell help specific for the La polypeptide fragment is able to provide helper signals to B cells reactive to other portions of the La molecule. This occurs because non-tolerized La-specific B cells remain in the normal B-cell repertoire of healthy individuals. These specific B cells naturally capture endogenous La/Ro RNP complexes and present T-cell determinants from these proteins. Experimentally, it is not difficult to generate an anti-La autoantibody response in normal animals. Given that endogenous La is avail-

Fig. 19.2 Model showing HLA-restricted control of anti Ro/La autoantibody diversification. (A) DR3-DQ2 dependent anti-Ro and anti-La cognate intramolecular help. Anti-Ro (upper panel) and anti-La (lower panel) B cells selectively bind Ro or La, respectively, through their membrane Ig, which then undergoes receptor-mediated endocytosis leading to antigen processing and presentation. Peptide determinants derived from both La and Ro are efficiently presented by HLA DR3 or DQ2 molecules. High-affinity precipitating anti-Ro or anti-La autoantibody responses are driven by T cells providing efficient cognate helper signals to a broad range of La-specific or Ro-specific B cells recognizing multiple determinants of La or Ro. Ro-specific B cells can also present La peptides and vice versa, indicating a capacity of autoreactive B cells to receive intermolecular help signals as well as cognate helper signals as illustrated in more detail in Figure 19.4. This may explain why anti-La autoantibodies rarely occur in the absence of anti-Ro antibodies. (B) DR2-DQ1-dependent cognate intramolecular anti-Ro and intermolecular anti-La help. Anti-Ro autoimmunity is initiated by helper T cells recognizing Ro peptides presented by HLA DR2 or DQ1 molecules (upper panel). However, HLA DR2-DQ1 molecules fail to present peptides derived from La, and T-help signals for anti-La B cells are provided only through the presentation of Ro determinants as a result of capture of Ro protein associated with La in the Ro/La RNP complex (lower panel). Intermolecular help is limiting because only a proportion of La is associated with the Ro/La RNP and there is a free pool of La that restricts the number of anti-La B cells able to take up Ro and La together. This results in the production of low-titer, pauciclonal anti-La antibodies lacking the ability to form latticed precipitates. (Adapted from [19]).

(A)

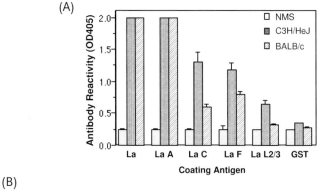

(B)

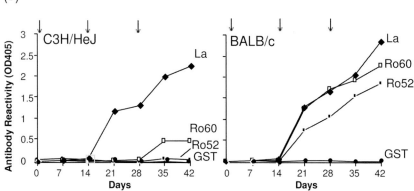

Fig. 19.3 Autoimmunity determinant spreading of the autoantibody response in mice immunized with recombinant La autoantigen. (A) Intramolecular spreading of the autoimmune response. C3H/HeJ and BALB/c mice were immunized with 100 µg recombinant 6× His-hLa A (aa 1–107) in Freund's complete adjuvant and were boosted twice at 10-day intervals with 50 µg antigen in incomplete Freund's adjuvant. Pooled sera from groups of six mice (diluted 1:250) were assayed for reactivity to GST-mLa (La) and GST-mLa sub-fragments (La A [aa 1–107], La C [aa 112–242], La F [aa 243–345], and La L2/3 [aa 346–415]) or GST alone by ELISA.

The reactivity of normal mouse sera (NMS) is also shown. (Adapted from [22].) (B) Kinetics of intermolecular spreading. Groups of C3H/HeJ or BALB/c mice were immunized with 100 µg of recombinant 6× His-hLa in complete Freund's adjuvant and boosted twice at 14-day intervals with 50 µg of antigen in incomplete Freund's adjuvant, as indicated by vertical arrows. Sera was collected at seven-day intervals from the initial immunization, pooled, and tested for reactivity with 6× His-mRo52 (Ro52 ■), 6× His-hRo60 (Ro60 □), 6× His-mLa (La ◆), or glutathione-S-transferase (GST ●). (Adapted from [23]).

able to autoreactive B cells for capture, processing, and presentation to T cells, then once La-specific T cells are activated, self-reactive B cells are potentially stimulated by the T_h cells.

In a similar fashion, the diversification of the immune response from one component of the Ro/La RNP to other members of the particle readily occurs. Thus, immunization with the full-length recombinant La protein initially elic-

Table 19.2 Intermolecular determinant spreading generates auto-antibodies to physically associated molecules in mice following immunization.

Immunogen	Antibody to immunogen	Autoantibodies generated by determinant spreading				
		La	Ro60	Ro52	Grp78	Calreticulin
La	✓		✓	✓		
Ro60	✓	✓		✓	✓	✓
Ro52	✓	✓	✓		✓	✓
Grp78	✓			✓		✓

ited antibodies to the La antigen followed by autoantibodies to the associated Ro60 [22] and Ro52 [23] proteins. In reciprocal experiments, immunization with Ro proteins resulted in recruitment of antibodies to Ro and La proteins as well as to chaperone proteins, including calreticulin and Grp78 [24, 25], that are believed to associate with the Ro proteins (Table 19.2). The mechanism of intermolecular diversification of the B-cell and T-cell responses is modeled in Figure 19.4. Here we hypothesize that La-specific T cells are able to provide T-helper signals to both anti-La B cells through cognate help as well as providing T-helper signals to Ro-specific B cells that have captured, processed, and presented La peptides because of the linked nature of the components within the Ro/La RNP complex (Fig. 19.4 A). In addition, the diversification of the T-cell responses to linked proteins may be orchestrated despite limited B-cell specificities (Fig 19.4 B). B cells with anti-La specificity capture and present processed peptide antigens in association with MHC class II molecules from physically associated components of the Ro/La RNP complex and associated chaperone proteins. This allows the activation of a diversified population of T cells, resulting in recruitment of additional antigen targets through the provision of cognate help.

Intriguingly, following immunization with recombinant Ro or La proteins, the antibody responses of different mouse strains are not identical, suggesting an influence of the genetic background in selecting and presenting La determinants. This is illustrated in Figure 19.3 B, where the magnitude, kinetics, and pattern of autoantibodies generated through determinant spreading differ in two inbred mouse strains (C3H/HeJ and BALB/c) following immunization with La [23]. This observation mirrors the findings in patients as discussed above, where the degree of autoantibody intra- and intermolecular spreading is limited by the HLA class II genes of the individual.

Thus, in experimental mouse models, the initiation of a restricted immune response rapidly results in the spontaneous intra- and intermolecular spreading of autoimmunity, driven by the self-antigen and/or antigenic particle. The autoimmune response in normal non-autoimmune-prone mice in this experimental model implies that a poor level of immune tolerance to the Ro/La complex is the normal state of affairs. The data also confirm the importance of polymorphic host genes in controlling the autoantibody diversification.

(A) B cell epitope spreading

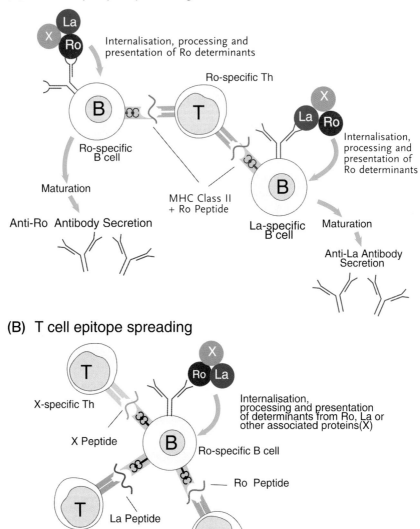

(B) T cell epitope spreading

Fig. 19.4 Model showing the mechanisms of B- and T-cell epitope spreading.
(A) Spreading of the B-cell response may be orchestrated by a single T-cell determinant. T cells specific for a single Ro epitope may provide help to B cells with multiple specificities on the same polypeptide (intramolecular) or on other physically associated compo-
nents of the Ro/La RNP complex such as La, Ro52, calreticulin, or heat shock proteins. B cells specific for Ro determinants internalize, process, and present the Ro determinant in association with MHC class II to a Ro-specific T cell. Ro-specific T cells provide cognate help to Ro-specific B cells, resulting in maturation and production of anti-Ro

19.6
Tolerance to Nuclear Antigens

Little is known about immune tolerance to nuclear antigens. The nature of the ribonucleoprotein particles, their restricted localization and sequestration within the cell, their relatively low abundance but ubiquitous expression, their redistribution during apoptosis, and their association with viral RNA transcripts may all influence the generation of tolerance and autoimmunity. As such, insights gained from data on mechanisms of tolerance observed for nominal neo-autoantigens such as ovalbumin and hen egg lysosome, or autoantigens such as cytochrome c and DNA, may have limited applicability to understanding the situation for the Ro/La RNP antigens. Therefore, we chose to study immune tolerance to La itself by exploiting the difference between the human and mouse La molecules in a transgenic experimental mouse model. La is a highly conserved molecule, such that human and mouse La share 77% amino acid sequence identity [26]. Not surprisingly, human autoantibodies to La antigen generally cross-react with the mouse autoantigen. We have used two approaches to examine tolerance of both B and T cells to La autoantigen. Firstly, a comparison of antibody response to human La versus mouse La in mice immunized with each of these antigens allows a true comparison of "autoantibody" response versus a xenogeneic antibody response. In these experiments we observed an increased immunogenicity of human La over mouse La, implying a degree of foreignness of the homologous human La antigen, while revealing some constraints (tolerance) on the immune response to the mouse La autoantigen [22]. There are limits to how far this conclusion may be drawn; thus, to explore this idea further we generated mice that expressed the full-length, functional human La protein under the control of the human La promoter [27, 28]. By comparing the relative immune response to human La in the presence (hLa-Tg) or absence (non-Tg) of endogenously expressed human La protein, we were able to evaluate the impact of self-tolerance to this nuclear autoantigen on subsequent immune responses.

---

antibodies. Similarly, B cells specific for other determinants on linked proteins in the Ro/La RNP complex (e.g., La) selectively bind and internalize the Ro/La RNP via La-specific membrane Ig. The T-cell determinant from the Ro polypeptide is processed and presented by MHC class II to the activated Ro-specific T_h, which provides help for B-cell maturation and production of anti-La antibodies.

(B) Spreading of the T-cell response may be orchestrated by a single B-cell determinant. B cells with specificity for a single epitope of the Ro/La RNP (e.g., Ro) selectively and efficiently bind and internalize the Ro/La RNP through their membrane Ig. Epitopes from Ro, La, and other physically associated polypeptides, such as Ro52, calreticulin, or heat shock proteins (X), are processed and presented in association with MHC class II to recruit a diverse array of autoreactive T cells.

19.7
Lack of Tolerance in the B-cell Compartment

In many systems B-cell tolerance is measured by the inability to generate auto-antibodies following immunization with antigen. Indeed, immune self-tolerance to self-antigens such as cytochrome c [29] and histones [30] is well established, and in our hands immunization of mice with purified histones failed to generate detectable autoantibodies [22]. However, following immunization with recombinant La, antibodies to La are readily elicited, and the antibody response diversifies through determinant spreading as discussed above. These data demonstrate the limited B-cell tolerance to the members of the Ro/La particle.

When mice were immunized with equivalent amounts of recombinant human La or mouse La, they generated anti-La antibodies that were cross-reactive in both species. In several inbred mouse strains, we have observed a more vigorous antibody response to the heterologous hLa molecule with more rapid epitope diversification than observed when immunizing with mLa, presumably due to the presence of foreign B- and/or T-cell determinants in hLa [22]. In addition, in mice that are transgenic for the human La protein, the antibody response to human La is now diminished and is equivalent to that observed for mouse La in both non-transgenic and human La transgenic mice (Fig. 19.5) [28]. These findings indicate that anti-La B cells are not efficiently tolerized by endogenously expressed La; however, there is a degree of self-tolerance to endogenous La even though this is incomplete. The mechanism for partial immune tolerance to La may reside in the T-cell compartment, B-cell compartment, or both.

B-cell tolerance is known to be mediated by a number of mechanisms that result in a continuum of tolerogenic outcomes. The efficiency and nature of B-cell tolerance are dependent upon variable signaling thresholds that are dependent upon the affinity of the B-cell antigen receptor, antigen abundance, and the ability of antigen to induce B-cell receptor cross-linking [31]. Clonal deletion of self-reactive B cells in the bone marrow results from strong B-cell signals during bone marrow development, whereas weaker signals induce anergy or developmental arrest. Autoimmune B cells that escape tolerogenic mechanisms still require T-helper signals for their full development; therefore, the T-helper compartment may be the final checkpoint in B-cell self-tolerance. Natural tolerance to several lupus-associated antigens has been examined using immunoglobulin-transgenic mice. Anti-ssDNA and anti-dsDNA were found to be tolerized by a combination of mechanisms, including receptor editing, B-cell deletion, developmental arrest, and anergy [32–34]. In contrast, anti-Sm B cells are tolerized by developmental arrest followed by their deletion or shunting into the B-1 compartment, although some Sm-specific B cells may remain autoantigen ignorant [35–37].

To further examine tolerance to La in the B-cell compartment, anti-hLa B-cell transgenic mice were generated expressing the IgM heavy chain from a monoclonal antibody (A3; [38]) specific for a xenogeneic epitope within the human La

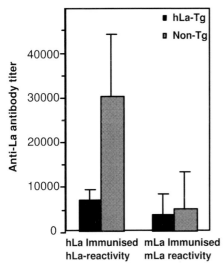

Fig. 19.5 Partial tolerance to endogenous La antigen. Groups of mice ($n=6$) were immunized with 50 µg of recombinant 6× His-hLa or 6× His-mLa in complete Freund's adjuvant and boosted twice at 14-day intervals with 25 µg of antigen in incomplete Freund's adjuvant. Sera from individual mice were assayed for reactivity with recombinant hLa-GST or mLa-GST. The average endpoint titer and standard deviation of the antibody response are shown. The autoantibody response to La autoantigen, either mLa or hLa in hLa-Tg mice, is significantly diminished ($P<0.01$, Mann-Whitney U-test) when compared to the antibody response to xenogeneic hLa, which shares 77% amino acid homology with mLa. (Adapted from [28]).

protein. The development of anti-hLa B cells could then be measured in both the presence and absence of cognate human La antigen by crossing the anti-hLa immunoglobulin transgenics to mice transgenically bearing the human La antigen [39]. This experiment found no evidence for induction of specific B-cell tolerance when the anti-hLa B cells developed in the presence of human La antigen; the findings of this work are summarized in Table 19.3. Thus, between 5% and 15% of transgenic B cells developing in the absence of hLa were specific for hLa, and these cells were neither deleted nor developmentally arrested in the presence of endogenous hLa expression. Instead, these autoreactive B cells matured normally and differentiated into antibody-forming cells, capable of secreting high-titer autoantibody in response to *in vitro* stimulation. Additionally, the lifespan of autoreactive hLa-specific B cells was not reduced, as is the case in anergic B cells. Instead, the anti-hLa B cells were phenotypically and functionally indistinguishable from naïve non-autoreactive hLa-specific B cells developing in the absence of hLa. Together these data suggest a lack of intrinsic tolerance for anti-La B cells involving any known mechanisms. In light of the diminished autoantibody response observed following immunization of hLa transgenic mice, we concluded that tolerance to the La autoantigen in the B-cell compartment appears to be mediated through regulation of T-cell help.

Table 19.3 Anti-hLa B cells show no evidence of tolerance when they develop in the presence of hLa antigen.

	Anti-hLa Tg	Anti-hLa×hLa-Tg	Conclusions
Number of B cells (spleen)	1.7×10^7	1.5×10^7	Not delected
Percentage splenic anti-hLa B cells	5–15	5–15	
Phenotype			
Mature in periphery (CD23$^+$, CD24$^-$)	✓	✓	Not developmen-
Increase in pre-B cells	×	×	tally arrested
Expression of activation markers *in vivo* (CD69$^+$, CD80$^+$, CD86$^-$, MHC class II^{high})	✓	✓	Not activated
Basal anti-La titer *in vivo*	✓	✓	Not anergic
Signaling through BCR	✓	✓	
In vitro antibody secretion following activation	✓	✓	
Expression of activation markers following stimulation with LPS	✓	✓	
Turnover *in vivo* (percentage BrdU incorporation in 8 days)	14.5 ± 1.9	14.8 ± 1.6	
Percentage anti-hLa B-1 cells in peritoneum	30–50	30–50	No differentiation to B-1 B cells

19.8
Tolerance in the T-cell Compartment

The above data suggest that control of autoantibody production rests with the T_h cells and that the regulation of autoreactivity in these cells will be critical to regulating autoimmune disease. It has not been possible to map the T-cell determinants to autoantigens such as La in patients due to the low precursor frequencies in the peripheral blood of normal individuals and to the apparent clonal exhaustion in affected individuals by the time of diagnosis. However, by exploiting the sequence differences between human and mouse La following immunization with recombinant human La, subsequent CD4$^+$ T-cell epitope mapping identified a hierarchy of peptide responses in the T_h compartment of mice immunized with hLa antigen [40].

This approach identified two immunodominant xenogeneic determinants (hLa$_{288-302}$ and hLa$_{61-84}$) that both differ from the mouse homologue by a single amino acid in their core epitope ([40]; A.D. Farris, personal communication) (Fig. 19.6A). In addition, several weaker and more variable T-cell responses were detected to a number of autologous and xenogeneic determinants. The I-A^k-restricted T-cell determinant of human La (hLa$_{288-302}$) dominated the immune response to hLa in that following immunization strong T-cell responses were gen-

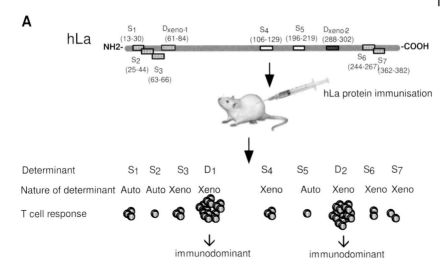

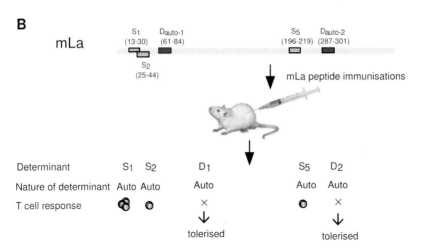

Fig. 19.6 Only the immunodominant determinants of endogenous mouse La induce T_h cell tolerance.

(A) Tolerance to endogenous mLa determinants was deduced by comparing T_h immunity to the xenogeneic human La (hLa) antigen versus the autoantigen mouse La (mLa). Mapping of T_h epitopes in hLa was carried out in A/J (H-2^a) mice following immunization with recombinant hLa. Two xenogeneic peptides dominated the T_h response (D_{xeno-1} and D_{xeno-2}). Subdominant T_h responses to several autologous (Auto) or xenogeneic (Xeno) determinants were observed (S_1–S_7). These were characterized by weaker and variable proliferative responses.

(B) T-cell tolerance to the homologous immunodominant determinants of mLa. Immunization of A/J mice with the homologous mouse peptides corresponding to the immunodominant regions of hLa (D_{auto-1} and D_{auto-2}) fails to stimulate T-cell activation and proliferation in A/J mice following immunization. Weak and variable T_h responses are once again observed in the subdominant self-determinants.

erated. However, the homologous mouse La$_{287-301}$ determinant was tolerogenic in that immunization with the mLa$_{287-301}$ peptide failed to induce either T-cell responses or autoantibody production (Fig. 19.6 B). This contrasted with the presence of responses in mice immunized with subdominant determinants from the mLa autoantigen. Although T$_h$ responses to subdominant determinants were observed less frequently and with lower potency, immunization with just a single autologous subdominant peptide resulted in the production of diverse autoantibodies to several regions on the La protein as well as intermolecular spreading to the associated Ro52 protein. Thus, these findings indicate that CD4$^+$ T-cell tolerance to La determinants is limited to dominant determinants and that reactivity to subdominant epitopes may be sufficient to trigger B-cell autoimmunity driven by T-helper responses.

To support the direct comparison of the immune responses to human and mouse La homologues, efficient MHC class II binding and presentation of the mLa$_{287-301}$ peptide were demonstrated by inhibition binding studies and specific antagonism of the hLa$_{288-302}$ responses by mouse T cells. However, immunodominance of a particular determinant in one species cannot be assumed for homologous determinants across species [41]. Therefore, we examined tolerance to the immunodominant hLa determinants (hLa$_{288-302}$ and hLa$_{61-84}$) in mice transgenically expressing the human La protein where the previously dominant xenoepitopes were now rendered self-determinants comparable to the mLa$_{287-301}$ and mLa$_{61-84}$ epitopes (illustrated in Fig. 19.7). In this experiment T cells in normal mice were raised to intact human La or to the immunodominant hLa$_{288-302}$ or hLa$_{61-84}$ peptides. Transfer of these immune T cells into mice expressing transgenic human La resulted in the production of anti-hLa autoantibodies, presumably by activating self-reactive anti-La B cells [28]. Anti-La autoantibodies did not develop following transfer of hLa-specific T cells into non-transgenic recipients, reflecting the lack of antigen presentation of any human La-specific determinants in these mice. However, transfer of T cells generated by identical immunization of hLa-Tg mice with hLa did not elicit an autoantibody response in host mice, reflecting CD4$^+$ T-cell tolerance to the immunodominant La epitopes in the donor hLa-Tg mice [28].

In addition, tolerance in the CD4$^+$ T-cell compartment to these immunodominant determinants was demonstrated by comparing the ability to generate peptide-specific T cells in hLa-Tg or non-Tg mice. Following immunization of hLa-Tg or non-Tg mice with dominant hLa peptide, the ability of the resulting T cells to proliferate or secrete cytokines *in vitro* was measured. T cells purified from hLa-Tg mice primed with hLa$_{288-302}$ did not proliferate in response to hLa$_{288-302}$, while T cells from non-Tg mice were activated to proliferate under the same circumstances. Moreover, T cells from hLa-Tg mice primed with hLa$_{288-302}$ or hLa$_{61-84}$ failed to secrete IL-10, IL-2, or IFN-γ upon restimulation with peptide *in vitro* when compared to non-Tg littermates (A. D. Farris, personal communication).

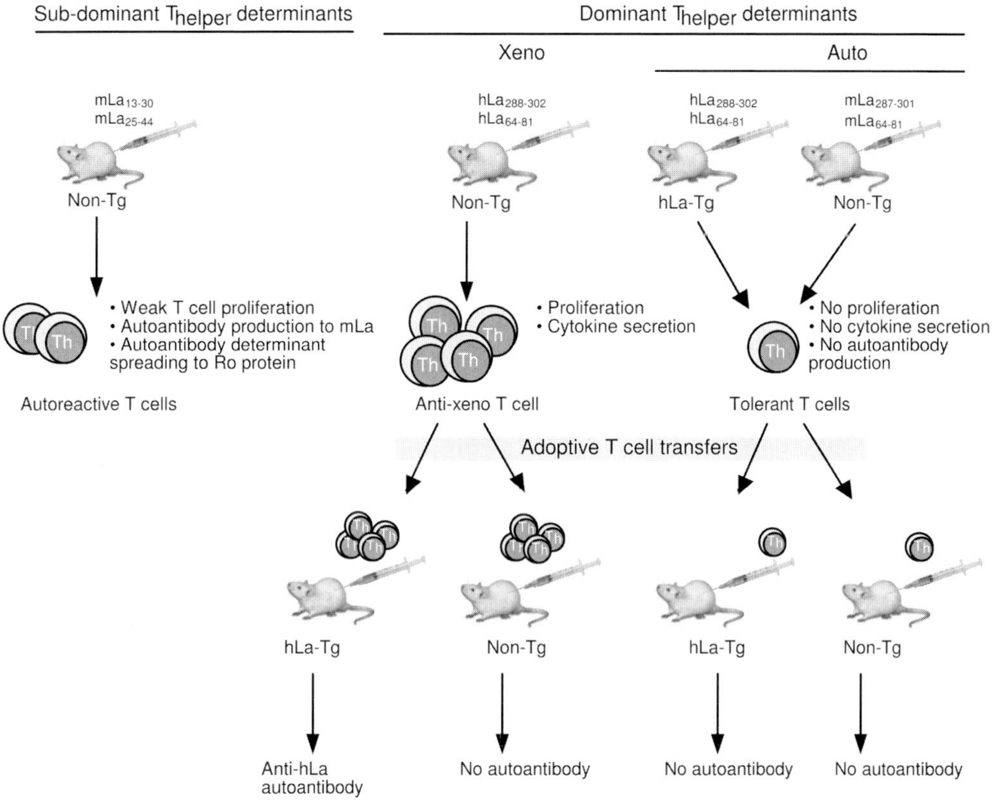

Fig. 19.7 Immunization of normal, non-transgenic A/J (Non-Tg) mice with subdominant autologous La peptide results in weak and variable activation of the CD4$^+$ T cell. These autoreactive T cells are capable of providing T help to autoreactive anti-La and anti-Ro B cells and induce autoantibody production and determinant spreading. Immunization of Non-Tg A/J mice with the dominant H-2^a-restricted determinants of human La generates a strong T-helper response to hLa peptide. Transfer of these activated T cells into human La transgenic mice (hLa-Tg) provides cognate help to autoreactive hLa-specific B cells and elicits anti-La autoantibodies without any further intervention. The transfer of these cells to Non-Tg mice cannot induce antibodies due to the absence of endogenous human La antigen. Immunization of mice with the dominant auto-determinants (either hLa peptides into hLa-Tg mice or mLa peptides into Non-Tg, A/J mice) fails to elicit autoreactive T cells. Transfer of T cells from mice primed with autologous, dominant determinants fails to elicit autoantibodies to human or mLa.

These results confirmed both the immunodominance of these determinants and the functional immune tolerance mediated through the CD4$^+$ T-cell compartment. Thus, it is the T-B axis that controls the vulnerability to autoimmunity in this model of La autoimmunity. From a detailed study of the immune response to the La autoantigen in mice, we have demonstrated that in the absence of any detectable B-cell tolerance, a diversified antibody profile can be generated following the priming of T cells to a single T-helper determinant, provided that this is the right determinant. Therefore, although the anti-La antibody observed in human autoimmunity is driven by self-antigen, the initiator of this autoantibody response remains unknown and could potentially result from a single T_h epitope mimic to a poorly tolerized determinant on the Ro or La molecule.

In this body of work we have demonstrated conclusively that the Ro/La RNP is not invisibly sequestered from the immune system. Instead, the Ro/La RNP is readily recognized by specific lymphocytes and can trigger autoreactive B cells when given sufficiently strong T-cell help. Mapping of the T-cell determinants on human La has revealed tolerance to a dominant determinant of La in H-2^a mice. On the other hand, whereas T cells specific for the dominant T-cell determinants are likely to be tolerized, suboptimal T-cell determinants are poorly tolerogenic, perhaps because antigen presentation is below the threshold of recognition for self-reactive T cells. This reveals a window of vulnerability in the control of autoimmunity to La. Once T_h cells are generated, potentially through antigen mimicry of subdominant determinants, cognate autoantibody production may be triggered, with determinant spreading to involve associated proteins that may become self-sustaining.

19.9
Induction of Disease

So what predisposes patients to develop anti-Ro and anti-La autoantibodies? The linkage of anti-Ro/La immunity with particular MHC class II haplotypes argues strongly for a restricted T-cell epitope involvement. Clearly, the animal studies demonstrating intermolecular spreading suggest that in normal non-autoimmune-prone individuals an antibody response to La will eventually develop following induction of immunity to associated Ro proteins and given the correct MHC class II restriction elements. However, in the experimental mouse models described, we found no evidence of pathology. Defects in apoptosis, clearance of apoptotic debris, B-cell signaling pathways, impaired complement regulation, or generation of neo-epitopes through post-translational modifications could still play a role in the initiation and maintenance of anti-Ro autoimmunity, but these are not essential for developing autoantibody in our model system. Notably, SLE and pSS, as well as animal models of systemic autoimmunity (MRL and lpr mice), are known to be associated with defects in apoptosis and the clearance of apoptotic material. This suggests that ANAs might be triggered or sustained in these disorders due to abundant antigen turnover, potentially in an altered form due to the redistribution of cellular components in apoptosis [42]. Apoptosis occurs constantly *in vivo*, and proteins such as La and Ro are constantly redistributed, degraded, and modified by molecules such as caspases [43], granzymes [44], and phosphatases [45]. Accordingly, altered regulation of defects in these processes could expose the immune system to autoimmunity through the mechanisms operating in our experimental models.

Sjögren's syndrome is associated not only with the presence of anti-La but also with other indicators of aberrant B-cell function, including polyclonal hypergammaglobulinemia, production of rheumatoid factor, lymphocytic infiltrates of the lung and kidneys, occasional purpura, and an increase incidence of B-cell lymphomas. Recently, excess production of B cell–activating factor (BAFF) has been associated with pSS and SLE. BAFF belongs to the TNF family and is a B-cell survival factor essential for B-cell maturation that contributes to autoimmunity when overexpressed in mice [46]. In addition to developing features of SLE, mice transgenic for BAFF develop a secondary pathology reminiscent of pSS, manifested by severe sialadenitis, decreased saliva production, and destruction of submaxillary salivary glands, although anti-Ro/La antibodies are not secreted in these mice [47]. To translate these findings to humans with pSS, levels of BAFF were measured in sera from a cohort of patients with pSS and were found to be significantly higher than in healthy controls. Furthermore, the levels of BAFF were higher in pSS than in SLE and rheumatoid arthritis, consistent with the observation that B-cell hyperactivity is generally more marked in pSS than in other systemic rheumatic diseases. The higher levels of BAFF in patients with pSS may also explain why pSS is associated with the development of B-cell malignancies. While the levels of serum BAFF in this initial study did not correlate with the presence of anti-Ro or anti-La precipitins, a second study has reported that BAFF levels correlate with anti-Ro antibody titers [48]. Further studies are required to determine whether BAFF levels correlate with specific autoantibody production in pSS, most notably anti-La antibody secretion, and whether BAFF is a determinant of anti-Ro/La intermolecular epitope spreading in these patients. Overall, the impressive elevation of BAFF levels in pSS identifies this common autoimmune disease as a prime candidate for trials with BAFF antagonist or neutralizing therapies.

Thus, in our concept of anti-La/Ro autoimmunity functional immune tolerance is balanced upon the fulcrum of limited tolerance to La in both the B- and T-cell compartments. This is characterized by constitutive antigen presentation but without induction of autoimmunity (Fig. 19.8). In the absence of an initiating insult, this balance is maintained and the natural state of immune tolerance prevails. Following activation of the anti-Ro/La response, potentially by an environmental trigger such as a viral infection, this balance is upset and in genetically susceptible individuals the balance tilts towards autoimmunity. The genes known to confer susceptibility may act to lower the threshold of responsiveness to these antigens, increase the antigenic load, and amplify and diversify the autoantibody response. This results in persistent autoantibody production and disease. In autoimmune-resistant individuals, the same environmental triggers may fail to generate sufficiently strong autoimmune responses, and any autoimmunity and autoantibody production are transient, as the propensity for hyperactivity is absent, the endogenous antigen load is limited through efficient clearance of apoptotic debris, and the autoimmune response is not amplified or sustained. As the environmental insult clears, the natural balance of immune tolerance is reestablished and autoimmunity wanes.

Abbreviations

ANA   antinuclear antibody
BAFF   B cell–activating factor
h   human
hLa-Tg   human La transgenic mice
La   48-kDa La/SS-B protein
m   mouse
non-Tg   non-transgenic mice
pSS   primary Sjögren's syndrome
RNP   ribonucleoprotein complex
Ro60   60-kDa Ro protein
Ro52   52-kDa Ro protein
RRM   RNA recognition motif
SLE   systemic lupus erythematosus
T_h CD4$^+$ helper T cells
Y   small cytoplasmic RNA

References

1 Tan, E. M. (1989) Antinuclear antibodies: diagnostic markers for autoimmune diseases and probes for cell biology, *Adv. Immunol.* **44**, 93–151.

2 Fox, R. I., Robinson, C. A., Curd, J. G., Kozin, F. and Howell, F. V. (1986) Sjögren's syndrome: proposed criteria for classification, *Arthritis Rheum.* **29**, 577–585.

3 Anderson, J. R., Gray, K. G. and Beck, J. S. (1961) Precipitating autoantibodies in Sjögren's syndrome, *Lancet* **2**, 456–460.

4 Slobbe, R. L., Pruijn, G. J. M. and van Venrooij, W. J. (1991) Ro(SS-A) and La(SS-B) ribonucleoprotein complexes: structure, function and antigenicity, *Ann. Med. Interne.* **142**, 592–600.

5 Maraia, R. J., Kenan, D. J. and Keene, J. D. (1994) Eukaryotic transcription termination factor La mediates transcript release and facilitates reinitiation by RNA polymerase III, *Mol. Cell. Biol.* **14**, 2147–2158.

6 Maraia, R. J., Kenan, D. J. and Keene, J. D. (1996) Transcription termination factor La is also and initiation factor for RNA polymerase III, *Proc. Natl. Acad. Sci.* **93**, 3383–3387.

7 Gottlieb, E. and Steitz, J. (1989) Function of mammalian La protein: evidence for its action in transcription termination by RNA polymerase III, *EMBO J.* **8**, 851–861.

8 Gottlieb, E. and Steitz, J. (1989) The RNA binding protein La influences both the accuracy and efficiency of RNA polymerase III transcription *in vitro*, *EMBO J.* **8**, 841–850.

9 Weser, S., Bachmann, M., Seifart, K. H. and Meisner, W. (2000) Transcription efficiency of human polymerase II genes *in vitro* does not depend on the RNP-forming autoantigen La, *Nucleic Acids Res.* **28**, 3935–3942.

10 Wolin, S. and Cedervall, T. (2002) The La protein, *Annu. Rev. Biochem.* **71**, 375–403.

11 Bachmann, M. (1989) The La antigen shuttles between the nucleus and the cytoplasm in CV-1 cells, *Mol. Cell. Biochem.* **85**, 103–114.

12 St. Clair, E. W. (1992) Anti-La antibodies, *Rheum. Dis. Clin. North Am.* **18**, 359–377.

13 McNeilage, L. J., MacMillan, E. and Whittingham, S. (1990) Mapping of epi-

topes on the La (SS-B) autoantigen of primary Sjögren's syndrome: identification of a cross-reactive epitope, *J. Immunol.* **145**, 3829–3835.

14 Tzoufas, A. G., Yiannaki, E., Sakarellos, C. and Moutsopoulos, H. M. (1997) Fine specificity of autoantibodies to La/SSB epitope mapping and characterisation, *Clin. Exp. immunol.* **108**, 191–198.

15 McNeilage, L. J., Umpathysivam, K., Macmillan, E., Guidolin, A., Whittingham, S. and Gordon, T. (1992) Definition of a discontinuous immunodominant epitope at the NH$_2$ terminus of the La/SS-B ribonucleoprotein autoantigen, *J. Clin. Invest.* **89**, 1652–1656.

16 Weng, Y.-M., McNeilage, J., Topfer, F., McCluskey, J. and Gordon, T. (1993) Identification of a human-specific epitope in a conserved region of the La/SS-B autoantigen, *J. Clin. Invest.* **92**, 1104–1108.

17 Rischmueller, M., McNeilage, L. J., McCluskey, J. and Gordon, T. (1995) Human autoantibodies directed against the RNA recognition motif of La (SS-B) bind to a conformational epitope present on the intact La (SS-B)/Ro (SS-A) ribonucleoprotein particle, *Clin. Exp. Immunol.* **101**, 39–44.

18 Beer, R. G., Rischmueller, M., Coates, T., Purcell, A. W., Keech, C. L., McCluskey, J. and Gordon, T. P. (1996) Nonprecipitating anti-La(SS-B) autoantibodies in primary Sjögren's syndrome, *Clin. Immunol. Immunopath.* **79**, 314–318.

19 Rischmueller, M., Lester, S., Chen, Z., Champion, G., Vandenberg, R., Beer, R., Coates, T., McCluskey, J. and Gordon, T. (1998) HLA Class II phenotype controls diversification of the autoantibody response in primary Sjögren's syndrome (PSS), *Clin Exp Immunol* **111**, 365–371.

20 Tzoufas, A. G., Wassmuth, R., Dafni, U. G., Guialis, A., Haga, H.-J., Isenberg, D. A., Jonsson, R., Kalden, J. R., Keiener, H., Sakarellos, C., Smolen, J. S., Sutcliffe, N., Vitali, C., Yiannaki, E. and Moutsopoulos, H. M. (2002) Clinical, immunological, and immunogenetic aspects of autoantibody production against Ro/SSA, La/SSB and their linear epitopes in primary Sjögren's syndrome

(pSS): a European multicentre study, *Ann Rheum Dis* **61**, 398–404.

21 McCluskey, J., Farris, A. D., Keech, C. L., Purcell, A. W., Rischmueller, M., Kinoshita, G., Reynolds, P. and Gordon, T. P. (1998) Determinant spreading: lessons from animal models and human disease, *Immunol. Rev.* **164**, 209–229.

22 Topfer, F., Gordon, T. and McCluskey, J. (1995) Intra- and inter-molecular spreading of autoimmunity involving the nuclear self-antigens La (SS-B) and Ro (SS-A). *Proc. Natl. Acad. Sci. USA* **92**, 875–879.

23 Keech, C. L., Gordon, T. P. and McCluskey, J. (1996) The immune response to 52-kDa and 60-kDa Ro is linked in experimental autoimmunity, *J. Immunol.* **157**, 3694–3699.

24 Kinoshita, G., Keech, C. L., Sontheimer, R. D., Purcell, A., McCluskey, J. and Gordon, T. P. (1998) Spreading of the immune response from 52 kDa Ro and 60 kDa Ro to calreticulin in experimental autoimmunity, *Lupus* **7**, 7–11.

25 Kinoshita, G., Purcell, A. W., Keech, C. L., Farris, A. D., McCluskey, J. and Gordon, T. P. (1999) Molecular chaperones are targets of autoimmunity in Ro(SS-A) immune mice, *Clin. Exp. immunol.* **11**, 268–274.

26 Topfer, F., Gordon, T. and McCluskey, J. (1993) Characterisation of the mouse autoantigen La (SS-B): Identification of conserved RNA binding motifs, a putative ATP binding site and reactivity of recombinant protein with poly(U) and human autoantibodies., *J. Immunol.* **150**, 3091–3100.

27 Keech, C. L., Gordon, T. P., Reynolds, P. and McCluskey, J. (1993) Expression and functional conservation of the human La(SS-B) nuclear autoantigen in murine cell lines., *J. Autoimmunity* **6**, 543–555.

28 Keech, C. L., Farris, A. D., Beroukas, D., Gordon, T. P. and McCluskey, J. (2001) Cognate T cell help is sufficient to trigger antinuclear autoantibodies in naive mice, *J. Immunol.* **166**, 5826–5835.

29 Lin, R. H., Mamula, M. J., Hardin, J. A. and Janeway, C. A. (1991) Induction of autoreactive B Cells allows priming of autoreactive T cells, *J Exp Med* **173**, 1433–1439.

30 Rubin, R. L., Tang, F. L., Tsay, G. and Pollard, K. M. (1990) Pseudoautoimmunity in normal mice: anti-histone antibodies elicited by immunization versus induction during graft-versus-host reaction, *Clin. Immunol. Immunopath.* **54**, 320–332.

31 Goodnow, C. C. (1996) Balancing immunity and tolerance: deleting and tuning lymphocyte repertoires, *Proc. Natl. Acad. Sci.* **93**, 2264–2271.

32 Erikson, J., Radic, M. Z., Camper, S. A., Hardy, R. R., Carmack, C. and Weigery, M. (1991) Expression of anti-DNA immunoglobulin transgenes in nonautoimmune mice, *Nature* **349**, 331–334.

33 Chen, C., Nagy, Z., Radic, M. Z., Hardy, R. R., Huszar, D, Camper, S. A. and Weigert, M. (1995) The site and stage of anti-DNA B cell deletion., *Nature* **373**, 252–255.

34 Mandik-Nayak, L., Bui, A., Noorchashm, H., Eaton, A. and Erikson, J. (1997) Regulation of anti-double-stranded DNA B cells in nonautoimmune mice: localization to the T-B interface of the splenic follicle, *J. Exp. Med.* **186**, 1257–1267.

35 Santulli-Marotto, S., Retter, M. W., Gee, R., Mamula, M. J. and Clarke, S. H. (1998) Autoreactive B cell regulation: peripheral induction of development arrest by lupus associated autoantigens, *Immunity* **8**, 209–219.

36 Qian, Y., Santiago, C., Borrero, M., Tedder, T. F. and Clarke S. H. (2001) Lupus-specific antiribonucleoprotein B cell tolerance in nonautoimmune mice is maintained by differentiation to B-1 and governed by B cell receptor signaling thresholds, *J. Immunol* **166**, 2412–2419.

37 Santulli-Marotto, S., Qian, Y., Ferguson, S. and Clarke, S. H. (2001) Anti-Sm B cell differentiation in Ig transgenic MRL/Mp-lpr/lpr mice: altered differentiation and an accelerated response, *J. Immunol.* **166**, 5292–5299.

38 Chan, E. K. L. and Tan, E. M. (1987) Human autoantibody-reactive epitopes of SS-B/La are highly conserved in comparison with epitopes recognized by murine monoclonal antibodies, *J. Exp. Med.* **166**, 1627–1640.

39 Aplin, B. D., Keech, C. L., de Kauwe, A. L., Gordon, T. P., Cavill, D. and McCluskey, J. (2003) Tolerance through indifference: autoractive B cells t the nuclear antigen La show no evidence of tolerance in a transgenic model, *J. Immunol.* **171**, 5890–5900.

40 Reynolds, P., Gordon, T. P., Purcell, A. W., Jackson, D. C. and McCluskey, J. (1996) Hierarchical self-tolerance to T cell determinants within the ubiquitous nuclear self antigen La (SS-B) permits induction of systemic autoimmunity in normal mice, *J. Exp. Med.* **184**, 1–14.

41 Sercarz, E. E., Lehmann, P. V., Ametani, A., Benichou, G., Miller, A. and Moudgil, K. (1993) Dominance and crypticity of T cell antigenic determinants, *Annu. Rev. Immunol.* **11**, 729–766.

42 Casciola-Rosen, L. A., Anhalt, G. and Rosen, A. (1994) Autoantigens targeted in systemic lupus erythematosus are clustered in two populations of surface structures on apoptotic keratinocytes, *J. Exp. Med.* **179**, 1317–1330.

43 Rosen, A., Casciola-Rosen, L. and Ahearn, J. (1995) Novel packages of viral and self-antigens are generated during apoptosis, *J. Exp. Med.* **181**, 1557–1561.

44 Casciola-Rosen, L. A., Andrade, F., Ulanet, D., Wong, W. B. and Rosen, A. (1999) Clevage by granzyme B is strongly predictive of autoantigen status: implications for initiation of autoimmunity, *Immunity* **190**, 815–825.

45 Rutjes, S. A., Utz, P. J., van der Heijden, A., Broekhuis, C., van Venrooij, W. and Pruijn, G. J. M. (1999) The La(SS-B) autoantigen, a key protein in RNA biogenesis is dephoshorylated and cleaved early during apoptosis, *Cell Death Differ* **6**, 976–986.

46 Mackay, F. and Browning, J. L. (2002) BAFF: a fundamental survival factor for B cells, *Nat Rev Immunol.* **2**, 465–475.

47 Groom, J., Kalled, S., Cutler, A., Olson, C., Woodcock, S., Schneider, P., Tschopp, J., Cachero, T., Batten, M., Wheway, J., Mauri, D., Cavill, D., Gordon, T., Mackay, C. and Mackay, F. (2002) Association of BAFF/BLyS overexpression and altered B

cell differentiation with Sjogren's syndrome, *J Clin Invest* **109**, 59–68.

48 Mariette, X., Roux, S., Zhang, J., Bengoufa, D., Lavie, F., Zhou, T. and Kimberly, R. (2003) The level of BLyS (BAFF) correlates with the titre of autoantibodies in human Sjögren's syndrome, *Ann Rheum Dis* **62**, 168–171.

49 Miranda-Carus, M., Askanase, A., Clancy, R., Di Donato, F., Chou, T., Libera, M., Chan, E. and Buyon, J. (2000) Anti-SSA/Ro and anti-SSB/La autoantibodies bind the surface of apoptotic fetal cardiocytes and promote secretion of TNF-alpha by macrophages, *J. Immunol.* **165**, 5345–5351.

50 Tran, H., Macardle, P., Hiscock, J., Cavill, D., Bradley, J., Buyon, J. and Gordon, T. (2002) Anti-La/SSB antibodies transported across the placenta bind apoptotic cells in fetal organs targeted in neonatal lupus, *Arthritis Rheum* **46**, 1572–1579.

51 Xiao, G., Qu, Y., Hu, K. and Boutjdir, M. (2001) Down-regulation of L-type calcium channel in pups born to 52 kDa SSA/Ro immunized rabbits, *FASEB J.* **15**, 1539–1545.

52 Buyon, J. and Clancy, R. (2003) Maternal autoantibodies and congenital heart block: mediators, markers, and therapeutic approach, *Semin Arthritis Rheum* **33**, 140–154.

20
Autoantibody Recognition of Functional Sites

Carlo Selmi, Sabine Oertelt, Pietro Invernizzi, Mauro Podda,
and M. Eric Gershwin

20.1
Introduction

A large number of autoantibodies react against functional structures of the cell, particularly nuclear components. Although in most cases the autoepitopes have been mapped, the inhibitory power of autoantibodies *in vivo* remains incompletely defined. Among the identified autoantigens, functional sites are found within chromatin, nucleoli, and ribonucleoproteins (RNPs), as well as in mitochondrial proteins and cellular receptors.

DNA molecules and the bound histones are among the most common nuclear autoantigens, being recognized in up to 65% of sera from patients with systemic lupus erythematosus (SLE). These antinuclear autoantibodies (ANAs) react with the sugar-phosphate backbone of the double-stranded molecule as well as with single bases of the single-stranded DNA, while anti-histone antibodies directed against H2A and H2B more specifically characterize drug-induced lupus. Other autoantibodies are directed against nuclear proteins expressed or activated during specific phases of the cell cycle. For example, anti-centromere antibodies (ACAs) target CENP-A, -B, and -C centromeric proteins during the metaphase. Similarly, anti-Scl70 antibodies are directed against topoisomerase I (Scl-70), a nuclear non-histone protein that uncoils condensed chromatin during mitosis (Tamby et al. 2003). Moreover, the nucleus presents other autoepitopes, such as extractable nuclear antigens (ENAs) associated with RNA molecules. Small nuclear RNAs (snRNAs) catalyze RNA splicing; in this process, while U1 and U2 particles bind to the extremities of an intron, the "spliceosome" (U4, U5, and U6 particles) leads to intron removal. Interestingly, the spliceosome is highly conserved in vertebrates and insects and represents one of the recognized antigens by SLE-specific anti-Smith (anti-Sm) autoantibodies (Zieve and Khusial 2003). The peculiarity of this serum autoantibody pattern is the combination of recognized snRNPs: the U1 particle is targeted by autoantibodies in mixed connective tissue, while anti-Sm antibodies react less specifically with all

Autoantibodies and Autoimmunity: Molecular Mechanisms
in Health and Disease. Edited by K. Michael Pollard
Copyright © 2006 WILEY-VCH Verlag GmbH & Co. KGaA, Weinheim
ISBN: 3-527-31141-6

snRNP particles. We also note that the major epitope is located within the C-terminus of the B protein and shares homology with an Epstein-Barr virus antigen. Finally, eukaryotic RNA polymerase III, responsible for tRNA, 5S RNA, and snRNA synthesis, is the autoantigen recognized by SS-B (or La) antibodies found in Sjögren's syndrome and SLE.

Other autoantibodies show reactivity to membrane receptors and active molecules. Thyroid peroxidase (TPO) and thyrotropin receptor (TSHR) are recognized by autoantibodies in autoimmune thyroid disease and are localized on the cell membrane. Known TPO epitopes present large overlapping regions, while the epitopes of TSHR are as yet undefined. Although the identified sites remain obscure in the latter case, the effects of autoantibody binding to TSHR are better known, resulting in either hyper- or hypothyroidism due to a TSH-like mimic action and a consequent enhancing or inhibitory effect. Curiously, both molecules require expression in mammalian cells to be recognized as autoantigens (Rapoport and McLachlan 2001).

Lupus anticoagulant, or antiphospholipid antibodies, is an example of extracellular protein interference resulting in a systemic clinical syndrome. In this case, autoantibodies recognize phospholipid-binding plasma proteins, such as prothrombin, annexin V, and beta-2-glycoprotein, and elicit a procoagulant effect along with additional endothelial cell activation. As the target molecule is shared by a large number of clotting factors, the disease clinical expression involves a multifactorial process (Mackworth-Young 2004).

While the previously discussed autoantigens are clearly characterized in their cellular or extracellular localization, the main issue of autoreactivity against intracellular antigens is linked to their potential aberrant expression. The question of whether autoepitopes are expressed on the cell surface triggering the autoimmune response or are extruded by cells undergoing apoptosis remains unsolved. Anti-mitochondrial autoantibodies (AMAs), the serum hallmark of primary biliary cirrhosis (PBC), are directed against specific intramitochondrial enzymes and present an as yet undefined etiological role. We will discuss in this chapter the available evidence and the current hypotheses regarding the induction, perpetuation, effects, and pathogenetic role of AMAs in PBC as a paradigm of autoantibodies directed against functional sites.

20.2
Anti-mitochondrial Antibodies in Primary Biliary Cirrhosis

Primary biliary cirrhosis (PBC) summarizes several unknown aspects of autoimmunity, being both a model and a paradox for autoimmune conditions (Gershwin and Mackay 1991). The former is indicated by the characteristics of PBC that are common to other conditions, such as the female predominance (Selmi et al. 2004a), the genetic predisposition (Selmi et al. 2004b, 2004c), and the presence of specific autoantibodies in the vast majority of cases. However, in the case of PBC, such autoantibodies also constitute the basis for the disease being a paradox, as their direct pathogenetic role is still poorly defined (Gershwin et al. 2000). Immunological attention to PBC was raised 10 years after its clinical definition (Ahrens et al. 1950) when patient sera were found to react by complement fixation with tissue extracts (Mackay 1958), later identified as mitochondria by indirect immunofluorescence (Walker et al. 1965). It was only in 1987 that molecular cloning showed that PBC-specific AMA recognized a family of components of 48–74 kDa that had previously been shown by immunoblotting (Frazer et al. 1985). The serum reactivity was further demonstrated as directed against the subunits of the 2-oxoacid dehydrogenase complex (2-OADC) (Gershwin et al. 1987).

20.2.1
Biochemistry of the 2-Oxoacid Dehydrogenase Complex

As mentioned above, the application of molecular biological techniques led to great progress in PBC, allowing molecular cloning of the cDNAs that encode the major mitochondrial autoantigens, i.e., the 2-oxoacid dehydrogenase complexes (2-OADCs). The 2-OADCs are multi-enzyme complexes that are essential in energy metabolism (Reed and Hackert 1990). This enzyme family comprises the pyruvate dehydrogenase complex (PDC), the 2-oxo-glutarate dehydrogenase complex (OGDC), and the branched chain 2-oxoacid dehydrogenase complex (BCOADC). Each of the three complexes consists of three subunits, i.e., E1, E2, and E3. All subunits are proteins separately encoded in the nucleus and imported through the cytoplasm into mitochondria for assembly into high-molecular-weight multimers located on the inner membrane. Each 2-OADC occupies a central position in intermediary metabolism, and the activity of each complex within mitochondria is under strict control by dietary factors and hormones. Table 20.1 summarizes the molecular weights and functions of the 2-OADC subunits. PDC links glycolysis to the citric acid cycle (Krebs cycle); OGDC works within the citric acid cycle; and BCOADC catalyzes an irreversible step in the catabolism of several essential amino acids, including the branched-chain amino acids valine, leucine, and isoleucine. The overall structure of each of the 2-OADCs is similar in that each consists of multiple copies of three functionally equivalent subunit enzymes. For each multi-enzyme complex, the E2 component forms a symmetrical core around which the E1 and E3 components are arranged (Patel and Roche 1990). The E2 components consist of several functional domains: the inner catalytic domain containing the active site, one or more lipoyl domains containing the lysine residue to which the essential cofactor lipoic acid is attached, and an E3-binding domain.

As explained in more detail below, PDC-E2 and E3BP are the major autoantigens for serum AMAs. Thus, it is crucial to illustrate their structure more fully. It has been demonstrated that both PDC-E2 and E3BP fold into distinct domains linked by flexible regions rich in alanine and proline residues; interestingly, such flexibility is important for the enzyme catalytic function. Moreover, both polypeptides have a central core region, responsible for binding to other

Table 20.1 Molecular weights and functions of the 2-oxo-acid dehydrogenase complexes.

Enzymes	MW (kDa)	Function
Pyruvate dehydrogenase complexes		
E1a decarboxylase	41	Decarboxylates pyruvate with thiamine pyrophosphate (TTP) as a cofactor
E1b decarboxylase	36	Decarboxylates pyruvate with TTP as a cofactor
E2 acetyltransferase	74	Transfers acetyl group from E1 to coenzyme A (CoA)
E3 lipoamide dehydrogenase	55	Regenerates disulphide of E2 by oxidation of lipoic acid
E3-binding protein (protein X)	56	Anchors E2 to the E2 core of pyruvate dehydrogenase complex
2-oxoglutarate dehydrogenase complexes		
E1 oxoglutarate dehydrogenase	113	Decarboxylates a-ketoglutarate with TTP as a cofactor
E2 succinyl transferase	48	Transfers succinyl group from E2 to CoA
E3 lipoamide dehydrogenase	55	Regenerates disulphide of E2 by oxidation of lipoic acid
Branched-chain 2-oxo-acid dehydrogenase complexes		
E1a decarboxylase	46	Decarboxylates a-keto acids
E1b decarboxylase	38	Is derived from leucine, isoleucine, and valine with TTP as a cofactor
E2 acyltransferase	52	Transfers acyl group from E1 to CoA
E3 lipoamide dehydrogenase	55	Regenerates disulphide of E2 by oxidation of lipoic acid

polypeptides. The E2 core, moreover, contains the residues essential for its catalytic activity and is linked to a binding domain, which accounts for the binding to E1 (and possibly E3). On the other hand, the corresponding E3BP region binds E3 only. Further, both polypeptides include at their amino terminals compact domains containing the covalently attached lipoic acid cofactor (Reed and Hackert 1990). PDC-E2 has two and E3BP a single lipoylated domain (Neagle et al. 1989). These domains are exposed on the surface of the E2 core, thus likely contributing to the antigenicity of the molecules (see Section 20.3). In all three cases, the domain is composed by a single lipoic acid residue covalently attached to a lysine residue in a constant DKA sequence motif. The three-dimensional structure of the inner lipoyl domain of human PDC-E2 has recently been determined and is illustrated in Figure 20.1 (Howard et al. 1998).

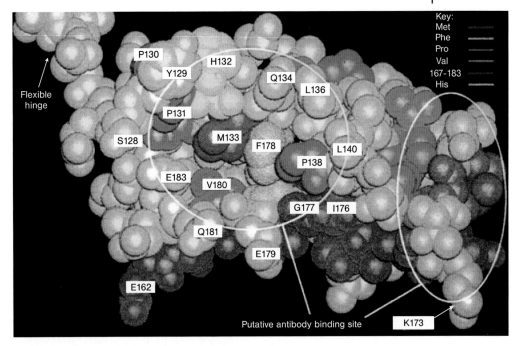

Fig. 20.1 Three-dimensional structure of the PDC-E2 inner lipoylated domain based on published NMR structure (Howard et al. 1998)

20.2.2
Epitopes in Biliary Epithelia

Biliary epithelial cells (BECs) constitute a heterogeneous cell population (Katayanagi et al. 1999), with those that line large extrahepatic bile ducts being distinct from those that line small intrahepatic bile ducts. The identification of specific characteristics of BECs (by the differential expression of cell adhesion molecules, response to cytokines, growth factors, and the like) may explain the strict organ specificity of the immune-mediated injury in PBC. In particular, intrahepatic BECs may express target molecules not expressed in the large bile ducts. Mechanisms involved in the disruption of the biliary epithelium in PBC, especially the association between AMAs and bile duct damage, remain poorly understood, although several hypotheses have been proposed. These include, but are not limited to, a T-cell-mediated cytotoxicity and/or an intracellular interaction between the IgA class of AMAs and mitochondrial autoantigens in BECs during the intracellular transport, resulting in cytotoxicity. Several studies suggest that BECs are antigenically distinct since they express molecules that are associated with immune recognition of target cells, such as adhesion molecules, antigens of the major histocompatibility complex (MHC), and costimulatory molecules. However, these molecules are not specific for PBC, having been described in other inflammatory liver diseases, and are therefore considered secondary events. Interestingly, PDC-E2 and E3BP, the two major autoantigens associated with PBC, are upregulated in PBC when BECs are examined immunohistochemically (Joplin et al. 1991, 1994; Van de Water et al. 1991). Furthermore, this upregulation is present at early stages in the natural history of the disease (Tsuneyama et al. 1995) and can also be found in BECs from allografts of patients with recurrent PBC following orthotopic liver transplantation (Van de Water et al. 1996). The latter observation strongly suggests a role for these antigens in the pathogenesis and/or progression (and recurrence) of PBC. Immunohistochemically, PDC-E2 also appears to be localized to the apical region of the BECs in the PBC liver. We can hypothesize that the increased focal expression of PDC-E2 by intrahepatic BECs in PBC might be secondary to enhanced synthesis, impaired degradation, and abnormal targeting of the PDC-E2 to the plasma membrane of BECs. It is not clear at present, however, whether the molecule that is detected at this special location is the whole PDC-E2 molecule, a part of PDC-E2, or possibly a non-2-OADC molecule that is cross-reactive with PDC-E2. The finding that PDC-E2 messenger RNA is undetectable in PBC BECs argues against simple enhanced synthesis with overspill to the cytoplasm and/or the surface (Harada et al. 1997 b); however, it does not rule out the possibility of a trafficking defect, in which PDC-E2 is aberrantly transported to the cytoplasmic membrane. This alteration might occur as a result of a point mutation in the mitochondrial presequence, in a manner analogous to the mistargeting of alanine in primary hyperoxaluria (Danpure 1998). Our study with specific monoclonal antibodies and human combinatorial antibodies indicated that a molecule cross-reactive with PDC-E2, but not PDC-E2 itself, is expressed at high levels at the lumenal region of bile ducts in PBC patients (Cha et al. 1994; Van de Water et al. 1993). Further, the analysis of AMA binding to the membrane fraction of purified BECs has suggested that AMAs in patients with PBC may react with PDC-E3BP rather than PDC-E2 (Joplin et al. 1997); similar to what was inferred from other expression studies, it is not clear at present which mechanism may lead to this alteration. Apoptosis is a widely studied player in this scenario. BECs undergo apoptosis in PBC as indicated by *in situ* nick-end labeling methods for the detection of DNA fragmentation (Harada et al. 1997 a; Koga et al. 1997). More recently, experimental evidence has further defined apoptosis in PBC and has demonstrated that such a process has unique features in PBC bile duct cells (Odin et al. 2001), and that PDC-E2 is released without caspase cleavage from apoptotic cells (Matsumura et al. 2002). The latter observations might in turn be responsible for the liberation from BECs undergoing apoptosis of intact PDC-E2 that could account for the appearance of AMA-IgG immunocomplexes. We also note that related studies have shown not only increased expression of perforin and granzymes in PBC, but, in addition, Fas (CD95) has also been shown to be upregulated on the BEC membrane. It is thus possible that both of these pathways might be involved (Harada et al. 1997 a; Kuroki et al. 1996). Similarly, BECs from PBC patients overexpress IL-6 and TNF-alpha compared to other hepatobiliary diseases (Yasoshima et al.

1998). The finding that TNF receptor and IL-6 receptor are also detected on damaged bile ducts clearly suggests an autocrine effect (Yasoshima et al. 1998). Accordingly, the increased expression of IL-6 and TNF-alpha could affect the proliferation, maturation, and regulation of B-cell and T-cell lineage infiltrates around bile ducts (Jelinek and Lipsky 1987). IL-6 promotes terminal differentiation of B cells, leading to immunoglobulin secretion. TNF-alpha, on the other hand, has been shown to induce the expression of adhesion molecules, HLA-DR, and a variety of other antigens on the bile ducts. It may also increase the cytotoxic activities of T cells. We may then surmise that IL-6 is responsible for BEC proliferation via an autocrine pathway (Matsumoto et al. 1994), while TNF-alpha may be directly involved in BEC damage. The autocrine role of TNF-alpha on cell damage, including apoptosis, has already been shown in renal epithelial cells and hepatitis B– and C virus–infected hepatocytes (Gonzalez-Amaro et al. 1994). TNF-alpha is also known to interfere with the barrier function of the bile ducts, which may lead to leakage of toxic substances into the bile, resulting in a local inflammatory process and cholangitis (Mano et al. 1996). The same process could also account for an increased circulation of chemicals, thus contributing to the xenobiotic story in PBC (see Section 20.9).

Extensive studies have mapped the autoimmune response to epitopes recognized by immune effectors. Among 2-OADCs, the antigenic determinants in PDC-E2 have been best characterized. For fine epitope mapping of the human PDC-E2, truncated constructs of PDC-E2 were generated, and assays of multiple overlapping recombinant proteins from human PDC-E2 cDNA indicated there were at least three AMA autoepitopes (Surh et al. 1990). Specifically, AMAs were demonstrated to bind the cross-reactive outer and inner lipoyl domains and a site surrounding the region that binds the E1 and E3 subunits, with the dominant epitope localized to the inner lipoyl region. The outer lipoyl region presents weaker reactivity, and only a minority of PBC sera reacted with the E1/E3-binding region. Analysis of recombinant fusion proteins expressed from a cDNA encoding the inner lipoyl domain revealed a minimal requirement of 76 amino acids (residues 146–221) for detectable autoantibody binding and of 94 amino acids (residues 128–221) for strong binding. This requirement for such a large peptide region for immunoreactivity is of interest and indicates that the autoepitope for the B-cell response is conformational (Rowley et al. 1991). PDC-E1a differs from PDC-E2 in that it lacks any covalently bound lipoic acid. The autoepitope of PDC-E1a is located at the region that contains the enzyme functional sites, the phosphorylation, and the TTP-binding sites (Iwayama et al. 1991). The antigenic determinants of BCOADC-E2 and OGDC-E2 have also been characterized using expressed fragments of BCOADC-E2 and OGDC-E2. Autoantibody reactivity to BCOADC-E2 mapped within residues 1–115 with strong binding and residues 1–84 (lipoyl domain) with weaker binding. Only the full-length recombinant protein (residues 1–421) is sufficient to remove all detectable anti-BCOADC-E2 reactivity (Leung et al. 1995). This suggested that the BCOADC-E2 epitopes are highly conformational. Similarly, a minimum of 81 amino acids (residues 67–147) corresponding to the lipoyl domain of OGDC-

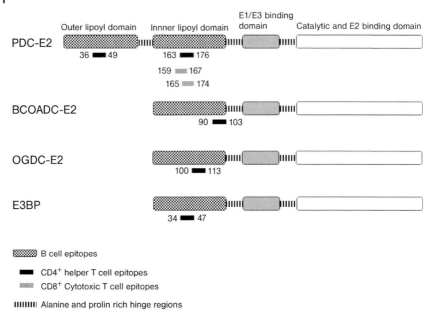

Fig. 20.2 Structure of 2-OADC proteins and the overlapping T-cell and B-cell epitopes in PBC.

E2 is necessary for anti-OGDC-E2 reactivity (Moteki et al. 1996b; Palmer et al. 1999). Recently, the epitope of the E3-binding protein recognized by AMAs was also determined as the lipoic acid–binding domain. There was little IgM response to the E3BP lipoyl domain, suggesting that this immune response is a secondary phenomenon, probably because of antigen-determinant spreading (Dubel et al. 1999). Interestingly, the immunodominant epitopes of PDC-E2, OGDC-E2, and BCOADC-E2 are all conformational lipoate-binding sites, and antibodies against them do not cross-react. Although it is beyond the scope of the present chapter, we also note that the epitopes recognized by autoreactive T cells in PBC have been identified and that they overlap partially with the amino acid sequences reacting with AMAs. Figure 20.2 illustrates the AMA and T-cell epitopes thus far demonstrated in PBC (Ishibashi et al. 2003).

Following AMA epitope-mapping studies, a triple-expression hybrid clone consisting of three different lipoyl domains, PDC-E2 (residues 91–128), OGDC-E2 (67–147), and BCOADC-E2 (1–118), was constructed and tested in immunoblotting and ELISA. Of 186 sera from patients with PBC, 152 (81.7%) reacted with recombinant PDC-E2, whereas 171 sera (91.9%) showed positive reactivity when probed by immunoblotting against the recombinant triple-hybrid protein (Moteki et al. 1996a). Table 20.2 illustrates the specific AMA pattern observed in PBC sera. Accordingly, ELISA or immunoblotting using this recombinant protein seems to be a powerful and specific method that will replace classical immunofluorescence for the detection of AMAs. Recent studies based on such recombi-

Table 20.2 Mitochondrial autoantigens recognized by PBC sera.

Antigen	Prevalence (%)
PDC-E2	90–95
PDC-E3-binding protein	90–95
OGDC-E2	39–88
BCOADC-E2	53–55
PDC-E1alpha	41–66
PDC-E1beta	1–7

nant antigens have provided similar results (Miyakawa et al. 2001) and allowed us to estimate that less than 5% of PBC sera lack AMAs when tested with the most sensitive technique available. Accordingly, the detection of AMAs is one of the criteria currently necessary for the diagnosis of PBC in the clinical management of intrahepatic cholestasis, along with an increased alkaline phosphatase plasma level and a compatible liver histology (Talwalkar and Lindor 2003).

The role of lipoic acid in AMA reactivity warrants particular attention, as previously indicated. In all AMA major autoantigens, in fact, epitopes contain the motif DKA, with lipoic acid covalently bound to the lysine (K) residue. It is not clear what the role of lipoic acid is in epitope recognition by AMAs; in fact, apparently conflicting results indicated that AMAs bind to both the lipoylated and unlipoylated forms of PDC-E2 (Quinn et al. 1993), while they can also bind to lipoic acid attached to a non-2-OADC peptide (Bruggraber et al. 2003). The role of lipoic acid in the breakdown of tolerance in PBC is further stressed by the xenobiotic theory; according to this theory, in fact, lipoic acid would be the most likely target to modification by chemicals to induce neo-antigens (see Section 20.4).

20.3
Enzyme Inhibition

As explained elsewhere in this chapter, AMAs from patients with PBC react against several 2-OADC enzymes and subunits. Within such molecules, moreover, different amino acid sequences can constitute the major epitope, thus making the humoral autoimmune response observed with routine methods (i.e., indirect immunofluorescence, immunoblotting) widely variable and, possibly, poorly specific with regard to the pathogenesis of the disease. Based on this theory, several studies have investigated the inhibitory effects of AMAs on PDC-E2 to provide a better definition of the recognized epitopes and to define the resulting effect from the antibody binding. Moreover, such assays were proven to be less subjective compared to routine methods in the interpretation of results (Jensen et al. 2000). As also indicated from the epitope mapping, AMAs share the capability of inhibiting the enzymatic activity of 2-OADCs, with most evidence gathered for PDC-E2. Quite expectedly, AMA titers also correlate with the enzyme inhibition capacity of these autoantibodies; interestingly, however, the common fluctuations in AMA titers observed in PBC could be best determined when using enzyme assay kits rather than immunoblotting using bovine heart mitochondria (Hazama et al. 2000). Other researchers compared the diagnostic sensitivity of the former assay with indirect immunofluorescence and estimated it to be 82%, thus lower than indirect immunofluorescence but accompanied by a specificity higher than 99% (Jois et al. 2000). Similar results were obtained in a study on 71 PBC sera that also indicated that the stage of disease did not influence the enzyme inhibition assay (Teoh et al. 1994b). We also note that the comparison of the AMA inhibition capacity on mammalian PDC-E2 and PDC-E2 from *E. coli* and *Saccharomyces cerevisiae* demonstrated that the enzyme inhibition was significantly lower in bacteria and yeasts than in mammalian molecules (Teoh et al. 1994a). These data could be interpreted as militating against a role for the two specific microorganisms in the induction of PBC through molecular mimicry (see Section 20.5).

20.4
Xenobiotics and AMA

The hypothesis that PBC might be caused by exposure to chemicals was first based on the geoepidemiology data on the prevalence of the disease, which in some cases indicated a role for water supplies or other environmental vectors (Selmi et al. 2004a). Xenobiotics are foreign compounds that may either alter or complex to defined self-proteins, inducing a change in the molecular structure of the native protein sufficient to induce an immune response. Such immune responses may then result in the recognition of not only the modified or altered protein but also the unmodified native protein (Rose 2000). The chronic presence of the self-protein serves to perpetuate the immune response initiated by the xenobiotic-induced adduct, thus leading to autoimmunity. Interestingly, most chemicals are transported to the liver through the portal system where they are also metabolized, thereby increasing the potential for liver-specific alteration of proteins. In fact, a liver-specific autoimmune disease was observed in some patients exposed to chlorofluorohydrocarbon anesthetics, while immunization with halothane, whose trifluoroacetyl (TFA) metabolite covalently links to lysine on cytochrome p450 2E1, induces the formation of antibodies that cross-react with not only the haptenated (TFA) immunogen but also lipoylated PDC-E2 (Sasaki et al. 2000). This finding has several potential implications in the pathogenesis of PBC; in fact, one of the major working hypotheses is currently that potential modifications of self-proteins by agents such as xenobiotics may alter such self-proteins enough to cause a breakdown of tolerance. In this scenario, the immune response would be perpetuated by the chronic low level of turnover for the self-protein, which is the case for PDC-E2, being essential for the function of mitochondria to change between an oxidized and reduced state. Perhaps the preference for enzymes, containing substituents like lipoic acid, can be explained because the functional site of the enzymes is more accessible and therefore more susceptible to modification by exogenous agents (e.g., xenobiotics), thus providing neoantigens that can be recognized by the immune system (Steinman 1999). To address this hypothesis, we therefore took advantage of *ab initio* quantum chemistry and synthesized the inner lipoyl domain of PDC-E2, replacing the lipoic acid moiety with a large number of synthetic structures designed to mimic a xenobiotically modified lipoyl hapten (Long et al. 2001). We then quantitated the reactivity of sera from PBC patients to these structures. Interestingly, AMAs reacted against three of the 18 organic modified autoepitopes with significantly higher affinity than to the native lipoylated domain. By structural analysis, the features that correlated with autoantibody binding included synthetic domain peptides with a halide or methyl halide in the *meta* or *para* position containing no strong hydrogen bond–accepting groups on the phenyl ring of the lysine substituents, and synthetic domain peptides with a relatively low rotation barrier about the linkage bond. More recently, it was reported that immunization of rabbits with a halogenated compound, i.e., 6-bromohexanoate, led to AMA appearance in the absence of a PDC-E2-like peptide backbone (Leung et al. 2003) and that such serum reactivity was reversible when the stimulus was suspended (Amano et al. 2004). However, no signs of liver disease were achieved with these animal models. It is intriguing that many common products, including pharmaceuticals and household detergents, have the potential to produce closely related halogenated derivatives as intermediate or end-stage metabolites. Moreover, a large number of common pharmaceuticals, including diuretic agents, also share halogenated structures. In fact, halogens are common substituents in pharmaceuticals that modulate binding, activity, and metabolism. The resulting thesis states that people genetically predisposed to PBC have inherited such predisposition based on either the cytochrome p450 pathway or another metabolic process responsible for degrading halogenated compounds. We note, however, that an association study of genetic polymorphisms influencing xenobiotic transport or metabolism (including CYP2E1 and 2D6) in a large series of patients with PBC and controls did not suggest a role for such variants in susceptibility to PBC (Kimura et al. 2005). Estrogens have also been shown to modulate the expression of many liver metabolic pathways, and this may explain the female predominance of PBC. Finally, the presence of primarily small bile duct destruction may be reflective of the local mucosal immune response, which is more prominent on epithelial surfaces (Reynoso-Paz et al. 2000).

20.5
Microorganisms and AMAs

The ability of infectious agents, particularly bacteria, to induce autoimmune responses in experimental settings has been documented, and molecular mimicry is the most widely studied mechanism to account for these phenomena (Van de

Water et al. 2001). This paradigm suggests that microorganisms present peptides sharing different degrees of similarity with self-proteins, thus leading to a promiscuous antibody- and cell-mediated immune response capable of reacting with both microbial and self-epitopes. T-cell activation produces cross-reacting T cells, leading to self-tissue destruction and thus perpetuating the autoimmune response, possibly through the corruption of the T-cell receptor and cross-priming (Selmi and Gershwin 2004). Of the bacterial strains potentially involved in PBC through molecular mimicry, most evidence has been reported for *Escherichia coli*, as suggested by reports of an increased incidence of urinary tract infections in patients with PBC (Parikh-Patel et al. 2001). Other microorganisms have been identified as potential mimics. *Chlamydia pneumoniae* persists in many human tissues and has a putative role in coronary disease and thus could be related to epithelial cell reactivity (Abdulkarim 2004); association with *Helicobacter pylori* is controversial, being identified by some, due to a higher incidence of gastritis type A among PBC patients, but not confirmed by others (Dohmen 2001; Floreani 1997). Finally, none of the mentioned microorganisms could be proven to have a definite association with disease development.

Our group has recently investigated the role in PBC of the newly defined bacterial strain *Novosphingobium aromaticivorans* (Selmi et al. 2003). This unique bacterium appears to be the best candidate to induce molecular mimicry in PBC for several reasons. First, the amino acid sequences of two different proteins from *N. aromaticivorans* present the highest degree of homology with the main PDC-E2 autoepitope (amino acids 208–237) recognized by AMAs and T cells. This degree of similarity, albeit not unique to *N. aromaticivorans*, is significantly higher compared to candidate proteins from other strains previously studied in PBC, such as *E. coli* or *Chlamydia pneumoniae*. Second, the bacterium is ubiquitous, has not been found to be pathogenic to humans, and shares the ability to activate 17-beta estradiol (Fujii et al. 2002). Further, we note that a role for halogenated xenobiotics has been proposed by our group in the induction of PBC (see Section 20.4), and the capability of *N. aromaticivorans* to metabolize a growing number of chemical compounds (Fredrickson et al. 1995) suggests that this bacterium, as well as other strains with similar characteristics, might be the missing link between xenobiotics and bacteria in PBC. In our first study, we analyzed a large number of sera from patients with PBC and controls using recombinant mitochondrial antigens and bacterial proteins from *N. aromaticivorans* homogenates. Reactivity against two lipoylated proteins with molecular weights of 47 kDa and 50 kDa was observed in 100% of anti-PDC-E2–positive sera and also in a fraction of AMA-negative sera. In contrast with what was reported for other bacterial species, the pattern was observed in patients with both early and advanced disease, and, in one case, it suggested the diagnosis of PBC in a previously considered healthy sister of a known patient. The reactivity was specific for PBC sera, as no samples from first-degree relatives of patients (with the exception of the previously mentioned specific case) or controls with other autoimmune diseases were found positive against such proteins. Moreover, we estimated that the reactivity against *N. aromaticivorans* was 100- to 1000-fold higher than against *E. coli*, being still detectable at 10^{-6} dilution in 23% of anti-PDC-E2–positive sera. To further address our hypothesis, we also searched for molecular evidence of the bacterium in fecal samples from patients with PBC and non-PBC controls living in the same household. Results showed that approximately 25% of specimens, regardless of the diagnosis, had detectable 16S rRNA target sequences, thus demonstrating for the first time the presence of *N. aromaticivorans* in humans.

For purposes of completeness, we also note that a novel human beta retrovirus has been suggested in the etiology of PBC (Xu et al. 2003); however, we were unable to confirm such data in an independent approach (Selmi et al. 2004d).

20.6
AMAs in the Pathogenesis of PBC

As stated above, several clinical and experimental findings strongly imply an autoimmune pathogenesis for PBC (Selmi et al. 2004a). Common features of other autoimmune conditions seem to apply only in part to PBC. First, autoantibodies should be present in patients with the disease. PBC is characterized by the presence of detectable AMAs in approximately 90–95% of affected individuals, although we note that patients lacking AMAs can present with a disease picture and progression similar to that found in AMA-positive subjects (Invernizzi et al. 1997), thus seemingly arguing against a pathogenic role for these autoantibodies. Autoreactive T cells, both CD4 and CD8, have been identified in AMA-negative PBC, and such lymphocytes and AMAs recognize overlapping epitopes within the mitochondrial antigens (Ishibashi et al. 2003) (Fig. 20.2). Second, autoantibodies should interact with the target antigen, the passive transfer of autoantibodies should reproduce the clinical features, and experimental immunization with the antigen should produce a model disease. No direct proof has yet been provided for a direct pathogenic role of AMAs in the bile duct injury observed in PBC. Similarly, no convincing animal model has been described, although AMAs can be generated in experimental animals following immunization with several antigens. Third, in autoimmune diseases the reduction of autoantibody levels should ameliorate the disease; this criterion is also poorly fulfilled in PBC where there is no correlation between the pattern or titer of AMAs and the progression of the disease (Bogdanos et al. 2003).

Finally, it is well established that most autoimmune diseases are responsive to immunosuppressive therapy. In PBC, all immunosuppressive agents have proven to be relatively ineffective (Talwalkar and Lindor 2003). In conclusion, therefore, the pathogenic role of AMAs still remains to be elucidated, similar to many other aspects in PBC pathogenesis. In fact, we cannot rule out, at present, that the specific humoral autoimmunity might not play a central role in the organ-specific injury of PBC.

20.7
Other Autoantibodies in PBC

The absence of detectable serum AMAs in 5–10% of patients with PBC has prompted the search for other noninvasive markers. Two distinct ANA patterns at immunofluorescence have been proven to be specific for PBC, i.e., multiple nuclear dots and rim-like patterns (Worman and Courvalin 2003). The autoantibodies producing the former pattern are directed against Sp100 and promyelocytic leukemia proteins and are detected in about 30% of PBC cases (Szostecki et al. 1997). Rim-like ANAs, on the other hand, react against proteins of the nuclear pore complexes, supramolecular structures that include gp210 (a 210-kDa transmembrane glycoprotein involved in the attachment of nuclear pore complex constituents within the nuclear membrane), p62 (a nuclear pore glycoprotein), and the inner nuclear membrane protein lamin B receptor. Serum anti-gp210 ANAs are detected in about 25% (10–40%) of AMA-positive and up to 50% of AMA-negative patients (in both cases with high specificity) (Invernizzi et al. 2001). Autoantibodies reacting with p62 or lamin B receptor are found in about 13% and 1% of patients with PBC, respectively. Interestingly, the presence of anti-gp210 and anti-p62 ANAs in the same serum is rare.

Other less-specific autoantibodies can be detected in PBC sera, directed against centromere proteins, histone, spliceosome components, and single-stranded DNA (Chou et al. 1995). In some cases, these autoantibodies reflect other autoimmune conditions that often coexist with PBC.

20.8
Concluding Remarks and Future Directions

Our knowledge of the "destructive" arm in the pathogenesis of PBC is still largely incomplete. Specific autoantibodies have been widely studied and defined, despite the incomplete understanding of their pathogenic role. Interestingly, epitopes recognized by the cellular and humoral immune system in the autoimmunity leading to PBC present significant overlapping, and this suggests that both compartments contribute to the pathogenesis of the disease. We have described herein the known and unknown aspects of the rise in AMAs and their role in the pathogenesis of PBC as a paradigm of autoantibodies against functional sites possibly leading to clinical disease. We note that similar findings are being reported in other autoimmune diseases in which autoantibodies are directed against critical enzymes. In all of these conditions, only a wider effort capable of studying both humoral and cellular autoreactivity, as well as better immunological definition in light of the proposed etiologic factors, can provide further insight into the pathogenetic mechanisms of these autoimmune diseases, thus allowing novel and more focused therapeutic approaches for autoimmunity.

References

Abdulkarim, A. S., Petrovic, L. M., Kim, W. R., Angulo, P., Lloyd, R. V., Lindor, K. D. (2004). Primary biliary cirrhosis: an infectious disease caused by Chlamydia pneumoniae? J Hepatol **40(3)**: 380–384.

Ahrens, E. H., Jr., Payne, M. A., Kunkel, H. G., Eisenmenger, W. J. and Blondheim, S. H. (1950). Primary biliary cirrhosis. Medicine (Baltimore) **29**: 299–364.

Amano, K., Leung, P. S., Xu, Q., Marik, J., Quan, C., Kurth, M. J., Nantz, M. H., Ansari, A. A., Lam, K. S., Zeniya, M., Coppel, R. L. and Gershwin, M. E. (2004). Xenobiotic-induced loss of tolerance in rabbits to the mitochondrial autoantigen of primary biliary cirrhosis is reversible. J Immunol **172**: 6444–6452.

Bogdanos, D. P., Baum, H. and Vergani, D. (2003). Antimitochondrial and other autoantibodies. Clin Liver Dis **7**: 759–777, vi.

Bruggraber, S. F., Leung, P. S., Amano, K., Quan, C., Kurth, M. J., Nantz, M. H., Benson, G. D., Van de Water, J., Luketic, V., Roche, T. E., Ansari, A. A., Coppel, R. L. and Gershwin, M. E. (2003). Autoreactivity to lipoate and a conjugated form of lipoate in primary biliary cirrhosis. Gastroenterology **125**: 1705–1713.

Cha, S., Leung, P. S., Coppel, R. L., Van de Water, J., Ansari, A. A. and Gershwin, M. E. (1994). Heterogeneity of combinatorial human autoantibodies against PDC-E2 and biliary epithelial cells in patients with primary biliary cirrhosis. Hepatology **20**: 574–583.

Chou, M. J., Lee, S. L., Chen, T. Y. and Tsay, G. J. (1995). Specificity of antinuclear antibodies in primary biliary cirrhosis. Ann Rheum Dis **54**: 148–151.

Danpure, C. J. (1998). The molecular basis of alanine: glyoxylate aminotransferase mistargeting: the most common single cause of primary hyperoxaluria type 1. J Nephrol **11 Suppl 1**: 8–12.

Dohmen, K. (2001). Primary biliary cirrhosis and pernicious anemia. J Gastroenterol Hepatol **16(12)**: 1316–1318.

Dubel, L., Tanaka, A., Leung, P. S., Van de Water, J., Coppel, R., Roche, T., Johanet, C., Motokawa, Y., Ansari, A. and Gershwin, M. E. (1999). Autoepitope mapping and reactivity of autoantibodies to the dihydrolipoamide dehydrogenase-binding protein (E3BP) and the glycine cleavage proteins in primary biliary cirrhosis. Hepatology **29**: 1013–1018.

Floreani, A., Biagini, M. R., Zappala, F., Farinati, F., Plebani, M., Rugge, M., Surrenti, C., Naccarato, R. (1997). Chronic atrophic gastritis and Helicobacter pylori infection in primary biliary cirrhosis: a cross-sectional study with matching. Ital J Gastroenterol Hepatol **29(1)**: 13–17.

Frazer, I. H., Mackay, I. R., Jordan, T. W., Whittingham, S. and Marzuki, S. (1985). Reactivity of anti-mitochondrial autoantibodies in primary biliary cirrhosis: definition of two novel mitochondrial polypeptide autoantigens. J Immunol **135**: 1739–1745.

Fredrickson, J. K., Balkwill, D. L., Drake, G. R., Romine, M. F., Ringelberg, D. B. and White, D. C. (1995). Aromatic-degrading Sphingomonas isolates from the deep subsurface. Appl Environ Microbiol **61**: 1917–1922.

Fujii, K., Kikuchi, S., Satomi, M., Ushio-Sata, N. and Morita, N. (2002). Degradation of 17beta-estradiol by a gram-negative bacterium isolated from activated sludge in a sewage treatment plant in Tokyo, Japan. Appl Environ Microbiol **68**: 2057–2060.

Gershwin, M. E., Ansari, A. A., Mackay, I. R., Nakanuma, Y., Nishio, A., Rowley, M. J. and Coppel, R. L. (2000). Primary biliary cirrhosis: an orchestrated immune response against epithelial cells. Immunol Rev **174**: 210–225.

Gershwin, M. E. and Mackay, I. R. (1991). Primary biliary cirrhosis: paradigm or paradox for autoimmunity. Gastroenterology **100**: 822–833.

Gershwin, M. E., Mackay, I. R., Sturgess, A. and Coppel, R. L. (1987). Identification and specificity of a cDNA encoding the 70 kd mitochondrial antigen recognized in primary biliary cirrhosis. J Immunol **138**: 3525–3531.

Gonzalez-Amaro, R., Garcia-Monzon, C., Garcia-Buey, L., Moreno-Otero, R., Alonso, J. L., Yague, E., Pivel, J. P., Lopez-Cabrera,

M., Fernandez-Ruiz, E., Sanchez-Madrid, F. (1994). Induction of tumor necrosis factor alpha production by human hepatocytes in chronic viral hepatitis. J Exp Med **179**: 841–848.

Harada, K., Ozaki, S., Gershwin, M. E. and Nakanuma, Y. (1997 a). Enhanced apoptosis relates to bile duct loss in primary biliary cirrhosis. Hepatology **26**: 1399–1405.

Harada, K., Van de Water, J., Leung, P. S., Coppel, R. L., Nakanuma, Y. and Gershwin, M. E. (1997 b). In situ nucleic acid hybridization of pyruvate dehydrogenase complex-E2 in primary biliary cirrhosis: pyruvate dehydrogenase complex-E2 messenger RNA is expressed in hepatocytes but not in biliary epithelium. Hepatology **25**: 27–32.

Hazama, H., Omagari, K., Masuda, J., Kinoshita, H., Ohba, K., Sakimura, K., Matsuo, I., Isomoto, H., Murase, K., Murata, I. and Kohno, S. (2000). Serial changes in enzyme inhibitory antibody to pyruvate dehydrogenase complex during the course of primary biliary cirrhosis. J Clin Lab Anal **14**: 208–213.

Howard, M. J., Fuller, C., Broadhurst, R. W., Perham, R. N., Tang, J. G., Quinn, J., Diamond, A. G. and Yeaman, S. J. (1998). Three-dimensional structure of the major autoantigen in primary biliary cirrhosis. Gastroenterology **115**: 139–146.

Invernizzi, P., Crosignani, A., Battezzati, P. M., Covini, G., De Valle, G., Larghi, A., Zuin, M. and Podda, M. (1997). Comparison of the clinical features and clinical course of antimitochondrial antibody-positive and -negative primary biliary cirrhosis. Hepatology **25**: 1090–1095.

Invernizzi, P., Podda, M., Battezzati, P. M., Crosignani, A., Zuin, M., Hitchman, E., Maggioni, M., Meroni, P. L., Penner, E. and Wesierska-Gadek, J. (2001). Autoantibodies against nuclear pore complexes are associated with more active and severe liver disease in primary biliary cirrhosis. J Hepatol **34**: 366–372.

Ishibashi, H., Nakamura, M., Shimoda, S. and Gershwin, M. E. (2003). T cell immunity and primary biliary cirrhosis. Autoimmun Rev **2**: 19–24.

Iwayama, T., Leung, P. S., Coppel, R. L., Roche, T. E., Patel, M. S., Mizushima, Y., Nakagawa, T., Dickson, R. and Gershwin, M. E. (1991). Specific reactivity of recombinant human PDC-E1 alpha in primary biliary cirrhosis. J Autoimmun **4**: 769–778.

Jelinek, D. F. and Lipsky, P. E. (1987). Enhancement of human B cell proliferation and differentiation by tumor necrosis factor-alpha and interleukin 1. J Immunol **139**: 2970–2976.

Jensen, W. A., Jois, J. A., Murphy, P., De Giorgio, J., Brown, B., Rowley, M. J. and Mackay, I. R. (2000). Automated enzymatic mitochondrial antibody assay for the diagnosis of primary biliary cirrhosis. Clin Chem Lab Med **38**: 753–758.

Jois, J., Omagari, K., Rowley, M. J., Anderson, J. and Mackay, I. R. (2000). Enzyme inhibitory antibody to pyruvate dehydrogenase: diagnostic utility in primary biliary cirrhosis. Ann Clin Biochem **37 (Pt 1)**: 67–73.

Joplin, R., Lindsay, J. G., Hubscher, S. G., Johnson, G. D., Shaw, J. C., Strain, A. J. and Neuberger, J. M. (1991). Distribution of dihydrolipoamide acetyltransferase (E2) in the liver and portal lymph nodes of patients with primary biliary cirrhosis: an immunohistochemical study. Hepatology **14**: 442–447.

Joplin, R. E., Johnson, G. D., Matthews, J. B., Hamburger, J., Lindsay, J. G., Hubscher, S. G., Strain, A. J. and Neuberger, J. M. (1994). Distribution of pyruvate dehydrogenase dihydrolipoamide acetyltransferase (PDC-E2) and another mitochondrial marker in salivary gland and biliary epithelium from patients with primary biliary cirrhosis. Hepatology **19**: 1375–1380.

Joplin, R. E., Wallace, L. L., Lindsay, J. G., Palmer, J. M., Yeaman, S. J. and Neuberger, J. M. (1997). The human biliary epithelial cell plasma membrane antigen in primary biliary cirrhosis: pyruvate dehydrogenase X? Gastroenterology **113**: 1727–1733.

Katayanagi, K., Van de Water, J., Kenny, T., Nakanuma, Y., Ansari, A. A., Coppel, R. and Gershwin, M. E. (1999). Generation of monoclonal antibodies to murine bile duct epithelial cells: identification of annexin V as a new marker of small intrahepatic bile ducts. Hepatology **29**: 1019–1025.

Kimura, Y., Selmi, C., Leung, P. S., Mao, T. K., Schauer, J., Watnik, M., Kuriyama, S., Nishioka, M., Ansari, A. A., Coppel, R. L., Invernizzi, P., Podda, M. and Gershwin, M. E. (2005). Genetic polymorphisms influencing xenobiotic metabolism and transport in patients with primary biliary cirrhosis. Hepatology **41(1)**: 55–63.

Koga, H., Sakisaka, S., Ohishi, M., Sata, M. and Tanikawa, K. (1997). Nuclear DNA fragmentation and expression of Bcl-2 in primary biliary cirrhosis. Hepatology **25**: 1077–1084.

Kuroki, T., Seki, S., Kawakita, N., Nakatani, K., Hisa, T., Kitada, T. and Sakaguchi, H. (1996). Expression of antigens related to apoptosis and cell proliferation in chronic nonsuppurative destructive cholangitis in primary biliary cirrhosis. Virchows Arch **429**: 119–129.

Leung, P. S., Chuang, D. T., Wynn, R. M., Cha, S., Danner, D. J., Ansari, A., Coppel, R. L. and Gershwin, M. E. (1995). Autoantibodies to BCOADC-E2 in patients with primary biliary cirrhosis recognize a conformational epitope. Hepatology **22**: 505–513.

Leung, P. S., Quan, C., Park, O., Van de Water, J., Kurth, M. J., Nantz, M. H., Ansari, A. A., Coppel, R. L., Lam, K. S. and Gershwin, M. E. (2003). Immunization with a xenobiotic 6-bromohexanoate bovine serum albumin conjugate induces antimitochondrial antibodies. J Immunol **170**: 5326–5332.

Long, S. A., Quan, C., Van de Water, J., Nantz, M. H., Kurth, M. J., Barsky, D., Colvin, M. E., Lam, K. S., Coppel, R. L., Ansari, A. and Gershwin, M. E. (2001). Immunoreactivity of organic mimeotopes of the E2 component of pyruvate dehydrogenase: connecting xenobiotics with primary biliary cirrhosis. J Immunol **167**: 2956–2963.

Mackay, I. R. (1958). Primary biliary cirrhosis showing a high titer of autoantibody; report of a case. N Engl J Med **258**: 185–188.

Mackworth-Young, C. G. (2004). Antiphospholipid syndrome: multiple mechanisms. Clin Exp Immunol **136**: 393–401.

Mano, Y., Ishii, M., Okamoto, H., Igarashi, T., Kobayashi, K. and Toyota, T. (1996). Effect of tumor necrosis factor alpha on intrahepatic bile duct epithelial cell of rat liver. Hepatology **23**: 1602–1607.

Matsumoto, K., Fujii, H., Michalopoulos, G., Fung, J. J. and Demetris, A. J. (1994). Human biliary epithelial cells secrete and respond to cytokines and hepatocyte growth factors in vitro: interleukin-6, hepatocyte growth factor and epidermal growth factor promote DNA synthesis in vitro. Hepatology **20**: 376–382.

Matsumura, S., Van De Water, J., Kita, H., Coppel, R. L., Tsuji, T., Yamamoto, K., Ansari, A. A. and Gershwin, M. E. (2002). Contribution to antimitochondrial antibody production: cleavage of pyruvate dehydrogenase complex-E2 by apoptosis-related proteases. Hepatology **35**: 14–22.

Miyakawa, H., Tanaka, A., Kikuchi, K., Matsushita, M., Kitazawa, E., Kawaguchi, N., Fujikawa, H. and Gershwin, M. E. (2001). Detection of antimitochondrial autoantibodies in immunofluorescent AMA-negative patients with primary biliary cirrhosis using recombinant autoantigens. Hepatology **34**: 243–248.

Moteki, S., Leung, P. S., Coppel, R. L., Dickson, E. R., Kaplan, M. M., Munoz, S. and Gershwin, M. E. (1996 a). Use of a designer triple expression hybrid clone for three different lipoyl domain for the detection of antimitochondrial autoantibodies. Hepatology **24**: 97–103.

Moteki, S., Leung, P. S., Dickson, E. R., Van Thiel, D. H., Galperin, C., Buch, T., Alarcon-Segovia, D., Kershenobich, D., Kawano, K., Coppel, R. L. and et al. (1996 b). Epitope mapping and reactivity of autoantibodies to the E2 component of 2-oxoglutarate dehydrogenase complex in primary biliary cirrhosis using recombinant 2-oxoglutarate dehydrogenase complex. Hepatology **23**: 436–444.

Neagle, J., De Marcucci, O., Dunbar, B. and Lindsay, J. G. (1989). Component X of mammalian pyruvate dehydrogenase complex: structural and functional relationship to the lipoate acetyltransferase (E2) component. FEBS Lett **253**: 11–15.

Odin, J. A., Huebert, R. C., Casciola-Rosen, L., LaRusso, N. F. and Rosen, A. (2001). Bcl-2-dependent oxidation of pyruvate dehydrogenase-E2, a primary biliary cirrhosis autoantigen, during apoptosis. J Clin Invest **108**: 223–232.

Palmer, J. M., Jones, D. E., Quinn, J., McHugh, A. and Yeaman, S. J. (1999). Characterization of the autoantibody responses to recombinant E3 binding protein (protein X) of pyruvate dehydrogenase in primary biliary cirrhosis. Hepatology **30**: 21–26.

Parikh-Patel, A., Gold, E. B., Worman, H., Krivy, K. E. and Gershwin, M. E. (2001). Risk factors for primary biliary cirrhosis in a cohort of patients from the united states. Hepatology **33**: 16–21.

Patel, M. S. and Roche, T. E. (1990). Molecular biology and biochemistry of pyruvate dehydrogenase complexes. Faseb J **4**: 3224–3233.

Quinn, J., Diamond, A. G., Palmer, J. M., Bassendine, M. F., James, O. F. and Yeaman, S. J. (1993). Lipoylated and unlipoylated domains of human PDC-E2 as autoantigens in primary biliary cirrhosis: significance of lipoate attachment. Hepatology **18**: 1384–1391.

Rapoport, B. and McLachlan, S. M. (2001). Thyroid autoimmunity. J Clin Invest **108**: 1253–1259.

Reed, L. J. and Hackert, M. L. (1990). Structure-function relationships in dihydrolipoamide acyltransferases. J Biol Chem **265**: 8971–8974.

Reynoso-Paz, S., Leung, P. S., Van De Water, J., Tanaka, A., Munoz, S., Bass, N., Lindor, K., Donald, P. J., Coppel, R. L., Ansari, A. A. and Gershwin, M. E. (2000). Evidence for a locally driven mucosal response and the presence of mitochondrial antigens in saliva in primary biliary cirrhosis. Hepatology **31**: 24–29.

Rose, N. R. (2000). Viral damage or "molecular mimicry"-placing the blame in myocarditis. Nat Med **6**: 631–632.

Rowley, M. J., McNeilage, L. J., Armstrong, J. M. and Mackay, I. R. (1991). Inhibitory autoantibody to a conformational epitope of the pyruvate dehydrogenase complex, the major autoantigen in primary biliary cirrhosis. Clin Immunol Immunopathol **60**: 356–370.

Sasaki, M., Ansari, A., Pumford, N., van de Water, J., Leung, P. S., Humphries, K. M., Szweda, L. I., Nakanuma, Y., Roche, T. E., Coppel, R. L., Bach, J. F. and Gershwin, M. E. (2000). Comparative immunoreactivity of anti-trifluoroacetyl (TFA) antibody and anti-lipoic acid antibody in primary biliary cirrhosis: searching for a mimic. J Autoimmun **15**: 51–60.

Selmi, C., Balkwill, D. L., Invernizzi, P., Ansari, A. A., Coppel, R. L., Podda, M., Leung, P. S., Kenny, T. P., Van De Water, J., Nantz, M. H., Kurth, M. J. and Gershwin, M. E. (2003). Patients with primary biliary cirrhosis react against a ubiquitous xenobiotic-metabolizing bacterium. Hepatology **38**: 1250–1257.

Selmi, C. and Gershwin, M. E. (2004). Bacteria and human autoimmunity: the case of primary biliary cirrhosis. Curr Opin Rheumatol **16**: 406–410.

Selmi, C., Invernizzi, P., Keeffe, E. B., Coppel, R. L., Podda, M., Rossaro, L., Ansari, A. A., Gershwin, M. E. and Keefe, E. B. (2004 a). Epidemiology and pathogenesis of primary biliary cirrhosis. J Clin Gastroenterol **38**: 264–271.

Selmi, C., Invernizzi, P., Miozzo, M., Podda, M. and Gershwin, M. E. (2004 b). Primary biliary cirrhosis: does X mark the spot? Autoimmun Rev **3**: 493–499.

Selmi, C., Mayo, M. J., Bach, N., Ishibashi, H., Invernizzi, P., Gish, R. G., Gordon, S. C., Wright, H. I., Zweiban, B., Podda, M. and Gershwin, M. E. (2004 c). Primary biliary cirrhosis in monozygotic and dizygotic twins: genetics, epigenetics, and environment. Gastroenterology **127(2)**: 485–492.

Selmi, C., Ross, S. R., Ansari, A. A., Invernizzi, P., Podda, M., Coppel, R. L. and Gershwin, M. E. (2004 d). Lack of immunological or molecular evidence for a role of mouse mammary tumor retrovirus in primary biliary cirrhosis. Gastroenterology **127**: 493–501.

Steinman, L. (1999). Absence of "original antigenic sin" in autoimmunity provides an unforeseen platform for immune therapy. J Exp Med **189**: 1021–1024.

Surh, C. D., Coppel, R. and Gershwin, M. E. (1990). Structural requirement for autoreactivity on human pyruvate dehydrogenase-E2, the major autoantigen of primary biliary cirrhosis. Implication for a conformational autoepitope. J Immunol **144**: 3367–3374.

Szostecki, C., Guldner, H. H. and Will, H. (1997). Autoantibodies against "nuclear dots" in primary biliary cirrhosis. Semin Liver Dis **17**: 71–78.

Talwalkar, J. A. and Lindor, K. D. (2003). Primary biliary cirrhosis. Lancet **362**: 53–61.

Tamby, M. C., Chanseaud, Y., Guillevin, L. and Mouthon, L. (2003). New insights into the pathogenesis of systemic sclerosis. Autoimmun Rev **2**: 152–157.

Teoh, K. L., Mackay, I. R., Rowley, M. J. and Fussey, S. P. (1994a). Enzyme inhibitory autoantibodies to pyruvate dehydrogenase complex in primary biliary cirrhosis differ for mammalian, yeast and bacterial enzymes: implications for molecular mimicry. Hepatology **19**: 1029–1033.

Teoh, K. L., Rowley, M. J., Zafirakis, H., Dickson, E. R., Wiesner, R. H., Gershwin, M. E. and MacKay, I. R. (1994b). Enzyme inhibitory autoantibodies to pyruvate dehydrogenase complex in primary biliary cirrhosis: applications of a semiautomated assay. Hepatology **20**: 1220–1224.

Tsuneyama, K., Van de Water, J., Leung, P. S., Cha, S., Nakanuma, Y., Kaplan, M., De Lellis, R., Coppel, R., Ansari, A. and Gershwin, M. E. (1995). Abnormal expression of the E2 component of the pyruvate dehydrogenase complex on the luminal surface of biliary epithelium occurs before major histocompatibility complex class II and BB1/B7 expression. Hepatology **21**: 1031–1037.

Van de Water, J., Ansari, A. A., Surh, C. D., Coppel, R., Roche, T., Bonkovsky, H., Kaplan, M. and Gershwin, M. E. (1991). Evidence for the targeting by 2-oxo-dehydrogenase enzymes in the T cell response of primary biliary cirrhosis. J Immunol **146**: 89–94.

Van de Water, J., Gerson, L. B., Ferrell, L. D., Lake, J. R., Coppel, R. L., Batts, K. P., Wiesner, R. H. and Gershwin, M. E. (1996). Immunohistochemical evidence of disease recurrence after liver transplantation for primary biliary cirrhosis. Hepatology **24**: 1079–1084.

Van de Water, J., Ishibashi, H., Coppel, R. L. and Gershwin, M. E. (2001). Molecular mimicry and primary biliary cirrhosis: premises not promises. Hepatology **33**: 771–775.

Van de Water, J., Turchany, J., Leung, P. S., Lake, J., Munoz, S., Surh, C. D., Coppel, R., Ansari, A., Nakanuma, Y. and Gershwin, M. E. (1993). Molecular mimicry in primary biliary cirrhosis. Evidence for biliary epithelial expression of a molecule cross-reactive with pyruvate dehydrogenase complex-E2. J Clin Invest **91**: 2653–2664.

Walker, J. G., Doniach, D., Roitt, I. M. and Sherlock, S. (1965). Serological Tests in Diagnosis of Primary Biliary Cirrhosis. Lancet **39**: 827–831.

Worman, H. J. and Courvalin, J. C. (2003). Antinuclear antibodies specific for primary biliary cirrhosis. Autoimmun Rev **2**: 211–217.

Xu, L., Shen, Z., Guo, L., Fodera, B., Keogh, A., Joplin, R., O'Donnell, B., Aitken, J., Carman, W., Neuberger, J. and Mason, A. (2003). Does a betaretrovirus infection trigger primary biliary cirrhosis? Proc Natl Acad Sci USA **100**: 8454–8459.

Yasoshima, M., Kono, N., Sugawara, H., Katayanagi, K., Harada, K. and Nakanuma, Y. (1998). Increased expression of interleukin-6 and tumor necrosis factor-alpha in pathologic biliary epithelial cells: in situ and culture study. Lab Invest **78**: 89–100.

Zieve, G. W. and Khusial, P. R. (2003). The anti-Sm immune response in autoimmunity and cell biology. Autoimmun Rev **2**: 235–240.

Part 5
Autoantibodies in Experimental Models of Autoimmunity

Autoantibodies and Autoimmunity: Molecular Mechanisms
in Health and Disease. Edited by K. Michael Pollard
Copyright © 2006 WILEY-VCH Verlag GmbH & Co. KGaA, Weinheim
ISBN: 3-527-31141-6

action and interdependency between autoAbs and T-cell immunity. Indeed, their symbiotic relationship is evident in the inductive phase as well as the effector phase of disease. In addition, studies on these unique models have identified an unexpected mechanism of how autoAbs are induced and regulated, and how the Ab causes immunopathology and disease. In this chapter, we will present our findings, whereas only a limited review of the pertinent literature will be provided.

21.2
The Autoimmune Ovarian Disease (AOD) Models

21.2.1
The ZP3 Model

ZP3 is a glycoprotein of the zona pellucida (ZP) matrix that surrounds growing and mature ovarian oocytes. It is accessible by circulating Abs and functions as the primary sperm receptor in fertilization [3]. The autoAg is the murine ZP3 peptide (330–342) (NSSSSQFQIHGPR; pZP3) (Table 21.1), which induces severe AOD when injected with complete Freund's adjuvant (CFA) [4]. Disease induction is major histocompatibility complex (MHC)-restricted: thus, inbred and H-2 congenic mice of the k, a, u, and s haplotypes are responders, whereas those of the b, d, and q haplotypes are non-responders [5]. However, (C57BL/6×A/J) F_1 (B6AF1) mice are most susceptible, and therefore they have been used in most of our studies.

B6AF1 mice immunized with pZP3 in CFA develop a pZP3-specific T-cell response and produce mixed Th1- and Th2-type cytokines. They also develop auto-Abs to the ZP, detectable in serum and bound to the ovarian ZP. The truncated ZP3 (330–340) peptide has two nested T-cell epitopes, and they overlap with an 8-mer native ZP3 B-cell epitope (335–342) (QFQIHGPR) [5, 6] (Table 21.1). The phenylalanine in position 336 is a critical residue of the T-cell epitopes, but it is not required for the integrity of the native B epitope (335–342) [5]. The pZP3-specific CD4+ T cells are pivotal and sufficient to cause AOD because disease can be adoptively transferred by regional lymph node CD4+ (but not CD8+) T cells of pZP3-immunized mice. AOD is also transferred by pZP3-specific CD4+ T-cell lines and T-cell clones [4, 7]. Both T-cell clones that produce Th1- and Th2-dominant cytokines transfer severe granulomatous inflammation in the ovaries of normal recipients; however, eosinophilic infiltration is detected only in the granuloma induced by the Th2 clones (Alard and Tung, unpublished). In contrast to T-cell transfer, passively transferred ZP3 Ab forms immune complex with the ovarian ZP, but this has no associated C3 deposition and does not cause ovarian pathology.

The finding in ZP3-induced AOD is similar to many other organ-specific autoimmune disease (experimental autoimmune encephalomyelitis [EAE], diabetes in non-obese diabetic (NOD) mice, etc.), with the exception that in AOD, the Ab is a well-defined component of the ZP3 autoimmune response and the ovarian ZP is a well-defined target that permits precise visualization of autoAb binding *in vivo*.

21.2.2
The Day-3 Thymectomy AOD Model

Day-3 thymectomy (d3tx) in different inbred mice results in frequent and severe spontaneous autoimmune disease. Although the incidence of disease is the highest in the ovary, it also targets the stomach, thyroid, lachrymal gland, prostate, and testis. The diseased mice produce respective organ-specific autoAbs and pathogenic T-cell response [8–12]. The autoAbs from d3tx mice have been used successfully to identify the dominant cognate autoAgs in autoimmune gastritis ($H^+K^+ATPase$) [13, 14], AOD (Mater) [15], and autoimmune prostatitis (Ohno, Setiady, and Tung, unpublished). The CD4$^+$ effector T cells from the d3tx mice can transfer the donor disease; however, the role of the autoAb has not been fully investigated. An imbalance of effector and regulatory T cells created by d3tx is likely responsible for the induction of autoimmune disease and autoAbs. The CD4$^+$ T cells that express CD25 (IL2Ra) have been shown to be critical in maintaining self-tolerance; also, the infusion of CD4$^+$CD25$^+$ spleen T cells or CD4$^+$CD8-CD25$^+$ thymocytes from normal syngeneic adults completely inhibits d3tx disease [16–18]. In addition, thymus-derived CD4$^+$CD25$^+$ T cells are detected in the spleen after day 3 of life, and they would be depleted or reduced by d3tx [19]. The lack of CD25$^+$ regulatory T-cell function in 3-day-old mice is also supported by the finding that CD4$^+$ T cells from 3-day-old, but not adult, euthymic BALB/c donors induced autoimmune diseases in syngeneic *nu/nu* recipients [20]. However, mechanisms other than CD4$^+$CD25$^+$ T-cell depletion are also operative in d3tx disease because CD25$^+$ T-cell depletion per se does not induce autoimmune disease in normal mice and because d3tx mice exhibit severe lymphopenia that is critical for disease induction [21].

21.2.3
The Neonatal AOD Model

Although adult females with autoAb response to the ZP3 B-cell epitope (335–342) are free of AOD, the progeny of the autoAb-positive dams developed severe AOD [22]. This model of AOD documented for the first time the differential pathogenicity of autoAb in adult versus neonatal mice. It also recalls the clinical observation of congenital heart block in infants of mothers with circulating autoAbs to Ro and La but free of cardiac problems themselves. Unlike other forms of neonatal autoimmune disease induced by maternal autoAbs, which are transient, neonatal AOD (nAOD), just like the congenital heart block, is severe and progressive, with inflammation and loss of functional tissues, oocytes in AOD and the conduction system in heart block disease. As we will describe later, autoAbs to ZP3 do not cause nAOD directly; instead, they form immune complex with ovarian ZP3 and induce *do novo* activation of pathogenic T cells in the neonatal mice.

In summary, the three models of AOD illustrate three different mechanisms of autoimmune disease pathogenesis. In the pZP3 model, activation of Ag-presenting cells (APC) by adjuvant facilitates the induction of pathogenic autoimmune response to the pZP3 in individuals with an intact immune system and illustrates how infection may participate in autoimmune disease pathogenesis. AOD and autoAb response occur in the d3tx mice because of perturbation of the normal immune system, and the autoimmune response is stimulated by endogenous Ags. This model strongly supports the existence of potentially pathogenic T cells in normal individuals, which are normally kept in check by the regulatory T cells. The nAOD model describes a unique autoimmune disease that affects neonatal mice but spares adult mice, and it provides an excellent opportunity for investigation of the properties of neonatal immune response *in vivo*. The AOD models have permitted investigation of autoimmune response to well-defined T- and B-cell epitopes and the study of T cells and autoAb response in isolation or combined. Moreover, because ovarian Ags are gender specific, studies of male and female responses also permit comparison between the response to the same peptide perceived as foreign or as self. Moreover, endogenous Ag can be depleted by ovariectomy, and ovarian graft can provide the target organ for "autoimmune" disease in animals deficient in ovaries. These useful properties of the AOD models have allowed us to study the induction and maintenance of tolerance to organ-specific, non-sequestered autoAgs and to discover unexpected mechanisms of autoAb response.

21.3
Mechanism of Induction and Antigen Specificity of Autoantibodies

21.3.1
T-cell Peptide of a Self-protein Elicits Autoantibodies to Distant Sites of the Protein Antigen

This phenomenon of amplified autoAb response was first described in AOD study. In 1993, when we immunized female mice with pZP3 (330–340), the self-peptide that lacked the native B-cell epitope sequence (335–342), the animals produced an Ab response against native ZP3 (Fig. 21.1). We called the phenomenon an "amplified" Ab response, also known as the diversified Ab response. The amplified ZP-binding Ab did not react with the immunizing peptide, but it was removed by absorption with ZP that contains intact ZP3. Moreover, the amplified Ab was found to react with B-cell epitopes distant from the ZP3 (335–342) epitope, including pZP3 (171–180), pZP3 (301–310), and pZP3 (411–430) epitopes [23]. This study described for the first time that T to B epitope spreading can occur in an autoimmune response, namely, the induction of

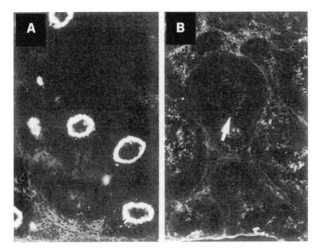

Fig. 21.1 T to B epitope spreading: spontaneous Ab response to native ZP3 in female mice immunized with a T-cell peptide of ZP3. (A) IgG bound to the ovarian ZP detected by direct immunofluorescence in mice immunized with pZP3 (330–340) that contained known T-cell but not B-cell epitopes. Zona-bound IgG was not detected in mice immunized with pZP3 (331–339) that was devoid of demonstrable T and B epitopes. The arrow in (B) points to the unstained ZP (×200).

Ab to a distant native B-cell epitope of a protein that follows immunization with a pure T-cell epitope of that protein.

Epitope spreading has been found in many other autoimmune diseases (for a review of this topic, see *Immunological Review*, Vol. 164). In a model of glomerulonephritis, injection of rats with a single pathogenic T-cell epitope of the non-collagen domain 1 of the collagen type IV $a3$ chain (29–39) induced Abs against basement membrane proteins [24]. We have recently observed that epitope spreading occurs against autoAgs of the eye and the testis (Agersborg, Gonzales, and Tung, unpublished), providing evidence that challenges the dogma of complete Ag sequestration in these organs. Experimental models of SLE also revealed epitope spreading in autoimmune response to the Ro60 [25, 26], the La Ags [27], and a peptide that mimics DNA [28]. The occurrence of epitope spreading in patients with autoimmune disease has been documented in patients with SLE against the SmB/B' Ag [29]. However, the studies based on human autoAbs were based largely on serological analysis, and it is important to consider Ag cross-reaction between different B-cell epitopes as an alternate mechanism of "epitope spreading" [26].

An important message derived from studies on amplified autoAb responses is that the Ag specificity of a natural autoAb (in patients or experimental animals) need not mirror the immunogen that elicits the autoimmune disease. This argument is also supported by studies on the Ab responses in mice injected with T-cell epitopes of the murine acetylcholine receptor (ACR) peptide [30] and mice injected with murine cytochrome *c* [31].

21.3.2
Mechanism of the Amplified Autoantibody Response

The mechanism of the amplified autoAb response detectable by indirect immunofluorescence on ovary section has been investigated most extensively in AOD induced by pZP3 immunization. Amplified autoAb induction is surprisingly rapid. It was detected on day 7 following immunization with the ZP3 T-cell epitope (330–340), only three days after a detectable T-cell response to the immunogen. In contrast, autoAb response to the peptidic B-cell epitope in ZP3 (330–340) was not evident until two weeks later. The rapid induction of the amplified autoAb response by endogenous Ag strongly argues against the existence of intrinsic B-cell tolerance to the peripheral tissue Ags that do not have access to developing B cells. Instead, control of the autoAb response to the peripheral tissue Ag occurs via silencing of the autoreactive helper T-cell response.

The endogenous ovarian Ag is responsible for induction of the amplified autoAb. Immunization of mice without ovaries (ovariectomized female) by pZP3 (330–340) did not elicit amplified autoAb, although the mice produced Ab to the nonnative, peptidic B-cell epitope present in the immunizing peptide. To strengthen the requirement of endogenous Ag in amplified autoAb induction, we recently observed that male mice also did not produce amplified Ab to pZP3; however, they would do so after they were implanted with ovarian grafts from normal mice but not from *zp3* knockout mice (Pramoonjago, Sharp, and Tung, unpublished). Interestingly, the amplified Ab induced by the ZP3 T-cell epitope reacted with the ZP in ovaries from normal mice as well as with the ovaries of *zp3* knockout mice. This finding provides evidence for the occurrence of intermolecular epitope spreading (from ZP3 T-cell epitope to ZP2 and/or ZP1 B-cell epitopes) in the AOD system.

Induction of the amplified autoAb response is not a consequence of ovarian injury for the following reasons. First, AOD and the autoAb response appeared simultaneously on day 7 after immunization. Second, immunization with low doses of pZP3 (330–340) induced a ZP Ab response in mice without oophoritis. Additional support comes from experiments on mice with timed ovariectomy (Ag depletion) around the time of ZP3 T-cell epitope immunization. When mice were ovariectomized at two weeks or one day before immunization, they did not produce ZP Abs. However, when the ovariectomy was delayed to day 2, day 4, or day 6 (when oophoritis was absent), the immunized mice still produced amplified ZP Abs. As control, all ovariectomized mice produced a comparable level of Abs to the peptide epitope of ZP3 (330–340). Therefore, amplified Ab induction is a highly sensitive component of an autoimmune response. Unlike the phenomenon of T to T epitope spreading, described in experimental autoimmune encephalomyelitis (EAE) [32], ovarian injury is not required for the induction of the amplified Ab response.

The induction of amplified autoAb likely occurs in the regional lymph node since B220+ B cells and plasma cells were undetectable in ovaries of immunized mice. Recent studies [33, 34] have shown that, in steady state, dendritic cells

(DCs) continually internalize Ag derived from apoptotic cells in peripheral tissues and carry this Ag to the lymph node, where the Ag is presented to the T cell to induce peripheral tolerance. In the case of a cycling ovary, a cohort of 40–50 primordial oocytes enters the growth phase every 4–5 days, and 80–90% of the developing oocytes enter an apoptotic pathway and their follicles undergo atresia [35]. The ZP Ag was detectable in atretic follicles and inside MHC II–positive phagocytes, providing a continuous supply of the ZP Ag. In the lymph node, the ZP-loaded DCs may present the Ag to the T cells and may also "share" the Ag with the ZP-specific B cells. Normally, B-cell activation and Ab production do not occur because appropriate T-cell help is lacking. However, pZP3 immunization overrides the tolerance mechanism and activates pZP3-specific T cells that can recognize the endogenous ZP3 peptide presented by B cells in their MHC II and stimulate ZP3 Ab production through cognate help. Indeed, inhibition of the costimulatory molecules CD40 ligand and B7 by monoclonal Ab to CD40 ligand and/or CTLA4-Ig fusion protein completely blocked the amplified ZP3 Ab response [36] and inhibited the autoAb effect on disease retargeting (see Section 21.4.2).

21.3.3
Amplified Autoantibody Response Also Occurs in Response to a Foreign T-cell Epitope That Mimics a Self T-cell Epitope

Ag mimicry has long been proposed as a potential mechanism by which infectious agents induce autoimmune disease, and there have been tantalizing associations between infectious agents and autoimmunity, e.g., beta-hemolytic streptococci with rheumatic fever, coxsackie B3 viruses with myocarditis, diverse viruses with multiple sclerosis, herpes simplex virus with myasthenia gravis, and *Compylobacter jejuni* with Guillain-Barré syndrome. Until recently, most studies on molecular mimicry have examined cross-reaction between B-cell epitopes of foreign and self-Ags. In the AOD study, we investigated the cross-reaction of T-cell epitopes between ZP3 and non-ovarian self- or foreign proteins. Indeed, such cross-reactivity can be found frequently; moreover, the response to every cross-reactive T-cell epitope also led to the production of an amplified autoAb response to ZP3.

Studies of pZP3 (330–338) peptide with a single alanine substitution have defined two nested T-cell epitopes with slightly different motifs, each containing four critical residues. This result was confirmed by the study of polyalanine peptides that contained the four critical residues in the correct registers. The substituted polyalanine peptide stimulated the proliferation of pZP3-specific oophoritogenic T-cell clones and induced severe AOD and ZP autoAb response *in vivo*.

A search in the protein library sequence for non-ovarian peptides that shared homology with the two pZP3 critical residue motifs yielded many peptide sequences. A murine acetylcholine receptor (ACR) peptide (ACRδ; 120–128) that fit with one pZP3 residue motif was found to stimulate oophoritogenic T-cell

Table 21.1 The functional domains of the ZP3 (330–342) peptide.

Peptide	Amino acid sequence	Immunologic functions
ZP3 (330–342)	NSSSSQFQIHGPR	Self T + self native B epitopes
ZP3 (330–340)	NSSSSQFQIHG	Self T + peptidic B epitopes
ZP3 (330–338)	NSSSSQFQI	Minimum self T epitope 1
ZP3 (332–340)	SSSQFQIHG	Minimum self T epitope 2
ZP3 (335–342)	QFQIHGPR	Self native B epitope
ZP3 (330–334)	NSSSS	Anchor residues for O-linked carbohydrate that functions as sperm receptor
CP2	Bovine RNase (94–104)-QAQIHGPR	Foreign T epitope + modified self native B epitope

have allowed us to identify two novel mechanism by which autoAbs influence autoimmune disease pathogenesis: (1) AutoAbs can modify effector T-cell homing within the target organ of adult mice, and (2) AutoAbs can induce severe AOD in neonatal mice but spares adult mice.

21.4.2
ZP Antibodies Cause Organ Failure by Retargeting T Cell-induced Inflammation to the Functional Target

Although proinflammatory T cells can induce tissue inflammation, inflammation alone does not always result in functional loss of the target organ. For example, perivascular cuffing of mononuclear cells is found in non-paralytic EAE [41], and peri-insulitis is the hallmark of pre-diabetic NOD mice [42].

In ovary, the ZP3 Ag is found in two distinct anatomical locations. It is expressed in the ZP matrix that surrounds viable oocytes in the growing and mature ovarian follicles, which support gamete interactions and are the functional reproductive units in the ovaries. In addition, ZP3 protein is found within the degenerating oocytes of the atretic follicles. During oocyte development in the ovaries, the majority of ZP3-positive oocytes undergo apoptosis and they become the content of atretic follicles that are present in the ovarian interstitium. Some of the ZP3 in the atretic follicles is detectable in MHC class II–positive, F4/80+ cells. Following adoptive transfer, ZP3-specific T cells were found to home exclusively to the atretic follicles but not to the viable ovarian follicles (Fig. 21.3 B, C). This was followed by recruitment and activation of leukocytes, expression of adhesion molecules, and the formation of numerous large granulomas that exist exclusively in the ovarian interstitium. The granulomatous interstitial oophoritis of the T-cell recipients can be severe and may occupy up to 80% of the interstitial space. Despite the intense interstitial ovarian inflammation, the animals remained fertile and retained normal ovarian function with respect to follicular growth, follicular maturation, ovulation, production of normal oocytes, and support of normal pregnancy [7].

However, when T-cell recipients mounted a ZP3 Ab response induced by CP2 immunization, the ovarian ZP3 immune complex was found to dramatically alter the distribution of the T cell–induced inflammation from the interstitial space into the normal ovarian follicles (Fig. 21.3 E, G). The retargeting of T cell–mediated inflammation was also induced by passively transferred ZP3 Ab (Fig. 21.3 F). The leukocytes migrated through the granulosa cell layer, adhered to the ZP, and penetrated the ZP matrix to reach and destroy the oocytes (Fig. 21.3 E, F). Thus, while recipients of T cells or autoAbs alone retained normal ovarian function, recipients of both T cells and autoAbs exhibited loss of oocytes and ovarian function. The new mechanism of autoAb action, "T-cell retargeting", does not depend on the specificity of the ZP Abs. Thus, Abs against different ZP3 epitopes or ZP2 epitopes can retarget T cells. Moreover, both Th1 and Th2 T cells against pZP3 can be retargeted by ZP3 autoAbs [43]. And as indicated earlier, blockade of costimulators including CD28/B7 and CD40L/CD40 also inhibits retargeting of T-cell injury by autoAbs to ZP3 [36].

The retargeting phenomenon has led to the concept that autoAbs can influence the clinical outcome of a T cell–mediated autoimmune disease by focusing tissue destruction to the functional unit of the diseased organ. It is possible that T-cell retargeting can explain the synergistic effect of autoAbs in other models of autoimmunity. Transfer of serum Abs to myelin oligodendrocyte glycoprotein (MOG) have been shown to reconstitute EAE in B cell–deficient mice that are resistant to EAE induction by MOG immunization [44]. Abs to myelin basic protein have also been found to enhance murine EAE severity, and it was postulated that autoAbs enhanced Ag processing and presentation [45–47]. Alternatively, T cell–associated inflammation may injure endothelial cells, reduce the blood-brain barrier, and facilitate the entrance of demyelinating Abs to the central nervous system [45, 48]. In collagen-induced arthritis, although Abs alone transfer synovitis to normal mice, severe and erosive arthritis occurs only when both T cells and Abs are present [49]. A similar situation has been reported in mice with tubulointerstitial nephritis induced by immune response to a renal tubular basement membrane Ag [50, 51]. In Figure 21.4, we have summarized the interactions among endogeneous antigen, T cell response and autoantibody response in autoimmune disease pathogenesis.

21.4.3
Autoantibodies That Are Non-pathogenic in Adults Can be Pathogenic in Neonatal Mice (nAOD)

As mentioned above, autoAbs to ZP3 (335–342) elicited by CP2 immunization formed ovarian immune complex but did not cause AOD in adult mice. Strikingly, B6AF1 female progenies of CP2-immunized dams developed severe AOD by week 2 (Fig. 21.5). This new disease, called neonatal AOD (nAOD), can also be induced by injection of serum or purified serum IgG from adult female or male mice immunized with CP2 in CFA, or by the transfer of a mouse monoclonal Ab to ZP3 (335–342). Therefore, autoAb is the cause of nAOD, and dis-

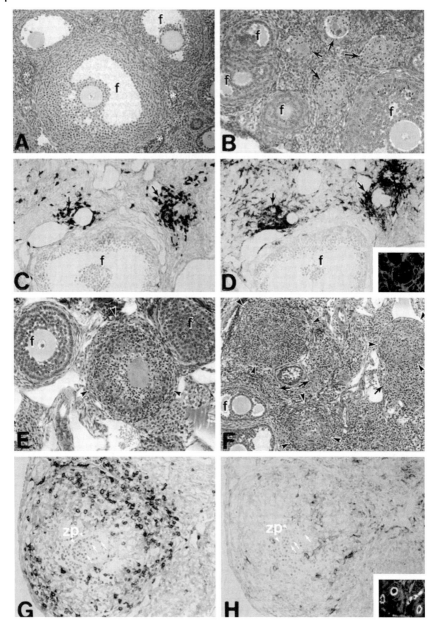

Fig. 21.3 Retargeting of pZP3-specific T cell-mediated ovarian inflammation by ZP3 auto-Abs in adult mice.
(A) Histology of a normal B6AF1 mouse ovary that contains growing and mature follicles (f) and atretic follicles (asterisks).
(B) Ovarian histology of a mouse injected with pZP3-specific T cells, with numerous monocytic granulomas (arrows) located in atretic follicles of the interstitium, sparing the growing and mature follicles (f).
(C, D) Immunoperoxidase staining that colocalizes T cells (CD3) (C) and MHC II+ cells (D) in two atretic follicles (arrows) on adja-

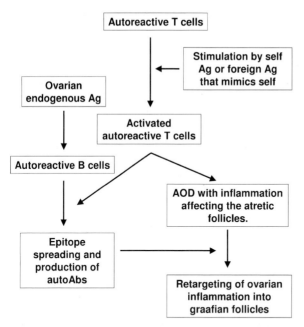

Fig. 21.4 Diagrammatic description of cellular events that may be responsible for the induction of pathogenic autoreactive T cells, autoAb responses, and immunopathology through T-cell epitope mimicry in adult mice.

ease induction is independent of maternal lymphocytes or other pregnancy-associated factors.

Maternal Abs can be transmitted to the progenies during gestation and also through milk at postpartum. To determine the transmission route of the pathogenic ZP3 Ab, pups from CP2-immunized dams were delivered by caesarean section and fostered by CFA-immunized dams. These pups did not contain any circulating ZP3 Abs, the ovaries were free of immune complex, and they did not develop nAOD. In contrast, B6AF1 pups born from unimmunized dams

cent sections of an ovary from a pZP3-specific T-cell recipient. The normal follicle (f) is unaffected. The inset in (D) shows negative immunofluorescence staining for mouse IgG in the ovarian ZP of the T-cell recipient. (E) Ovarian histology of a mouse injected with CP2 in CFA and later receiving pZP3-specific T cells, with inflammation that affects a growing follicle (arrowhead) and spares two other growing follicles (f). (F) Ovarian histology of a mouse that received both mouse polyclonal Abs to ZP3 and a pZP3-specific T-cell line. Inflammation affected three growing follicles (arrowheads) but spared two other follicles (f). (G, H) Immunoperoxidase staining that co-localizes T cells (CD3) (G) and MHC II$^+$ cells (H) in mature ovarian follicles from a mouse that received both murine Abs to pZP3 and pZP3-specific T cells. Leukocytes (arrows) have replaced the oocytes inside the ZP (arrowheads). The inset in (H) shows binding of mouse IgG in the ovarian ZP in this ovary by direct immunofluorescence. Hematoxylin and eosin, (A), (B), (E), (F) ×100; toluidine blue stain, (C), (D), (G), (H), ×200. (Reproduced from [43], with permission from the Journal of Immunology).

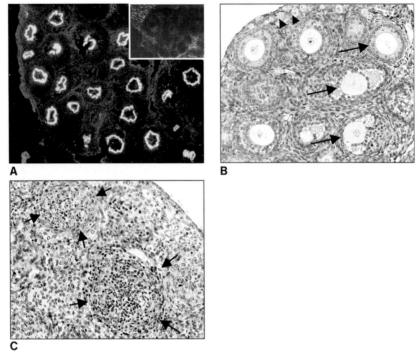

Fig. 21.5 Ovarian histopathology of nAOD in neonatal B6AF1 mice induced by CP2 autoAbs.
(A) *In vivo* IgG binding to ovarian ZP in progeny of CP2 Ab–positive dam (direct immuno-fluorescence, ×100). The inset shows negative IgG binding to ovarian ZP in control ovary.

(B) Normal ovarian histology of 14-day-old mice (×200). Note growing follicles (long arrow) and primordial follicles (arrowhead) in the ovary free of inflammation.
(C) Ovary from CP2 Ab recipients shows loss of oocytes and heavy mononuclear infiltration (arrow) (×200).

but fostered by CP2-immunized dams developed severe nAOD. Therefore, the pathogenic maternal ZP3 Ab is transmitted to the progeny through milk.

21.4.4
Mechanism of nAOD I: Autoantibody Induction of *de novo* Neonatal Pathogenic T-cell Response by Formation of the Autoantigen-antibody Complex

To understand the nAOD pathogenic mechanism, we question whether neonatal ovaries are uniquely more susceptible to immune injury than adult ovaries. Neonatal and adult ovaries were engrafted under the renal capsule of postpartum females that had been previously immunized with CP2 in CFA. Despite the presence of ZP immune complex, all ovarian grafts were free of AOD. In contrast, normal pups that were fostered by the graft recipients developed severe AOD. Therefore, the predisposition to nAOD does not depend on chronological age of the ovary; instead, it depends on the unique immune response of neonatal mice.

Immune complex can induce inflammatory response in several ways, including through (1) activation of the complement cascade involving proinflammatory C5a, (2) Ab-mediated cell cytotoxicity (ADCC) mediated by FcγR, and (3) T-cell activation mediated by FcγR and/or complement receptor–positive APC. Monoclonal Abs to C5 had no effect, but blockade of FcγRs completely inhibited nAOD (see Section 21.4.7). ADCC is a rapid process, while inflammation induced by pathogenic T cells is of late onset. Although the ovarian ZP-IgG complex was readily detectable after transfer of ZP3 Ab, oophoritis did not emerge until after a lag period of seven days. Moreover, the ovarian infiltrating cells were composed of lymphocytes/monocytes with the immunophenotype of T cells, B cells, and MHC II–positive macrophages and only occasional clusters of neutrophils/eosinophils. We therefore looked for evidence that T cell–mediated response may occur in nAOD. When we depleted CD4$^+$ and CD8$^+$ T cells or blocked the T-cell costimulation with anti-B7.1 and -B7.2 monoclonal Abs, nAOD was completely inhibited. Furthermore, when the CD4$^+$ T cells from mice with nAOD were adoptively transferred to normal pups, they induced severe AOD in the neonatal recipients. Therefore, the ZP3 Ab forms immune complex with the endogenous Ag and, through the FcγR pathway, triggers *de novo* neonatal pathogenic T-cell response [22].

The nAOD model is the first *in vivo* demonstration that an autoAb, by interacting with endogenous Ag, can induce *de novo* T-cell activation leading to autoimmune disease. Many *in vitro* studies have predicted this possibility by showing that Ab forms immune complex with Ag and significantly affects T-cell response. Engagement of immune complex with Fc receptors on APC results in an over 1000-fold increase in Ag uptake [52] and induces maturation and cytokine production by DCs [53, 54], thus promoting T-cell response. There is some evidence that auto-Abs from humans with autoimmune diseases can stimulate autoreactive T-cell response *in vitro* [55–57]. Thus, the nAOD model has revealed the hidden significance of autoAbs in triggering T cell–based autoimmune disease.

21.4.5
Mechanism of nAOD II: Disease Induction is Influenced by the B-cell Epitope Specificity of the Autoantibody

Analysis of the immune complex that induces T-cell response *in vitro* has revealed that the fine specificity of Abs can influence the Ag processing and epitope selection by the APC. This also determines the outcome and specificity of the attendant T-cell response [58]. We therefore compared monospecific polyclonal murine Abs to two distinct native ZP3 B-cell epitopes. The CP3 is a chimeric peptide that induces polyclonal Abs to the native B-cell epitope ZP3 (171–180). Abs to ZP3 (171–180) do not react with the ZP3 (335–342) epitope and vice versa. However, both Abs can retarget the T-cell inflammation in adult ovaries. Adult female B6AF1 mice immunized with CP2 and CP3 produced Abs of comparable IgG isotypes, and they both reacted strongly with the ZP in neonatal ovaries without concomitant C3 binding. However, in contrast to the CP2

Ab, the CP3 Ab did not induce nAOD. This finding suggests that the capacity of the ZP3 autoAb to elicit pathogenic T-cell response is dependent on the epitope specificity of the autoAb.

21.4.6
Mechanism of nAOD III: Neonatal Time Window of Disease Susceptibility that is Partially Influenced by the CD4$^+$CD25$^+$ Regulatory T Cells

nAOD development requires exposure to ZP3 Abs during the first five days of life. nAOD developed only when the feeding of ZP3 Ab–positive milk began at days 3 or 5 but not at days 7 or 9. Pups of CP2-immunized dams that were delivered by caesarian section, and therefore were not exposed to ZP3 Ab–containing milk, had no disease, while those that were exposed for 2–3 days after birth still developed nAOD. nAOD also occurred when exposure to the ZP3 Ab was limited to the 1–6 neonatal days. This phenomenon is independent of the ontogeny of intestinal neonatal FcR (FcRn) required for transport of maternal IgG from the gut lumen because the activity of neonatal rodent FcRn increases from day of birth, peaks at day 14, and afterwards decreases and disappears at time of weaning (day 21) [59].

As we discussed in the d3tx model of AOD, the CD4$^+$CD25$^+$ T cells that maintain self-tolerance and prevent autoimmune disease occurrence may have a late ontogeny (see Section 21.3.4). To address whether the belated emergence of CD4$^+$CD25$^+$ regulatory T-cell function was responsible for prevention of nAOD in the older mice, we studied the effect of CD25$^+$ T-cell depletion on nAOD. When neonatal mice were treated with CD25 Abs and fed ZP3 Ab–positive milk from postnatal day 9, 90% of them developed severe nAOD. In contrast, mice that received ZP3 Ab from day 9, or those that received CD25 Ab alone, were free of nAOD. Therefore, the emergence of CD4$^+$CD25$^+$ regulatory T-cell function readily explains the resistance to nAOD in mice older than seven days.

If the neonatal time window of disease susceptibility was due to immaturity or preferential deficiency of CD4$^+$CD25$^+$ T cells, one might expect the transfer of adult CD25$^+$ regulatory T cells to close the neonatal window. However, the infusion of CD4$^+$CD25$^+$ T cells from 9-day-old or adult mice, with or without co-transfer of adult APCs, failed to change the course of nAOD. These results suggest that the neonatal mice are resistant to suppression by CD4$^+$CD25$^+$ T cells. Because innate cells (including natural killer [NK] cells), macrophages, and DCs are known to influence adaptive immune response, but also to inhibit the function of regulatory CD4$^+$CD25$^+$ T cells [60], we investigated the neonatal innate system in nAOD, in particular the neonatal NK cells.

21.4.7
Mechanism of nAOD IV: Requirement of NK Cells, FcR, and Proinflammatory Cytokines in Disease Pathogenesis

Currently, very little is known about the function of NK cells in neonatal mice. They have been described to have different properties from adult NK cells. *In vi-*

tro studies suggest that neonatal NK cells are immature and few in number. Purified neonatal NK cells are barely cytotoxic against the classical NK cell targets and do not reach adult activity until 2–3 weeks of age [61, 62]. The progenitors of neonatal NK cells divide more rapidly than adult NK cells [63]. Expression of receptors for the MHC class I or class I–like molecule on neonatal NK cells is more restricted; they express predominantly CD94/NKG2A [64, 65], and the Ly49 receptors are not detected before one week [66].

In view of the data on the immaturity of neonatal NK cells, we were surprised to detect NK1.1$^+$ TCRVβ^- (but not NK1.1$^+$ TCRVβ^+) cells in the neonatal spleen and lymph node of B6AF1 mice. Moreover, it was found that the neonatal NK cells produced as much IFNγ as adult mice *in vivo*, in response to lipopolysaccharide injection. Most importantly, when NK cells were depleted by monoclonal Abs, the neonatal mice no longer developed nAOD [67]. The neonatal NK cells were required in both the induction phase and the effector phase of nAOD. Thus, in adoptive transfer of nAOD, the disease of the T-cell recipient was ameliorated when NK cells were depleted from either the T-cell donor or the T-cell recipient.

The NK cells can be directly activated by ZP immune complex through FcγR. As indicated above, monoclonal Abs to FcγRIIB and FcγRIII completely inhibited nAOD development [22]. FcγRIII and the FcγRIIB share similar specificities, but they transmit signals that lead to opposing cellular responses; FcγRIII elicits a proinflammatory response, whereas FcγRIIB inhibits the stimulatory signal [68]. Both FcγRs are widely expressed in various leukocytes, with the exception that NK cells express FcγRIII but not FcγRIIB. Intriguingly, mice deficient in FcγRIII or the common Fc receptor's γ-subunit failed to develop nAOD, while the lack of FcγRIIB aggravated the disease [67]. Therefore, the balance of FcγRIII and FcγRIIB determined the outcome of nAOD induction. This finding is in agreement with previous reports on other immune complex–mediated diseases such as lupus glomerulonephritis [69].

How do NK cells influence T-cell response to immune complexes? Adult NK cells can induce maturation and cytokine production by DCs, which in turn can activate nave T cells [70–74]. In nAOD, neonatal NK cells may function by promoting the APC function of neonatal DCs or by stimulating neonatal T cells directly through engagement of 2B4 with CD48 on T cells [75]. The interaction between NK cells and DC or T cells is bidirectional; thus, both DC and T cells, when activated, can reciprocally induce the proliferation, activation, and cytokine production of NK cells [70–72, 76, 77]. These cells may communicate by cell contact or via cytokines such as IL2 [78], IL15 [79], IFNγ, and TFNα [70–72, 76]. Indeed, the ovaries with nAOD expressed high levels of IFNγ and TNFα that correlated with disease severity. *In vivo*, nAOD was enhanced by recombinant IFNγ, and the disease was inhibited by anti-TFNα or anti-IFNγ Abs. Interestingly, when T-cell donors were treated with IFNγ Abs, adoptive transfer of nAOD was also inhibited; thus, IFNγ is likely operative during T-cell activation, and NK cells are a probable source of the IFNγ [67].

Neonatal mice have traditionally been considered immunologically immature. However, this view has been challenged recently by studies showing that foreign

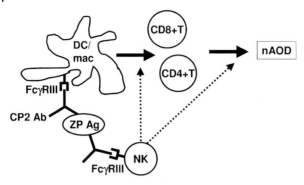

Fig. 21.6 Schematic diagram of the cellular mechanism of nAOD. The ZP autoAg-Ab complex, through FcRIII, activates NK cells and APC such as DC and macrophages. APC, with the help of soluble cytokines from NK cells, induces activation of ovarian-specific CD4$^+$ and CD8$^+$ T cells, which then recruit proinflammatory cells such as NK cells to generate ovarian inflammation.

or self-peptides and -proteins administered to neonates can elicit responses similar to adult responses [80–82]. In AOD, we have accrued evidence that neonatal mice are actually more responsive to autoAgs and environmental stimuli and more prone to autoimmune disease than adult animals (reviewed in [83]). The nAOD study has extended this paradigm by showing that maternal Abs, as an environmental factor, can evoke autoimmune response in neonates but not in adults. The cellular interactions leading to neonatal AOD is illustrates in Fig. 21.6.

Abbreviations

Ab	antibody
ACR	acetylcholine receptor
Ag	antigen
AOD	autoimmune ovarian disease
APC	antigen-presenting cell
B6AF1	(C57BL/6×A/J) F$_1$ mice
CFA	complete Freund's adjuvant
CP	chimeric peptide
d3tx	thymectomy on day 3 of life
DC	dendritic cell
EAE	experimental autoimmune encephalomyelitis
FcγR	Fcγ receptor
IFA	incomplete Freund's adjuvant
IFNγ	interferon γ
MHC	major histocompatibility complex

MOG	myelin oligodendrocyte glycoprotein
nAOD	neonatal AOD
NK	natural killer
NOD	non-obese diabetic
pZP3	murine ZP3 peptide (330–342)
SLE	systemic lupus erythematosus
TNFα	tumor necrosis factor α
ZP	zona pellucida

References

1 Matsumoto, I., Maccioni, M., Lee, D.M., Maurice, M., Simmons, B., Brenner, M., Mathis, D., Benoist, C., How antibodies to a ubiquitous cytoplasmic enzyme may provoke joint-specific autoimmune disease. *Nat.Immunol.* **2002**, 3: 360–365.

2 Sakaguchi, N., Takahashi, T., Hata, H., Nomura, T., Tagami, T., Yamazaki, S., Sakihama, T., Matsutani, T., Negishi, I., Nakatsuru, S., Sakaguchi, S., Altered thymic T-cell selection due to a mutation of the ZAP-70 gene causes autoimmune arthritis in mice. *Nature* **2003**, 426: 454–460.

3 Wassarman, P.M., Zona pellucida glycoproteins. *Annu.Rev.Biochem.* **1988**, 57: 415–442.

4 Rhim, S.H., Millar, S.E., Robey, F., Luo, A.M., Lou, Y.H., Yule, T., Allen, P., Dean, J., Tung, K.S., Autoimmune disease of the ovary induced by a ZP3 peptide from the mouse zona pellucida. *J. Clin. Invest* **1992**, 89: 28–35.

5 Lou, Y., Ang, J., Thai, H., McElveen, F., Tung, K.S., A zona pellucida 3 peptide vaccine induces antibodies and reversible infertility without ovarian pathology. *J.Immunol.* **1995**, 155: 2715–2720.

6 Garza, K.M., Tung, K.S., Frequency of molecular mimicry among T cell peptides as the basis for autoimmune disease and autoantibody induction. *J.Immunol.* **1995**, 155: 5444–5448.

7 Bagavant, H., Adams, S., Terranova, P., Chang, A., Kraemer, F.W., Lou, Y., Kasai, K., Luo, A.M., Tung, K.S., Autoimmune ovarian inflammation triggered by proinflammatory (Th1) T cells is compatible

with normal ovarian function in mice. *Biol.Reprod.* **1999**, 61: 635–642.

8 Kojima, A., Tanaka-Kojima, Y., Sakakura, T., Nishizuka, Y., Spontaneous development of autoimmune thyroiditis in neonatally thymectomized mice. *Lab Invest* **1976**, 34: 550–557.

9 Taguchi, O., Nishizuka, Y., Autoimmune oophoritis in thymectomized mice: T cell requirement in adoptive cell transfer. *Clin.Exp.Immunol.* **1980**, 42: 324–331.

10 Taguchi, O., Nishizuka, Y., Experimental autoimmune orchitis after neonatal thymectomy in the mouse. *Clin.Exp.Immunol.* **1981**, 46: 425–434.

11 Tung, K.S., Smith, S., Matzner, P., Kasai, K., Oliver, J., Feuchter, F., Anderson, R.E., Murine autoimmune oophoritis, epididymoorchitis, and gastritis induced by day 3 thymectomy. Autoantibodies. *Am.J.Pathol.* **1987**, 126: 303–314.

12 Tung, K.S., Smith, S., Teuscher, C., Cook, C., Anderson, R.E., Murine autoimmune oophoritis, epididymoorchitis, and gastritis induced by day 3 thymectomy. Immunopathology. *Am.J.Pathol.* **1987**, 126: 293–302.

13 Jones, C.M., Callaghan, J.M., Gleeson, P.A., Mori, Y., Masuda, T., Toh, B.H., The parietal cell autoantigens recognized in neonatal thymectomy-induced murine gastritis are the alpha and beta subunits of the gastric proton pump. *Gastroenterology* **1991**, 101: 287–294.

14 Kontani, K., Taguchi, O., Takahashi, T., Involvement of the H+/K(+)-ATPase alpha subunit as a major antigenic protein in autoimmune gastritis induced by neo-

natal thymectomy in mice. *Clin.Exp.Immunol.* **1992**, 89: 63–67.

15 Tong, Z. B., Nelson, L. M., A mouse gene encoding an oocyte antigen associated with autoimmune premature ovarian failure. *Endocrinology* **1999**, 140: 3720–3726.

16 Sakaguchi, S., Sakaguchi, N., Asano, M., Itoh, M., Toda, M., Immunologic self-tolerance maintained by activated T cells expressing IL-2 receptor alpha-chains (CD25). Breakdown of a single mechanism of self-tolerance causes various autoimmune diseases. *J.Immunol.* **1995**, 155: 1151–1164.

17 Suri-Payer, E., Amar, A. Z., Thornton, A. M., Shevach, E. M., CD4+CD25+ T cells inhibit both the induction and effector function of autoreactive T cells and represent a unique lineage of immunoregulatory cells. *J.Immunol.* **1998**, 160: 1212–1218.

18 Itoh, M., Takahashi, T., Sakaguchi, N., Kuniyasu, Y., Shimizu, J., Otsuka, F., Sakaguchi, S., Thymus and autoimmunity: Production of CD25(+)CD4(+) naturally anergic and suppressive T cells as a key function of the thymus in maintaining immunologic self-tolerance. *J.Immunol.* **1999**, 162: 5317–5326.

19 Asano, M., Toda, M., Sakaguchi, N., Sakaguchi, S., Autoimmune disease as a consequence of developmental abnormality of a T cell subpopulation. *J. Exp. Med.* **1996**, 184: 387–396.

20 Smith, H., Lou, Y. H., Lacy, P., Tung, K. S., Tolerance mechanism in experimental ovarian and gastric autoimmune diseases. *J.Immunol.* **1992**, 149: 2212–2218.

21 McHugh, R. S., Shevach, E. M., Cutting edge: depletion of CD4+CD25+ regulatory T cells is necessary, but not sufficient, for induction of organ-specific autoimmune disease. *J.Immunol.* **2002**, 168: 5979–5983.

22 Setiady, Y. Y., Samy, E. T., Tung, K. S., Maternal autoantibody triggers de novo T cell-mediated neonatal autoimmune disease. *J.Immunol.* **2003**, 170: 4656–4664.

23 Lou, Y. H., McElveen, M. F., Garza, K. M., Tung, K. S., Rapid induction of autoantibodies by endogenous ovarian antigens

and activated T cells: implication in autoimmune disease pathogenesis and B cell tolerance. *J.Immunol.* **1996**, 156: 3535–3540.

24 Wu, J., Arends, J., Borillo, J., Zhou, C., Merszei, J., McMahon, J., Lou, Y. H., A self T cell epitope induces autoantibody response: mechanism for production of antibodies to diverse glomerular basement membrane antigens. *J.Immunol.* **2004**, 172: 4567–4574.

25 Deshmukh, U. S., Lewis, J. E., Gaskin, F., Kannapell, C. C., Waters, S. T., Lou, Y. H., Tung, K. S., Fu, S. M., Immune responses to Ro60 and its peptides in mice. I. The nature of the immunogen and endogenous autoantigen determine the specificities of the induced autoantibodies. *J.Exp.Med.* **1999**, 189: 531–540.

26 Deshmukh, U. S., Lewis, J. E., Gaskin, F., Dhakephalkar, P. K., Kannapell, C. C., Waters, S. T., Fu, S. M., Ro60 peptides induce antibodies to similar epitopes shared among lupus-related autoantigens. *J. Immunol.* **2000**, 164: 6655–6661.

27 Topfer, F., Gordon, T., McCluskey, J., Intra- and intermolecular spreading of autoimmunity involving the nuclear self-antigens La (SS-B) and Ro (SS-A). *Proc. Natl. Acad. Sci. USA* **1995**, 92: 875–879.

28 Putterman, C., Diamond, B., Immunization with a peptide surrogate for double-stranded DNA (dsDNA) induces autoantibody production and renal immunoglobulin deposition. *J. Exp. Med.* **1998**, 188: 29–38.

29 James, J. A., Gross, T., Scofield, R. H., Harley, J. B., Immunoglobulin epitope spreading and autoimmune disease after peptide immunization: Sm B/B'-derived PPPGMRPP and PPPGIRGP induce spliceosome autoimmunity. *J. Exp. Med.* **1995**, 181: 453–461.

30 Yeh, T. M., Krolick, K. A., T cells reactive with a small synthetic peptide of the acetylcholine receptor can provide help for a clonotypically heterogeneous antibody response and subsequently impaired muscle function. *J.I mmunol.* **1990**, 144: 1654–1660.

31 Lin, R. H., Mamula, M. J., Hardin, J. A., Janeway, C. A., Jr., Induction of autoreactive B cells allows priming of autoreac-

tive T cells. *J. Exp. Med.* **1991**, 173: 1433–1439.

32 Miller, S. D., Eagar, T. N., Functional role of epitope spreading in the chronic pathogenesis of autoimmune and virus-induced demyelinating diseases. *Adv. Exp. Med. Biol.* **2001**, 490: 99–107.

33 Huang, F. P., Platt, N., Wykes, M., Major, J. R., Powell, T. J., Jenkins, C. D., Mac-Pherson, G. G., A discrete subpopulation of dendritic cells transports apoptotic intestinal epithelial cells to T cell areas of mesenteric lymph nodes. *J. Exp. Med.* **2000**, 191: 435–444.

34 Hawiger, D., Inaba, K., Dorsett, Y., Guo, M., Mahnke, K., Rivera, M., Ravetch, J. V., Steinman, R. M., Nussenzweig, M. C., Dendritic cells induce peripheral T cell unresponsiveness under steady state conditions in vivo. *J. Exp. Med.* **2001**, 194: 769–779.

35 Kaipia, A., Hsueh, A. J., Regulation of ovarian follicle atresia. *Annu. Rev. Physiol* **1997**, 59: 349–363.

36 Griggs, N. D., Agersborg, S. S., Noelle, R. J., Ledbetter, J. A., Linsley, P. S., Tung, K. S., The relative contribution of the CD28 and gp39 costimulatory pathways in the clonal expansion and pathogenic acquisition of self-reactive T cells. *J. Exp. Med.* **1996**, 183: 801–810.

37 Luo, A. M., Garza, K. M., Hunt, D., Tung, K. S., Antigen mimicry in autoimmune disease sharing of amino acid residues critical for pathogenic T cell activation. *J. Clin. Invest* **1993**, 92: 2117–2123.

38 Alard, P., Thompson, C., Agersborg, S. S., Thatte, J., Setiady, Y., Samy, E., Tung, K. S., Endogenous oocyte antigens are required for rapid induction and progression of autoimmune ovarian disease following day-3 thymectomy. *J. Immunol.* **2001**, 166: 4363–4369.

39 Suri-Payer, E., Amar, A. Z., McHugh, R., Natarajan, K., Margulies, D. H., Shevach, E. M., Post-thymectomy autoimmune gastritis: fine specificity and pathogenicity of anti-H/K ATPase-reactive T cells. *Eur. J. Immunol.* **1999**, 29: 669-677.

40 Florman, H. M., Wassarman, P. M., O-linked oligosaccharides of mouse egg ZP3 account for its sperm receptor activity. *Cell* **1985**, 41: 313–324.

41 Moore, G. R., Traugott, U., Stone, S. H., Raine, C. S., Dose-dependency of MBP-induced demyelination in the guinea pig. *J. Neurol. Sci.* **1985**, 70: 197–205.

42 Garchon, H. J., Bedossa, P., Eloy, L., Bach, J. F., Identification and mapping to chromosome 1 of a susceptibility locus for periinsulitis in non-obese diabetic mice. *Nature* **1991**, 353: 260–262.

43 Lou, Y. H., Park, K. K., Agersborg, S., Alard, P., Tung, K. S., Retargeting T cell-mediated inflammation: a new perspective on autoantibody action. *J. Immunol.* **2000**, 164: 5251–5257.

44 Lyons, J. A., Ramsbottom, M. J., Cross, A. H., Critical role of antigen-specific antibody in experimental autoimmune encephalomyelitis induced by recombinant myelin oligodendrocyte glycoprotein. *Eur. J. Immunol.* **2002**, 32: 1905–1913.

45 Lassmann, H., Suchanek, G., Kitz, K., Stemberger, H., Schwerer, B., Bernheimer, H., Antibodies in the pathogenesis of demyelination in chronic relapsing EAE (cr-EAE). *Prog. Clin. Biol. Res.* **1984**, 146: 165–170.

46 Hashim, G. A., Day, E. D., Carvalho, E., Abdelaal, A., Experimental allergic encephalomyelitis (EAE): role of B cell and T cell epitopes in the development of EAE in Lewis rats. *J. Neurosci. Res.* **1987**, 17: 375–383.

47 Myers, K. J., Sprent, J., Dougherty, J. P., Ron, Y, Synergy between encephalitogenic T cells and myelin basic protein-specific antibodies in the induction of experimental autoimmune encephalomyelitis. *J. Neuroimmunol.* **1992**, 41: 1–8.

48 Linington, C., Engelhardt, B., Kapocs, G., Lassman, H., Induction of persistently demyelinated lesions in the rat following the repeated adoptive transfer of encephalitogenic T cells and demyelinating antibody. *J. Neuroimmunol.* **1992**, 40: 219–224.

49 Wang, Y., Rollins, S. A., Madri, J. A., Matis, L. A., Anti-C5 monoclonal antibody therapy prevents collagen-induced arthritis and ameliorates established disease. *Proc. Natl. Acad. Sci. USA* **1995**, 92: 8955–8959.

50 Bannister, K. M., Ulich, T. R., Wilson, C. B., Induction, characterization, and cell transfer of autoimmune tubulointerstitial nephritis. *Kidney Int.* **1987**, 32: 642–651.

51 Wilson, C. B., Study of the immunopathogenesis of tubulointerstitial nephritis using model systems. *Kidney Int.* **1989**, 35: 938–953.

52 Amigorena, S. Bonnerot, C., Fc receptors for IgG and antigen presentation on MHC class I and class II molecules. *Semin.Immunol.* **1999**, 11: 385–390.

53 Kalergis, A. M., Ravetch, J. V., Inducing Tumor Immunity through the Selective Engagement of Activating Fcgamma Receptors on Dendritic Cells. *J.Exp.Med.* **2002**, 195: 1653–1659.

54 Schuurhuis, D. H., Ioan-Facsinay, A., Nagelkerken, B., van Schip, J. J., Sedlik, C., Melief, C. J., Verbeek, J. S., Ossendorp, F., Antigen-antibody immune complexes empower dendritic cells to efficiently prime specific CD8+ CTL responses in vivo. *J.Immunol.* **2002**, 168: 2240–2246.

55 Reijonen, H., Daniels, T. L., Lernmark, A., Nepom, G. T., GAD65-specific autoantibodies enhance the presentation of an immunodominant T-cell epitope from GAD65. *Diabetes* **2000**, 49: 1621–1626.

56 Dai, Y., Carayanniotis, K. A., Eliades, P., Lymberi, P., Shepherd, P., Kong, Y., Carayanniotis, G., Enhancing or suppressive effects of antibodies on processing of a pathogenic T cell epitope in thyroglobulin. *J.Immunol.* **1999**, 162: 6987–6992.

57 Kita, H., Lian, Z. X., Van de, W. J., He, X. S., Matsumura, S., Kaplan, M., Luketic, V., Coppel, R. L., Ansari, A. A., Gershwin, M. E., Identification of HLA-A2-restricted CD8(+) cytotoxic T cell responses in primary biliary cirrhosis: T cell activation is augmented by immune complexes cross-presented by dendritic cells. *J. Exp. Med.* **2002**, 195: 113–123.

58 Antoniou, A. N., Watts, C., Antibody modulation of antigen presentation: positive and negative effects on presentation of the tetanus toxin antigen via the murine B cell isoform of FcgammaRII. *Eur. J. Immunol.* **2002**, 32: 530–540.

59 Martin, M. G., Wu, S. V., Walsh, J. H., Hormonal control of intestinal Fc receptor gene expression and immunoglobulin transport in suckling rats. *J. Clin. Invest* **1993**, 91: 2844–2849.

60 Pasare, C., Medzhitov, R., Toll pathway-dependent blockade of CD4+CD25+ T cell-mediated suppression by dendritic cells. *Science* **2003**, 299: 1033–1036.

61 Dussault, I., Miller, S. C., Suppression of natural killer cell activity in infant mice occurs after target cell binding. *Nat. Immun.* **1995**, 14: 35–43.

62 Hackett, J., Jr., Tutt, M., Lipscomb, M., Bennett, M., Koo, G., Kumar, V., Origin and differentiation of natural killer cells. II. Functional and morphologic studies of purified NK-1.1+ cells. *J. Immunol.* **1986**, 136: 3124–3131.

63 Jamieson, A. M., Isnard, P., Dorfman, J. R., Coles, M. C., Raulet, D. H., Turnover and proliferation of NK cells in steady state and lymphopenic conditions. *J.Immunol.* **2004**, 172: 864–870.

64 Sivakumar, P. V., Gunturi, A., Salcedo, M., Schatzle, J. D., Lai, W. C., Kurepa, Z., Pitcher, L., Seaman, M. S., Lemonnier, F. A., Bennett, M., Forman, J., Kumar, V., Cutting edge: expression of functional CD94/NKG2A inhibitory receptors on fetal NK1.1+Ly-49- cells: a possible mechanism of tolerance during NK cell development. *J.Immunol.* **1999**, 162: 6976–6980.

65 Kubota, A., Kubota, S., Lohwasser, S., Mager, D. L., Takei, F., Diversity of NK cell receptor repertoire in adult and neonatal mice. *J. Immunol.* **1999**, 163: 212–216.

66 Ortaldo, J. R., Winkler-Pickett, R., Wiegand, G., Activating Ly-49D NK receptors: expression and function in relation to ontogeny and Ly-49 inhibitor receptors. *J. Leukoc. Biol.* **2000**, 68: 748–756.

67 Setiady, Y. Y., Pramoonjago, P., Tung, K. S., Requirements of NK cells and proinflammatory cytokines in T cell-dependent neonatal autoimmune ovarian disease triggered by immune complex. *J. Immunol.* **2004**, 173: 1051–1058.

68 Ravetch, J. V., Lanier, L. L., Immune inhibitory receptors. *Science* **2000**, 290: 84–89.

69 Bolland, S., Ravetch, J.V., Spontaneous autoimmune disease in Fc(gamma)RIIB-deficient mice results from strain-specific epistasis. *Immunity.* **2000**, 13: 277–285.

70 Ferlazzo, G., Tsang, M.L., Moretta, L., Melioli, G., Steinman, R.M., Munz, C., Human dendritic cells activate resting natural killer (NK) cells and are recognized via the NKp30 receptor by activated NK cells. *J.Exp.Med.* **2002**, 195: 343–351.

71 Piccioli, D., Sbrana, S., Melandri, E., Valiante, N.M., Contact-dependent stimulation and inhibition of dendritic cells by natural killer cells. *J. Exp. Med.* **2002**, 195: 335–341.

72 Gerosa, F., Baldani-Guerra, B., Nisii, C., Marchesini, V., Carra, G., Trinchieri, G., Reciprocal activating interaction between natural killer cells and dendritic cells. *J.Exp.Med.* **2002**, 195: 327–333.

73 Mocikat, R., Braumuller, H., Gumy, A., Egeter, O., Ziegler, H., Reusch, U., Bubeck, A., Louis, J., Mailhammer, R., Riethmuller, G., Koszinowski, U., Rocken, M., Natural killer cells activated by MHC class I(low) targets prime dendritic cells to induce protective CD8 T cell responses. *Immunity.* **2003**, 19: 561–569.

74 Mailliard, R.B., Son, Y.I., Redlinger, R., Coates, P.T., Giermasz, A., Morel, P.A., Storkus, W.J., Kalinski, P., Dendritic cells mediate NK cell help for Th1 and CTL responses: two-signal requirement for the induction of NK cell helper function. *J.Immunol.* **2003**, 171: 2366–2373.

75 Assarsson, E., Kambayashi, T., Schatzle, J.D., Cramer, S.O., von Bonin, A., Jensen, P.E., Ljunggren, H.G., Chambers, B.J., NK cells stimulate proliferation of T and NK cells through 2B4/CD48 interactions. *J. Immunol.* **2004**, 173: 174–180.

76 Fernandez, N.C., Lozier, A., Flament, C., Ricciardi-Castagnoli, P., Bellet, D., Suter, M., Perricaudet, M., Tursz, T., Maraskovsky, E., Zitvogel, L., Dendritic cells directly trigger NK cell functions: crosstalk relevant in innate anti-tumor immune responses in vivo. *Nat.Med.* **1999**, 5: 405–411.

77 Ferlazzo, G., Morandi, B., D'Agostino, A., Meazza, R., Melioli, G., Moretta, A., Moretta, L., The interaction between NK cells and dendritic cells in bacterial infections results in rapid induction of NK cell activation and in the lysis of uninfected dendritic cells. *Eur.J.Immunol.* **2003**, 33: 306–313.

78 Granucci, F., Zanoni, I., Pavelka, N., Van Dommelen, S.L., Andoniou, C.E., Belardelli, F., Degli Esposti, M.A., Ricciardi-Castagnoli, P., A contribution of mouse dendritic cell-derived IL-2 for NK cell activation. *J. Exp. Med.* **2004**, 200: 287–295.

79 Koka, R., Burkett, P., Chien, M., Chai, S., Boone, D.L., Ma, A., Cutting edge: murine dendritic cells require IL-15R alpha to prime NK cells. *J.Immunol.* **2004**, 173: 3594–3598.

80 Forsthuber, T., Yip, H.C., Lehmann, P.V., Induction of TH1 and TH2 immunity in neonatal mice. *Science* **1996**, 271: 1728–1730.

81 Ridge, J.P., Fuchs, E.J., Matzinger, P., Neonatal tolerance revisited: turning on newborn T cells with dendritic cells. *Science* **1996**, 271: 1723–1726.

82 Sarzotti, M., Robbins, D.S., Hoffman, P.M., Induction of protective CTL responses in newborn mice by a murine retrovirus. *Science* **1996**, 271: 1726–1728.

83 Tung, K.S., Agersborg, S.S., Alard, P., Garza, K.M., Lou, Y.H., Regulatory T-cell, endogenous antigen and neonatal environment in the prevention and induction of autoimmune disease. *Immunol. Rev.* **2001**, 182: 135–148.

22
Environmental Factors That Contribute to Autoimmunity

Per Hultman

22.1
Relation Between Genetic and Environmental Factors in Autoimmunity

Autoimmune diseases, divided into at least 80 diseases or syndromes, play a distinct role in the spectrum of human diseases. Close to 10 million Americans are affected [1], and autoimmune diseases are among the leading causes of death for women under the age of 65 [2]. While the etiologic factors responsible for autoimmune diseases are still largely unknown, the cause has to be sought among genetic and environmental factors. A combination of these factors is usually necessary for autoimmune diseases to develop, and it is likely that stochastic events in the immune system may also play a role in deciding if an individual will be the subject of autoimmune disease.

The role of genetic factors in development of autoimmune diseases is clearly demonstrated by comparing the concordance rate for autoimmune disease in monozygous and dizygous twins. Monozygous twins are from birth genetically identical, while dizygous twins share on average only 50% of their genes. The concordance rate for autoimmune diseases is substantially higher in monozygous twins (30–50%) than in dizygous twins (5–20%), which demonstrates a strong influence of genetic factors on disease susceptibility [3].

A few very rare autoimmune diseases are *monogenic*. First, the autoimmune polyendocrine syndrome type I (APS-I) has a mutation in the autoimmunity regulatory gene (AIRE-I) on chromosome 21 and shows a recessive inheritance pattern with near 100% penetrance. The clinical manifestations include autoimmune hypoparathyroidism, Addison's disease, and mucocutaneous candidiasis [4]. Secondly, the X-linked polyendocrinopathy, immune dysfunction, and diarrhea (IPEX) syndrome with a mutation in the FOXP3 gene (analogue to the mouse scurfy gene) is characterized by severe allergic as well as autoimmune manifestations and a marked T-helper type 2 skewed immune system [5].

The possibility of *oligogenic* inheritance has been discussed in autoimmune diseases, especially in type 1 diabetes (T1D), with human leukocyte antigen (HLA) loci genes in combination with a few diabetogenes [6]. However, recent studies indicate that autoimmune diseases are *polygenic*, i.e., linked to a number of susceptibility (and resistance) genes. Evidence for a polygenic inheritance mood of autoimmune diseases stems from both animal models and humans, and it has been concluded that 65% of the genes regulating autoimmune disease may be mapped into 18 different clusters [7]. These genetic polymorphisms are present in 5% or more of the population. Development of autoimmunity may depend on epistatic interaction of these autoimmune-predisposing genes and environmental factors. Furthermore, when a specific environmental factor interacts with different genetic profiles, a number of phenotypic responses and clinical conditions may ensue. Therefore, it is not necessary or even likely that a specific environmental exposure will result in a fixed autoimmune manifestation.

22.2
Environmental Factors in Autoimmunity

Since the concordance rate for autoimmune diseases even in monozygous twins is only 30–50% [3], non-genetic factors must play an important role in the development of autoimmunity. These non-genetic factors are summarized here under the term environmental factors. What is an environmental factor? In a broad sense, environmental factors include everything non-genetic, from the intrauterine environment, to physical and chemical effects, to behavioral and social aspects [8]. However, this review will be limited to the following groups of etiologic agents: xenobiotics subdivided into drugs, biological agents, and environmental agents and, in addition, microbial agents and hormones. The effects on the postnatal immune system of prenatal exposure to environmental agents poses a special problem [9].

22.3
Xenobiotics

22.3.1
Drug-related Autoimmune Diseases/Syndromes

The first drug to be associated with autoimmunity was sulfadiazine, reported by Hoffman in 1945 to cause a lupus-like disease [10]. The increasing use of drugs during the following decade resulted in an increased number of drug-related hypersensitivity cases including autoimmune diseases. In 1954 the antihypertensive drug hydralazine was identified as an inductor of lupus [11]. In 1962 the antiarrhythmic drug procainamide was firmly associated with lupus-like disease [12], with up to 90% of patients showing antinuclear antibodies (ANA) within a year of starting treatment and up to 30% subsequently developing a lupus-like syndrome. Today, the following drugs have been more firmly associated with de-

velopment of lupus: chlorpromazine, hydralazine, isoniazid, methyldopa, mino-
cycline, procainamide, and quinidine. Case reports make it likely that many
more drugs may occasionally induce lupus [13].

The limited number of susceptible individuals among those exposed to a specific agent indicates that genetic factors are also important for drug-induced lupus (DIL). While there are as yet no generally accepted criteria for DIL, the condition seems to show a less distinct preponderance for females and occurs less
often in African Americans than does idiopathic SLE. Furthermore, the disease
symptoms are somewhat milder in DIL, renal and CNS manifestations being
less common than in idiopathic disease. Serositis and pleuro-pulmonary involvement is more common in DIL [14]. Many patients have polyarthralgia or
polyarthritis in small joints. The symptoms are often aborted when the offend-
ing drug is stopped. While ANAs are present in virtually all cases, antibodies to
double-stranded (ds) DNA and anti-Sm antibodies are quite unusual. In contrast, antibodies to single-stranded (ss) DNA are frequently found, and almost
all cases show antibodies to histones. These antibodies are preferably directed to
the H2A-H2B dimer after procainamide exposure and against H3 and H4 in hydralazine-induced lupus [15]. Antiphospholipid antibodies and lupus anticoagulants, often of the IgM isotype, are present in some cases.

22.3.2
Biological Agents

Biological agents first include many cytokines and anti-cytokine antibodies. Of
special importance is IFN-a, which has been associated with a number of autoimmune disorders, ranging from lupus erythematosus, rheumatoid arthritis,
diabetes mellitus, immune-mediated thrombocytopenia, and hemolytic anemia
to myasthenia gravis [16]. Up to 30% of the patients develop autoantibodies during treatment with IFN-a, but progress to autoimmune disease is limited and
the clinical relevance usually uncertain. However, autoimmune thyroid disorders
are a common side effect of IFN-a therapy, clinical or subclinical thyroid abnormalities being reported in up to 34% of chronic hepatitis C patients treated with
IFN-a for 6–12 months [17], and genetic factors seem to determine whether
autoimmunity will develop or not. Anti-TNF-a therapy has been associated with
rare occurrences of anti-dsDNA antibodies and/or DIL [18].

Another class of biological agents is vaccines. Both increased [19] and reduced
[20, 21] incidences of autoimmune diseases have been reported in studies using
experimental models, differences that may be related to the type of vaccine and
the experimental model used. There are also a number of case reports suggesting induction of autoimmune disease by vaccination [22]. However, epidemiological studies have not shown a link between vaccinations and autoimmune
diseases [23, 24]. Although systemic autoimmune diseases are generally considered a relative contraindication for vaccination, there is actually little evidence to
suggest that vaccination would in general lead to flares in autoimmune diseases, such as SLE [25, 26].

Not only vaccines themselves but also additives in vaccines have been implicated as having adverse immunological effects. In this respect, comments should be made on thimerosal, an organic mercury compound, and hydrocarbon oil. Thimerosal was until very recently a disinfectant in many vaccines. The active component of thimerosal is ethyl mercury, which is slowly de-ethylated to inorganic mercury in the body. Data on the toxicokinetics of ethyl mercury in humans are scarce [27], but recent studies in mice have increased the available knowledge [28, 29]. While the amount of thimerosal present in the individual vaccine dose is small, the extensive vaccination program used in infants combined with the small mass of these recipients was found to lead to more extensive Hg exposure than expected. In 2001 the National Academy discouraged the use of thimerosal in vaccines [30], leading to a dramatic reduction in the use of thimerosal in vaccines in the U.S. However, thimerosal is still used in other parts of the world. The possibility of health effects, especially autism [31], has been discussed, but there are no convincing data to support this theory [32, 33]. With regard to effects on the immune system, there is no evidence of an adverse effect of thimerosal when used in vaccines; this is also supported by animal studies taking into account the high susceptibility to autoimmune disease of some mouse strains [28]. Another vaccine component is adjuvants (hydrocarbon oils). Incomplete Freunds's adjuvant (IFA) is the classical compound, which has been replaced by the oil squalene (MF59), the only adjuvant approved by the Food and Drug Administration for use in vaccines together with alum [34]. Since epidemiological studies have not been able to show an accelerating effect of vaccination on autoimmune disease development, there is *a priori* no reason to suspect such an effect from the adjuvants used. It should, however, be noted that a single intraperitoneal injection of the adjuvant oils pristane, IFA, or squalene is able to induce lupus-related autoantibodies to nRNP/Sm- and Su-antigen in non-autoimmune BALB/c mice, but the relevance for human vaccination is not proven [35].

22.3.3
Environmental Agents

22.3.3.1 Chemicals

Hydrazine and its metabolite tartrazine have been associated with DIL [36]. The hair-drying agent phenylenediamine has been epidemiologically associated with connective tissue disease [37]. Silica dust has been associated with lupus as well as scleroderma-like disease in humans [38] and in animal models [39]. Pesticides have often appeared in tabulations of agents inducing autoimmunity. However, there are few data linking most of the pesticides to autoimmunity. A recent review on pesticides and autoimmunity [40] concluded that there is epidemiological and experimental evidence for an immunostimulatory effect of the pesticide hexachlorobenzene, which may contribute to autoimmunity. This possibility was reinforced by a recent epidemiological study showing a significant association between SLE and mixing pesticides for agricultural work [41]. Recent data indicate phthalates (softeners used in plastics) as an inductor of autoreactive B cells in autoimmune-prone NZBWF1 mice [42]. Organic solvents have been associated with autoimmunity both as *de novo* initiators in humans [43] and as an exacerbator of autoimmunity in MRL-+/+ mice [44]. Exposure to organic solvents regularly consists of a mix of aromatic and aliphatic hydrocarbons, as well as chlorinated compounds, and has been associated with systemic sclerosis, especially in patients with autoantibodies to Scl-70 (DNA polymerase I) having the diffuse form of the disease [45]. Another compound with a proven association to scleroderma-like disease is the synthetic resin vinyl chloride $CH2=CHCl$, which is used in the manufacturing of plastics. A scleroderma-like syndrome linked to cumulative vinyl chloride exposures over time occurs in >3% of the exposed individuals [46]. Further studies have revealed an increased prevalence of HLA-DR3 and HLA-DR3/B8 haplotypes in the affected individuals [47].

22.3.3.2 Metals

Exposure to mercury, gold, and silver has been unequivocally associated with autoimmune reactions in humans and animals. The documentation for mercury includes case reports on systemic autoimmunity [48, 49], as well as immune-mediated membranous glomerulonephritis, following accidental or occupational exposure and therapeutic use [50]. A recent epidemiological study [41] supported these observations by showing a significant association between SLE and self-reported mercury exposure, as well as between SLE and dental work. Extensive experimental studies have been performed on mercury-induced autoimmune and hypersensitivity reactions since 1971, when Bariety first reported immune-complex (IC) disease in a fraction of outbred rats treated with Hg [51]. Sapin et al. subsequently described Hg-induced biphasic autoimmune disease in the genetically susceptible Brown Norway rat strain [52]. These observations were further elaborated with the first reports on Hg-induced autoimmune conditions in inbred and outbred mice [53, 54]. A biphasic systemic autoimmune condition also has been found following Hg treatment in rabbits [55].

Gold compounds, mainly the anti-rheumatic drug sodium aurothiomalate, have caused autoimmune reactions [56] characterized by cytotoxic effects, especially thrombocytopenia [57], but also systemic immune-mediated renal diseases [58, 59], and antinuclear antibodies [60]. Studies in rats and mice lend support to the autoimmune potential of gold [61–63].

Silver has been shown to induce autoantibodies targeting the 34-kDa nucleolar protein fibrillarin in mice [64]. The autoantibody specificity and the genetic susceptibility [65] is the same as in murine mercury-induced autoimmunity.

During the last decade additional metals have been indicated as being able to induce autoimmunity [66]. Lithium has been associated with autoimmune thyroid disease, and a weak correlation was reported between thyroid peroxidase antibodies and lithium intake [67]. However, in other studies increased frequency of antibodies to thyroid peroxidase and the T1D-associated GAD65A was associated with bipolar disease [68] but not with lithium [69].

The search for a primary autoimmune effect of lead in mice has not met with success, but the autoimmune-prone ZBWF1 hybrid shows enhanced development of autoimmune manifestations during lead treatment [70, 71]. Cadmium has been shown to induce ANA in outbred mice [72], and cadmium was recently shown to exacerbate spontaneous autoimmunity in ZBWF1 mice [73].

22.3.3.3 Primarily Dietary Factors

In 1981 an epidemic outbreak of acute respiratory illness, now known as the "toxic oil syndrome" (TOS), occurred in Spain. The acute phase was later found to include fever, rash, eosinophilia, hyper-IgE, and myalgia developing one to two months after consumption of the oil in question, followed after two to four months by an intermediate phase in some 60% of the affected individuals and a chronic phase occurring four months after exposure in 10–20% of the exposed subjects [74].The syndrome afflicted more than 20,000 individuals, and around 2% died. The autoimmune-like condition that developed in the chronic phase of TOS showed similarities with scleroderma, including sicca, Raynaud's phenomenon, and ANA [75]. The etiologic agent has not been unequivocally identified, but the vehicle was aniline-denatured industrial oil diverted to human consumption. An increased prevalence of HLA-DR3, -DR4, -DR2, and -DR8 has been suggested in TOS patients, but a recent study showed a significant association only between TOS and HLA-DR2 [76]. Interestingly, this association was found only in patients who succumbed to the disease.

A number of animal studies have been carried out to find a relevant model for TOS, but so far no species or strain studied has mimicked the entire spectrum of the human disease [77]. However, the original oil was recently reported to accelerate the spontaneous autoimmune condition in MRL-*lpr* mice [78].

In 1989 another epidemic outbreak occurred in the U.S. that had a clinical picture similar to that of TOS, namely, eosinophilia, myalgia, urticaria, fasciitis, elevated C-reactive protein, and ANA, which was found to be associated with ingestion of L-tryptophan [79]. Carriers of HLA-DR4 experienced an increased risk for contracting this so called "eosinophilic-myalgic syndrome" [80]. The death rate was almost 3% among the 1370 identified cases. Interestingly, it has been reported that at least two contaminants in the process of tryptophan production was the same as in the oil related to TOS [81].

Intake of canavanine (an analogue of L-arginine) from alfalfa seed sprouts has been associated with SLE-like syndromes in both humans and monkeys [80].

Iodide has long been discussed as a factor in thyroid autoimmunity. A recent review summarized that iodide may be an immunogenic factor for thyroid autoimmunity, but only in predisposed subjects [82].

22.3.3.4 Ultraviolet Radiation

Photosensitivity is common in autoimmune diseases such as lupus erythematosus [83] and dermatomyositis [84]. Furthermore, UV radiation has been shown to accelerate spontaneous autoimmunity and mortality in BXSB mice [85]. Surprisingly, exposure to UVA and/or UVB causes immunosuppression, which is experimentally linked to certain strains of inbred mice and to polymorphism in the TNF region [86]. Studies have focused on the ability of different doses of UV radiation to cause inflammation, apoptosis, and/or necrosis of keratinocytes and redistribution to lupus autoantigens [87]. This has led to the suggestion that immunosuppression following UV radiation has a teleological meaning, namely, to reduce the likelihood of inducing autoimmune conditions in the UV-radiated, autoantigen-enriched skin. However, while UV radiation is one of the most prevalent environmental factors, its importance for induction of autoimmunity remains unknown.

22.4
Microbial Agents in Autoimmunity

Infections have long been connected with autoimmune diseases – either as a primary inducer of the disease or as the cause of flare-ups in established disease. Two diseases more definitely associated with microbials are rheumatic fever (RF) and Guillain-Barré syndrome (GBS). The identification in heart muscle from patients with rheumatic disease of T-cell clones recognizing both cardiac myosin proteins and epitopes in streptococcal M proteins [88] strongly supports molecular mimicry as important in RF. In GBS there is evidence that infection with *Campylobacter jejuni*, cytomegalovirus, Epstein-Barr virus, and *Mycoplasma pneumoniae* (in order of prevalence) precedes GBS symptoms more often than in controls. The prevalence of these presymptomatic infections range from 5% for *Mycoplasma pneumoniae* to 60% for *Campylobacter jejuni* [89].

Extensive studies have been undertaken to try to link T1D to infections. The picture emerging from epidemiological and animal studies is complicated. For example, there is now evidence that microbial agents such as *Mycobacteria* spp., *Salmonella typhimurium*, and *Schistosoma mansoni* may actually prevent T1D [90], while mumps, human cytomegalovirus, rotavirus, retrovirus, and rubella virus have all been implicated as important factors in human T1D. There is conclusive epidemiological and experimental evidence for congenital rubella as a harbinger to T1D, since up to 25% of the children with congenital rubella will develop T1D [91]. However, these children also have other autoimmune diseases [92], which indicates that the congenital infection may cause a basic defect in the immune system. The lesson of rubella might in addition be of limited interest for the etiology of T1D since rubella has largely been eradicated in developed countries due to vaccination, while the incidence of T1D is increasing. Enterovirus infections as a cause of T1D have received much interest [93]. A recent review summarized that "the evidence for the enteroviruses (in causing type 1 diabetes) is stronger than for most other environmental agents, but still final proof is lacking" [94].

Another autoimmune condition in which infectious agents have long been implicated is SLE. Among the viruses and their viral proteins linked to SLE are endogenous retroviruses, hepatitis C virus, Epstein-Barr virus, human polyoma virus, human cytomegalovirus, human papillomaviruses, human parvovirus, and varicella-zoster virus [95, 96]. Endogenous retroviruses, while present as proviruses in the genome of all individuals and potentially able to modulate cellular gene expression, are often not intact and incapable of protein expression. The possible association between SLE and retroviruses is founded on four observations. First, retrovirus infections in humans (HIV and HTLV1) give rise to manifestations that are similar to some of the leading symptoms in SLE, and similar observations have been made in animals. Secondly, mouse strains with spontaneous lupus-like disease, e.g., the ZBWF1 model, produce high amounts of an *env*-coded protein, gp70, and these animals have high-titer anti-gp70 antibodies. Immune complexes composed of gp70-anti-gp70 are present in the circulation, and their presence correlates with the amount of IC deposits in the glomeruli [97]. Third, the *Fas* gene defect in the spontaneous autoimmune MRL-*lpr* strain is caused by insertion of a retrovirus element into the *Fas* gene [98]. Finally, a number of different endogenous and exogenous retroviral antigens share sequences with autoantigens, opening the possibility for a molecular mimicry mechanism [99]. However, the actual importance of retroviruses for development of SLE remains unknown.

A possible influence of microbial agents has also been discussed in other autoimmune diseases, such as multiple sclerosis (Epstein-Barr, herpes simplex, HHV-6, and varicella-zoster virus), myasthenia gravis (hepatitis C virus), and autoimmune hepatitis (Epstein-Barr and hepatitis A virus) [96], but final proof is lacking. Finally, as noted above for T1D, there are indications that microbial agents may in some instances actually reduce the prevalence of autoimmune disease. A striking modification of the autoimmune response in experimental encephalomyelitis has been noted during helminthic infections [100]. The mechanisms discussed include a Th2 polarization, due to the ability of helminths to evoke a Th2 response, or an activation of regulatory T cells.

22.5
Hormones in Autoimmunity

Autoimmune diseases are with few exceptions much more common in females than in males [1]. Androgens and estrogens have strong immunomodulating effects in both the thymus and the bone marrow, with androgens acting suppressively and estrogens stimulating [101]. The difference in autoimmune disease prevalence is commonly believed to be related to the action of sex hormones, although gonadotropin-releasing hormones may have the potential for exacerbating experimental systemic autoimmune diseases independently of sex hormones [102]. It cannot be formally excluded that other mechanisms such as X-chromosomal activation are also operative [103]. What is, therefore, the evidence for a role of sex hormones in the induction, development, and persistence of autoimmune diseases? First, alteration of sex hormones during pregnancy [104], ovarian failure [105], and intake of oral contraceptives [106] have all been associated with variations in lupus diseases. These observations in humans are supported by acceleration of the spontaneous lupus-like disease in ZBWF1 and MRL-*lpr* mice using exogenous estrogens [107, 108]. However, a recent epidemiological study offered little support for the concept of an increased risk for SLE in individuals exposed to estrogen or prolactin [109]. In a recent review [110] the authors stated that "a clear understanding of relationships between serum estradiol concentrations, steroid enzymes, metabolite effects, and disease activity in SLE remains elusive."

A recently discovered but potentially serious factor is the exposure to sex hormones not only from endogenous sources, or exogenous sources such as oral contraceptives and replacement therapy, but also in the form of endocrine disrupters in the environment. Environmental estrogens are present in plastics, detergents, surfactants, industrial chemicals, pesticides, phytoestrogens, and as natural plant estrogens as well as mycoestrogens, which may contaminate food intake. These substances are often chemically stable, may accumulate in body fat, and are released during starvation or are vertically transmitted during pregnancy and with the colostrum/milk. Recently, endocrine disruptors were shown to increase autoantibody production by B1 cells [111]. However, the effect, if any, of environmental estrogens on the development of autoimmunity in humans is unknown [112].

22.6
Prenatal Exposure and Postnatal Autoimmune Effects

It would be inappropriate to discuss the possible autoimmune effects of environmental agents on the human immune system without mentioning the concept of prenatal exposure and postnatal aberration of the immune system. The effect observed is predominantly one of immunosuppression. However, the *in utero* exposure to diethylstilbestrol of 1.5 million women in the U.S. not only caused genital tract abnormalities and reproductive problems but also made them more susceptible to autoimmune disease [113]. Recent studies have shown a marked increase in the exposed women's response to T-cell mitogens, possibly due to a lifelong developmental arrest [114], while exposure to polyhalogenated aromatic hydrocarbons (TCDD) caused long-lasting postnatal immunosuppression in rats [115]. However, there is presently no convincing evidence for an effect of prenatal exposure on development of autoimmunity. A recent meeting summarized the knowledge about TCDD and similar agents on the immune system [116].

22.7
Acceleration and Aggravation of Autoimmunity by Environmental Agents

As mentioned above, each environmental agent will probably be able to cause a number of phenotypic expressions of autoimmune diseases due to interaction with different genotypes. One possibility is that the agents do not cause an autoimmune disease *de novo*, but instead accelerate and aggravate autoimmune conditions with other primary genetic or non-genetic etiology. The most instructive observations on this subject have recently emerged from the use of certain metals in mice. Hg is a potent *de novo* inductor of a systemic autoimmune disease condition in rodents with a mainly MHC (H-2) class II gene-related susceptibility [117, 118]. While these rodent models continue to be very useful for elucidating immunological mechanisms in systemic autoimmunity, dose-response studies applied to humans have indicated that *de novo* induction of autoimmunity by metals may occur mainly in hazardous work places or by accidental or voluntary ingestion. However, there is now firm experimental evidence that Hg may act in a much more insidious way by accelerating the onset and aggravating autoimmune diseases with other primary etiologies. Furthermore, there is some evidence that this might occur at a dose that is comparable with existing limits for occupational exposure and substantially lower than the exposure needed to induce autoimmunity *de novo*.

22.7.1
Acceleration of Spontaneous Autoimmune Diseases by Hg

In experimental models, the polyclonal B cell–activating agent lipopolysaccharide–lipid A portion [119], UV radiation [85], halothane [120], and polyinosinic-polycytidylic acid [121] accelerate spontaneous autoimmune disease manifestations. Recently, inorganic Hg was shown to have similar effects. Hg accelerates the spontaneous autoimmune manifestations occurring in the ZBWF1 mouse hybrid as evidenced by lymphoid hyperplasia [122], polyclonal B-cell activation [123], hyperimmunoglobulinemia [122, 123], anti-chromatin antibodies [122], and immune-complex deposits [122, 123]. Hg treatment of the MRL-+/+ strain and the autoimmune-prone MRL-*lpr/lpr* (*Fas*-deficient) strain caused severely and slightly accelerated autoimmune manifestations, respectively [122]. However, recent studies have shown that the autoimmunity may be severely aggravated also in the MRL-*lpr/lpr* strain, provided that a lower dose of Hg is administered [124]. Using the AKR strain, which is H-2 congenic with the MRL strains, non-MHC genes were shown to be responsible for the more extensive disease in the MRL strains [122]. Studies in the autoimmune-prone BXSB and the non-autoimmune C57BL/6 strains, which share the *H-2^b* haplotype, showed that Hg triggers the *Yaa* gene–dependent lupus-like autoimmune disease in BXSB mice by aggravating lymphoid hyperplasia, anti-chromatin antibodies, and glomerulonephritis, but had little effect on the C57BL/6J strain, linking the genetic susceptibility to non-MHC genes [125]. Interestingly, a short course of

Hg to BXSB mice was sufficient to cause a lifelong increase in the autoimmune response. Furthermore, a dose of Hg that was relatively lower than the dose accepted in the occupational setting accelerated the spontaneous autoimmune disease.

While the above observations may give the impression that Hg given in a sufficient dose always accelerates spontaneous autoimmune diseases, we have found [166] that Hg treatment for more than one year in the spontaneous autoimmune $(SWR \times SJL)F_1$ mouse model [126] neither accelerated the onset nor increased the severity of the systemic autoimmune manifestations. The conclusion is that the SWR strain possesses non-MHC genes that can suppress Hg-induced exacerbation of autoimmunity. This shows that it is necessary to examine the effect of environmental agents like Hg on all available spontaneous models of autoimmune disease, since a specific interaction takes place between genetics (also outside the MHC), the spontaneous autoimmune conditions, and the environmental agents.

These studies on the accelerating effect of Hg exposure have all been performed in models with a distinct and known genetic predisposition. Recently, Silbergeld et al. examined whether an autoimmune disease caused by a primarily non-genetic mechanism might also be accelerated by Hg [127]. A lupus-like chronic graft-versus-host disease (GVHD) was induced using F_1 hybrids of two strains resistant to Hg (C57BL/6 and DBA/2) and DBA/2 donor cells. A two-week exposure to host and donor mice of low-dose Hg (20 µg/kg body weight every other day) ending one week before GVHD induction aggravated the lupus-like GVHD condition.

22.7.2
Acceleration of Spontaneous Autoimmune Diseases by Cadmium and Lead

Recent studies have expanded the above findings using Hg. Cadmium in a high dose increases the ANA in autoimmune-prone ZBWF1 mice during the first month's treatment, while a lower dose increased the IgG2a serum level and the proteinuria but did not increase glomerular IC deposits [73]. As mentioned above, lead enhances the autoimmune manifestations in the autoimmune-prone ZBWF1 hybrid [70]. A recent study in four New Zealand mixed strains revealed a complex relation between the spontaneous autoimmune disease, lead exposure, genetics, and gender, with different phenotypic expression of the susceptibility to, or in some instances even attenuation of, the autoimmune process [71].

22.8
Comments on the Accelerating Effect of Metals on Autoimmunity

Understanding the ability of metals to accelerate and aggravate genetically as well as non-genetically determined autoimmune disease processes is an important advance in the area of environmental agents and autoimmunity. While some of the studies included limited dose-response data, the potential importance for human conditions warrants further dose-response studies in all these models. An additional major task will be to examine by which mechanism(s) the metals are able to accelerate the autoimmune process. Hopefully, such studies will also be able to catalyze the understanding of the pathogenic mechanisms involved in spontaneous autoimmune diseases.

22.8.1
Mechanisms for Induction of Autoimmunity by Environmental Agents

For many of the environmental agents discussed in this review, the association with autoimmune diseases is derived mainly from case reports and epidemiological studies. As indicated above, experimental studies have been used in many instances to try to unravel the mechanisms underlying the autoimmune effects of environmental agents, but the data obtained have often been of limited help in understanding the mechanisms involved. The following sections will briefly review the mechanisms in some areas of environmentally induced autoimmunity that have been of special importance for increasing our understanding of autoimmune disease mechanisms.

22.8.2
Lessons from Procainamide and Hydralazine

Procainamide and hydralazine are among the oldest drugs connected to drug-induced systemic autoimmunity (lupus) (see Section 22.3.1), and experimental studies using these drugs have shed light on important mechanisms that may be operating in xenobiotics-induced autoimmunity. A prerequisite for these effects is the *in vivo* generation from the drugs of metabolites with new properties, an effect that takes place not only in hepatic microsomal systems in the liver [128] but also in peripheral blood neutrophils utilizing myeloperoxidase and hydrogen peroxide, leading to formation of the unstable product procainamide hydroxylamine (PAHA) [129]. Importantly, not only are all the major classes of lupus-inducing drugs able to undergo transformation to reactive products by exposure to activated neutrophils, but the degree to which this transformation takes place correlates with the potency of the drug to induce lupus [130]. By injecting PAHA into the thymus of normal mice, an autoantibody profile mimicking that seen in procainamide-induced lupus in humans (IgM antibodies to denatured DNA after the first injection and high levels of IgG anti-chromatin antibodies after the second injection) was elicited [131]. Furthermore, anti-chromatin-reactive T cells simultaneously appeared in the peripheral immune organs, and transfer studies indicated the likelihood that flooding the periphery with these cells overwhelmed the peripheral tolerance system [132]. These elegant studies so far have not been validated for the human situation, but the very similar autoantibody specificity in PAHA-injected mice and procainamide-induced human lupus strongly supports this mechanism as being important in humans.

Procainamide and hydralazine are also able to induce autoimmunity by another mechanism, primarily affecting the peripheral lymphoid system, by causing hypomethylation of DNA. Procainamide is a competitive inhibitor of the nuclear DNA methyltransferase activity [133], while hydralazine causes hypomethylation by inhibiting the ERK signaling pathway, which prevents upregulation of Dnmt1 and Dnmt3a in stimulated T cells [134]. This hypomethylation seems to be able to induce hyperexpression of the adhesion molecule LFA-1, increasing the T-cell reactivity to a level where class II molecules might present inappropriate antigens, similar to the mechanism for chronic graft-versus-host disease [134, 135]. Interestingly, patients with idiopathic lupus have been shown to have hypomethylated lupus T cells and an autoreactive T-cell subset hyperexpressing LFA-1 [135, 136]. However, to what extent this mechanism is responsible for human SLE, and the reason that T cells should be hypomethylated in these patients, remains unknown.

22.8.3
Lessons from Metal-induced Autoimmunity

Another area in which new data have recently been derived is autoimmunity induced by metals. The effect of Hg on the immune system can be divided into lymphoproliferation, hypergammaglobulinemia, and autoimmunity manifested as specific autoantibody production and immune-complex disease [118].

In rats, the major advances with regard to Hg- and Au-induced autoimmunity have recently been summarized [117]. Briefly, rat T cells exhibit upon contact with these metals a stimulation of the early steps in T-cell activation, mimicking the effect of TCR cross-linking and leading to a polyclonal activation of both T and B cells. The frequency of autoreactive anti-MHC class II T cells increases drastically in the susceptible Brown Norway strain, which also shows a defective IFN-γ production but enhanced IL-4-production in the CD8 compartment, while the resistant Lewis strain exhibits a reciprocal cytokine pattern. These reactions lead to lymphoproliferation and hyperimmunoglobulinemia (of mainly the Th2 type) in the BN strains, producing anti-basement membrane (anti-laminin) and anti-DNA antibodies. The manifestations might be severe, including fatalities, but in the surviving rats the disease subsides within a month, first going through a quiescent state with systemic IC deposits, even if injections of Hg are pursued.

While there are phenotypic similarities between the autoimmune reaction to Hg in rats and that in mice, it is now clear that the underlying mechanisms are very different. The ability of mercury to cause lymphoproliferation in mice is virtually strain-independent, since the DBA/2 strain was the only strain out of 22 lacking lymphoproliferation, which also included strains with the same MHC haplotype as DBA/2 [137]. These *in vivo* findings correlate with the species-independent, Hg-induced lymphocyte proliferation demonstrated *in vitro* 35 years ago [138] and now identified as a cell- and concentration-dependent proliferation of adult T cells (but not B cells or immature T cells, or thymocytes)

[139–141]. The *in vitro* proliferation is linked to MHC class II [142] and costimulatory molecules, especially IL-1 [140], and there is evidence of an oligoclonal T-cell proliferation both *in vitro* [143] and *in vivo* [144]. Mercury may cause cell proliferation by perturbating lymphocyte signaling [145, 146], but also by attenuating lymphocyte apoptosis [147] due to interference with the Fas–Fas ligand interaction *in vitro* [148]. Exaggerated proliferation and defective apoptosis might not only cause expansion of peripheral lymphocytes but also allow autoreactive T cells to escape IFN-γ-dependent activation-induced cell death. This unspecific lymphoproliferative response to Hg is complemented by a specific proliferation occurring as part of an autoantigen-specific response.

The other main characteristic in Hg-induced murine autoimmunity, hyperimmunoglobulinemia, is not likely to be due to a direct effect of Hg on B cells, which are *in vitro* 10-fold more sensitive to the cytotoxic effect of Hg than T cells [149]. Instead, an initial polyclonal activation of both T helper type 1 and T helper type 2 cells induces B cell–stimulating and -switching factors such as IFN-γ and IL-4 [150], which leads to B-cell proliferation and Ig production [151].

The third murine response to metals is the induction of autoantibodies against the 34-kDa U3 small nucleolar ribonucleoprotein particle component fibrillarin using Hg [152, 153], Ag [64], and Au (Hultman and Pollard, unpublished observations). Intriguingly, the molecular specificity of the metal-induced anti-fibrillarin antibodies (AFA) is similar to that of AFA in a subset of patients with systemic sclerosis [154]. The restricted AFA response in Hg-treated mice is critically dependent on certain MHC class II (H-2) haplotypes [155] – specifically, the A locus genes –, T cells [156], and the IFN-γ cytokine [157] – but the exact mechanisms underlying the reaction are still unknown. However, a number of observations have been made. First, Hg may interact directly with fibrillarin-fibrillarin peptides, causing a physically altered molecule [158]. Secondly, non-apoptotic cell death, for example, by Hg, modifies the cleavage pattern for fibrillarin, resulting in neo-peptides of fibrillarin and exposing cryptic epitopes [158], which may be the target for T cells [159]. Since exposure to Hg is able to create a 19-kDa immunogenic fragment of fibrillarin even without direct molecular interaction between fibrillarin and Hg, the new cleavage pattern is likely to be of prime importance [160]. Finally, the immunopathology of Hg-induced autoimmunity is derived from deposition in the renal glomerular mesangium and systemically in the vessel walls of immune complexes consisting of IgG and a complement [161]. The mice exhibit a mild glomerulonephritis with mild proteinuria but not vasculitis or severe signs of tissue damage. AFA have been eluted from kidneys with deposits [162]. The lack of tissue IC deposits after treatment with silver [64] and Au (Hultman and Pollard, unpublished) indicates that the mere presence of serum AFA is not sufficient to induce IC deposits, and that other antigen-antibody systems than fibrillarin–anti-fibrillarin antibodies may also be involved.

22.9
Concluding Remarks

In conclusion, environmental factors are on theoretical grounds likely to be a major determinant of autoimmune diseases. However, only a limited (usually small) fraction of individuals exposed to a sufficient dose of an environmental agent will experience an autoimmune disease condition. This observation of individual susceptibility to environmental agents was made in 1962 by Kazantzis, who described four occupationally mercury-exposed workers with nephrotic syndrome and noted that there were other workers excreting equal or even larger amounts of mercury who were not affected [163]. The explanation lies in the genotype of the exposed person. To some extent and in some situations, this might be related to the toxicokinetics of the substance, but in most cases it is likely to depend on genes regulating the immune response [164].

The genotype-dependent susceptibility, the high degree of ignorance regarding the specific genes involved, and lack of knowledge regarding the genotype in many of the individuals who experience an autoimmune reaction to the different compounds make it a challenging task to link autoimmune diseases with environmental agents. Further increasing these difficulties is the possibility that the same environmental agent interacting with different genotypes may result in a number of different phenotypic disease expressions, including a mere acceleration and aggravation of autoimmune diseases with another primary etiology. However, a better recognition of environmental factors among clinicians taking care of patients with autoimmune diseases, and improved integration between studies in animals and humans leading to a "bench-to-bedside" concept of translational research, should enable a better understanding of the mechanisms involved in development of autoimmune diseases, including the complex interaction between genetic and environmental factors [165].

References

1 Jacobson D. L., Gange S. J., Rose N. R., Graham N. M., Epidemiology and estimated population burden of selected autoimmune diseases in the United States. Clin Immunol Immunopathol 1997, 84: 223–243.

2 Walsh S. J., Rau L. M., Autoimmune diseases: a leading cause of death among young and middle-aged women in the United States. Am J Public Health 2000, 90: 1463–1466.

3 Cooper G. S., Miller F. W., Pandey J. P., The role of genetic factors in autoimmune disease: implications for environmental research. Environ Health Perspect 1999, 107 Suppl 5: 693–700.

4 Myhre A. G., Halonen M., Eskelin P., Ekwall O., Hedstrand H., Rorsman F., Kampe O., Husebye E. S., Autoimmune polyendocrine syndrome type 1 (APS I) in Norway. Clin Endocrinol (Oxf) 2001, 54: 211–217.

5 Torgerson T. R., Ochs H. D., Immune dysregulation, polyendocrinopathy, enteropathy, X-linked syndrome: a model of immune dysregulation. Curr Opin Allergy Clin Immunol 2002, 2: 481–487.

6 Moriyama H., Eisenbarth G. S., Genetics and environmental factors in endocrine/organ-specific autoimmunity: have there been any major advances? Springer Semin Immunopathol 2002, 24: 231–242.

7 Becker K.G., Simon R.M., Bailey-Wilson J.E., Freidlin B., Biddison W.E., McFarland H.F., Trent J.M., Clustering of non-major histocompatibility complex susceptibility candidate loci in human autoimmune diseases. Proc Natl Acad Sci USA 1998, 95: 9979–9984.

8 Corvalan C.F., Kjellstrom T., Smith K.R., Health, environment and sustainable development: identifying links and indicators to promote action. Epidemiology 1999, 10: 656–660.

9 Holladay S.D., Prenatal immunotoxicant exposure and postnatal autoimmune disease. Environ Health Perspect 1999, 107 Suppl 5: 687–691.

10 Hoffman B., Sensitivity to sulfadiazine resembling acute disseminated lupus erythematosus. Archives of Dermatology Syphilis 1945, 51: 190–192.

11 Dustan H.P., Taylor R.D., Corcoran A.C., Rheumatic and febrile syndrome during prolonged hydralazine treatment. J Am Med Assoc 1954, 154: 23–29.

12 Ladd A.T., Procainamide-induced lupus erythematosus. N Engl J Med 1962, 267: 1357–1358.

13 Hess E.V., Are there environmental forms of systemic autoimmune diseases? Environ Health Perspect 1999, 107 Suppl 5: 709–711.

14 Antonov D., Kazandjieva J., Etugov D., Gospodinov D., Tsankov N., Drug-induced lupus erythematosus. Clin Dermatol 2004, 22: 157–166.

15 Burlingame R.W., Cervera R., Anti-chromatin (anti-nucleosome) autoantibodies. Autoimmun Rev 2002, 1: 321–328.

16 Vial T., Descotes J., Clinical toxicity of cytokines used as haemopoietic growth factors. Drug Saf 1995, 13: 371–406.

17 Preziati D., La Rosa L., Covini G., Marcelli R., Rescalli S., Persani L., Del Ninno E., Meroni P.L., Colombo M., Beck-Peccoz P., Autoimmunity and thyroid function in patients with chronic active hepatitis treated with recombinant interferon alpha-2a. Eur J Endocrinol 1995, 132: 587–593.

18 Khanna D., McMahon M., Furst D.E., Safety of tumour necrosis factor-alpha antagonists. Drug Saf 2004, 27: 307–324.

19 Classen J.B., The timing of immunization affects the development of diabetes in rodents. Autoimmunity 1996, 24: 137–145.

20 Serreze D.V., Chapman H.D., Post C.M., Johnson E.A., Suarez-Pinzon W.L., Rabinovitch A., Th1 to Th2 cytokine shifts in nonobese diabetic mice: sometimes an outcome, rather than the cause, of diabetes resistance elicited by immunostimulation. J Immunol 2001, 166: 1352–1359.

21 Gazda L.S., Baxter A.G., Lafferty K.J., Regulation of autoimmune diabetes: characteristics of non-islet-antigen specific therapies. Immunol Cell Biol 1996, 74: 401–407.

22 Maillefert J.F., Sibilia J., Toussirot E., Vignon E., Eschard J.P., Lorcerie B., Juvin R., Parchin-Geneste N., Piroth C., Wendling D., Kuntz J.L., Tavernier C., Gaudin P., Rheumatic disorders developed after hepatitis B vaccination. Rheumatology (Oxford) 1999, 38: 978–983.

23 Offit P.A., Hackett C.J., Addressing parents' concerns: do vaccines cause allergic or autoimmune diseases? Pediatrics 2003, 111: 653–659.

24 Chen R.T., Pool V., Takahashi H., Weniger B.G., Patel B., Combination vaccines: postlicensure safety evaluation. Clin Infect Dis 2001, 33 Suppl 4: S327–333.

25 Battafarano D.F., Battafarano N.J., Larsen L., Dyer P.D., Older S.A., Muehlbauer S., Hoyt A., Lima J., Goodman D., Lieberman M., Enzenauer R.J., Antigen-specific antibody responses in lupus patients following immunization. Arthritis Rheum 1998, 41: 1828–1834.

26 Klippel J.H., Karsh J., Stahl N.I., Decker J.L., Steinberg A.D., Schiffman G., A controlled study of pneumococcal polysaccharide vaccine in systemic lupus erythematosus. Arthritis Rheum 1979, 22: 1321–1325.

27 Magos L., Review on the toxicity of ethylmercury, including its presence as a preservative in biological and pharmaceutical products. J Appl Toxicol 2001, 21: 1–5.

28 Havarinasab S., Lambertsson L., Qvarnstrom J., Hultman P., Dose-response study of thimerosal-induced murine systemic autoimmunity. Toxicol Appl Pharmacol 2004, 194: 169–179.

29 Qvarnstrom J., Lambertsson L., Havarinasab S., Hultman P., Frech W., Determination of methylmercury, ethylmercury, and inorganic mercury in mouse tissues, following administration of thimerosal, by species-specific isotope dilution GC-inductively coupled plasma-MS. Anal Chem 2003, 75: 4120–4124.

30 Stratton K., Gable A., McCormick M.C.: Thimerosal-containing vaccines and neurodevelopmental disorders. Institute of Medicine, Washington D.C., 2001.

31 Blaxill M.F., Redwood L., Bernard S., Thimerosal and autism? A plausible hypothesis that should not be dismissed. Med Hypotheses 2004, 62: 788–794.

32 Nelson K.B., Bauman M.L., Thimerosal and autism? Pediatrics 2003, 111: 674–679.

33 Stehr-Green P., Tull P., Stellfeld M., Mortenson P.B., Simpson D., Autism and thimerosal-containing vaccines: lack of consistent evidence for an association. Am J Prev Med 2003, 25: 101–106.

34 Singh M., O'Hagan D., Advances in vaccine adjuvants. Nat Biotechnol 1999, 17: 1075–1081.

35 Kuroda Y., Nacionales D.C., Akaogi J., Reeves W.H., Satoh M., Autoimmunity induced by adjuvant hydrocarbon oil components of vaccine. Biomed Pharmacother 2004, 58: 325–337.

36 Reidenberg M.M., Adverse drug reactions: further controversy. Hosp Pharm 1976, 11: 376, 378.

37 Freni-Titulaer L.W., Kelley D.B., Grow A.G., McKinley T.W., Arnett F.C., Hochberg M.C., Connective tissue disease in southeastern Georgia: a case-control study of etiologic factors. Am J Epidemiol 1989, 130: 404–409.

38 Parks C.G., Conrad K., Cooper G.S., Occupational exposure to crystalline silica and autoimmune disease. Environ Health Perspect 1999, 107 Suppl 5: 793–802.

39 Brown J.M., Pfau J.C., Holian A., Immunoglobulin and lymphocyte responses following silica exposure in New Zealand mixed mice. Inhal Toxicol 2004, 16: 133–139.

40 Holsapple M.P., Developmental immunotoxicity testing: a review. Toxicology 2003, 185: 193–203.

41 Cooper G.S., Parks C.G., Occupational and environmental exposures as risk factors for systemic lupus erythematosus. Curr Rheumatol Rep 2004, 6: 367–374.

42 Lim S.Y., Ghosh S.K., Autoreactive responses to an environmental factor: 1. phthalate induces antibodies exhibiting anti-DNA specificity. Immunology 2003, 110: 482–492.

43 Kilburn K.H., Warshaw R.H., Prevalence of symptoms of systemic lupus erythematosus (SLE) and of fluorescent antinuclear antibodies associated with chronic exposure to trichloroethylene and other chemicals in well water. Environ Res 1992, 57: 1–9.

44 Griffin J.M., Blossom S.J., Jackson S.K., Gilbert K.M., Pumford N.R., Trichloroethylene accelerates an autoimmune response by Th1 T cell activation in MRL +/+ mice. Immunopharmacology 2000, 46: 123–137.

45 Nietert P.J., Sutherland S.E., Silver R.M., Pandey J.P., Knapp R.G., Hoel D.G., Dosemeci M., Is occupational organic solvent exposure a risk factor for scleroderma? Arthritis Rheum 1998, 41: 1111–1118.

46 Johnston E.N., Vinyl chloride disease. Br J Dermatol 1978, 99: 45–48.

47 Black C.M., Welsh K.I., Walker A.E., Bernstein R.M., Catoggio L.J., McGregor A.R., Jones J.K., Genetic susceptibility to scleroderma-like syndrome induced by vinyl chloride. Lancet 1983, 1: 53–55.

48 Schrallhammer-Benkler K., Ring J., Przybilla B., Meurer M., Landthaler M., Acute mercury intoxication with lichenoid drug eruption followed by mercury contact allergy and development of antinuclear antibodies. Acta Derm Venereol 1992, 72: 294–296.

49 Röger J., Zillikens D., Hartmann A.A., Burg G., Gleichmann E., Systemic autoimmune disease in a patient with longstanding exposure to mercury. European Journal of Dermatology 1992, 2.

50 Enestrom S., Hultman P., Does amalgam affect the immune system? A con-

troversial issue. Int Arch Allergy Immunol 1995, 106: 180–203.

51 Bariety J., Druet P., Laliberte F., Sapin C., Glomerulonephritis with γ- and BIC-globulin deposits induced in rats by mercuric chloride. Am J Pathol 1971, 65: 293–302.

52 Sapin C., Druet E., Druet P., Induction of antiglomerular basement membrane antibodies in the Brown-Norway rat by mercuric chloride. Clin Exp Immunol 1977, 28: 173–179.

53 Enestrom S., Hultman P., Immune-mediated glomerulonephritis induced by mercuric chloride in mice. Experientia 1984, 40: 1234–1240.

54 Robinson C. J., Abraham A. A., Balazs T., Induction of anti-nuclear antibodies by mercuric chloride in mice. Clin Exp Immunol 1984, 58: 300–306.

55 Roman-Franco A. A., Turiello M., Albini B., Ossi E., Milgrom F., Andres G. A., Anti-basement membrane antibodies and antigen–antibody complexes in rabbits injected with mercuric chloride. Clin Immunol Immunopathol 1978, 9: 464–481.

56 Bigazzi P. E., Autoimmunity and heavy metals. Lupus 1994, 3: 449–453.

57 Kosty M. P., Hench P. K., Tani P., McMillan R., Thrombocytopenia associated with auranofin therapy: evidence for a gold-dependent immunologic mechanism. Am J Hematol 1989, 30: 236–239.

58 Hall C. L., Fothergill N. J., Blackwell M. M., Harrison P. R., MacKenzie J. C., MacIver A. G., The natural course of gold nephropathy: long term study of 21 patients. Br Med J (Clin Res Ed) 1987, 295: 745–748.

59 Quarenghi M. I., Del Vecchio L., Casartelli D., Manunta P., Rossi R., MPO antibody-positive vasculitis in a patient with psoriatic arthritis and gold-induced membranous glomerulonephritis. Nephrol Dial Transplant 1998, 13: 2104–2106.

60 Tishler M., Nyman J., Wahren M., Yaron M., Anti-Ro (SSA) antibodies in rheumatoid arthritis patients with gold-induced side effects. Rheumatol Int 1997, 17: 133–135.

61 Robinson C. J., Balazs T., Egorov I. K., Mercuric chloride-, gold sodium thiomalate-, and D-penicillamine-induced antinuclear antibodies in mice. Toxicol Appl Pharmacol 1986, 86: 159–169.

62 Tournade H., Guery J. C., Pasquier R., Nochy D., Hinglais N., Guilbert B., Druet P., Pelletier L., Experimental gold-induced autoimmunity. Nephrol Dial Transplant 1991, 6: 621–630.

63 Qasim F. J., Thiru S., Gillespie K., Gold and D-penicillamine induce vasculitis and up-regulate mRNA for IL-4 in the Brown Norway rat: support for a role for Th2 cell activity. Clin Exp Immunol 1997, 108: 438–445.

64 Hultman P., Enestrom S., Turley S. J., Pollard K. M., Selective induction of anti-fibrillarin autoantibodies by silver nitrate in mice. Clin Exp Immunol 1994, 96: 285–291.

65 Hultman P., Ganowiak K., Turley S. J., Pollard K. M., Genetic susceptibility to silver-induced anti-fibrillarin autoantibodies in mice. Clin Immunol Immunopathol 1995, 77: 291–297.

66 Zelikoff J. T., Smialowicz R., Bigazzi P. E., Goyer R. A., Lawrence D. A., Maibach H. I., Gardner D., Immunomodulation by metals. Fundam Appl Toxicol 1994, 22: 1–7.

67 Prummel M. F., Strieder T., Wiersinga W. M., The environment and autoimmune thyroid diseases. Eur J Endocrinol 2004, 150: 605–618.

68 Padmos R. C., Bekris L., Knijff E. M., Tiemeier H., Kupka R. W., Cohen D., Nolen W. A., Lernmark A., Drexhage H. A., A high prevalence of organ-specific autoimmunity in patients with bipolar disorder. Biol Psychiatry 2004, 56: 476–482.

69 Kupka R., Nolen W., Post R., McElroy S., Althsuler L., Frye M., Keck P., Leverich G., Rush A., Suppes T., Pollio C., High rate of autoimmune thyroiditis in bipolar disorder:lack of association with lithium exposure. Biol Psychiatry 2002, 51: 305–311.

70 Rudofsky U. H., Lawrence D. A., New Zealand mixed mice: a genetic systemic lupus erythematosus model for assessing environmental effects. Environ Health Perspect 1999,07 Suppl 5: 713–721.

71 Hudson C.A., Cao L., Kasten-Jolly J., Kirkwood J.N., Lawrence D.A., Susceptibility of lupus-prone NZM mouse strains to lead exacerbation of systemic lupus erythematosus symptoms. J Toxicol Environ Health A 2003, 66: 895–918.

72 Ohsawa M., Takahashi K., Otsuka F., Induction of anti-nuclear antibodies in mice orally exposed to cadmium at low concentrations. Clin Exp Immunol 1988, 73: 98–102.

73 Leffel E.K., Wolf C., Poklis A., White K.L., Jr., Drinking water exposure to cadmium, an environmental contaminant, results in the exacerbation of autoimmune disease in the murine model. Toxicology 2003, 188: 233–250.

74 Lahoz C., del Pozo V., Gallardo S., Cardaba B., Jurado A., Cortegano I., del Amo A., Arrieta I., Palomino P., Immunological aspects of the toxic oil syndrome. Arch Toxicol Suppl 1997, 19: 65–73.

75 Bell S., Brand K., Meurer M., [Toxic oil syndrome – an example of an exogenously-induced autoimmune disease]. Hautarzt 1992, 43: 339–343.

76 Cardaba B., Ezendam J., Gallardo S., del Pozo V., Izquierdo M., Martin C., Cortegano I., Aceituno E., Rojo M., Arrieta I., Palomino P., Posada M., Lahoz C., DR2 antigens are associated with severity of disease in toxic oil syndrome (TOS). Tissue Antigens 2000,5: 110–117.

77 Weatherill A.R., Stang B.V., O'Hara K., Koller L.D., Hall J.A., Investigating the onset of autoimmunity in A.SW mice following treatment with "toxic oils". Toxicol Lett 2003, 136: 205–216.

78 Koller L.D., Stang B.V., Hall J.A., Posada de la Paz M., Ruiz Mendez M.V., Immunoglobulin and autoantibody responses in MRL/lpr mice treated with "toxic oils". Toxicology 2002, 178: 119–133.

79 Philen R.M., Hill R.H., Jr., Flanders W.D., Caudill S.P., Needham L., Sewell L., Sampson E.J., Falk H., Kilbourne E.M., Tryptophan contaminants associated with eosinophilia-myalgia syndrome. The Eosinophilia-Myalgia Studies of Oregon, New York and New Mexico. Am J Epidemiol 1993, 138: 154–159.

80 Yoshida S., Gershwin M.E., Autoimmunity and selected environmental factors of disease induction. Semin Arthritis Rheum 1993, 22: 399–419.

81 Philen R.M., Hill R.H., Jr., 3-(Phenylamino)alanine – a link between eosinophilia – algia syndrome and toxic oil syndrome? Mayo Clin Proc 1993, 68: 197–200.

82 Bournaud C., Orgiazzi J.J., Iodine excess and thyroid autoimmunity. J Endocrinol Invest 2003, 26: 49–56.

83 Lehmann P., Holzle E., Kind P., Goerz G., Plewig G., Experimental reproduction of skin lesions in lupus erythematosus by UVA and UVB radiation. J Am Acad Dermatol 1990, 22: 181–187.

84 Dourmishev L., Meffert H., Piazena H., Dermatomyositis: comparative studies of cutaneous photosensitivity in lupus erythematosus and normal subjects. Photodermatol Photoimmunol Photomed 2004, 20: 230–234.

85 Ansel J.C., Mountz J., Steinberg A.D., DeFabo E., Green I., Effects of UV radiation on autoimmune strains of mice: increased mortality and accelerated autoimmunity in BXSB male mice. J Invest Dermatol 1985, 85: 181–186.

86 Aubin F., Mechanisms involved in ultraviolet light-induced immunosuppression. Eur J Dermatol 2003,3: 515–523.

87 Caricchio R., McPhie L., Cohen P.L., Ultraviolet B radiation-induced cell death: critical role of ultraviolet dose in inflammation and lupus autoantigen redistribution. J Immunol 2003, 171: 5778–5786.

88 Cunningham M.W., Autoimmunity and molecular mimicry in the pathogenesis of post-streptococcal heart disease. Front Biosci 2003, 8: 533–543.

89 Hartung H.P., Infections and Guillan-Barré syndrome. Journal of Neurology, Neurosurgery and Psychiatry 1999,6: 277–279.

90 Cooke A., Zaccone P., Raine T., Phillips J.M., Dunne D.W., Infection and autoimmunity:are we winning the war, only to lose the peace? Trends in Parasitology 2004, 20: 316–321.

91 Shaver K.A., Boughman J.A., Nance W.E., Congenital rubella syndrome and

diabetes: a review of epidemiologic, genetic, and immunologic factors. Am Ann Deaf 1985. 130: 526–532.

92 Clarke W. L., Shaver K. A., Bright G. M., Rogol A. D., Nance W. E., Autoimmunity in congenital rubella syndrome. J Pediatr 1984, 104: 370–373.

93 Varela-Calvino R., Peakman M., Enteroviruses and type 1 diabetes. Diabetes Metab Res Rev 2003. 19: 431–441.

94 Tauriainen S., Salminen K., Hyoty H., Can enteroviruses cause type 1 diabetes? Ann NY Acad Sci 2003, 1005: 13–22.

95 Van Ghelue M., Moens U., Bendiksen S., Rekvig O. P., Autoimmunity to nucleosomes related to viral infection: a focus on hapten-carrier complex formation. J Autoimmun 2003, 20: 171–182.

96 Flodstrom-Tullberg M., Viral infections: their elusive role in regulating susceptibility to autoimmune disease. Microbes Infect 2003, 5: 911–921.

97 Rigby R. J., Rozzo S. J., Gill H., Fernandez-Hart T., Morley B. J., Izui S., Kotzin B. L., Vyse T. J., A novel locus regulates both retroviral glycoprotein 70 and anti-glycoprotein 70 antibody production in New Zealand mice when crossed with BALB/c. J Immunol 2004, 172: 5078–5085.

98 Adachi M., Watanabe-Fukunaga R., Nagata S., Aberrant transcription caused by the insertion of an early transposable element in an intron of the Fas antigen gene of lpr mice. Proc Natl Acad Sci USA 1993, 90: 1756–1760.

99 Nelson P. N., Carnegie P. R., Martin J., Davari Ejtehadi H., Hooley P., Roden D., Rowland-Jones S., Warren P., Astley J., Murray P. G., Demystified. Human endogenous retroviruses. Mol Pathol 2003, 56: 11–18.

100 Sewell D. L., Reinke E. K., Hogan L. H., Sandor M., Fabry Z., Immunoregulation of CNS autoimmunity by helminth and mycobacterial infections. Immunol Lett 2002, 82: 101–110.

101 Tanriverdi F., Silveira L. F., MacColl G. S., Bouloux P. M., The hypothalamic-pituitary-gonadal axis: immune function and autoimmunity. J Endocrinol 2003, 176: 293–304.

102 Jacobson J. D., Gonadotropin-releasing hormone and G proteins: potential roles in autoimmunity. Ann NY Acad Sci 2000, 917: 809–818.

103 Stewart J. J., The female X-inactivation mosaic in systemic lupus erythematosus. Immunol Today 1998, 19: 352–357.

104 Petri M., Prospective study of systemic lupus erythematosus pregnancies. Lupus 2004, 13: 688–689.

105 Mok C.C., Wong R.W., Lau C.S., Ovarian failure and flares of systemic lupus erythematosus. Arthritis Rheum 1999, 42: 1274–1280.

106 Sanchez-Guerrero J., Villegas A., Mendoza-Fuentes A., Romero-Diaz J., Moreno-Coutino G., Cravioto M. C., Disease activity during the premenopausal and postmenopausal periods in women with systemic lupus erythematosus. Am J Med 2001, 111: 464–468.

107 Greenstein B. D., Dhaher Y. Y., Bridges Ede F., Keser G., Khamashta M. A., Etherington J., Greenstein A. S., Coates P. J., Hall P. A., Hughes G. R., Effects of an aromatase inhibitor on thymus and kidney and on oestrogen receptors in female MRL/MP-lpr/lpr mice. Lupus 1993, 2: 221–225.

108 Apelgren L. D., Bailey D. L., Fouts R. L., Short L., Bryan N., Evans G. F., Sandusky G. E., Zuckerman S. H., Glasebrook A., Bumol T. F., The effect of a selective estrogen receptor modulator on the progression of spontaneous autoimmune disease in MRL lpr/lpr mice. Cell Immunol 1996, 173: 55–63.

109 Cooper G. S., Dooley M. A., Treadwell E. L., St Clair E. W., Gilkeson G. S., Hormonal and reproductive risk factors for development of systemic lupus erythematosus: results of a population-based, case-control study. Arthritis Rheum 2002, 46: 1830–1839.

110 McMurray R. W., May W., Sex hormones and systemic lupus erythematosus: review and meta-analysis. Arthritis Rheum 2003, 48: 2100–2110.

111 Yurino H., Ishikawa S., Sato T., Akadegawa K., Ito T., Ueha S., Inadera H., Matsushima K., Endocrine disruptors (environmental estrogens) enhance autoantibody production by B1 cells. Toxicol Sci 2004, 81: 139–147.

112 Ansar-Ahmed S., The immune system as a potential target for environmental estrogens (endocrine disrupters): a new emerging field. Toxicology 2000, 150: 191–206.

113 Noller K. L., Blair P. B., O'Brien P. C., Melton L. J., 3rd, Offord J. R., Kaufman R. H., Colton T., Increased occurrence of autoimmune disease among women exposed in utero to diethylstilbestrol. Fertil Steril 1988, 49: 1080–1082.

114 Burke L., Segall-Blank M., Lorenzo C., Dynesius-Trentham R., Trentham D., Mortola J. F., Altered immune response in adult women exposed to diethylstilbestrol in utero. Am J Obstet Gynecol 2001, 185: 78–81.

115 Forawi H. A., Tchounwou P. B., McMurray R. W., Xenoestrogen modulation of the immune system: effects of dichlorodiphenyltrichloroethane (DDT) and 2,3,7,8-tetrachlorodibenzo-p-dioxin (TCDD). Rev Environ Health 2004, 19: 1–13.

116 Holsapple M. P., Paustenbach D. J., Charnley G., West L. J., Luster M. I., Dietert R. R., Burns-Naas L. A., Symposium summary: children's health risk–what's so special about the developing immune system? Toxicol Appl Pharmacol 2004, 199: 61–70.

117 Fournie G. J., Saoudi A., Druet P., Pelletier L., Th2-type immunopathological manifestations induced by mercury chloride or gold salts in the rat: signal transduction pathways, cellular mechanisms and genetic control. Autoimmun Rev 2002, 1: 205–212.

118 Pollard K. M., Hultman P., Effects of mercury on the immune system. In Siegel A, Siegel S (eds): Metal Ions in Biological Systems 1997, 34: 421–440.

119 Hang L., Slack J. H., Amundson C., Izui S., Theofilopoulos A. N., Dixon F. J., Induction of murine autoimmune disease by chronic polyclonal B cell activation. J Exp Med 1983, 157: 874–883.

120 Lewis R. E., Jr., Cruse J. M., Johnson W. W., Mohammad A., Histopathology and cell-mediated immune reactivity in halothane-associated lymphomagenesis

and autoimmunity to BXSB/Mp and MRL/Mp mice. Exp Mol Pathol 1982, 36: 378–395.

121 Carpenter D. F., Steinberg A. D., Schur P. H., Talal N., The pathogenesis of autoimmunity in New Zealand mice. II. Acceleration of glomerulonephritis by polyinosinic-polycytidylic acid. Lab Invest 1970. 23: 628–634.

122 Pollard K. M., Pearson D. L., Hultman P., Hildebrandt B., Kono D. H., Lupus-prone mice as models to study xenobiotic-induced acceleration of systemic autoimmunity. Environ Health Perspect 1999, 107 Suppl 5: 729–735.

123 Abedi-Valugerdi M., Hu H., Moller G., Mercury-induced renal immune complex deposits in young (NZB x NZW)F1 mice: characterization of antibodies/autoantibodies. Clin Exp Immunol 1997, 110: 86–91.

124 Pollard K. M., Hultman P., Kono D. H.: Immunology and genetics of xenobiotic-induced autoimmunity. Autoimmunity Reviews 2005, 4: 282–288.

125 Pollard K. M., Pearson D. L., Hultman P., Deane T. N., Lindh U., Kono D. H., Xenobiotic acceleration of idiopathic systemic autoimmunity in lupus-prone bxsb mice. Environ Health Perspect 2001, 109: 27–33.

126 Vidal S., Gelpi C., Rodriguez-Sanchez J. L., (SWR x SJL)F1 mice: a new model of lupus-like disease. J Exp Med 1994, 179: 1429–1435.

127 Via C. S., Nguyen P., Niculescu F., Papadimitriou J., Hoover D., Silbergeld E. K., Low-dose exposure to inorganic mercury accelerates disease and mortality in acquired murine lupus. Environ Health Perspect 2003, 111: 1273–1277.

128 Michalets E. L., Update: clinically significant cytochrome P-450 drug interactions. Pharmacotherapy 1998, 18: 84–112.

129 Rubin R. L., Curnutte J. T., Metabolism of procainamide to the cytotoxic hydroxylamine by neutrophils activated in vitro. J Clin Invest 1989, 83: 1336–1343.

130 Jiang X., Khursigara G., Rubin R. L., Transformation of lupus-inducing

drugs to cytotoxic products by activated neutrophils. Science 1994, 266: 810–813.

131 Kretz-Rommel A., Duncan S. R., Rubin R. L., Autoimmunity caused by disruption of central T cell tolerance. A murine model of drug-induced lupus. J Clin Invest 1997, 99: 1888–1896.

132 Kretz-Rommel A., Rubin R. L., Disruption of positive selection of thymocytes causes autoimmunity. Nat Med 2000, 6: 298–305.

133 Scheinbart L. S., Johnson M. A., Gross L. A., Edelstein S. R., Richardson B. C., Procainamide inhibits DNA methyltransferase in a human T cell line. J Rheumatol 1991, 18: 530–534.

134 Deng C., Lu Q., Zhang Z., Rao T., Attwood J., Yung R., Richardson B., Hydralazine may induce autoimmunity by inhibiting extracellular signal-regulated kinase pathway signaling. Arthritis Rheum 2003, 48: 746–756.

135 Richardson B. C., Strahler J. R., Pivirotto T. S., Quddus J., Bayliss G. E., Gross L. A., O'Rourke K. S., Powers D., Hanash S. M., Johnson M. A., Phenotypic and functional similarities between 5-azacytidine-treated T cells and a T cell subset in patients with active systemic lupus erythematosus. Arthritis Rheum 1992, 35: 647–662.

136 Takeuchi T., Amano K., Sekine H., Koide J., Abe T., Upregulated expression and function of integrin adhesive receptors in systemic lupus erythematosus patients with vasculitis. J Clin Invest 1993, 92: 3008–3016.

137 Stiller-Winkler R., Radaszkiewicz T., Gleichmann E., Immunopathological signs in mice treated with mercury compounds – I. Identification by the popliteal lymph node assay of responder and nonresponder strains. Int J Immunopharmacol 1988, 10: 475–484.

138 Pauly J. L., Caron G. A., Suskind R. R., Blast transformation of lymphocytes from guinea pigs, rats, and rabbits induced by mercuric chloride in vitro. J Cell Biol 1969, 40: 847–850.

139 Jiang Y., Moller G., In vitro effects of HgCl2 on murine lymphocytes. I. Preferable activation of CD4+ T cells in a responder strain. J Immunol 1995, 154: 3138–3146.

140 Pollard K. M., Landberg G. P., The in vitro proliferation of murine lymphocytes to mercuric chloride is restricted to mature T cells and is interleukin 1 dependent. Int Immunopharmacol 2001, 1: 581–593.

141 Reardon C. L., Lucas D. O., Heavy-metal mitogenesis: Zn++ and Hg++ induce cellular cytotoxicity and interferon production in murine T lymphocytes. Immunobiology 1987, 175: 455–469.

142 Hu H., Abedi-Valugerdi M., Moller G., Pretreatment of lymphocytes with mercury in vitro induces a response in T cells from genetically determined low-responders and a shift of the interleukin profile. Immunology 1997, 90: 198–204.

143 Jiang Y., Moller G., In vitro effects of HgCl2 on murine lymphocytes. II. Selective activation of T cells expressing certain V beta TCR. Int Immunol 1996, 8: 1729–1736.

144 Heo Y., Lee W. T., Lawrence D. A., In vivo the environmental pollutants lead and mercury induce oligoclonal T cell responses skewed toward type-2 reactivities. Cell Immunol 1997, 179: 185–195.

145 Nakashima I., Pu M. Y., Nishizaki A., Rosila I., Ma L., Katano Y., Ohkusu K., Rahman S. M., Isobe K., Hamaguchi M., et al., Redox mechanism as alternative to ligand binding for receptor activation delivering disregulated cellular signals. J Immunol 1994, 152: 1064–1071.

146 McCabe M. J., Jr., Santini R. P., Rosenspire A. J., Low and nontoxic levels of ionic mercury interfere with the regulation of cell growth in the WEHI-231 B-cell lymphoma. Scand J Immunol 1999, 50: 233–241.

147 Whitekus M. J., Santini R. P., Rosenspire A. J., McCabe M. J., Jr., Protection against CD95-mediated apoptosis by inorganic mercury in Jurkat T cells. J Immunol 1999, 162: 7162–7170.

148 McCabe M. J., Jr., Whitekus M. J., Hyun J., Eckles K. G., McCollum G., Rosenspire A. J., Inorganic mercury attenu-

ates CD95-mediated apoptosis by interfering with formation of the death inducing signaling complex. Toxicol Appl Pharmacol 2003, 190: 146–156.

149 Daum J. R., Shepherd D. M., Noelle R. J., Immunotoxicology of cadmium and mercury on B-lymphocytes – I. Effects on lymphocyte function. Int J Immunopharmacol 1993, 15: 383–394.

150 Haggqvist B., Hultman P., Murine metal-induced systemic autoimmunity: baseline and stimulated cytokine mRNA expression in genetically susceptible and resistant strains. Clin Exp Immunol 2001, 126: 157–164.

151 Johansson U., Hansson-Georgiadis H., Hultman P., The genotype determines the B cell response in mercury-treated mice. Int Arch Allergy Immunol 1998, 116: 295–305.

152 Hultman P., Enestrom S., Pollard K. M., Tan E. M., Anti-fibrillarin autoantibodies in mercury-treated mice. Clin Exp Immunol 1989, 78: 470–477.

153 Reuter R., Tessars G., Vohr H. W., Gleichmann E., Luhrmann R., Mercuric chloride induces autoantibodies against U3 small nuclear ribonucleoprotein in susceptible mice. Proc Natl Acad Sci USA 1989, 86: 237–241.

154 Arnett F. C., Reveille J. D., Goldstein R., Pollard K. M., Leaird K., Smith E. A., Leroy E. C., Fritzler M. J., Autoantibodies to fibrillarin in systemic sclerosis (scleroderma). An immunogenetic, serologic, and clinical analysis. Arthritis Rheum 1996, 39: 1151–1160.

155 Hultman P., Johansson U., Strain differences in the effect of mercury on murine cell-mediated immune reactions. Food Chem Toxicol 1991, 29: 633–638.

156 Hultman P., Johansson U., Dagnaes-Hansen F., Murine mercury-induced autoimmunity: the role of T-helper cells. J Autoimmun 1995, 8: 809–823.

157 Kono D. H., Balomenos D., Pearson D. L., Park M. S., Hildebrandt B., Hultman P., Pollard K. M., The prototypic Th2 autoimmunity induced by mercury is dependent on IFN-gamma and not Th1/Th2 imbalance. J Immunol 1998, 161: 234–240.

158 Pollard K. M., Lee D. K., Casiano C. A., Bluthner M., Johnston M. M., Tan E. M., The autoimmunity-inducing xenobiotic mercury interacts with the autoantigen fibrillarin and modifies its molecular and antigenic properties. J Immunol 1997, 158: 3521–3528.

159 Kubicka-Muranyi M., Griem P., Lubben B., Rottmann N., Luhrmann R., Gleichmann E., Mercuric-chloride-induced autoimmunity in mice involves up-regulated presentation by spleen cells of altered and unaltered nucleolar self antigen. Int Arch Allergy Immunol 1995, 108: 1–10.

160 Pollard K. M., Pearson D. L., Bluthner M., Tan E. M., Proteolytic cleavage of a self-antigen following xenobiotic-induced cell death produces a fragment with novel immunogenic properties. J Immunol 2000, 165: 2263–2270.

161 Hultman P., Turley S. J., Enestrom S., Lindh U., Pollard K. M., Murine genotype influences the specificity, magnitude and persistence of murine mercury-induced autoimmunity. J Autoimmun 1996, 9: 139–149.

162 Hultman P., Enestrom S., Mercury induced antinuclear antibodies in mice: characterization and correlation with renal immune complex deposits. Clin Exp Immunol 1988, 71: 269–274.

163 Kazantzis G., Schiller K. F., Asscher A. W., Drew R. G., Albuminuria and the nephrotic syndrome following exposure to mercury and its compounds. Q J Med 1962, 31: 403–418.

164 Nielsen J. B., Hultman P., Mercury-induced autoimmunity in mice. Environ Health Perspect 2002, 110 Suppl 5: 877–881.

165 Hood E., The Environment-Autoimmune link. Environ Health Perspect 2003, 111: A274–276.

166 Hultman P., Taylor A., Yang J. M., Pollard K. M., The effect of xenobiotic exposure on spontaneous autoimmunity in (SWR×SJL)F1 hybrid mice. J Toxicol Env Health 2005, in press.

23
Genetics of Autoantibody Production in Mouse Models of Lupus

Dwight H. Kono and Argyrios N. Theofilopoulos

23.1
Introduction

Systemic lupus erythematosus (SLE) is a chronic autoimmune disease that most commonly affects the skin, kidney, and the hematologic, musculoskeletal, and central nervous systems, although virtually any organ can be involved. It is associated with extensive clinical heterogeneity with considerable variability in the severity and course of disease, as well as in the type and extent of tissue involvement. Disease manifestations are mediated by autoantibodies that, directly or through immune complex deposition, result in cell or tissue destruction. The level, specificity, and other characteristics of autoantibodies are thought to largely determine the clinical presentation of individual patients. Importantly, despite the aforementioned clinical heterogeneity, a common hallmark of lupus is the presence of autoantibodies to nuclear antigens, particularly ribonuclear proteins (RNPs) and nucleosome components, which have been increasingly implicated in disease pathogenesis. In more recent support for this, such antibodies were found to predate the onset of SLE [1] and to play a role in the activation of self-reactive B cells and dendritic cells via a TLR-dependent mechanism [2, 3]. Thus, there is substantial interest in identifying the etiopathogenic basis for their production.

Susceptibility to antinuclear antibodies and SLE has been shown to depend on a combination of genetic, environmental, and stochastic factors; genetic predisposition is likely an important prerequisite for disease development in the majority of cases. Similar to most common diseases, inheritance of lupus is polygenic, with each genetic alteration contributing to only a portion of the total autoimmune trait variance. Disease manifestations are also dependent on the specific combination of disease-predisposing as well as disease-suppressing genes (epistasis). Studies in human SLE have identified a number of candidate genes as well as several promising loci [4–6]. Overall, however, despite substantial progress, identification of the specific genetic alterations has remained elusive in large part because of the difficulty of characterizing complex inheritance.

Autoantibodies and Autoimmunity: Molecular Mechanisms in Health and Disease. Edited by K. Michael Pollard
Copyright © 2006 WILEY-VCH Verlag GmbH & Co. KGaA, Weinheim
ISBN: 3-527-31141-6

A complementary approach has been to use spontaneous and induced mouse models to define the genetic basis for lupus susceptibility. By utilizing the power of homogeneous backgrounds and defined genetic manipulation, significant inroads have been made toward identifying predisposing genes and in defining their roles in autoimmune susceptibility. Two different types of genetic approaches have yielded significant new insights. The first uses reverse genetics to determine whether an alteration in a specific gene enhances susceptibility to lupus. Although most reported cases have occurred serendipitously, a substantial number of lupus-promoting single-gene mutations have nonetheless been identified. These have suggested a number of common and unique pathways that can lead to loss of tolerance and the development of systemic autoimmune manifestations, including autoantibody production. This topic is covered in Chapter 24. The more traditional approach has been to identify predisposing genes by mapping autoimmune traits to chromosomal locations and then screening for the responsible polymorphisms (forward genetics). This chapter will review progress in this area with emphasis on susceptibility to autoantibodies.

23.2
Identifying Genes Predisposing to Systemic Autoimmunity

Advances over the past 10 years have made possible identification of disease susceptibility genes with only modest effects. Prior to this, attempts to find susceptibility genes were generally limited to either a candidate approach, wherein genes are screened based on specific characteristics, or, if traits are transmitted by simple Mendelian inheritance, by high-resolution mapping and cloning. Previous studies were able to identify two predisposing genes by screening candidates, the *H-2* (polymorphic variants) [7–9] and the *Fasl* (gld mutation) [10, 11], and two others, the *Fas* (*lpr* mutations) [12] and the *Hcph* (hemopoietic cell phosphatase or SHP-1, motheaten mutations) [13, 14], by a combination of mapping and candidate screening. The dominant *Yaa* gene that promotes B-cell activation and autoimmunity in male BXSB mice was also shown to exhibit Mendelian transmission, but it has not been cloned because of its location on the Y-chromosome, which cannot be mapped by conventional methods [15]. Details of these genes and their roles in autoantibody production and systemic autoimmunity have been previously reviewed [7].

The strategy for identifying genes with smaller quantitative effects, which constitute the majority of lupus susceptibility genes, has some variations but can be typically divided into four main steps. The first entails mapping traits to specific chromosomal regions by either regional or genome-wide scans using microsatellite or single-nucleotide polymorphisms. The intervals are generally 20–40 cM in size and typically contain tens to hundreds of possible candidate genes. In the next step, interval-specific congenic strains that each contain a single introgressed genomic fragment encompassing the relevant chromosomal region are generated and characterized. This permits confirmation of the initial mapping study as well as more precise definition of the contributions of individual predisposing genes. Clues about the identity of susceptibility genes and where they might be expressed are also obtained. The third step involves narrowing the interval to as small a size as possible, typically 0.5–2.0 Mb. This is critical for reducing the number of potential candidate genes that need to be screened and serves to eliminate with certainty adjacent polymorphic genes from consideration. Alternatively, microarray analysis comparing expression profiles of tissues from interval congenic and wild-type mice has been successfully applied to identify possible candidate genes in congenic mice with large introgressed intervals. A well-known example is the *Ifi202* gene within the NZB *Nba2* locus on chromosome 1, which was identified by this approach [16]. Verification of genes identified by this microarray approach, however, may still require the generation and testing of smaller interval congenic sublines. This is definitely true for *Ifi202*, since others have subsequently reported multiple lupus susceptibility loci within the *Nba2* interval [17]. Another potential drawback is that detection of expression polymorphisms requires testing the appropriate tissues and cells and may depend on activation state and developmental stage, which in most cases are not known. The final step consists of screening candidate genes within the fragment for structural and/or expression polymorphisms that are consistent with the observed component phenotypes. The recently completed sequence of the mouse genome has greatly facilitated this process.

23.3
Mouse Models of SLE in Mapping Studies

A large number of different strains have been used to map loci predisposing to SLE-related traits (Table 23.1). These include not only the major lupus-prone mice [15, 18], the NZB, NZW, MRL-*Fas*[lpr], and BXSB, but also the NZM2410, NZM2328, and BXD2 recombinant inbred lines and C57BL/6 (B6)×129 mixed background mice, which also develop significant spontaneous disease. Several other induced or genetically manipulated models of systemic autoimmune disease – such as mercury-induced autoimmunity [19], thrombin-exposed galactose-alpha1-3-galactose–deficient mice [20], *M. bovis*–induced lupus in NOD mice [21], and FcγRIIb-deficient mice – have also been analyzed (Table 23.1).

With regard to the relatedness of these strains, a recent study [22] has largely verified through single-nucleotide polymorphism (SNP) analysis the historical origin of inbred mice [23]. Roughly 67% of the haplotypes were found to be derived from *Mus musculus domesticus* and 21% from Asian mice (mainly *Mus musculus musculus* and *molossinus* subspecies). When compared with the B6, other inbred strains were found to exhibit, albeit in different regions, low rates of polymorphism in about two-thirds of the genome, with the remaining third having considerable divergence, most often from one strain having the *domesticus* and the other the *musculus* background. Furthermore, more careful analysis

Table 23.1 Susceptible lupus-prone strains and other mouse
models used to map susceptibility genes.

Strains or mixed backgrounds susceptible to spontaneous lupus	Induced and mutant models
NZB	Mercury-induced autoimmunity (DBA/2 resistance)
NZW	*M. bovis*–induced systemic autoimmunity (NOD susceptible)
NZM2410	FcγRIIb-deficient mice (B6 susceptible)
NZM2328	
MRL-*Fas*^lpr	
BXSB	
BXD2	
C57BL/6×129	

suggested that the genomic makeup of inbred strains represents the effects of recent breeding practices that created mosaics of two major ancestral strains. Thus, the genomic heterogeneity of lupus-predisposing genes in inbred strains will be limited by this common derivation, and many of the predisposing genetic alterations will likely be present in non-autoimmune strains if the predisposing mutations were derived from the original founders.

23.4
Lupus Quantitative Trait Loci

Currently, at least 113 loci linked to one or more lupus traits have been identified with distribution over all 19 autosomal chromosomes (Table 23.2, listed by chromosomal location). Of these, 72 were found to affect levels of autoantibodies, including antinuclear antibodies (ANAs), rheumatoid factors (RFs), and antibodies to DNA, chromatin, histone, cardiolipin, gp70, red blood cells, and platelets. Autoantibody-related loci were located on all autosomal chromosomes except 15. Lupus traits were mapped not only to lupus-prone strains but also, in some crosses, to non-autoimmune mice. These strains include the B6, B10, C57L, BALB/c, 129, SWR, DBA/2, and the diabetes-prone NOD. The large number of lupus-related loci, however, is likely somewhat overestimated since this number includes loci with only suggestive linkages. Furthermore, several overlapping or adjacent loci mapped in different studies may in fact be identical since some of these are linked to similar trait(s) and the same strain background. Nonetheless, despite these considerations it is evident that there is considerable heterogeneity and complexity in the genetics of lupus and autoantibody production among inbred mice. Overall, the inheritance of lupus in all spontaneous mouse models examined has been shown to be polygenic and dependent on the number and specific combination of susceptibility loci. Similarly, it appears that many of the autoimmune manifestations in lupus, including autoantibody specificities, are also to a large extent determined by specific loci [24–27].

23.5
Loci in NZB, NZW, and NZB×NZW Recombinant Inbred Mice

Significant progress has been made in delineating the role of quantitative trait loci (QTL) in disease pathogenesis and in identifying candidate genes for NZB and NZW mice and their recombinants, NZM2410 and NZM2328. Mapping studies involving a variety of crosses to autoimmune and normal strains have identified at least 21 NZB and 19 NZW susceptibility loci, as well as lupus-predisposing loci in several non-autoimmune strains, including BALB/c, SWR, C57BL/6, C57BL/10, and C57L (Table 23.2). Furthermore, four chromosomal regions in NZW mice linked to disease suppression, termed Sles1–4, have also been described [27]. In this case, loci were considered to be lupus-suppressing NZW genes since pure NZW mice develop only mild lupus despite having the NZW Sle1, Sle2, and Sle3 loci, which in the B6 background results in severe lethal autoimmunity. This interpretation, however, depends on the point of view since it is also possible that lupus-predisposing genes in the B6 might be responsible. Ultimately, designation of loci as disease promoting or inhibiting will depend on the structure and function of the polymorphic alleles.

Several non-MHC loci identified in NZB and NZW mice have been confirmed in more than one mapping study. These include Sle1/Cgnz1/Agnz1 (NZW-derived) and Lbw7/Nba2 (NZB-derived) loci on chromosome 1, Lbw2/Sle2/nba1/Imh1/Mott/Spm1 (NZB-derived) on chromosome 4, Lbw5/Sle3S/Sle5 (NZW-derived) and Nba5/Aem2 (NZB-derived) on chromosome 7, Lbw8 (NZB-derived) on proximal chromosome 8, Sgp3 on chromosome 13 (NZB- and NZW-derived), and nwa1 (NZW-derived) on chromosome 16 (Table 23.2). Loci on chromosomes 1, 4, 7, and 13 have been confirmed by interval congenic lines.

There is particular interest in defining the NZ chromosome 1 susceptibility loci since they overlap with homologous regions on human chromosome 1 linked to SLE in several independent studies [5, 6, 28]. For both the NZW and NZB intervals on chromosome 1, congenic mice have been characterized and several promising candidate genes have been identified. With regard to the NZW loci, Sle1 was initially shown in B6 congenics (B6.NZMc1) to enhance the production of IgG antinuclear antibodies, particularly to the H2A/H2B/DNA nucleosomal components [29–31]. Although mice with this single locus did not develop glomerulonephritis (GN), bi- or triple-locus congenic mice with combinations of Sle1 with Sle2 (chromosome 4) and Sle3 (chromosome 7) developed varying degrees of GN and early mortality depending on the specific combination [31, 32]. Other studies using bone marrow transfers with various combinations of B6.NZMc1, wild-type B6, and mice deficient for B cells or T cells showed that Sle1 is functionally expressed in both B and T cells [33]. Interval-specific NZM2328 congenic mice containing the non-autoimmune Cgnz1 interval from the C57L strain (NZMC57Lc1, NZW-derived) were also generated and demonstrated significant reductions in anti-dsDNA and related antibodies as well as GN [34]. This essentially reciprocal congenic to B6.*Sle1* shows quite nicely that the lack of a single interval can have a significant impact on disease.

More precise delineation of the *Sle1* locus using subinterval congenic mice has subsequently shown that *Sle1* is a cluster of at least four (*Sle1a–d*) loci, each conferring varying degrees of loss of tolerance to chromatin and enhancement of systemic autoimmunity [35]. The most potent appears to be *Sle1b*, which leads to ANA production in B6.*Sle1b* congenics and fatal GN when combined with either the *Fas^{lpr}* or *Yaa* autoimmune-accelerating mutations [36]. Individually, however, *Sle1a–c* do not induce severe GN when combined with other *Sle* loci, indicating the additive nature of their contributions and demonstrating the complexity that may exist within a locus originally thought to consist of a single susceptibility gene. Moreover, this finding raises the specter of other loci being similarly composed of clusters of predisposing genes with individually weak effects.

Physical mapping and cloning of the 900-kb genomic segment of *Sle1b* (NZM2410/NZW) revealed the presence of 24 expressed genes and two pseudogenes, among which 19 were expressed in the spleen and therefore considered possible candidates [37]. Furthermore, this interval contained the SLAM/ CD2 family genes, which encode surface molecules on hematopoietic lineage cells that mediate stimulatory or inhibitory signals. Strikingly, there was extensive polymorphism between the B6.*Sle1b* (*Sle1b* haplotype) and B6 genomes that involved 10 genes: *Usp23, Nit1, Refbp2, Cd229, Cs1, CD48, CD84, Ncstn, Copa,* and *Pxf.* Interestingly, *Cd224* was expanded in B6 mice to a four-locus cluster, of which transcripts from three of the genes were detected in spleen cDNA. Among these genes, *CD48, CD150, CD84,* and *Ly108* appear to be the strongest candidates, although it is possible that the entire haplotype contributes to susceptibility. In this regard, the *Sle1b* haplotype is also present in most inbred strains, including 129/SvJ, A/J, AKR/J, BALB/cJ, C3H/HeJ, CBA/J, CE/J, DBA/ 2J, DDY, Jc1, LP/J, MRL/MpJ, NOD/Lt, NZB/B1WJ, NZW, P/J, PL/J, SB/Le, SEA/GnJ, SJL/J, SM/J, WB/Re, PERA/EiJ, PERA/RkJ, PERC/EiJ, SK/CamEiJ, and SF/CamEiJ. In contrast, the B6 haplotype is limited to B6, C57BR/cdJ, C57L/M, RF/J, MOLF/EiJ, and MOLE/EiJ. Thus, the *Sle1b* and B6 haplotypes appear to be of ancestral origin. Recently, a 129 locus on chromosome 1 overlapping with *Sle1b* was shown to promote lupus-like disease when present on the B6 background [38] (see below). This could be due to the *Sle1b* haplotype and suggests that chromosome 1 intervals from any of the strains with the *Sle1b*-haplotype including NZB mice would have a similar effect.

The complement receptor 2 (*Cr2*) gene has been identified as a candidate gene for *Sle1c* [39]. Comparison of the *Cr2* alleles of NZM2410/NZW and B6 strains revealed considerable polymorphism, with differences in 16 nucleotide residues (11 resulting in amino acid changes) and a three-nucleotide insertion/ deletion [39]. Most significant was a C → A (His → Asn) mutation at residue 1342 located in either the external domain short consensus repeat 7 (SCR7) of

CR1 or the SCR1 of CR2, which introduced a new N-linked glycosylation site within the ligand-binding domain. This mutation caused reduced C3dg binding, CR1/CR2-mediated signaling, and IgG response to T-dependent antigens. Based on the known structure of CR1/CR2, it appeared that glycosylation of the Asn residue altered the function of CR2 by inhibiting its dimerization [39]. Similarly, reduced levels of CR1/CR2 in SLE have also been found [40]. The *Cr2* gene in mice encodes by alternative splicing both CR1 and CR2 glycoproteins [41, 42]. CR1/CR2 is expressed primarily on the surfaces of mature B cells and follicular dendritic cells and binds C3 and C4 split products on antigens or immune complexes. CR2 reduces the B-cell activation threshold and plays a role in both B-cell apoptosis and antigen processing/presentation, particularly within the germinal center. Mice lacking *Cr2* have reduced T-dependent responses, generation of memory B cells, and germinal center formation. CR2 appears to help establish tolerance by enhancing the presentation of self-antigens, as suggested by the accelerated disease observed in *Fas^{lpr}* mice when combined with *Cr2*-deficiency [43, 44]. However, to what extent transfer of the *Sle1b* SLAM/CD2 haplotype (present in the 129 genome where the knockout of *Cr2* was generated) plays a role in the lupus-like disease attributed to Cr2 deficiency remains to be determined.

B6 congenic mice containing the NZB chromosome 1 interval (B6.*Nba2*) have also been generated and characterized [16]. These mice, similar to the *Sle1* congenics, spontaneously produce increased levels of IgG anti-DNA and anti-chromatin autoantibodies, but do not develop GN. Furthermore, combining this interval with the *Yaa* also leads to higher levels of autoantibodies, including those to DNA, chromatin, and gp70, as well as the development of severe lethal GN. At least part of this effect must be due to the *Sle1b* SLAM/CD2 haplotype present in NZB mice. In this regard, other studies attempting to more precisely map alterations in B-cell activation induced by the NZB chromosome 1 interval suggest that the *Nba2* interval is also composed of more than one susceptibility gene [17].

Analysis of microarray expression profiles of spleen cells from B6 and B6.*Nba2* congenic mice recently identified *Ifi202* as a potential candidate gene for the *Nba2* [16]. In mice containing the NZB *Nba2* interval, there was a more than 10-fold increase in *Ifi202* and a decrease in *Ifi203* (both within the Ifi200 cluster), and, impressively, out of 11,000 genes these were the only differences detected. Increased expression of Ifi202 at both the RNA and protein levels was also demonstrated in NZB spleen cells compared with NZW. The specific polymorphism responsible for the increased expression is not known, although several differences identified in the promoter region of the *Ifi202* gene are suspected. *Ifi202* is an interferon-inducible family of two genes (*Ifi202a* and *Ifi202b*) that has been suggested to play a role in cell survival, proliferation, and differentiation [45]. *Ifi202* is also upregulated by IL-6 through STAT3 activation [46].

Another candidate for *Nba2* is the FcγRIIb, which in NZB mice has two deletions in the promoter region [47]. These changes are associated with lower lev-

els of FcγRII expression in germinal centers and with hypergammaglobulinemia. FcγRIIb on B cells normally inhibits B-cell antigen receptor signaling by
recruiting SHIP and possibly to a lesser extent SHP-1 to the antigen receptor
[48, 49]. Lack of FcγRIIb enhances humoral responses and in B6 mice leads to
the development of lupus-like disease [50]. However, similar to *Nba2*, to what
extent this is due to the *Sle1b* SLAM/CD3 haplotype will need to be determined.

Congenic mice for the chromosome 4 loci have also been studied. B6.NZMc4
congenic mice, which contain a mixture of NZW genome on the acromeric portion and NZB genome on the telomeric part of the interval, were found to develop generalized B-cell hyperactivity, expansion of B1 cells, and increased polyclonal IgM levels, but no increase in IgG antinuclear antibodies or GN [51]. It
was suggested that the expanded B1 cell population, which expresses higher levels of costimulatory molecules such as B7, might promote autoimmunity by enhancing self-antigen presentation T cells [52]. More recently, BWF1 congenics
that contain one or no copies of the NZW chromosome 4 interval (*Lbw2*)
showed reduced B-cell activation to LPS, decreased IgM levels and autoantibodies, less glomerular immune complex deposits and GN, and reduced mortality,
but, unexpectedly, no difference in levels of IgG autoantibodies [53]. Nevethe-
less, spontaneous IgG autoantibody-secreting cells were significantly reduced,
and the number of these cells correlated with the amount of kidney deposits
but not serum levels. Furthermore, kidney eluates did not demonstrate significant difference in the autoantibody repertoire in deposits from BWF1 mice with
one or no copy of the NZB *Lbw2* locus. Thus, it was concluded that serum levels of IgG autoantibodies did not reflect the actual differences in production of
autoantibodies and that the primary defect of *Lbw2* is B-cell hyperactivity. Interestingly, congenic NZM2328 mice with replacement of the *Adnz1* chromosome
4 interval that overlaps *Sle2* and *Lbw2* (NZM.C57Lc4) developed severe GN similar to wild-type NZM2328, but had markedly reduced to normal levels of anti-
dsDNA antibodies [34]. This model is particularly interesting since elucidation
of the responsible genetic alteration should yield significant insights about the
etiopathogenesis of antinuclear antibodies. Overall, findings in these various interval congenic mice suggest the presence of multiple subloci within the NZW
chromosome 4 interval and/or considerable influence of background genes.

A NZB C1q polymorphism located within the *Nba1/Lbw2/Imh1/Mott* interval
on chromosome 4 that downregulates C1q levels was recently reported and suggested to be a potential candidate [54]. This is an attractive possibility since deficiencies of the early complement components (C1q–s, C2, or C4) predispose to
SLE in humans. Moreover, homozygous C1q knockout mice develop a strain
background–dependent loss of tolerance to nuclear antigens and abnormal accumulation of apoptotic bodies in the kidney glomeruli, suggesting that C1q may
prevent systemic autoimmunity by playing a non-redundant role in the clearance of apoptosis byproducts [55, 56]. More recent fine-mapping, however, has
indicated that C1q is not within the *Lbw2* interval [53].

The chromosome 7 interval is similar to chromosome 1 in that both NZW
and NZB loci have been mapped to this region. In terms of the NZW locus, the

B6 congenic for *Sle3/Sle5* (B6.NZMc7) was found to develop elevated, but low, levels of antinuclear antibodies and a low incidence of GN, but when combined with other *Sle* loci, it promoted severer lupus manifestations, depending on the combinations [32, 57]. *Sle3* was initially thought to promote generalized T-cell activation because of a marked increase in activated T cells, elevated CD4 : CD8 ratios, and resistance to activation-induced cell death in congenic mice [57]. More recently, however, using bone marrow chimera experiments with allotype-labeled B and T cells from B6 and B6.Sle3/5 mice, it was shown that the susceptibility genes were expressed in a non-lymphocyte bone marrow–derived population that affected T-cell selection, survival, or both [58].

B6.*Yaa* mice congenic for the NZB chromosome 7 locus (B6.*Nba5*) have also been generated and characterized [59]. Compared with B6.*Yaa* mice, congenics develop increased gp70 immune complexes and severer GN, although the incidence was low and the onset delayed compared with B6.Yaa congenic for the *Nba2* (NZB chromosome 1) locus. Remarkably, *Nba5* had no effect on either anti-DNA or anti-chromatin IgG autoantibodies. Thus, *Nba5* represents another locus that affects autoantibody specificity.

A CD22^a variant, present in NZW and NZB mice and located within the *Sle5* and *Lbw5* intervals, has been suggested as a possible candidate [60]. CD22^a has a 794-bp insertion within the second intron of a cluster of short interspersed nucleotide elements, which leads to aberrant alternative splicing. This is associated with reduced LPS-stimulated expression of CD22 in B cells to about half the level observed with the CD22^b (B6 mice) allele. The CD22 is a candidate gene for *Sle5*, but it is not a candidate for *Lbw5*, since congenic NZB mice containing the NZW *Lbw5* interval have enhanced disease (unpublished observations).

The *Sgp3* locus on chromosome 13 has also been confirmed in B6 mice containing either the relevant NZW or NZB intervals [59, 61]. *Sgp3* was primarily associated with increased production of gp70; however, in autoimmune-prone *Yaa* mice *Sgp3* also enhanced GN and in some cases autoantibodies to DNA and chromatin.

23.6
Loci Identified in Crosses of MRL-*Fas^{lpr}* Mice

Although the *Fas^{lpr}* mutation promotes loss of tolerance and autoimmunity, the development of lupus depends on background susceptibility genes. In fact, in humans, the majority of individuals with deficiencies of Fas or molecules related to the same pathway (FasL, caspase 10) develop ALPS or Canale-Smith syndrome with lymphoproliferation, but little to no evidence of SLE [62]. This suggests that the frequency of such lupus-enhancing variants is relatively rare in humans and that the genes involved in promoting autoimmunity must have special characteristics. Several groups have identified lupus-related QTL in a variety of crosses with the highly lupus-susceptible MRL-*Fas^{lpr}* mice (Table 23.2).

Table 23.2 QTL predisposing to autoantibodies and other lupus-related traits.

Name	Chr	cM	Trait	Strain allele	Ref.
Bxs4	1	7.7	LN	BXSB	72
–	1	19.5	**IgM RBC**	BALB/c	84
Bxs1	1	32.8	GN/ANA/spleen	BXSB	71
–	1	54.0	**IgM ssDNA/IgM histone**	BALB/c	85
Bana3	1	60.9	ANA (*M. bovis*)	NOD	79
Bxs2	1	63.1	GN/ANA/spleen	BXSB	71
–	1	65.0	Sialadenitis	MRL	66
Swrl1	1	87.9	**dsDNA/histone**	SWR	86
Sle1	1	87.9	dsDNA/GN/spleen	NZM2410 (NZW)	87, 88
Hmr1	1	87.9/92.3	glom dep (HgIA resistance)	DBA/2	19
–	1	87.9–95.8	ANA/chrom/dsDNA/ ssDNA	129	38
Cgnz1	1	92.3	Chronic GN	NZM2328 (NZW)	89
Lbw7	1	92.3	**chrom**/spleen	NZB	24
Nba2	1	92.3/94.2	ANA/gp70IC/GN	NZB	90–92
Bxs3	1	100.0	dsDNA	BXSB	71
Agnz1	1	101.0	Acute GN	NZM2328 (NZW)	89
–	1	106.3	ssDNA	NZW	85
–	2		ssDNA/dsDNA	MRL +/+,lpr/+	93
–	2	78	dsDNA/RF	DBA/2	77
Rends (Wbw1)	2	86.0	Mortality/GN	NZW	94
–	3	17	**IgG RBC**	NZB	84
Sles2	3	35.2	dsDNA/GN (resistance)	NZW	27
Bxs5	3	39.7	ANA/IgG3	BXSB	72
–	3	44–50.4	ANA/chrom/ssDNA	B6	38
Lprm2	3	66.2	Vasculitis (resistance)	MRL	64
–	4	7	**IgG RBC**	NZB	84
Arvm1	4	19.8	Vasculitis	MRL	67
Lprm1	4	32.5	Vasculitis	MRL	64
Acla2	4	40.0	aCL	BXSB	73
Sle2	4	44.5	GN	NZM2410 (NZW)	87
Spm1	4	45.9	Spleen	NZB	95
Adaz1	4	49.6	dsDNA	NZM2328	89
–	4	51.3–61.5	dsDNA	B6	38
–	4	53.5	dsDNA/RF	B6	77
Lbw2	4	55.6	Mortality/GN/spleen	NZB	24
Sles2	4	57.6	dsDNA/GN (resistance)	NZW	27
–	4	62.3	GN	NZB	90

Table 23.2 (continued)

Name	Chr	cM	Trait	Strain allele	Ref.
Arvm2	4	57.6	Vasculitis	MRL	67
Asm2	4	65.0	Sialadenitis	MRL female	66
nba1	4	65.7	GN	NZB	96
Lmb1	4	**69.8**	Lprn/**dsDNA**	B6	63
Imh1/Mott	4	**69/69.8**	Hyper IgM/GN/**dsDNA**	NZB	97, 98
Aia1	4	**75**	**RBC**	NZB	99
Sle6	5	20.0	GN	NZW	27
Lmb2	5	**41.0**	Lprn/**dsDNA**	MRL	63
Lprm4	5	54.0	Spleen	MRL	64
Lbw3	5	84.0	Mortality	NZW	24
–	6	**21.3**	**IgG RBC**	NZB	84
–	6	35.0	GN (resistance)	MRL	100
Lbw4	6	64.0	Mortality	NZB	24
–	6	**74.0**	**dsDNA**	B6	88
Sle5	7	**0.5**	**dsDNA**	NZM2410 (NZW)	88
Lrdm1	7	6.0	GN	MRL	65
Sle3	7	16.0	GN	NZM2410 (NZW)	88
Lbw5	7	**23.0**	Mortality	NZW	24
Nba5	7	**23.0**	gp70IC	NZB	59
Lmb3	7	**27.0**	Lprn/**dsDNA**	MRL	63
–	7	15–26.5	GN	129	38
Sle3	7	28.0	GN	NZM (NZW)	87
Aem2	7	**28.4**	**RBC**	NZB	84, 95
–	7	**51.5**	GN	NZB	90
–	7	**56.5**	**dsDNA**	NZB	101
Myo1	7	69.0	MI	BXSB	73
Pbat2	8	**11**	**Platelet**	BXSB	73
sbb1	9	17.0	Spleen (FcγRIIb ko)	BALB/c	82
baa1	9	**28.0**	**IgM ssDNA/IgM histone**	BALB/c	85
–	9	56	IgG dsDNA/ssDNA	BALB/c	102
Gp1	9	**57.9**	gp70IC	BXSB	103
Bana2	10	**0.0**	**ANA** (*M. bovis*)	BALB/c	79
Asm1	10	38/40	Sialadenitis	MRL	66
Aem3	10	**41.5**	**RBC**	NZB	95
Lmb4	10	51.0	Lprn/GN	MRL	63
–	10	69.0	GN	NZM or B6	88
–	**10**	**70.0**	**chrom**	B10	104

Table 23.2 (continued)

Name	Chr	cM	Trait	Strain allele	Ref.
–	11	2.0/17.0	GN	NZB	92
–	11	20.0	GN/dsDNA	NZM	88
Lbw8	11	28.0	chrom	NZB	24
–	11	28.5	ssDNA	NZW	85
–	11	54.0	dsDNA/ssDNA/aCL	MRL	93
–	12	1	IgM RBC	NZB	84
sbb2	12	6.0	ANA (FcγRIIb ko)	B6	82
–	12	2.3–6	gp70/gp70IC/chrom/ ssDNA/dsDNA/GN	NZB	102, 105
–	12	13	gp70/gp70IC/chrom/ ssDNA/dsDNA/GN	NZW	102, 105
Lrdm2	12	27.0	GN	MRL	65
–	12	28	chrom/GN	NZB	102
–	12	41	dsDNA/ssDNA	NZB	102
Bxs6	13	24.0	gp70/gp70IC	BXSB	103
Spg3	13	41.0	gp70IC/gp70	NZW, NZB	59, 61, 106
–	13	43.4–46	IgM RBC	NZB	84
–	13	59.0	gp70IC/GN	B10	104
–	13	71.0	dsDNA	NZM	87
–	13	71.0	GN	NZB	90
–	14	19.5	Histone	NZW	85
Swrl2	14	27.5	GN/dsDNA	SWR	86
Myo2	14	39.0	MI	BXSB	73
–	14	42.5/40.0	GN	NZB	92
Lprm3	14	44.0	GN (resistance)	MRL	64
Paam1	15	17.8	Arthritis in males	MRL	107
Lprm5	16	21.0	dsDNA	MRL	64
Bah2	16	34.6	RBC (*M. bovis*)	BALB/c	79
nwa1	16	38.0	histone	NZW	85
nwa1	16	38.0	GN/dsDNA	NZW	101
Bana1/Bah1	17	0.9	ANA/RBC (*M. bovis*)	NOD	79
sbb3	17	16.0	ANA/spleen (FcγRIIb ko)	BALB/c	82
Acla1	17	18.2	aCL	NZW/BXSB	73
Sles1	17	18.8	GN/dsDNA (resistance)	NZW	27
Phat1	17	18.9	Platelet	NZW/BXSB	73
Wbw2	17	24.0	Mortality/GN	NZW	94
Agnz2	17	55.7	Acute GN	C57L	89
Swrl3	18	20	dsDNA/histone	SWR	86
–	18	22.0	Sialadenitis	MRL	66
Lbw6	18	47.0	Mortality/GN	NZW	24

Table 23.2 (continued)

Name	Chr	cM	Trait	Strain allele	Ref.
nwa2	19	41.0	ssDNA	NZW	85
–	19	50.0	dsDNA	NZM	87

Autoantibody QTLs and specificity are indicated by boldface type. Loci with linkages $P<0.01$ or lod>1.9 are included. Chromosome (Chr) and locations in cM (Mouse Genome Informatics, Jackson Laboratory) are based on the estimated peak or the marker with the highest association. Traits are disease manifestations that mapped to loci.

chrom = anti-chromatin autoantibody; aCL = anticardiolipin autoantibody; dsDNA = anti-dsDNA autoantibody; glom dep = glomerular IgG deposits; GN = glomerulonephritis; gp70IC = gp70 immune complexes (represents levels of anti-gp70 autoAbs); histone: anti-histone autoantibody, LN = lymphadenopathy; Lprn = lymphoproliferation; MI = myocardial infarct, platelet = anti-platelet autoantibody and thrombocytopenia; RBC = anti-RBC autoantibody; spleen = splenomegaly.

In the trait column, induced or genetically modified models are indicated in parentheses as follows: FcγRIIbko = FcγRIIb-deficient mice; HgIA = mercury-induced autoimmunity; *M. bovis* = M. bovis i.v.–induced model.

Nineteen QTL for one or more autoimmune trait have been identified in at least 14 of the autosomal chromosomes. The number of loci is in part related to the different strains of crosses used and wide spectrum of traits examined, including GN, arthritis, sialadenitis, and vasculitis. A few of the loci, such as those on chromosomes 4 (Arvm1, Lprm1), 5 (*Lmb2, Lprm4*), 7 (*Lmb3, Ldrm1*), and 10 (*Lmb4, Asm1*) overlap and therefore may represent the same susceptibility gene [63–66]. Loci to several autoantibody specificities have been identified, including chromatin, dsDNA, ssDNA, and cardiolipin.

The CD72^c variant in MRL mice, which originated from the LG/J strain, has 13 amino acid substitutions, compared with the CD72^b allele (C3H strain), that include acidic, basic, and neutral changes and it is a candidate for the *Arvm1* locus [67]. CD72 is a member of the C-type lectin superfamily and is expressed on the surface of B cells [68]. It acts as a negative regulator of B-cell activation and also plays a role in B-cell development.

23.7
Loci in BXSB Crosses

The *Yaa* gene is responsible for the development of severe lupus-like disease in BXSB males, but, similar to the *Fas^{lpr}* mutation, susceptibility is also highly dependent on other BXSB background genes [15, 69, 70]. Genome-wide searches to define these genes have identified 13 BXSB-derived loci encompassing eight chromosomes in backcrosses of BXSB to C57BL/10 (B10) or to NZW strains (Table 23.2). In reciprocal male BXSB×B10 backcrosses, five QTL were found to be linked to one or more traits, including antinuclear antibodies, lymphoproliferation, and GN [71, 72]. Four were located in different regions on chromosome 1 and one was mapped to chromosome 3. Other loci with suggestive linkages were also identified on chromosomes 4, 10, and 13. By contrast, in a male BXSB×NZW backcross study, a completely different set of BXSB loci for other traits that included anticardiolipin antibodies, anti-platelet antibodies, thrombocytopenia, and myocardial infarction were found to map to chromosomes 4, 7, 8, 14, and 17 [73]. Finally, in another study of female (BXSB×NZW) F_2 mice, two BXSB loci were identified, one on chromosome 1 to splenomegaly and the other on chromosome 4 (*Lxw1*) to anti-chromatin autoantibodies [74]. Interestingly, although female (BXSB×NZW) F_1 and female (NZB×NZW) F_1 mice both developed accelerated disease compared with parental strains, the genetic contributions of BXSB and NZB loci to this additive effect were completely different. This suggests that at least some of the susceptibility gene variants in these strains may not be derived from the common ancestral Asian and European mouse strains.

BXSB loci (*Bxs1–4*) on chromosome 1 have also been somewhat confirmed with four congenic B10.*Yaa* mice containing large and overlapping chromosome 1 fragments of the BXSB genome [75]. Three of these intervals, however, contain more than one *Bxs* locus, and therefore more precise mapping will be required to verify the presence of these loci and to more precisely delineate their characteristics.

23.8
Loci in Other Spontaneous Lupus Crosses

A recent study documented lupus-like disease in (129×B6) hybrids and identified loci on chromosomes 1 (129-derived), 3 (B6-derived), and 4 (B6-derived) that promote autoantibodies to nuclear antigens, including DNA and chromatin [38] (Table 23.2). Furthermore, introgression of the 129 chromosome 1 interval in B6 congenic mice was sufficient to cause loss of tolerance to nuclear antigens and the production of autoantibodies. The 129 chromosome 1 region overlaps with *Sle1b*, and the findings may be related to the aforementioned polymorphisms of the SLAM/CD2 locus [37]. Since 129×B6 mixed backgrounds are often used to define characteristics of mice with gene knockouts, these results suggest caution in ascribing lupus manifestations solely to the deficient gene, particularly if the gene is located on chromosome 1 [76].

Another recently identified model of lupus and rheumatoid arthritis is the BXD2 recombinant inbred strain [77]. This line is one of approximately 80 B6×DBA/2 recombinant inbred strains originally developed at the Jackson Laboratory [78]. BXD2 mice spontaneously develop a systemic autoimmune disease, characterized by anti-DNA autoantibodies, rheumatoid factor (RF), immune complex GN, severe erosive arthritis, and a reduced lifespan of 14 months [77]. Mapping susceptibility loci using 20 recombinant BXD strains identified two loci: a DBA/2 locus on chromosome 2 that was linked to anti-DNA autoantibodies and a B6 locus on chromosome 4 linked to RF levels.

23.9
Loci Identified in Induced or Mutant Models of Lupus

Loci contributing to systemic autoimmunity have also been identified in several induced or mutant models of SLE. In mercury-induced autoimmunity, most strains are susceptible with the notable exception of the DBA/2. Mapping of F_2 crosses between the DBA/2 and susceptible SJL or NZB identified a single DBA/2 locus on chromosome 1 (*Hmr1*) that was linked to reduced glomerular immune complex deposition [19]. Interestingly, antibodies to nucleoli, a characteristic specificity observed in this disease, were affected only by the H-2^s haplotype and no other background genes.

Intravenous *Mycobacterium bovis* (bacillus Calmette-Guerin) given to type I diabetes mellitus–susceptible NOD mice prevents diabetes but, remarkably, induces systemic autoimmunity manifested by hemolytic anemia, antinuclear antibodies, immune complex–mediated GN, and exacerbation of sialadenitis [21]. When backcrosses to BALB/c mice were analyzed for predisposing loci, hemolytic anemia mapped to two loci on chromosomes 17 (*Bah1*) and 16 (*Bah2*) and ANAs to 17 (*Bana1*), 10 (*Bana2*), and 1 (*Bana3*). No locus was identified for GN. Interestingly, two of the four regions (*Bana3*, *Bah1/Bana1*) overlap with previously identified lupus-predisposing loci. Another interesting observation is that, other than the MHC region, none of the lupus-predisposing loci co-localized with diabetes loci. Thus, there is no evidence for common autoimmune-predisposing genes in NOD mice, although lupus- and diabetes-susceptibility genes shared by both NOD and BALB/c mice have not been ruled out [79].

Deficiency of FcγRIIb has been shown to enhance autoimmunity in several different disease models, including spontaneous lupus [50], type II collagen-induced arthritis [80], and type IV collagen-induced Goodpasture's syndrome [81]. Other complementation studies documented that the FcγRIIb knockout synergizes with the *Yaa* gene and, to a lesser extent, with the *Sle1* locus, but surprisingly not with the *Fas^{lpr}* defect [82]. In terms of lupus, background genes are also critically important as evidenced by the fact that lack of FcγRIIb in B6, but not in BALB/c, mice results in systemic autoimmunity. Genome-wide analysis to define the genetic basis for this difference in susceptibility revealed three regions, designated *sbb1–3* on chromosomes 9, 12, and 17, that were linked to ANAs, spleen weight, and/or proteinuria [82] (Table 23.2). One of these loci, *sbb1*, was derived from the non-susceptible BALB/c genome. Notably, none of the B6 loci identified in the (129×B6) cross (chromosomes 3 and 4) were found in this study. This suggests that the 129-gene segment may not contribute to the development of lupus in the FcγRIIb knockouts or may be a reflection of differences in the BALB/c and 129 genomes (different sets of susceptibility genes that overlap with B6).

23.10
Conclusions

The cumulative data suggest that susceptibility to lupus and the variation in disease manifestations among strains are due to the additive and epistatic contribution of diverse sets of susceptibility genes with any one strain generally having a few major predisposing loci. Even within the inbred strains, there is considerable genetic heterogeneity, with susceptibility genes derived from both recent and ancestral mutations/variants. There is not necessarily a clear-cut relationship of genotype to phenotype, and the observed effects may be highly dependent on what other susceptibility/resistance genes are present. To add further complexity, loci may be composed of a cluster of subloci and there may be several potential candidate genes within the narrowed intervals. Thus, a major difficulty in both mouse and human SLE will be how to determine the contribution of single polymorphisms.

Certain tentative conclusions can also be made about the nature of loci linked to the production of self-reactive antibodies. In different backgrounds, it is clearly evident that completely different sets of loci can predispose to similar autoantibody specificities. This genetic heterogeneity is consistent with different pathogenic mechanisms involved in loss of tolerance and autoantibody production. In contrast, certain loci can predispose to several autoantibody specificities, implying that these genes may affect common pathways of self-tolerance. Other loci are linked to only one autoantibody specificity in one or more different strains, which provides direct evidence that autoantibody specificity can be genetically imposed. In the case of *Sgp3* on chromosome 13 (NZB- and NZW-derived), the mechanism may simply be related to the production of the gp70 self-antigen. In contrast, the basis for *Adnz1*'s effect on anti-dsDNA autoantibodies is not clear, but it may be related to the TLR9 pathway [3] or degradation of DNA [83].

Overall, as presented in this review, there has been substantial progress in defining the genetics of lupus in multiple mouse models. Along with this, however, has come a greater appreciation of the large number of genes that mediate the various autoimmune traits, the complexity of the interplay between genetic elements that result in autoimmune manifestations, and the difficulties that will need to be surmounted in order to identify and verify predisposing mutations and variant alleles. Nevertheless, the foundation for further advancement has been laid for many of the major intervals and approaches to meet these challenges are being applied. These genetic studies will undoubtedly yield significant new and important insights into the etiopathogenesis of systemic autoimmunity and the factors that lead to autoantibody production.

Acknowledgments

This is publication number 17506-IMM from the Department of Immunology, The Scripps Research Institute, La Jolla, CA. The work herein was supported by National Institutes of Health grants AR42242, ES08666, AI059777, and AR39555.

References

1 M. R. Arbuckle, M. T. McClain, M. V. Rubertone, R. H. Scofield, G. J. Dennis, J. A. James, J. B. Harley. *N Engl J Med* 2003, 349, 1526–1533.

2 G. A. Viglianti, C. M. Lau, T. M. Hanley, B. A. Miko, M. J. Shlomchik, A. Marshak-Rothstein. *Immunity* 2003, 19, 837–847.

3 M. W. Boule, C. Broughton, F. Mackay, S. Akira, A. Marshak-Rothstein, I. R. Rifkin. *J Exp Med* 2004, 199, 1631–1640.

4 E. K. Wakeland, K. Liu, R. R. Graham, T. W. Behrens. *Immunity* 2001, 15, 397–408.

5 S. K. Nath, J. Kilpatrick, J. B. Harley. *Curr Opin Immunol* 2004, 16, 794–800.

6 B. P. Tsao. *Curr Opin Rheumatol* 2004, 16, 513–521.

7 D. H. Kono, R. Baccala, A. N. Theofilopoulos, Genes and genetics of murine lupus, in *Systemic Lupus Erythematosus*, R. G. Lahita (ed.), Academic Press, San Diego, 2004, 225–263.

8 B. Chiang, E. Bearer, A. Ansari, K. Dorshkind, M. E. Gershwin. *J Immunol* 1990, 145, 94–101.

9. R. Merino, L. Fossati, M. Lacour, R. Lemoine, M. Higaki, S. Izui. *Eur J Immunol* 1992, 22, 295–299.

10 D. H. Lynch, M. L. Watson, M. R. Alderson, P. R. Baum, R. E. Miller, T. Tough, M. Gibson, T. Davis-Smith, C. A. Smith, K. Hunter, D. Bhat, W. Din, R. G. Goodwin, M. F. Seldin. *Immunity* 1994, 1, 131–136.

11 T. Takahashi, M. Tanaka, C. I. Brannan, N. A. Jenkins, N. G. Copeland, T. Suda, S. Nagata. *Cell* 1994, 76, 969–976.

12 R. Watanabe-Fukunaga, C. I. Brannan, N. G. Copeland, N. A. Jenkins, S. Nagata. *Nature* 1992, 356, 314–317.

13 L. D. Shultz, P. A. Schweitzer, T. V. Rajan, T. Yi, J. N. Ihle, R. J. Matthews, M. L. Thomas, D. R. Beier. *Cell* 1993, 73, 1445–1454.

14 H. W. Tsui, K. A. Siminovitch, L. deSouza, F. W. L. Tsui. *Nature Genet* 1993, 4, 124–129.

15 A. N. Theofilopoulos, F. J. Dixon. *Adv Immunol* **1985**, 37, 269–390.

16 S. J. Rozzo, J. D. Allard, D. Choubey, T. J. Vyse, S. Izui, G. Peltz, B. L. Kotzin. *Immunity* 2001, 15, 435–443.

17 J. E. Wither, G. Lajoie, S. Heinrichs, Y. C. Cai, N. Chang, A. Ciofani, Y. H. Cheung, R. MacLeod. *J Immunol* 2003, 171, 1697–1706.

18 A. N. Theofilopoulos, D. H. Kono, Murine lupus models: gene-specific and genome-wide studies, in *Systemic Lupus Erythematosus*, R. G. Lahita (ed.), Academic Press, San Diego 1999, 145–181.

19 D. H. Kono, M. S. Park, A. Szydlik, K. M. Haraldsson, J. D. Kuan, D. L. Pearson, P. Hultman, K. M. Pollard. *J Immunol* 2001, 167, 2396–2403.

20 J. G. Schoenecker, R. K. Johnson, A. P. Lesher, J. D. Day, S. D. Love, M. R. Hoffman, T. L. Ortel, W. Parker, J. H. Lawson. *Am J Pathol* 2001, 159, 1957–1969.

21 P. A. Silveira, A. G. Baxter. *Autoimmunity* 2001, 34, 53–64.

22 C. M. Wade, E. J. Kulbokas, 3rd, A. W. Kirby, M. C. Zody, J. C. Mullikin, E. S. Lander, K. Lindblad-Toh, M. J. Daly. *Nature* 2002, 420, 574–578.

23 J. A. Beck, S. Lloyd, M. Hafezparast, M. Lennon-Pierce, J. T. Eppig, M. F. Festing, E. M. Fisher. *Nat Genet* 2000, 24, 23–25.

24 D. H. Kono, R. W. Burlingame, D. G. Owens, A. Kuramochi, R. S. Balderas,

D. Balomenos, A. N. Theofilopoulos. *Proc Natl Acad Sci USA* 1994, 91, 10168–10172.

25 T. J. Vyse, B. L. Kotzin. *Annu Rev Immunol* 1998, 16, 261–292.

26 L. Morel, E. K. Wakeland. *Curr Opin Immunol* 1998, 10, 718–725.

27 L. Morel, X. H. Tian, B. P. Croker, E. K. Wakeland. *Immunity* 1999, 11, 131–139.

28 P. M. Gaffney, K. L. Moser, R. R. Graham, T. W. Behrens. *Rheum Dis Clin North Am* 2002, 28, 111–126.

29 L. Morel, C. Mohan, Y. Yu, B. P. Croker, N. Tian, A. Deng, E. K. Wakeland. *J Immunol* 1997, 158, 6019–6028.

30 L. Morel, Y. Yu, K. R. Blenman, R. A. Caldwell, E. K. Wakeland. *Mamm Genome* 1996, 7, 335–339.

31 C. Mohan, E. Alas, L. Morel, P. Yang, E. K. Wakeland. *J Clin Invest* 1998, 101, 1362–1372.

32 L. Morel, B. P. Croker, K. R. Blenman, C. Mohan, G. Huang, G. Gilkeson, E. K. Wakeland. *Proc Natl Acad Sci USA* 2000, 97, 6670–6675.

33 E. S. Sobel, C. Mohan, L. Morel, J. Schiffenbauer, E. K. Wakeland. *J Immunol* 1999, 162, 2415–2421.

34 S. T. Waters, M. McDuffie, H. Bagavant, U. S. Deshmukh, F. Gaskin, C. Jiang, K. S. Tung, S. M. Fu. *J Exp Med* 2004, 199, 255–264.

35 L. Morel, K. R. Blenman, B. P. Croker, E. K. Wakeland. *Proc Natl Acad Sci USA* 2001, 98, 1787–1792.

36 B. P. Croker, G. Gilkeson, L. Morel. *Genes Immun* 2003, 4, 575–585.

37 A. E. Wandstrat, C. Nguyen, N. Limaye, A. Y. Chan, S. Subramanian, X. H. Tian, Y. S. Yim, A. Pertsemlidis, H. R. Garner, Jr., L. Morel, E. K. Wakeland. *Immunity* 2004, 21, 769–780.

38 A. E. Bygrave, K. L. Rose, J. Cortes-Hernandez, J. Warren, R. J. Rigby, H. T. Cook, M. J. Walport, T. J. Vyse, M. Botto. *PLoS Biol* 2004, 2, E243.

39 S. A. Boackle, V. M. Holers, X. Chen, G. Szakonyi, D. R. Karp, E. K. Wakeland, L. Morel. *Immunity* 2001, 15, 775–785.

40 H. V. Marquart, A. Svendsen, J. M. Rasmussen, C. H. Nielsen, P. Junker, S. E. Svehag, R. G. Leslie. *Clin Exp Immunol* 1995, 101, 60–65.

41 D. T. Fearon, M. C. Carroll. *Annu Rev Immunol* 2000, 18, 393–422.

42 M. C. Carroll. *Adv Immunol* 2000, 74, 61–88.

43 A. P. Prodeus, S. Goerg, L. M. Shen, O. O. Pozdnyakova, L. Chu, E. M. Alicot, C. C. Goodnow, M. C. Carroll. *Immunity* 1998, 9, 721–731.

44 X. Wu, N. Jiang, C. Deppong, J. Singh, G. Dolecki, D. Mao, L. Morel, H. D. Molina. *J Immunol* 2002, 169, 1587–1592.

45 D. Choubey, B. L. Kotzin. *Front Biosci* 2002, 7, 252–262.

46 R. Pramanik, T. N. Jorgensen, H. Xin, B. L. Kotzin, D. Choubey. *J Biol Chem* 2004, 279, 16121–16127.

47 Y. Jiang, S. Hirose, R. Sanokawa-Akakura, M. Abe, X. Mi, N. Li, Y. Miura, J. Shirai, D. Zhang, Y. Hamano, T. Shirai. *Int Immunol* 1999, 11, 1685–1691.

48 M. Ono, H. Okada, S. Bolland, S. Yanagi, T. Kurosaki, J. V. Ravetch. *Cell* 1997, 90, 293–301.

49 M. J. S. Nadler, B. Chen, J. S. Anderson, H. H. Wortis, B. G. Neel. *J Biol Chem* 1997, 272, 20038–20043.

50 S. Bolland, J. V. Ravetch. *Immunity* 2000, 13, 277–285.

51 C. Mohan, L. Morel, P. Yang, E. K. Wakeland. *J Immunol* 1997, 159, 454–465.

52 C. Mohan, L. Morel, P. Yang, E. K. Wakeland. *Arthritis Rheum* 1998, 41, 1652–1662.

53 M. K. Haraldsson, N. G. dela Pas, J. G. Kuan, M. L. Santiago-Raber, A. N. Theofilopoulos, D. H. Kono. *J Immuno*, in press,

54 Y. Miura-Shimura, K. Nakamura, M. Ohtsuji, H. Tomita, Y. Jiang, M. Abe, D. Zhang, Y. Hamano, H. Tsuda, H. Hashimoto, H. Nishimura, S. Taki, T. Shirai, S. Hirose. *J Immunol* 2002, 169, 1334–1339.

55 M. Botto, C. Dell'Agnola, A. E. Bygrave, E. M. Thompson, H. T. Cook, F. Petry, M. Loos, P. P. Pandolfi, M. J. Walport. *Nat Genet* 1998, 19, 56–59.

56 D. A. Mitchell, M. C. Pickering, J. Warren, L. Fossati-Jimack, J. Cortes-Hernandez, H. T. Cook, M. Botto, M. J. Walport. *J Immunol* 2002, 168, 2538–2543.

57 C. Mohan, Y. Yu, L. Morel, P. Yang, E. K. Wakeland. *J Immunol* 1999, 162, 6492–6502.

58 E. S. Sobel, L. Morel, R. Baert, C. Mohan, J. Schiffenbauer, E. K. Wakeland. *J Immunol* 2002, 169, 4025–4032.

59 S. Kikuchi, L. Fossati-Jimack, T. Moll, H. Amano, E. Amano, A. Ida, N. Ibnou-Zekri, C. Laporte, M. L. Santiago-Raber, S. J. Rozzo, B. L. Kotzin, S. Izui. *J Immunol* 2005, 174, 1111–1117.

60 C. Mary, C. Laporte, D. Parzy, M. T. Santiago, F. Stefani, F. Lajaunias, R. M. Parkhouse, T. L. O'Keefe, M. S. Neuberger, S. Izui, L. Reininger. *J Immunol* 2000, 165, 2987–2996.

61 C. Laporte, B. Ballester, C. Mary, S. Izui, L. Reininger. *J Immunol* 2003, 171, 3872–3877.

62 A. K. Vaishnaw, E. Toubi, S. Ohsako, J. Drappa, S. Buys, J. Estrada, A. Sitarz, L. Zemel, J. L. Chu, K. B. Elkon. *Arthritis Rheum* 1999, 42, 1833–1842.

63 S. Vidal, D. H. Kono, A. N. Theofilopoulos. *J Clin Invest* 1998, 101, 696–702.

64 Y. Wang, M. Nose, T. Kamoto, M. Nishimura, H. Hiai. *Am J Pathol* 1997, 151, 1791–1798.

65 M. L. Watson, J. K. Rao, G. S. Gilkeson, P. Ruiz, E. M. Eicher, D. S. Pisetsky, A. Matsuzawa, J. M. Rochelle, M. F. Seldin. *J Exp Med* 1992, 176, 1645–1656.

66 M. Nishihara, M. Terada, J. Kamogawa, Y. Ohashi, S. Mori, S. Nakatsuru, Y. Nakamura, M. Nose. *Arthritis Rheum* 1999, 42, 2616–2623.

67 W. Qu, T. Miyazaki, M. Terada, L. Lu, M. Nishihara, A. Yamada, S. Mori, Y. Nakamura, H. Ogasawara, C. Yazawa, S. Nakatsuru, M. Nose. *Eur J Immunol* 2000, 30, 2027–2037.

68 J. R. Parnes, C. Pan. *Immunol Rev* 2000, 176, 75–85.

69 C. C. Hudgins, R. T. Steinberg, D. M. Klinman, M. J. P. Reeves, A. D. Steinberg, M. J. Reeves. *J Immunol* 1985, 134, 3849–3854.

70 S. Izui, M. Higaki, D. Morrow, R. Merino. *Eur J Immunol* 1988, 18, 911–915.

71 M. B. Hogarth, J. H. Slingsby, P. J. Allen, E. M. Thompson, P. Chandler, K. A. Davies, E. Simpson, B. J. Morley, M. J. Walport. *J Immunol* 1998, 161, 2753–2761.

72 M. E. Haywood, M. B. Hogarth, J. H. Slingsby, S. J. Rose, P. J. Allen, E. M. Thompson, M. A. Maibaum, P. Chandler, K. A. Davies, E. Simpson, M. J. Walport, B. J. Morley. *Arthritis Rheum* 2000, 43, 349–355.

73 A. Ida, S. Hirose, Y. Hamano, S. Kodera, Y. Jiang, M. Abe, D. Zhang, H. Nishimura, T. Shirai. *Eur J Immunol* 1998, 28, 2694–2703.

74 D. H. Kono, M. S. Park, A. N. Theofilopoulos. *J Immunol* 2003, 171, 6442–6447.

75 M. E. Haywood, N. J. Rogers, S. J. Rose, J. Boyle, A. McDermott, J. M. Rankin, V. Thiruudaian, M. R. Lewis, L. Fossati-Jimack, S. Izui, M. J. Walport, B. J. Morley. *J Immunol* 2004, 173, 4277–4285.

76 J. D. Gillmore, W. L. Hutchinson, J. Herbert, A. Bybee, D. A. Mitchell, R. P. Hasserjian, K. Yamamura, M. Suzuki, C. A. Sabin, M. B. Pepys. *Immunology* 2004, 112, 255–264.

77 J. D. Mountz, P. Yang, Q. Wu, J. Zhou, A. Tousson, A. Fitzgerald, J. Allen, X. Wang, S. Cartner, W. E. Grizzle, N. Yi, L. Lu, R. W. Williams, H. C. Hsu. *Scand J Immunol* 2005, 61, 128–138.

78 B. A. Taylor, C. Wnek, B. S. Kotlus, N. Roemer, T. MacTaggart, S. J. Phillips. *Mamm Genome* 1999, 10, 335–348.

79 M. A. Jordan, P. A. Silveira, D. P. Shepherd, C. Chu, S. J. Kinder, J. Chen, L. J. Palmisano, L. D. Poulton, A. G. Baxter. *J Immunol* 2000, 165, 1673–1684.

80 T. Yuasa, S. Kubo, T. Yoshino, A. Ujike, K. Matsumura, M. Ono, J. V. Ravetch, T. Takai. *J Exp Med* 1999, 189, 187–194.

81 A. Nakamura, T. Yuasa, A. Ujike, M. Ono, T. Nukiwa, J. V. Ravetch, T. Takai. *J. Exp. Med.* 2000, 191, 899–906.

82 S. Bolland, Y. S. Yim, K. Tus, E. K. Wakeland, J. V. Ravetch. *J Exp Med* 2002, 195, 1167–1174.

83 K. Yasutomo, T. Horiuchi, S. Kagami, H. Tsukamoto, C. Hashimura, M. Urushihara, Y. Kuroda. *Nat Genet* 2001, 28, 313–314.

84 N. J. Lee, R. J. Rigby, H. Gill, J. J. Boyle, L. Fossati-Jimack, B. J. Morley, T. J. Vyse. *Clin Exp Immunol* 2004, 138, 39–46.

85 T. J. Vyse, L. Morel, F. J. Tanner, E. K. Wakeland, B. L. Kotzin. *J Immunol* 1996, 157, 2719–2727.

86 S. Xie, S. Chang, P. Yang, C. Jacob, A. Kaliyaperumal, S. K. Datta, C. Mohan. *J Immunol* 2001, 167, 7141–7149.

87 L. Morel, U.H. Rudofsky, J.A. Longmate, J. Schiffenbauer, E.K. Wakeland.
Immunity 1994, 1, 219–229.

88 L. Morel, C. Mohan, Y. Yu, J. Schiffen-
bauer, U.H. Rudofsky, N. Tian, J.A.
Longmate, E.K. Wakeland. *Mamm
Genome* 1999, 10, 176–181.

89 S.T. Waters, S.M. Fu, F. Gaskin, U.S.
Deshmukh, S.S. Sung, C.C. Kanna-
pell, K.S. Tung, S.B. McEwen,
M. McDuffie. *Clin Immunol* 2001, 100,
372–383.

90 C.G. Drake, S.J. Rozzo, H.F. Hirsch-
feld, N.P. Smarnworawong, E. Palmer,
B.L. Kotzin. *J Immunol* 1995, 154,
2441–2447.

91 T.J. Vyse, S.J. Rozzo, C.G. Drake,
S. Izui, B.L. Kotzin. *J Immunol* 1997,
158, 5566–5574.

92 S.J. Rozzo, T.J. Vyse, C.G. Drake, B.L.
Kotzin. *Proc Natl Acad Sci USA* 1996,
93, 15164–15168.

93 L. Gu, A. Weinreb, X.P. Wang,
D.J. Zack, J.H. Qiao, R. Weisbart,
A.J. Lusis. *J Immunol* 1998, 161,
6999–7006.

94 Z.S. Rahman, S.K. Tin, P.N. Buena-
ventura, C.H. Ho, E.P. Yap, R.Y. Yong,
D.R. Koh. *J Immunol* 2002, 168, 3042–
3049.

95 K. Ochiai, S. Ozaki, A. Tanino, S.
Watanabe, T. Ueno, K. Mitsui, J. Toei,
Y. Inada, S. Hirose, T. Shirai, H. Nishi-
mura. *Int Immunol* 2000, 12, 1–8.

96 C.G. Drake, S.K. Babcock, E. Palmer,
B.L. Kotzin. *Proc Natl Acad Sci USA*
1994, 91, 4062–4066.

97 S. Hirose, H. Tsurui, H. Nishimura,
Y. Jiang, T. Shirai. *Int Immunol* 1994,
6, 1857–1864.

98 Y. Jiang, S. Hirose, Y. Hamano, S. Kodera, H. Tsurui, M. Abe, K. Terashima,
S. Ishikawa, T. Shirai. *J Immunol* 1997,
158, 992–997.

99 J.G. Knight, D.D. Adams. *J Clin Lab
Immunol* 1981, 5, 165–170.

100 S. Nakatsuru, M. Terada, M. Nishihara,
J. Kamogawa, T. Miyazaki, W.M. Qu,
K. Morimoto, C. Yazawa, H. Ogasa-
wara, Y. Abe, K. Fukui, G. Ichien,
M.R. Ito, S. Mori, Y. Nakamura,
M. Nose. *Pathol Int* 1999, 49, 974–982.

101 T.J. Vyse, C.G. Drake, S.J. Rozzo,
E. Roper, S. Izui, B.L. Kotzin. *J Clin
Invest* 1996, 98, 1762–1772.

102 R.J. Rigby, S.J. Rozzo, J.J. Boyle, M.
Lewis, B.L. Kotzin, T.J. Vyse. *J Immunol* 2004, 172, 4609–4617.

103 M.E. Haywood, T.J. Vyse, A. McDermott, E.M. Thompson, A. Ida, M.J.
Walport, S. Izui, B.J. Morley. *J Immunol* 2001, 167, 1728–1733.

104 S.J. Rozzo, T.J. Vyse, K. Menze, S.
Izui, B.L. Kotzin. *J Immunol* 2000, 164,
5515–5521.

105 R.J. Rigby, S.J. Rozzo, H. Gill, T. Fernandez-Hart, B.J. Morley, S. Izui,
B.L. Kotzin, T.J. Vyse. *J Immunol* 2004,
172, 5078–5085.

106 M.L. Santiago, C. Mary, D. Parzy,
C. Jacquet, X. Montagutelli, R.M. Park-
house, R. Lemoine, S. Izui, L. Reininger.
Eur J Immunol 1998, 28, 4257–4267.

107 J. Kamogawa, M. Terada, S. Mizuki,
M. Nishihara, H. Yamamoto, S. Mori,
Y. Abe, K. Morimoto, S. Nakatsuru,
Y. Nakamura, M. Nose. *Arthritis
Rheum* 2002, 46, 1067–1074.

24
Genetic Manipulation

Matthew C. Pickering and Marina Botto

24.1
Introduction

Over the past 20 years considerable effort has been devoted to mapping the genetic loci associated with autoimmunity in spontaneous models of systemic lupus erythematosus (SLE) (see Chapter 23). Although this type of approach has been very fruitful in identifying several lupus-susceptibility linkage regions, the identification of the causative gene variants has proved to be more complex. In genetically complex diseases like SLE, many different loci appear to be contributing additively, epistatically, or heterogeneously to the autoimmune phenotype, and thus the correspondence between a predisposing genotype at one locus and the disease outcome is a weak signal to trace [1, 2]. An alternative strategy to analyze the contribution of individual alleles to a multigenic trait has been the development of animals carrying genetic manipulations of specific genes implicated in the pathogenesis of SLE [3]. This is a more synthetic approach that allows an *in vivo* assessment of the impact on the immune system of severe modifications in the expression (deficiency or overproduction) of genes suspected to play a role in the development of an autoimmune response. These genetically manipulated models have proved to be very useful to dissect effector mechanisms involved in disease pathogenesis and/or to delineate genetic mechanisms that may lead to systemic autoimmunity. However, these models have intrinsic problems that have become more apparent in the past few years. Firstly, they require careful controls to avoid possible misinterpretations. For example, in transgenic lines the piece of DNA carrying the gene of interest integrates randomly into the genome, and in doing so it can potentially alter the expression of other genes located in the chromosome region into which the DNA has been integrated. To control this potentially confounding effect, one usually compares several independent transgenic lines. More problematic is the interpretation of the results obtained with gene-targeted mice; this will be considered in more detail below. Secondly, a number of differences exist between the human and the rodent immune system [4]. Since immune dysfunctions are at the root of SLE,

Autoantibodies and Autoimmunity: Molecular Mechanisms in Health and Disease. Edited by K. Michael Pollard
Copyright © 2006 WILEY-VCH Verlag GmbH & Co. KGaA, Weinheim
ISBN: 3-527-31141-6

such differences may limit the extrapolations from animal models to human diseases. Nevertheless, genetically engineered animal models of SLE have proved to be an invaluable research tool to decipher disease mechanisms. In this chapter we will provide an overview of the most significant gene-targeted models of SLE and discuss how they contributed to our knowledge of the pathogenesis of SLE. In addition we will discuss the powerful influence of other unknown genes present in the genomes of mouse strains commonly used to generate genetically manipulated mice.

24.2
Genetic Pathways Leading to Autoimmunity: Lessons from Genetically Manipulated Models

The generation of genetically modified animals has been one of the most productive approaches to identify autoimmune regulatory genes and the mechanisms implicated in the development of SLE. Though this strategy tends to be biased toward a narrow band of candidate genes of known immunological relevance with a limited possibility of revealing new genetic factors contributing to the disease pathogenesis, it has led to the discovery of new roles for genes with known immune functions. The complement-deficient animals that will be discussed in more detail below are a typical example of this. In addition, from the analysis of genetically engineered models of SLE, there appear to be some common pathways leading to an abnormal immune response to self-antigens. One could classify the genes implicated in the development of autoimmunity into three main functional pathways: abnormalities in the immune response thresholds, imbalances in the lymphocyte homeostasis, and impairment in disposal mechanisms. Table 24.1 provides a summary of the genes involved in each pathway. It is worth noting that some genes may well contribute to SLE by operating in more than one pathway. For simplicity in describing some of the most significant mouse models of SLE, we will group the genes according to these functional pathways.

24.2.1
Dysregulation of the Immune Response

The immune system has developed complex and intriguing ways to maintain self-tolerance and prevent autoimmunity. Thus, it is not surprising that mutations of signaling molecules regulating the activation of B and T cells can lead to the development of an autoimmune disease. Enhanced cell signaling can be the result of mutations that compromise cell feedback inhibitory pathways or increase the activity of positive-acting receptors. The best-known examples of the first mechanism include targeted disruptions of three B-cell components that normally act in concert to attenuate B-cell receptor (BCR) signaling: Lyn, CD22, and the SH2 domain–containing protein tyrosine phosphatase (SHP)-1. Lyn is a

Table 24.1 Summary of the most significant genes and pathways implicated in SLE.

Disease pathway	Murine model of SLE	Ref.	Linkage to human SLE	Ref.
Dysregulation of immune system	Lyn knockout	5, 6		
	SHP-1 knockout	11		
	CD22 knockout	10		
	PD-1 knockout	14	PD-1 (PDCD1)	146
	CD45 E613R mutation	23		
	G2A knockout	147		
	Cr2 knockout	19		
	FcγRIIb knockout	13	FcγRIIa;	148
			FcγRIIIa	149
	Blys transgenic	34–36		
	CD19 transgene	24		
	Cbl-b knockout	26		
	PKCδ knockout	27		
Lymphocyte homeostasis	Fas knockout	29	ALPS [a]	33
	FasL knockout	30	ALPS	150
	p21 cyclin-dependent knockout	139, 151		
	Pten heterozygous deficiency	42		
	BIM knockout	45		
	TACI knockout	152		
	PKB transgenic	41		
Scavenger mechanisms	C1q knockout	62	C1q	81
	C4 knockout	91	C4	81
	DNAse 1 knockout	105	DNAse 1	106
	Serum IgM knockout	93, 94		
	Mer knockout	109		
	Ro antigen knockout	145		
	Transglutaminase 2 knockout	112		
	IFN-gamma transgenic	153		
	MFG-E8 [b] knockout	107		
Others	α-mannosidase II	154		

a) ALPS: autoimmune lymphoproliferative syndrome.
b) MFG-E8: milk fat globule epidermal growth factor (EGF) factor 8.

member of the Src-tyrosine kinase family and acts at the initial step in activating NK cell-activating receptors and BCR, T-cell receptor (TCR), and Fc receptor signaling by phosphorylating tyrosines in the immunoreceptor tyrosine-based activation motif (ITAM) sequences present in the cytoplasmatic domains of these multi-chain receptors. In addition to this positive role in activating ITAMs, Lyn engages feedback inhibitory pathways involving FcγRIIb and CD22. It phosphorylates tyrosines in their immunoreceptor tyrosine-based inhibitor motifs (ITIMs), which then recruit phosphatases such as SHP-1 that downregulate the BCR signaling reactions. Mice deficient in Lyn, CD22, or SHP-1 all produced varying levels of antinuclear antibodies [5–11]. Interestingly, compound-heterozygous mice in which Lyn, CD22, or SHP-1 were all partially compromised exhibited enhancement in BCR signaling, suggesting that combinations of partial loss-of-function mutations can contribute to the genetic susceptibility of autoimmune disease [12]. Similarly, mice deficient in FcγRIIb, a molecule involved in inhibiting the BCR signaling reactions, exhibited a lupus-like disease [13], though to a lesser degree than mice deficient in Lyn. Furthermore, in the FcγRIIb-deficient mice the autoantibody production strongly depended on the genetic background, and the interpretation of some of the autoimmune features described in these mice will require reviewing in light of some recent genetic findings described below in Section 24.3.

In addition to Lyn, CD22, or SHP-1, several other cell-surface negative regulators also participate in restraining autoantibody production. Programmed cell death 1 (PD-1) appears to function as a negative regulatory of both T and B cells [14]. PD-1 is a member of the Ig superfamily with a cytoplasmic domain that can recruit SHP-2, a close relative of SHP-1 [15]. It is expressed by activated T and B cells and by myeloid cells, and mice lacking PD-1 developed an autoimmune disease with arthritis and glomerulonephritis [14]. Again the expression of some phenotypic features was highly influenced by the strain background [14], and, as for the FcγRIIb gene, the absence of PD-1 might have contributed only in part to the production of autoantibodies.

Another molecule that may lead to autoimmunity by altering the B-cell signaling threshold is the Cr2 gene, which in mice encodes both complement receptors CR1 and CR2 [16, 17]. Though it is known that CR2 is a strong positive factor in promoting B-cell activation when an immune complex is present [18], there is also evidence, using the anti-lysozyme Ig model, that it participates in induction of B-cell tolerance. Lack of this function may explain the autoimmune phenotype observed in the CR1/2-deficient mice [19]. However, it is of note that the CR1/2-deficient mice on the C57BL/6 background developed a mild disease, and other unrelated genetic factors may contribute to this phenotype [20, 21].

Alterations in cell-surface molecules that positively act on antigen receptor signaling can also lead to breakdown in tolerance. An example of this type of molecule is CD45. CD45 is a transmembrane protein tyrosine phosphatase that participates positively in TCR and BCR signaling by removing inhibitory phosphorylations near the C-termini of Src family tyrosine kinases, thereby keeping them in an active state [22]. Recently, mice with a point mutation in CD45

(E613R) that induces an increase in its activity and in antigen receptor signaling have been shown to have several autoimmune symptoms, including antinuclear antibody production [23]. Another cell-surface molecule that regulates B-cell activity is CD19, a receptor that operates in close association with CR2. Expression of even low levels of human CD19 transgene in mice with normal levels of mouse CD19 results in hyperactive B cells and loss of tolerance to nuclear antigen [24, 25].

In addition to reduced cell-surface negative regulators or increased activity of positive-acting receptors, abnormalities in functions or amounts of intracellular signaling components can also induce loss of self-tolerance. For example, Cbl and Cbl-b are intracellular negative regulators of antigen receptors. Mice lacking Cbl-b developed a lupus-like disease with anti-DNA antibodies [26]. In these mice T cells display a hyperproliferative phenotype and produce more IL-2, suggesting that abnormalities in T-cell functions are the possible underlying mechanisms for the breakdown in tolerance. Similarly, animals deficient in one of the protein kinase C (PKC) isoforms (PKCδ) have been shown to have increased proliferation of B cells and autoimmunity [27]. The PKC isoforms were thought to be positive effectors of antigen receptor signaling downstream of phospholipase C (PLC)γ hydrolysis of phosphoinositides. However genetic ablation of PKCδ led to defects in B-cell anergy induction, indicating that PKCδ may be a mediator of BCR signaling that contributes selectively to tolerance reactions [28].

Taken collectively, the observations from murine models with engineered defects in one of the activation threshold genes indicate that alterations in the signaling pathways downstream of the lymphocyte antigen receptors predispose the mice to the development of autoimmune features. Though it seems logical to postulate that mutations compromising negative feedback mechanisms or increasing activity of positive-acting receptors can lead to increased numbers of activated B cells, plasma cells, and elevated serum Ig levels, the mechanisms causing a breakdown in B-cell tolerance to self-antigens remain to be elucidated.

24.2.2
Perturbations in Lymphocyte Homeostasis

The second pathway promoting the development of SLE includes a collection of genes with various roles in the regulation of lymphocyte survival. Among them the best known are the genes encoding either Fas or Fas ligand, which have been shown to be involved in the process of immune tolerance by deletion of unwanted autoreactive T cells and B cells [29, 30]. Depending upon the genetic background, mice with defects in the Fas (*lpr*) or the Fas ligand gene (*gld*) exhibit lymphadenopathy, splenomegaly, autoantibodies, and glomerulonephritis [31]. Interestingly, early treatment of *gld/gld* mice, deficient in functional Fas ligand, with an agonistic anti-Fas antibody protected the mice from the subsequent development of SLE by a mechanism that presumably involves Fas-dependent deletion of autoreactive lymphocytes [32]. It is of note that a small number of human patients have been described with mutations in the genes encoding either Fas or Fas ligand. These patients display an autoimmune lymphoproliferative syndrome (ALPS or Canale-Smith syndrome) characterized by lymphadenopathy, splenomegaly, and autoantibodies against red blood cells or platelets [33]. Affected individuals typically do not develop joint or renal disease, and therefore defects in the Fas pathway do not appear to be critical to the pathology in these organs but can contribute to autoantibody production.

Recently, autoimmune phenomena have been observed in mice overexpressing the TNF family member BAFF (B-cell activation factor belonging to the TNF family, also known as BlyS, TALL-1, and TNFSF13). These mice display lupus-like symptoms and a Sjögren's syndrome–like disease [34–37]. Although BAFF appears to play an important role in the survival of mature follicular B cells and marginal zone B cells [38, 39], the mechanisms by which it contributes to autoantibody production remain unclear.

Defects in the signaling pathways that are important for lymphocyte homeostasis have also been described in mice expressing active phosphatidylinositol 3-kinase (PI3K) [40, 41] or with reduced levels of phosphatase and tensin homologue (PTEN) [42], which regulates the levels of PtdIns $(3,4,5)P_3$. The PI3K pathway is activated downstream to a variety of receptors expressed on lymphocytes, including TCR, CD28, CD19, and IL2-R, and promotes cell survival via the serine threonine kinase protein kinase B/Akt (PKB) [43, 44]. Several experimental models with increased active PKB have been shown to have autoimmune features similar to the ones observed in animals with defective Fas or Fas ligand genes, indicating that untangling the signaling networks that lead to lymphocyte deletion and anergy versus activation is a key issue for understanding the underlying mechanisms of the disease [40–42].

There is also evidence that activation of the PI3K-PKB pathway promotes survival by inhibiting the expression of pro-apoptotic molecules such as the Bcl-2 family member BIM. Interestingly, mice deficient in this molecule had a defective negative selection of self-reactive T lymphocytes and developed a lupus-like syndrome [45–47]. Thus, considerable evidence indicates that enhanced signaling of PI3K-PKB pathways may alter lymphocyte homeostasis and lead to autoimmune traits.

24.2.3
Defects in the Scavenging Mechanisms

24.2.3.1 Introduction
The physiological processes through which damaged or dying cells are removed from tissues have become the focus of intense interest over recent years. Specifically, abnormalities in the clearance of cells dying by apoptosis (programmed cell death) have been linked closely to autoimmune and persistent inflammatory diseases. In the preceding sections we considered mechanisms that may result in the generation of autoreactive T and B cells independently of the antigens,

e.g., through mechanisms that disrupt the normal processes of central tolerance or failure to regulate normal lymphocyte survival. Now we consider an obvious alternative — but by no means mutually exclusive — hypothesis, namely, that an autoimmune response may develop in response to inappropriate presentation of self-antigens, i.e., the source of autoantigens is driving the immune response.

One of the unifying features of SLE is the presence of circulating antibodies to self-antigens, typically antinuclear antibodies. Autoantibodies in this condition may be directed at serum components (e.g., C1q, β2-glycoprotein 1), at cell-surface antigens (e.g., phospholipids like phosphatidylserine), and, perhaps most confusingly, at intracellular targets (e.g., chromatin, the spliceosome complex, and the Ro/La small cytoplasmic ribonucleoprotein complex). Two obvious questions follow from this. (1) How do antibodies develop to antigens normally found only within the nuclei of cells, a location obviously inaccessible to circulating antibodies? (2) Why do patients with SLE develop a relatively limited portfolio of antinuclear antibody responses compared with the theoretically huge numbers of possible intranuclear antigenic targets? One hypothesis proposed to answer these questions is that apoptotic cells are the source of the autoantigens that drive autoantibody production in patients with SLE. First we will discuss the mechanisms through which apoptotic cells are removed and then, using gene-targeted models of SLE, how alterations in this physiological process may result in autoimmunity.

24.2.3.2 Mechanisms of Apoptotic Cell Clearance

Apoptosis (from the ancient Greek for "falling, as leaves from a tree") is a rapid process characterized by cell shrinkage, condensation and fragmentation of the nucleus, cytoplasmic blebbing with maintenance of membrane integrity, and cell fragmentation into discrete apoptotic bodies. Apoptotic cells are rarely detected in healthy tissues as they are rapidly removed by both professional and nonprofessional phagocytes, followed by intracellular degradation. *Caenorhabditis elegans* has served as a model organism to identify genes regulating apoptosis. During development, dying cells are rapidly engulfed by neighboring cells. Approximately seven genes that encode two partially overlapping pathways for uptake and ingestion of apoptotic cells have been identified (reviewed in Ref. [48]). Unlike *C. elegans*, mammals have specialized phagocytic cells that ingest apoptotic cells, and these cells express a much larger number of receptors that have been implicated in the recognition and tethering of apoptotic cells. Examples of these receptors are the $a_v\beta_3$ vitronectin receptor [49], the phosphatidylserine receptor [50], CD36 [51], CD14 [52], scavenger receptor A [53], receptors for low-density lipoprotein [54–56], and complement receptors 3 and 4 [57]. The reason for the vast array of phagocytic receptors is unclear, although cell- and tissue-specific differences in receptor usage [58, 59] may provide a partial explanation. The trigger to cell death may also determine the efficiency with which the cells doomed to die are ingested [60], suggesting that receptor usage may vary according to the nature of the apoptotic meal. It is notable in this respect that

C1q-deficient mice, which spontaneously develop a lupus-like syndrome on a permissive genetic background (see below), although having defective clearance of apoptotic cells in the peritoneum [61] and kidney [62], showed no such defects in the skin [63] and developed normally *in utero*. This tissue-specific difference observed in gene-targeted animals might reflect variability in adaptation to clearance defects, (e.g., by the upregulation of expression of alternative phagocytic receptors) or differences in clearance mechanisms in various tissues.

There is also compelling evidence that engulfment of apoptotic cells depends on the presence of various soluble factors, which act as bridging molecules. These include thrombospondin [64], milk-fat globule epidermal growth factor 8 (MFG-E8) [65], and elements of the innate immune system such as collectins, complement [57, 61], and pentraxin [66–71]. The involvement of molecules of the innate immune system in the physiological clearance of dying cells implies that there are similarities between the recognition of unwanted (apoptotic) debris and non-self microorganisms. In this context, it is of particular interest that CD14, a molecule of the innate immune system known to bind lipopolysaccharide (LPS) and mediate inflammatory responses as part of the innate response to infection, has been shown to mediate apoptotic cell uptake by macrophages without inducing the release of proinflammatory cytokines [72]. The apoptotic cell ligand for CD14 remains unclear. It is distinct from phosphatidylserine since, although CD14 is able to bind to phospholipids, phosphatidylserine-containing liposomes failed to reduce CD14-dependent apoptotic cell uptake by macrophages [73].

24.2.3.3 Apoptotic Cells: A Potential Source of Lupus Autoantigens

There are several lines of evidence that apoptotic cells are the source of the autoantigens of lupus. Firstly, the structure of apoptotic cells is reorganized such that the "lupus autoantigens" become superficially accessible to recognition by antibodies. In a series of elegant studies, Rosen and his collaborators found that apoptotic cells express many of the nuclear autoantigens of SLE in surface blebs and apoptotic bodies [74, 75]. For example, in one-third of SLE patients, antiphospholipid antibodies are directed against the negatively charged phospholipid phosphatidylserine. This phospholipid is found in the inner part of the cell membrane of healthy cells and is actively translocated to the outer layer during apoptosis [76, 77]. It is thought to act as one of main recognition molecules for the physiological uptake and disposal of apoptotic cells. Secondly, injection of apoptotic cells into mouse strains normally not susceptible to the development of SLE induces an autoantibody response [78]. Thirdly, many lupus autoantigens undergo post-translational modification (e.g., phosphorylation) during the process of apoptosis. This process could generate neo-epitopes on self-antigens, which may facilitate the development of an immunogenic response [79, 80]. However, the specific binding of a lupus autoantibody to a neo-epitope on the surface of an antigen modified as part of the apoptotic process has not been demonstrated. Before discussing how gene-targeted mice, in particular complement-deficient animals, have led to the hypothesis that defects in the clearance of dying cells could enhance the chance of developing SLE, we will first summarize the link between complement deficiency and SLE.

24.2.3.4 Complement Deficiency and SLE

Although the etiology of SLE remains unclear and is likely to involve multiple genetic and environmental factors, it remains a striking observation that almost all cases of complete genetic deficiency of C1q (the first component in the classical pathway activation cascade) develop an SLE-like illness. Thus, genetic deficiency of C1q is still the strongest genetic susceptibility factor for SLE identified in humans. Furthermore, there appears to be a hierarchy of severity and susceptibility to the development of disease according to the position of the deficient complement protein in the activation sequence of the classical pathway of complement. Hence, 39 of the 42 (93%) described individuals with homozygous C1q deficiency had SLE, which was frequently very severe. Next in the hierarchy come C1r deficiency and C1s deficiency (usually combined) (SLE prevalence: 8 of 14 subjects [57%]) and then C4 deficiency (SLE prevalence: 18 out of 24 subjects [75%]). There is then a significant drop in the strength of the association of SLE with deficiency of the next protein in the classical pathway, C2. C2 deficiency is the commonest hereditary complement deficiency in western European Caucasian populations and is associated with the development of SLE in approximately 10% of cases. Finally, there is C3 deficiency, which, although strongly associated with the development of rashes and glomerulonephritis, typically is not associated with the development of lupus autoantibodies. The reported cases of complement-deficient patients have been analyzed in many reviews, and the interested reader is directed to [81].

These clinical observations strongly suggest that there is a physiological function of the classical pathway of complement activation that protects against the development of SLE. Furthermore, the hierarchy of susceptibility and severity of lupus, according to the missing classical pathway protein (C1q>C4≫C2), suggests that an activity of the early part of the classical pathway plays a key protective role against the disease. That a deficiency in these components results in SLE is paradoxical when one appreciates that complement activation is considered to be a major mediator of the tissue damage that one sees in non-complement-deficient SLE patients. There are currently two main hypotheses to explain the causal link between complement deficiency and the development of SLE, neither of which is mutually exclusive. One hypothesis, which we mentioned in the preceding sections, proposes that complement plays a role in determining the thresholds of activation of B and T lymphocytes and that complement deficiency causes autoantibody production and SLE by impairment of the normal mechanisms of tolerance induction and maintenance. The reports published to date testing this hypothesis are somewhat controversial [19, 82], and further studies are currently underway to test this using different experimental models.

The second hypothesis, which we discuss next, involves the role of complement in physiological waste-disposal mechanisms, in particular, the clearance of dying cells and immune complexes. It has been proposed that deficiency of complement impairs the normal mechanism of waste disposal and that dying cells and tissue injury provide a source of autoantigens and inflammatory cues that could drive the production of autoantibodies and further tissue inflammation.

24.2.3.5 Complement Promotes the Clearance of Dying Cells *in vitro* and *in vivo*

Complement was implicated first in the clearance of apoptotic cells by the observation by Korb and Ahearn that C1q could bind specifically and directly to the surface blebs of apoptotic keratinocytes [83]. This interaction is thought to be mediated via the globular heads of the C1q molecule [84] and to induce activation of the classical pathway [85]. Subsequent studies have demonstrated that collectins such as C1q, as well as MBL, can drive the ingestion of apoptotic cells through interaction with calreticulin (known as cC1qR) and CD91 on human phagocytes [86]. More recently it was also shown that opsonization of apoptotic cells with C1q and MBL targets these cells to dendritic cells as well as to macrophages and increases the efficiency of their uptake [87]. This led to the hypothesis that C1q may promote the clearance of apoptotic cells, and hence exposed autoantigens, preventing stimulation of the immune system. In addition, *in vitro* studies by Mevorach and colleagues using complement-depleted sera and human monocyte-derived macrophages supported a role for both the classical and alternative pathways of complement in the phagocytosis of apoptotic cells [57]. Blockade of complement receptors CR3 and CR4 impaired the phagocytosis of apoptotic cells. The presence of iC3b on the surface of apoptotic cells that had been incubated with serum suggested that the clearance was mediated by interactions between iC3b and CR3 (CD11B-CD18) and/or CR4 (CD11C-CD18) [57]. However, considerable caution is required when interpreting *in vitro* data. Cell culture models may not reflect physiological conditions, and different experimental conditions may explain controversial observations reported in the literature. For example, efficient uptake of apoptotic cells has also been observed when β2-integrins are blocked [88] or deleted [89]. For these reasons the study of gene-targeted complement-deficient mice has significantly advanced our understanding of the role of complement in the pathogenesis of SLE, which we will now review.

C1q-deficient (*C1qa*–/–) mice were generated by insertional mutagenesis of the first exon of the C1qA chain gene, *C1qa*, resulting in mice that had no *C1qa* transcripts detectable by Northern blot and no circulating C1q protein detectable by Western blot or ELISA [62]. As one would expect, these animals lacked classical pathway-mediated lytic activity and the ability to opsonize immune complexes with C3, but alternative pathway function was intact. Moreover, these mice spontaneously developed autoimmunity on the hybrid 129×C57BL/6 genetic background. At eight months of age, more than half of the C1q-deficient animals had detectable levels of ANA and 25% had histological evidence of proliferative glomerulonephritis [62]. The glomerulonephritis was associated with the presence of electron-dense subendothelial and subepithelial immune deposits and the glomeruli stained positively for IgG and C3, suggesting activation of complement via the alternative pathway. An unexpected but critical finding was the presence of a significantly increased number of glomerular apoptotic bodies in C1q-deficient mice without histological evidence of renal inflammation compared with the control animals. Unlike C1q-deficient humans where an SLE-like illness develops uniformly, the expression of autoimmunity in the C1q-deficient mice was found to be dependent on the genetic background of the animals [90], indicating that in mice C1q acts as a disease-modifying gene capable of accelerating the development of autoimmunity only on a permissive background. Similar findings have been reported for other complement-deficient mice [91].

Following the observation of increased numbers of apoptotic cells in the glomeruli of C1q-deficient mice, further analysis was performed to assess the *in vivo* clearance of apoptotic cells in these animals. Using a model of apoptotic cell phagocytosis during sterile peritonitis, the macrophage-mediated phagocytic uptake of intraperitoneally injected syngeneic apoptotic thymocytes was shown to be significantly impaired in both C1q- and C4-deficient mice compared to wild-type animals [61]. More importantly, the defect in phagocytosis was significantly greater in the C1q-deficient animals than in the C4-deficient mice [61]. These observations indicated the existence of a hierarchy within the classical pathway with regard to the role of the complement components in the phagocytosis of apoptotic cells, which mirrors the hierarchy of disease susceptibility in humans with complement deficiency.

In addition to the direct binding of C1q to apoptotic cells, a number of other molecules that can bind C1q and activate the classical complement pathway have been shown to recognize the modified cell membranes that form during the process of apoptosis. Among them, human C-reactive protein (CRP) [69] and natural IgM, but not IgG [92], have been shown to bind to apoptotic cells and activate the classical pathway of complement. In this context it is of note that mice lacking soluble IgM develop a lupus-like disease [93, 94]. In addition, the binding of CRP to apoptotic cells was shown to protect the cells from assembling the membrane attack complex and to mediate the non-inflammatory uptake of apoptotic cells, a mechanism dependent on the presence of C1q [69]. These accessory proteins may, in part, account for some of the complement deposition on dying cells, leading to their safe clearance by complement-dependent mechanisms.

It is interesting to note that the binding of complement components, as well as IgM and pentraxins, to apoptotic cells appears to occur only during a late phase of the process of apoptosis, and to cells that have undergone secondary necrosis [95]. This could suggest that there are sequential mechanisms in the clearance of apoptotic cells, with uptake by local macrophage representing a very early event and complement-mediated processes a rather late event. Under normal situations this should provide ample opportunity for efficient clearance

lipopolysaccharide (LPS) and pathogen-derived nucleic acids [122]. Cytokines produced by the host in response to infection may also play an important role in driving dendritic cell maturation, such as TNF-a and interferon-a [123]. In the context of inflammation, the maturation of dendritic cells into efficient antigen-presenting cells could allow apoptotic cell–derived antigen presentation. Indeed immature dendritic cells have been shown to be able to engulf apoptotic cells, via the $a_v\beta_3$ vitronectin receptor [119], and subsequently present apoptotic cell–derived antigens to MHC class I– and class II–restricted T cells [119, 124, 125]. In this context it is noteworthy that there is now a large body of evidence suggesting that in SLE patients there is an increased proportion of functionally active monocytes and that these monocytes, normally quiescent cells, when isolated from the blood of SLE patients, are able to induce a strong mixed lymphocyte reaction, a property usually used to define mature DCs [126]. In addition, it has been recently demonstrated by microarray technology that peripheral blood mononuclear cells from all SLE patients with active disease have a dysregulated expression of genes induced through the IFN pathway [127, 128]. Both of these observations suggest that DC maturation is abnormal in SLE; interestingly, the incubation of normal monocytes with serum of some SLE patients induced the differentiation of normal monocytes to DCs, with the factor in SLE serum responsible for this spontaneous maturation of DCs shown to be IFN-a [126]. It is also interesting to note that in addition to viral and bacteria infection, DNA-IgG immune complexes [129, 130] and UV can trigger secretion of excessive amounts of IFN-a. In conclusion, there is strong circumstantial evidence suggesting that chronic stimulation of DCs by "danger signals" can lead to a break in peripheral tolerance and the development of SLE.

A further mechanism that, in the setting of an impaired clearance of apoptotic cells, could increase the likelihood of immunogenicity occurring is the presence of a large number of bystander uncleared apoptotic cells that could become necrotic and be efficiently captured and presented by dendritic cells. It has been demonstrated that ingestion of high numbers of apoptotic cells by dendritic cells alone may be adequate to allow dendritic cell maturation with subsequent presentation of apoptotic cell–derived autoantigens [131]. The same scientists also found that autoantibodies (anti-β2-glycoprotein I) bound to apoptotic cells caused dendritic cells to secrete inflammatory cytokines, e.g., interleukin-1β and tumor necrosis factor-a, that may directly promote dendritic cell maturation [132]. The existence of such a balance between macrophage- and dendritic cell–mediated capture of apoptotic tumor cells that can influence the outcome of a subsequent immune response has also been demonstrated *in vivo* [133]. Ronchetti and colleagues showed that after immunizing mice with bone marrow–derived macrophages and dendritic cells that had been pulsed with apoptotic tumor cells, only the dendritic cells could induce a protective antitumor immune response. Importantly, the apoptotic cells were rendered more effective at protecting the mice from live tumor cells if animals were pretreated with carrageenan (to reduce phagocytosis by the peritoneal macrophages). Furthermore, if macrophage uptake was enhanced (through pretreatment of animals with granulocyte monocyte colony stimulating factor, GM-CSF), the animals were more susceptible to rechallenge with live tumor cells [133]. Despite these findings, very few studies so far have been able to demonstrate that apoptotic cells are directly immunogenic. The first *in vivo* data derived from a study that showed that exposure of normal mice to syngeneic apoptotic thymocytes by intravenous injection resulted in transient production of antinuclear, anticardiolipin, and anti-ssDNA antibodies [78]. Recently, the same investigators showed that immunization of mice with established autoimmunity (MRL/Mp.*lpr*/*lpr* mouse strain), using high doses of syngeneic late apoptotic cells, accelerated the production of antibodies (anticardiolipin and anti-dsDNA antibodies) and the extent of renal injury. No effect was seen, however, when a related autoimmune-prone strain (MRL/Mp) was used [134]. Another recent study by Manfredi and colleagues has demonstrated that immunization of (NZB×NZW) F_1 mice (a strain that spontaneously develops a lupus-like phenotype) with apoptotic thymocytes enhanced autoantibody production and renal inflammation only if co-administered with adjuvant [135]. The adjuvants used included incomplete Freund's adjuvant and dendritic cells that had been exposed to apoptotic cells *in vitro*. Interestingly, and related to previous work by Rovere and colleagues, was the finding that high numbers of apoptotic cells alone could produce the same effects.

In summarizing our current understanding of the pathogenesis of SLE, the data strongly argue that multiple abnormalities must be present in order for disease to occur. The data supporting the hypothesis that apoptotic cells are the source of lupus autoantigens is compelling, but evidently impaired clearance of such cells is, on its own, insufficient to produce autoimmunity. The data available emphasize that susceptibility to an autoimmune disease might depend on many factors in addition to the defective removal of dying cells. The subsequent production of autoantibodies, i.e., the break in tolerance, may require, for example, abnormalities in B-cell activation thresholds, impaired regulatory T-cell function, or disrupted mechanisms of B-cell tolerance. The challenge now is to test these hypotheses in experimental models that combine defects in apoptotic cell clearance with specific disorders of lymphocyte homeostasis.

24.3
Epistatic Effects of Background Genes on Gene-targeted Models of SLE: The Importance of Appropriate Controls

Epistasis is classically defined as a genetic interaction in which the genotype at one locus affects the phenotypic expression of the genotype at another locus. Evidence consistent with epistatic interactions among susceptibility alleles has been reported in both lupus-prone strains and animals with spontaneous mutations associated with a lupus-like disease. (NZB×NZW) F_1 hybrid mice are known to develop severe systemic autoimmunity, although both parental strains have a mild phenotype. Similarly, spontaneous mutations of Fas (*lpr*) and Fas ligand (*gld*) lost most of their autoimmune phenotype when crossed onto other genetic backgrounds different from the MRL/Mp [31]. Comparable findings were made with the yaa gene in the BXSB strain [136]. These observations clearly illustrate that the full expression of the autoimmune potential of a susceptibility allele depends on the presence of a permissive genome. There are now accumulating data that similar important epistatic interactions occur in genetically engineered animals in which the null mutation has been generated in embryonic stem cells derived from 129 strain mice and then backcrossed to the C57BL/6 or another mouse strain. In view of the relevance of these interactions in the expression of autoimmune traits in gene-targeted animals, this evidence will be discussed in more detail below.

Several targeted gene disruptions have been reported to have autoimmune traits only when crossed into a specific inbred strain or carried on the 129× C57BL/6 hybrid genetic background, the most common genome in gene-targeted models. Indeed, the 129×C57BL/6 hybrid genetic background has been shown to be spontaneously predisposed to the development of humoral autoimmunity with a low level of glomerulonephritis [62, 137–139]. A recent genome-wide scan analysis of this hybrid strain found multiple genetic loci, derived from both 129 and C57BL/6, contributing to the autoimmune traits. These findings demonstrate interacting loci between 129 and C57BL/6 mice that can cause the expression of a powerful autoimmune phenotype in these animals, in the absence of any gene-targeted mutations [140]. In addition, they indicate that some susceptibility genes can be inherited from the genome of "normal" parental strains, demonstrating that non-autoimmune strains often carry alleles that enhance disease susceptibility when integrated into a permissive genome.

Comparison of the genomic locations of susceptibility genes in the 129 and C57BL/6 hybrid strains with other lupus-prone strains demonstrated that the majority, although not all, of the intervals identified overlapped with intervals detected in other linkage studies, suggesting that at least some susceptibility may be shared among lupus-prone strains. Among these shared susceptibility loci, the most striking are loci on distal chromosome 1, for which important contributing genes have been found in New Zealand and BXSB models [141, 142]. This region—orthologous with a region on the long arm of human chromosome 1, which has been found to be linked to SLE in several studies—was of 129 origin. It is notable that several strains of mice with targeted mutations of genes encoded in this region have been reported to express lupus-like illness, including mice lacking Fc-gamma RIIb [13], serum amyloid P component [138, 143], complement receptor *Cr2* [21], decay-accelerating factor (CD55) [144], PD-1 [14], and Ro antigen [145]. In each case the autoimmune phenotype has been reported in mice in which the null mutation was generated in embryonic stem cells derived from 129 strain mice and then backcrossed onto the C57BL/6 or another mouse strain. While it is possible that the autoimmune phenotype in each of these mice is due wholly to the consequences of the targeted null mutation, there is an alternative possibility. It is possible that a 129-derived gene located in the flanking region of the targeted gene, when expressed on the C57BL/6 background, is sufficient to cause autoimmunity in its own right (in which case the effects of the targeted null gene may be irrelevant) or alternatively may modify the phenotype of the targeted null gene. To test this hypothesis, a congenic mouse strain bearing a portion of 129 chromosome 1 on a C57BL/6 background was generated. This wild-type congenic line expressed high levels of autoantibodies comparable with the ones detected in mice lacking the serum amyloid P component gene that is located in this chromosomal region, indicating that this gene is not implicated in the induction of antinuclear autoimmunity as originally suggested [140]. The same consideration applies to other genes located in the same chromosome 1 region that have been implicated in the development of SLE when inactivated by gene targeting in 129 embryonic stem cells and then backcrossed onto a pure genetic background [13, 14, 21, 144, 145]. For each of them, there has to be a question as to whether the antinuclear autoimmunity is due to the gene-targeted mutant gene or to the normal 129 genes expressed in the same region as the targeted gene.

Thus, though gene targeting has been an invaluable tool in understanding the mechanisms of immunologically mediated diseases such as SLE, using gene-targeted models has its pitfalls, and making appropriate controls is crucial for a meaningful interpretation of the findings. The data obtained from genetically modified models of SLE indicate that epistatic interactions between normal mouse genomes can significantly affect the development of autoimmunity. Thus, the potency of many susceptibility alleles is strongly influenced by the genomic context as a result of complex interactions with other alleles. Although the extent of epistasis in humans remains unclear, one could predict that interactions among functional polymorphisms will significantly contribute to disease susceptibility and expression.

24.4
Conclusions

Genetic engineering of mice has led to the identification of several genes that can contribute to an autoimmune diathesis when they are deleted or overexpressed. These genes encode antigen co-receptors, costimulatory molecules, antigen-signaling cascades, molecules involved in pathways that promote apoptosis and those that inhibit it, and molecules that clear antigen or antigen-antibody complexes. Several important observations have emerged from the genetically engineered models. First, whether a particular gene or mutation causes a disease depends on the host: both disease susceptibility and the disease phenotype that result from the alteration of a single gene depend on other genes. Second, some genetic defects may share common pathogenic pathways. As a result of this one could reasonable predict the possibility of developing common therapeutic strategies to treat this multifactorial complex condition. Finally, gene knockout strategies commonly aim to eliminate whole proteins, as opposed to natural sequence variations, which often yield missense alleles. Elimination of an entire protein can obscure key immunoregulatory functions, either because cell response is abolished altogether or because another related protein fills the vacant functional space. Nevertheless, as the pace of genetic analysis in human and in mice increases rapidly and more powerful tools are created to navigate between the mouse and the human genome, it is reasonable to predict that in the future the analysis of genetically manipulated animals will provide new insights into the mechanisms underlying autoimmunity and facilitate the development of new therapeutic approaches.

References

1 Wandstrat, A. and Wakeland, E., The genetics of complex autoimmune diseases: non-MHC susceptibility genes. *Nat Immunol* 2001, 2: 802–809.

2 Ermann, J. and Fathman, C.G., Autoimmune diseases: genes, bugs and failed regulation. *Nat Immunol* 2001, 2: 759–761.

3 Smithies, O., Animal models of human genetic diseases. *Trends Genet* 1993, 9: 112–116.

4 Mestas, J. and Hughes, C.C., Of mice and not men: differences between mouse and human immunology. *J Immunol* 2004, 172: 2731–2738.

5 Hibbs, M.L., Tarlinton, D.M., Armes, J., Grail, D., Hodgson, G., Maglitto, R., Stacker, S.A. and Dunn, A.R., Multiple defects in the immune system of Lyn-deficient mice, culminating in autoimmune disease. *Cell* 1995, 83: 301–311.

6 Nishizumi, H., Taniuchi, I., Yamanashi, Y., Kitamura, D., Ilic, D., Mori, S., Watanabe, T. and Yamamoto, T., Impaired proliferation of peripheral B cells and indication of autoimmune disease in lyn-deficient mice. *Immunity* 1995, 3: 549–560.

7 Chan, V.W., Meng, F., Soriano, P., DeFranco, A.L. and Lowell, C.A., Characterization of the B lymphocyte populations in Lyn-deficient mice and the role of Lyn in signal initiation and down-regulation. *Immunity* 1997, 7: 69–81.

8 Yu, C.C., Yen, T.S., Lowell, C.A. and DeFranco, A.L., Lupus-like kidney disease in mice deficient in the Src family tyrosine kinases Lyn and Fyn. *Curr Biol* 2001, 11: 34–38.

9 O'Keefe, T.L., Williams, G.T., Davies, S.L. and Neuberger, M.S., Hyperresponsive B cells in CD22-deficient mice. *Science* 1996, 274: 798–801.

10 O'Keefe, T.L., Williams, G.T., Batista, F.D. and Neuberger, M.S., Deficiency in CD22, a B cell-specific inhibitory receptor, is sufficient to predispose to development of high affinity autoantibodies. *J Exp Med* 1999, 189: 1307–1313.

11 Tsui, H.W., Siminovitch, K.A., de Souza, L. and Tsui, F.W., Motheaten and viable motheaten mice have mutations in the haematopoietic cell phosphatase gene. *Nat Genet* 1993, 4: 124–129.

12 Cornall, R.J., Cyster, J.G., Hibbs, M.L., Dunn, A.R., Otipoby, K.L., Clark, E.A. and Goodnow, C.C., Polygenic autoimmune traits: Lyn, CD22, and SHP-1 are limiting elements of a biochemical pathway regulating BCR signaling and selection. *Immunity* 1998, 8: 497–508.

13 Bolland, S. and Ravetch, J.V., Spontaneous autoimmune disease in Fc(gamma)RIIB-deficient mice results from strain-specific epistasis. *Immunity* 2000, 13: 277–285.

14 Nishimura, H., Nose, M., Hiai, H., Minato, N. and Honjo, T., Development of lupus-like autoimmune diseases by disruption of the PD-1 gene encoding an ITIM motif-carrying immunoreceptor. *Immunity* 1999, 11: 141–151.

15 Okazaki, T., Maeda, A., Nishimura, H., Kurosaki, T. and Honjo, T., PD-1 immunoreceptor inhibits B cell receptor-mediated signaling by recruiting src homology 2-domain-containing tyrosine phosphatase 2 to phosphotyrosine. *Proc Natl Acad Sci USA* 2001, 98: 13866–13871.

16 Holers, V.M. and Boackle, S.A., Complement receptor 2 and autoimmunity. *Curr Dir Autoimmun* 2004, 7: 33–48.

17 Boackle, S.A., Holers, V.M., Chen, X., Szakonyi, G., Karp, D.R., Wakeland, E.K. and Morel, L., Cr2, a candidate gene in the murine Sle1c lupus susceptibility locus, encodes a dysfunctional protein. *Immunity* 2001, 15: 775–785.

18 Dempsey, P.W., Allison, M.E., Akkaraju, S., Goodnow, C.C. and Fearon, D.T., C3d of complement as a molecular adjuvant: bridging innate and acquired immunity. *Science* 1996, 271: 348–350.

19 Prodeus, A.P., Goerg, S., Shen, L.M., Pozdnyakova, O.O., Chu, L., Alicot, E.M., Goodnow, C.C. and Carroll, M.C., A critical role for complement in maintenance of self-tolerance. *Immunity* 1998, 9: 721–731.

20 Chen, Z., Koralov, S.B. and Kelsoe, G., Complement C4 inhibits systemic autoimmunity through a mechanism independent of complement receptors CR1 and CR2. *J Exp Med* 2000, 192: 1339–1352.

21 Wu, X., Jiang, N., Deppong, C., Singh, J., Dolecki, G., Mao, D., Morel, L. and Molina, H.D., A role for the Cr2 gene in modifying autoantibody production in systemic lupus erythematosus. *J Immunol* 2002, 169: 1587–1592.

22 Hermiston, M.L., Xu, Z., Majeti, R. and Weiss, A., Reciprocal regulation of lymphocyte activation by tyrosine kinases and phosphatases. *J Clin Invest* 2002, 109: 9–14.

23 Majeti, R., Xu, Z., Parslow, T.G., Olson, J.L., Daikh, D.I., Killeen, N. and Weiss, A., An inactivating point mutation in the inhibitory wedge of CD45 causes lymphoproliferation and autoimmunity. *Cell* 2000, 103: 1059–1070.

24 Sato, S., Ono, N., Steeber, D.A., Pisetsky, D.S. and Tedder, T.F., CD19 regulates B lymphocyte signaling thresholds critical for the development of B-1 lineage cells and autoimmunity. *J Immunol* 1996, 157: 4371–4378.

25 Inaoki, M., Sato, S., Weintraub, B.C., Goodnow, C.C. and Tedder, T.F., CD19-regulated signaling thresholds control peripheral tolerance and autoantibody production in B lymphocytes. *J Exp Med* 1997, 186: 1923–1931.

26 Bachmaier, K., Krawczyk, C., Kozieradzki, I., Kong, Y.Y., Sasaki, T., Oliveira-dos-Santos, A., Mariathasan, S., Bouchard, D., Wakeham, A., Itie, A., Le, J., Ohashi, P.S., Sarosi, I., Nishina, H., Lipkowitz, S. and Penninger, J.M., Negative regulation of lymphocyte activation and autoimmunity by the molecular adaptor Cbl-b. *Nature* 2000, 403: 211–216.

27 Miyamoto, A., Nakayama, K., Imaki, H., Hirose, S., Jiang, Y., Abe, M., Tsukiyama, T., Nagahama, H., Ohno, S., Hatakeyama, S. and Nakayama, K.I., Increased proliferation of B cells and auto-immunity in mice lacking protein kinase Cdelta. *Nature* 2002, 416: 865–869.

28 Mecklenbrauker, I., Saijo, K., Zheng, N.Y., Leitges, M. and Tarakhovsky, A., Protein kinase Cdelta controls self-antigen-induced B-cell tolerance. *Nature* 2002, 416: 860–865.

29 Watanabe-Fukunaga, R., Brannan, C.I., Copeland, N.G., Jenkins, N.A., Nagata, S., Lymphoproliferation disorder in mice explained by defects in Fas antigen that mediates apoptosis. *Nature* 1992, 356: 314–317.

30 Takahashi, T., Tanaka, M., Brannan, C.I., Jenkins, N.A., Copeland, N.G., Suda, T. and Nagata, S., Generalized lymphoproliferative disease in mice, caused by a point mutation in the Fas ligand. *Cell* 1994, 76: 969–976.

31 Izui, S., Kelley, V.E., Masuda, K., Yoshida, H., Roths, J.B. and Murphy, E.D., Induction of various autoantibodies by mutant gene lpr in several strains of mice. *J Immunol* 1984, 133: 227–233.

32 Nishimura-Morita, Y., Nose, M., Inoue, T. and Yonehara, S., Amelioration of systemic autoimmune disease by the stimulation of apoptosis-promoting receptor Fas with anti-Fas mAb. *Int Immunol* 1997, 9: 1793–1799.

33 Fisher, G.H., Rosenberg, F.J., Straus, S.E., Dale, J.K., Middleton, L.A., Lin, A.Y., Strober, W., Lenardo, M.J. and Puck, J.M., Dominant interfering Fas gene mutations impair apoptosis in a human autoimmune lymphoproliferative syndrome. *Cell* 1995, 81: 935–946.

34 Khare, S.D., Sarosi, I., Xia, X.Z., McCabe, S., Miner, K., Solovyev, I., Hawkins, N., Kelley, M., Chang, D., Van, G., Ross, L., Delaney, J., Wang, L., Lacey,

68 Familian, A., Zwart, B., Huisman, H.G., Rensink, I., Roem, D., Hordijk, P.L., Aarden, L.A. and Hack, C.E., Chromatin-independent binding of serum amyloid P component to apoptotic cells. *J Immunol* 2001, 167: 647–654.

69 Gershov, D., Kim, S., Brot, N. and Elkon, K.B., C-Reactive protein binds to apoptotic cells, protects the cells from assembly of the terminal complement components, and sustains an antiinflammatory innate immune response: implications for systemic autoimmunity. *J Exp Med* 2000, 192: 1353–1364.

70 Rovere, P., Peri, G., Fazzini, F., Bottazzi, B., Doni, A., Bondanza, A., Zimmermann, V.S., Garlanda, C., Fascio, U., Sabbadini, M.G., Rugarli, C., Mantovani, A. and Manfredi, A.A., The long pentraxin PTX3 binds to apoptotic cells and regulates their clearance by antigen-presenting dendritic cells. *Blood* 2000, 96: 4300–4306.

71 Bijl, M., Horst, G., Bijzet, J., Bootsma, H., Limburg, P.C. and Kallenberg, C.G., Serum amyloid P component binds to late apoptotic cells and mediates their uptake by monocyte-derived macrophages. *Arthritis Rheum* 2003, 48: 248–254.

72 Gregory, C.D. and Devitt, A., CD14 and apoptosis. *Apoptosis* 1999, 4: 11–20.

73 Devitt, A., Pierce, S., Oldreive, C., Shingler, W.H. and Gregory, C.D., CD14-dependent clearance of apoptotic cells by human macrophages: the role of phosphatidylserine. *Cell Death Differ* 2003, 10: 371–382.

74 Casciola-Rosen, L.A., Anhalt, G. and Rosen, A., Autoantigens targeted in systemic lupus erythematosus are clustered in two populations of surface structures on apoptotic keratinocytes. *J Exp Med* 1994, 179: 1317–1330.

75 Rosen, A., Casciola-Rosen, L. and Ahearn, J., Novel packages of viral and self-antigens are generated during apoptosis. *J Exp Med* 1995, 181: 1557–1561.

76 Casciola-Rosen, L., Rosen, A., Petri, M. and Schlissel, M., Surface blebs on apoptotic cells are sites of enhanced procoagulant activity: implications for coagulation events and antigenic spread in sys-

temic lupus erythematosus. *Proc Natl Acad Sci USA* 1996, 93: 1624–1629.

77 Fadok, V.A., Voelker, D.R., Campbell, P.A., Cohen, J.J., Bratton, D.L. and Henson, P.M., Exposure of phosphatidylserine on the surface of apoptotic lymphocytes triggers specific recognition and removal by macrophages. *J Immunol* 1992, 148: 2207–2216.

78 Mevorach, D., Zhou, J.L., Song, X. and Elkon, K.B., Systemic exposure to irradiated apoptotic cells induces autoantibody production. *J Exp Med* 1998, 188: 387–392.

79 Rosen, A. and Casciola-Rosen, L., Autoantigens as substrates for apoptotic proteases: implications for the pathogenesis of systemic autoimmune disease. *Cell Death Differ* 1999, 6: 6–12.

80 Casciola-Rosen, L., Andrade, F., Ulanet, D., Wong, W.B. and Rosen, A., Cleavage by granzyme B is strongly predictive of autoantigen status: implications for initiation of autoimmunity. *J Exp Med* 1999, 190: 815–826.

81 Pickering, M.C., Botto, M., Taylor, P.R., Lachmann, P.J. and Walport, M.J., Systemic lupus erythematosus, complement deficiency, and apoptosis. *Adv Immunol* 2000, 76: 227–324.

82 Cutler, A.J., Cornall, R.J., Ferry, H., Manderson, A.P., Botto, M. and Walport, M.J., Intact B cell tolerance in the absence of the first component of the classical complement pathway. *Eur J Immunol* 2001, 31: 2087–2093.

83 Korb, L.C. and Ahearn, J.M., C1q binds directly and specifically to surface blebs of apoptotic human keratinocytes: complement deficiency and systemic lupus erythematosus revisited. *J Immunol* 1997, 158: 4525–4528.

84 Navratil, J.S., Wisnieski, J.J. and Ahearn, J.M., The globular heads of C1q bind specifically to surface blebs of apoptotic human endothelial cells: implications for immune tolerance (abstract). *Mol Immunol* 1998, 35: 398.

85 Nauta, A.J., Trouw, L.A., Daha, M.R., Tijsma, O., Nieuwland, R., Schwaeble, W.J., Gingras, A.R., Mantovani, A., Hack, E.C. and Roos, A., Direct binding of C1q to apoptotic cells and cell blebs induces complement activation. *Eur J Immunol* 2002, 32: 1726–1736.

86 Ogden, C.A., deCathelineau, A., Hoffmann, P.R., Bratton, D., Ghebrehiwet, B., Fadok, V.A. and Henson, P.M., C1q and mannose binding lectin engagement of cell surface calreticulin and CD91 initiates macropinocytosis and uptake of apoptotic cells. *J Exp Med* 2001, 194: 781–795.

87 Nauta, A.J., Castellano, G., Xu, W., Woltman, A.M., Borrias, M.C., Daha, M.R., van Kooten, C. and Roos, A., Opsonization with C1q and mannose-binding lectin targets apoptotic cells to dendritic cells. *J Immunol* 2004, 173: 3044–3050.

88 Savill, J.S., Henson, P.M. and Haslett, C., Phagocytosis of aged human neutrophils by macrophages is mediated by a novel "charge-sensitive" recognition mechanism. *J Clin Invest* 1989, 84: 1518–1527.

89 Ren, Y., Stuart, L., Lindberg, F.P., Rosenkranz, A.R., Chen, Y., Mayadas, T.N. and Savill, J., Nonphlogistic clearance of late apoptotic neutrophils by macrophages: efficient phagocytosis independent of beta 2 integrins. *J Immunol* 2001, 166: 4743–4750.

90 Mitchell, D.A., Pickering, M.C., Warren, J., Fossati-Jimack, L., Cortes-Hernandez, J., Cook, H.T., Botto, M. and Walport, M.J., C1q deficiency and autoimmunity: the effects of genetic background on disease expression. *J Immunol* 2002, 168: 2538–2543.

91 Paul, E., Pozdnyakova, O.O., Mitchell, E. and Carroll, M.C., Anti-DNA autoreactivity in C4-deficient mice. *Eur J Immunol* 2002, 32: 2672–2679.

92 Kim, S.J., Gershov, D., Ma, X., Brot, N. and Elkon, K.B., I-PLA(2) activation during apoptosis promotes the exposure of membrane lysophosphatidylcholine leading to binding by natural immunoglobulin M antibodies and complement activation. *J Exp Med* 2002, 196: 655–665.

93 Boes, M., Schmidt, T., Linkemann, K., Beaudette, B.C., Marshak-Rothstein, A. and Chen, J., Accelerated development of IgG autoantibodies and autoimmune disease in the absence of secreted IgM. *Proc Natl Acad Sci USA* 2000, 97: 1184–1189.

94 Ehrenstein, M.R., O'Keefe, T.L., Davies, S.L. and Neuberger, M.S., Targeted gene disruption reveals a role for natural secretory IgM in the maturation of the primary immune response. *Proc Natl Acad Sci USA* 1998, 95: 10089–10093.

95 Gaipl, U.S., Kuenkele, S., Voll, R.E., Beyer, T.D., Kolowos, W., Heyder, P., Kalden, J.R. and Herrmann, M., Complement binding is an early feature of necrotic and a rather late event during apoptotic cell death. *Cell Death Differ* 2001, 8: 327–334.

96 Herrmann, M., Voll, R.E., Zoller, O.M., Hagenhofer, M., Ponner, B.B. and Kalden, J.R., Impaired phagocytosis of apoptotic cell material by monocyte-derived macrophages from patients with systemic lupus erythematosus. *Arthritis Rheum* 1998, 41: 1241–1250.

97 Grootscholten, C., van Bruggen, M.C., van der Pijl, J.W., de Jong, E.M., Ligtenberg, G., Derksen, R.H. and Berden, J.H., Deposition of nucleosomal antigens (histones and DNA) in the epidermal basement membrane in human lupus nephritis. *Arthritis Rheum* 2003, 48: 1355–1362.

98 van Bruggen, M.C., Kramers, C., Walgreen, B., Elema, J.D., Kallenberg, C.G., van den Born, J., Smeenk, R.J., Assmann, K.J., Muller, S., Monestier, M. and Berden, J.H., Nucleosomes and histones are present in glomerular deposits in human lupus nephritis. *Nephrol Dial Transplant* 1997, 12: 57–66.

99 Baumann, I., Kolowos, W., Voll, R.E., Manger, B., Gaipl, U., Neuhuber, W.L., Kirchner, T., Kalden, J.R. and Herrmann, M., Impaired uptake of apoptotic cells into tingible body macrophages in germinal centers of patients with systemic lupus erythematosus. *Arthritis Rheum* 2002, 46: 191–201.

100 Amoura, Z., Piette, J.C., Chabre, H., Cacoub, P., Papo, T., Wechsler, B., Bach, J.F. and Koutouzov, S., Circulating plasma levels of nucleosomes in patients with systemic lupus erythematosus: correlation with serum antinucleosome antibody titers and absence of clear association with disease activity. *Arthritis Rheum* 1997, 40: 2217–2225.

apoptotic cells in vivo: role of antigen load, antigen-presenting cells, and cytokines. *J Immunol* 1999, 163: 130–136.

134 Shoshan, Y. and Mevorach, D., Accelerated autoimmune disease in MRL/MpJ-Fas(lpr) but not in MRL/MpJ following immunization with high load of syngeneic late apoptotic cells. *Autoimmunity* 2004, 37: 103–109.

135 Bondanza, A., Zimmermann, V.S., Dell'Antonio, G., Cin, E.D., Balestrieri, G., Tincani, A., Amoura, Z., Piette, J.C., Sabbadini, M.G., Rovere-Querini, P. and Manfredi, A.A., Requirement of dying cells and environmental adjuvants for the induction of autoimmunity. *Arthritis Rheum* 2004, 50: 1549–1560.

136 Merino, R., Shibata, T., De Kossodo, S. and Izui, S., Differential effect of the autoimmune Yaa and lpr genes on the acceleration of lupus-like syndrome in MRL/MpJ mice. *Eur J Immunol* 1989, 19: 2131–2137.

137 Obata, Y., Tanaka, T., Stockert, E. and Good, R.A., Autoimmune and lymphoproliferative disease in (B6-GIX+ X 129)F1 mice: relation to naturally occurring antibodies against murine leukemia virus-related cell surface antigens. *Proc Natl Acad Sci USA* 1979, 76: 5289–5293.

138 Bickerstaff, M.C., Botto, M., Hutchinson, W.L., Herbert, J., Tennent, G.A., Bybee, A., Mitchell, D.A., Cook, H.T., Butler, P.J., Walport, M.J. and Pepys, M.B., Serum amyloid P component controls chromatin degradation and prevents antinuclear autoimmunity. *Nat Med* 1999, 5: 694–697.

139 Santiago-Raber, M.L., Lawson, B.R., Dummer, W., Barnhouse, M., Koundouris, S., Wilson, C.B., Kono, D.H. and Theofilopoulos, A.N., Role of cyclin kinase inhibitor p21 in systemic autoimmunity. *J Immunol* 2001, 167: 4067–4074.

140 Bygrave, A.E., Rose, K.L., Cortes-Hernandez, J., Warren, J., Rigby, R.J., Cook, H.T., Walport, M., Vyse, T.J. and Botto, M., Spontaneous autoimmunity in 129 and C57BL/6 mice-implications for autoimmunity described in gene-targeted mice. *PLoS Biol* 2004, 2: E243.

141 Theofilopoulos, A.N. and Kono, D.H., The genes of systemic autoimmunity. *Proc Assoc Am Physicians* 1999, 111: 228–240.

142 Wakeland, E.K., Liu, K., Graham, R.R. and Behrens, T.W., Delineating the genetic basis of systemic lupus erythematosus. *Immunity* 2001, 15: 397–408.

143 Gillmore, J.D., Hutchinson, W.L., Herbert, J., Bybee, A., Mitchell, D.A., Hasserjian, R.P., Yamamura, K., Suzuki, M., Sabin, C.A. and Pepys, M.B., Autoimmunity and glomerulonephritis in mice with targeted deletion of the serum amyloid P component gene: SAP deficiency or strain combination? *Immunology* 2004, 112: 255–264.

144 Miwa, T., Maldonado, M.A., Zhou, L., Sun, X., Luo, H.Y., Cai, D., Werth, V.P., Madaio, M.P., Eisenberg, R.A. and Song, W.C., Deletion of decay-accelerating factor (CD55) exacerbates autoimmune disease development in MRL/lpr mice. *Am J Pathol* 2002, 161: 1077–1086.

145 Xue, D., Shi, H., Smith, J.D., Chen, X., Noe, D.A., Cedervall, T., Yang, D.D., Eynon, E., Brash, D.E., Kashgarian, M., Flavell, R.A., Wolin, S.L., A lupus-like syndrome develops in mice lacking the Ro 60-kDa protein, a major lupus autoantigen. *Proc Natl Acad Sci USA* 2003, 100: 7503–7508.

146 Prokunina, L., Padyukov, L., Bennet, A., de Faire, U., Wiman, B., Prince, J., Alfredsson, L., Klareskog, L. and Alarcon-Riquelme, M., Association of the PD-1.3A allele of the PDCD1 gene in patients with rheumatoid arthritis negative for rheumatoid factor and the shared epitope. *Arthritis Rheum* 2004, 50: 1770–1773.

147 Le, L.Q., Kabarowski, J.H., Weng, Z., Satterthwaite, A.B., Harvill, E.T., Jensen, E.R., Miller, J.F. and Witte, O.N., Mice lacking the orphan G protein-coupled receptor G2A develop a late-onset autoimmune syndrome. *Immunity* 2001, 14: 561–571.

148 Salmon, J. E., Millard, S., Schachter, L. A., Arnett, F. C., Ginzler, E. M., Gourley, M. F., Ramsey-Goldman, R., Peterson, M. G. and Kimberly, R. P., Fc gamma RIIA alleles are heritable risk factors for lupus nephritis in African Americans. *J Clin Invest* 1996, 97: 1348–1354.

149 Wu, J., Edberg, J. C., Redecha, P. B., Bansal, V., Guyre, P. M., Coleman, K., Salmon, J. E. and Kimberly, R. P., A novel polymorphism of FcgammaRIIIa (CD16) alters receptor function and predisposes to autoimmune disease. *J Clin Invest* 1997, 100: 1059–1070.

150 Wu, J., Wilson, J., He, J., Xiang, L., Schur, P. H. and Mountz, J. D., Fas ligand mutation in a patient with systemic lupus erythematosus and lymphoproliferative disease. *J Clin Invest* 1996, 98: 1107–1113.

151 Balomenos, D., Martin-Caballero, J., Garcia, M. I., Prieto, I., Flores, J. M., Serrano, M. and Martinez, A. C., The cell cycle inhibitor p21 controls T-cell proliferation and sex-linked lupus development. *Nat Med* 2000, 6: 171–176.

152 Seshasayee, D., Valdez, P., Yan, M., Dixit, V. M., Tumas, D. and Grewal, I. S., Loss of TACI causes fatal lymphoproliferation and autoimmunity, establishing TACI as an inhibitory BLyS receptor. *Immunity* 2003, 18: 279–288.

153 Seery, J. P., Carroll, J. M., Cattell, V. and Watt, F. M., Antinuclear autoantibodies and lupus nephritis in transgenic mice expressing interferon gamma in the epidermis. *J Exp Med* 1997, 186: 1451–1459.

154 Chui, D., Sellakumar, G., Green, R., Sutton-Smith, M., McQuistan, T., Marek, K., Morris, H., Dell, A., Marth, J., Genetic remodeling of protein glycosylation in vivo induces autoimmune disease. *Proc Natl Acad Sci USA* 2001, 98: 1142–1147.

using peripheral blood lymphocytes of lupus patients have identified groups of interferon-associated genes leading to the description of an interferon signature that shows correlation with disease activity [7, 8]. These studies have led to the suggestion that type 1 IFNs (IFN-α/β) contribute to early disease events, while IFN-γ (type II IFN) influences established disease [9]. However, this was not supported by gene expression studies in lupus nephritis, which suggested the involvement of type 1 IFN in organ pathology [10]. In addition, the importance of NK cells and IFN-γ production in eliciting T/B-cell responses in a model of myasthenia gravis [11] argues that INF-γ expression by cells of the innate immune system plays a significant role in autoimmunity. Additionally, the suggestion that NK cells may have divergent functions depending upon the stage of autoimmune disease [12, 13] suggests that care needs to be exercised in interpretation of studies focusing on the disease associations of IFNs. Contributing to this complicated picture is the diverse array of genes that are expressed in response to IFNs [7, 14].

A recent review by Theofilopoulos and colleagues [15] puts IFN-α/β at the heart of both systemic and organ-specific autoimmunity. The stimuli that elicit type I IFN production from plasmacytoid dendritic cells of the innate immune system are argued to be exogenous (bacterial and viral products) and endogenous (immune complexes and apoptotic/necrotic material) [3, 4, 15] factors. However, it remains to be determined how such stimulated IFN production results in autoimmunity. One argument is that IFN production leads to disease in genetically susceptible individuals [3], but the identity of the genetic elements required for susceptibility and the molecular/cellular mechanisms responsible are, as yet, poorly described. Although recent studies have identified some genes as being associated with type I IFN [16, 17], it is also being revealed that deficiency of proteins associated with innate immunity can result in hyperexpression of IFN-γ, hyper T-cell activity, and exacerbated autoimmunity [18]. On the other hand, it has been found that autoantibody responses can be dependent upon individual cytokines [19, 20], suggesting that certain facets of autoimmunity are subject to independent regulation. Given the broad range of genes that influence IFN expression and function, it will be important to determine how pervasively IFN-α/β and IFN-γ influence the different facets of organ-specific and systemic autoimmunity.

25.3
Autoantibodies as Diagnostic Markers

The epitopes recognized by autoantibodies are structurally diverse, ranging from linear peptide sequences to quaternary structures, and can be modified or hidden, or mimicked by other structures [21]. The ever-expanding diversity of autoantigens and their inherent epitopes is outgrowing conventional screening technologies and has spawned the development of multiplex assays [22] (see Chapter 8). While legal and ethical questions may require resolution before multiplex assays can be broadly accepted into clinical laboratories (see Chapter 8), it is clear that these new technologies offer the most appropriate platforms to screen autoantibody-containing sera against all possible autoepitopes (e.g., primary, secondary, tertiary, quaternary, cryptic, modified, and mimics) of one or more autoantigens. These assay systems have been validated for autoantibody detection using recombinant proteins, synthetic peptides, molecules with post-translational modifications, and nucleic acids as antigens [22]. The diversity of antigens that can be screened in multiplex assays should encourage rigorous testing of the hypothesis that autoantibody profiles, as opposed to an individual autoantibody response, provide superior diagnostic information [23].

Why is it important to know whether an autoantibody profile clusters with a particular autoimmune disease or with distinct clinical manifestations? While the observation that autoantibodies can have diagnostic, and even prognostic, significance has proven clinically useful, it has not helped to answer the most perplexing question regarding autoantibodies: Why are particular autoantibodies or sets of autoantibodies associated with certain autoimmune diseases? This question is of primary importance in the systemic autoimmune diseases because, unlike organ-specific autoimmunity, it is not clear whether many autoantibodies contribute to pathology, are "reporters" of the disease process, or are merely innocent bystanders. Multiplex assays provide, for the first time, the ability to test a single blood sample from a patient against thousands of biomarkers. Thus, a patient's autoantibody profile can be compared and contrasted with gene expression profiles of blood cells (e.g., either global or cell specific) [7, 24], with blood protein levels (e.g., cytokines, chemokines, immunoglobulins), and with intracellular proteins indicative of various states of cellular activity (e.g., intracellular signaling) [25]. Coupling such information with clinical markers has the potential to revolutionize associations between diseases and disease subsets, autoantibody profiles, and other biomarkers. In early studies the resulting molecular signatures have helped focus hypothesis-driven research [9, 16, 24]. However, there are significant hurdles to overcome before in-depth studies can be feasibly performed. They include collection of suitable clinical material, validation of methodologies, and development of bioinformatics and statistical approaches [26]. As these first tentative steps are taken towards the bioinformatics era of autoimmunity, it seems that autoantibodies will continue to buttress many of the experimental approaches.

25.4
Autoantibodies as Molecular and Cellular Probes

Many of the early contributions made by autoantibodies to molecular and cellular biology centered on identification of the molecular targets recognized by autoantibodies. This was most successfully achieved via cDNA cloning [27, 28], although classical biochemical purification procedures were also successful [29]. More recently the screening process has been reversed and cDNAs that have

6 Balomenos, D., R. Rumold, and A.N. Theofilopoulos (1998) Interferon-gamma is required for lupus-like disease and lymphoaccumulation in MRL-lpr mice. *J Clin Invest* 101:364–371.

7 Bennett, L., A.K. Palucka, E. Arce, V. Cantrell, J. Borvak, J. Banchereau, and V. Pascual. 2003. Interferon and granulopoiesis signatures in systemic lupus erythematosus blood. *J Exp Med* 197: 711–723.

8 Baechler, E.C., F.M. Batliwalla, G. Karypis, P.M. Gaffney, W.A. Ortmann, K.J. Espe, K.B. Shark, W.J. Grande, K.M. Hughes, V. Kapur, P.K. Gregersen, and T.W. Behrens (2003) Interferon-inducible gene expression signature in peripheral blood cells of patients with severe lupus. *Proc Natl Acad Sci USA* 100:2610–2615.

9 Crow, M.K., and K.A. Kirou (2004) Interferon-alpha in systemic lupus erythematosus. *Curr Opin Rheumatol* 16:541–547.

10 Peterson, K.S., J.F. Huang, J. Zhu, V. D'Agati, X. Liu, N. Miller, M.G. Erlander, M.R. Jackson, and R.J. Winchester (2004) Characterization of heterogeneity in the molecular pathogenesis of lupus nephritis from transcriptional profiles of laser-captured glomeruli. *J Clin Invest* 113:1722–1733.

11 Shi, F.D., H.B. Wang, H. Li, S. Hong, M. Taniguchi, H. Link, L. Van Kaer, and H.G. Ljunggren (2000) Natural killer cells determine the outcome of B cell-mediated autoimmunity. *Nat Immunol* 1:245–251.

12 Flodstrom, M., F.D. Shi, N. Sarvetnick, and H.G. Ljunggren (2002) The natural killer cell – friend or foe in autoimmune disease? *Scand J Immunol* 55:432-441.

13 Shi, F., H.G. Ljunggren, and N. Sarvetnick (2001) Innate immunity and autoimmunity: from self-protection to self-destruction. *Trends Immunol* 22:97–101.

14 Boehm, U., T. Klamp, M. Groot, and J.C. Howard (1997) Cellular responses to interferon-gamma. *Annu Rev Immunol* 15:749–795.

15 Theofilopoulos, A.N., R. Baccala, B. Beutler, and D.H. Kono (2005) Type I Interferons (/) in Immunity and Autoimmunity. *Annu Rev Immunol* 23:307–336.

16 Kirou, K.A., C. Lee, S. George, K. Louca, I.G. Papagiannis, M.G. Peterson, N. Ly, R.N. Woodward, K.E. Fry, A.Y. Lau, J.G. Prentice, J.G. Wohlgemuth, and M.K. Crow (2004) Coordinate overexpression of interferon-alpha-induced genes in systemic lupus erythematosus. *Arthritis Rheum* 50:3958–3967.

17 Sigurdsson, S., G. Nordmark, H.H. Goring, K. Lindroos, A.C. Wiman, G. Sturfelt, A. Jonsen, S. Rantapaa-Dahlqvist, B. Moller, J. Kere, S. Koskenmies, E. Widen, M.L. Eloranta, H. Julkunen, H. Kristjansdottir, K. Steinsson, G. Alm, L. Ronnblom, and A.C. Syvanen (2005) Polymorphisms in the tyrosine kinase 2 and interferon regulatory factor 5 genes are associated with systemic lupus erythematosus. *Am J Hum Genet* 76: 528–537.

18 Liu, J., T. Miwa, B. Hilliard, Y. Chen, J.D. Lambris, A.D. Wells, and W.C. Song (2005) The complement inhibitory protein DAF (CD55) suppresses T cell immunity in vivo. *J Exp Med* 201: 567–577.

19 Richards, H.B., M. Satoh, M. Shaw, C. Libert, V. Poli, and W.H. Reeves (1998) Interleukin 6 dependence of anti-DNA antibody production: evidence for two pathways of autoantibody formation in pristane-induced lupus. *J Exp Med* 188:985–990.

20 Bagenstose, L.M., P. Salgame, and M. Monestier (1998) IL-12 down-regulates autoantibody production in mercury-induced autoimmunity. *J Immunol* 160:1612–1617.

21 Mahler, M., M. Bluthner, and K.M. Pollard (2003) Advances in B-cell epitope analysis of autoantigens in connective tissue diseases. *Clin Immunol* 107:65–79.

22 Robinson, W.H., C. DiGennaro, W. Hueber, B.B. Haab, M. Kamachi, E.J. Dean, S. Fournel, D. Fong, M.C. Genovese, H.E. de Vegvar, K. Skriner, D.L. Hirschberg, R.I. Morris, S. Muller, G.J. Pruijn, W.J. van Venrooij, J.S. Smolen, P.O. Brown, L. Steinman, and P.J. Utz (2002) Autoantigen microarrays for multiplex characterization of autoantibody responses. *Nat Med* 8:295–301.

23 Tan, E.M (1989) Antinuclear antibodies: diagnostic markers for autoimmune diseases and probes for cell biology. *Adv Immunol* 44:93–151.

24 Banchereau, J., V. Pascual, and A.K. Palucka (2004) Autoimmunity through cytokine-induced dendritic cell activation. *Immunity* 20:539–550.

25 Utz, P.J. (2005) Protein arrays for studying blood cells and their secreted products. *Immunol Rev* 204:264–282.

26 Utz, P.J. (2004) Multiplexed assays for identification of biomarkers and surrogate markers in systemic lupus erythematosus. *Lupus* 13:304–311.

27 Pollard, K.M., E.K. Chan, B.J. Grant, K.F. Sullivan, E.M. Tan, and C.A. Glass (1990) In vitro posttranslational modification of lamin B cloned from a human T-cell line. *Mol Cell Biol* 10:2164–2175.

28 Chan, E.K., K.F. Sullivan, R.I. Fox, and E.M. Tan (1989) Sjogren's syndrome nuclear antigen B (La): cDNA cloning, structural domains, and autoepitopes. *J Autoimmun* 2:321-327.

29 Ogata, K., Y. Ogata, R.M. Nakamura, E.M. Tan (1985) Purification and N–terminal amino acid sequence of proliferating cell nuclear antigen (PCNA)/cyclin and development of ELISA for anti-PCNA antibodies. *J Immunol* 135:2623–2627.

30 Yang, J.M., Hildebrandt, B., Luderschmidt, C., Pollard, K.M. (2003) Human scleroderma sera contain autoantibodies to protein components specific to the U3 small nucleolar RNP complex. *Arthritis Rheum* 48:210–217.

31 Huguet, S., Labas, V., Duclos-Vallee, J.C., Bruneel, A., Vinh, J., Samuel, D., Johanet, C., Ballot, E. (2004) Heterogeneous nuclear ribonucleoprotein A2/B1 identified as an autoantigen in autoimmune hepatitis by proteome analysis. *Proteomics* 4:1341–1345.

32 Leung, A.K., Andersen, J.S., Mann, M., Lamond, A.I. (2003) Bioinformatic analysis of the nucleolus. *Biochem J* 376:553–569.

33 Schirmer, E.C., Florens, L., Guan, T., Yates, 3rd, J.R., Gerace, L. (2003) Nuclear membrane proteins with potential disease links found by subtractive proteomics. *Science* 301:1380–1382.

34 Andersen, J.S., Y.W. Lam, A.K. Leung, S.E. Ong, C.E. Lyon, A.I. Lamond, and M. Mann (2005) Nucleolar proteome dynamics. *Nature* 433:77–83.

35 Tan, E.M., and F.D. Shi (2003) Relative paradigms between autoantibodies in lupus and autoantibodies in cancer. *Clin Exp Immunol* 134:169–177.

36 Gires, O., M. Munz, M. Schaffrik, C. Kieu, J. Rauch, M. Ahlemann, D. Eberle, B. Mack, B. Wollenberg, S. Lang, T. Hofmann, W. Hammerschmidt, R. Zeidler (2004) Profile identification of disease-associated humoral antigens using AMIDA, a novel proteomics-based technology. *Cell Mol Life Sci* 61: 1198–1207.

37 Kono, D.H., R.W. Burlingame, D.G. Owens, A. Kuramochi, R.S. Balderas, D. Balomenos, and A.N. Theofilopoulos (1994) Lupus susceptibility loci in New Zealand mice. *Proc Natl Acad Sci USA* 91:10168–10172.

38 Rozzo, S.J., J.D. Allard, D. Choubey, T.J. Vyse, S. Izui, G. Peltz, and B.L. Kotzin (2001) Evidence for an interferon-inducible gene, Ifi202, in the susceptibility to systemic lupus. *Immunity* 15:435–443.

39 Kono, D.H., M.S. Park, and A.N. Theofilopoulos (2003) Genetic complementation in female (BXSB x NZW)F2 mice. *J Immunol* 171:6442–6447.

40 Morel, L., and E.K. Wakeland (2000) Lessons from the NZM2410 model and related strains. *Int Rev Immunol* 19: 423–446.

41 Vyse, T.J., and B.L. Kotzin (1998) Genetic susceptibility to systemic lupus erythematosus. *Annu Rev Immunol* 16: 261–292.

42 Seery, J.P., J.M. Carroll, V. Cattell, and F.M. Watt (1997) Antinuclear autoantibodies and lupus nephritis in transgenic mice expressing interferon gamma in the epidermis. *J Exp Med* 186:1451–1459.

43 Kono, D.H., D. Balomenos, D.L. Pearson, M.S. Park, B. Hildebrandt, P. Hultman, and K.M. Pollard (1998) The prototypic Th2 autoimmunity induced by mercury is dependent on IFN-gamma and not Th1/Th2 imbalance. *J Immunol* 161:234–240.

44 Simmonds, M.J., J.M. Heward, M.A. Kelly, A. Allahabadia, H. Foxall, C. Gordon, J.A. Franklyn, and S.C. Gough (2002) A nonsense mutation in exon 2 of the DNase I gene is not present in UK subjects with systemic lupus erythematosus and Graves' disease: Comment on the article by Rood et al. *Arthritis Rheum* 46:3109–3110.

45 Yasutomo, K., T. Horiuchi, S. Kagami, H. Tsukamoto, C. Hashimura, M. Urushihara, and Y. Kuroda (2001) Mutation of DNASE1 in people with systemic lupus erythematosus. *Nat Genet* 28:313–314.

46 Napirei, M., Karsunky, H., Zevnik, B., Stephan, H., Mannherz, H.G., Moroy, T. (2000) Features of systemic lupus erythematosus in Dnase1-deficient mice. *Nat Genet* 25:177–181.

47 Pollard, K.M., Hultman, P., Kono, D.H. (2003) Using Single-Gene Deletions to Identify Checkpoints in the Progression of Systemic Autoimmunity. *Ann NY Acad Sci* 987:236–239.

48 Vinuesa, C.G., Goodnow, C.C. (2004) Illuminating autoimmune regulators through controlled variation of the mouse genome sequence. *Immunity* 20:669–679.

Subject Index

*Autoantibodies and Autoimmunity: Molecular Mechanisms
in Health and Disease*. Edited by K. Michael Pollard
Copyright © 2006 WILEY-VCH Verlag GmbH & Co. KGaA, Weinheim
ISBN: 3-527-31141-6